Textbook of

Hospital Psychiatry

SECOND EDITION

Textbook of Hospital Psychiatry

SECOND EDITION

Edited by

Harsh K. Trivedi, M.D., M.B.A.

President and Chief Executive Officer, Sheppard Pratt Health System
Baltimore, Maryland

Steven S. Sharfstein, M.D., M.P.A.

President Emeritus, Sheppard Pratt Health System
Baltimore, Maryland

AMERICAN PSYCHIATRIC ASSOCIATION PUBLISHING

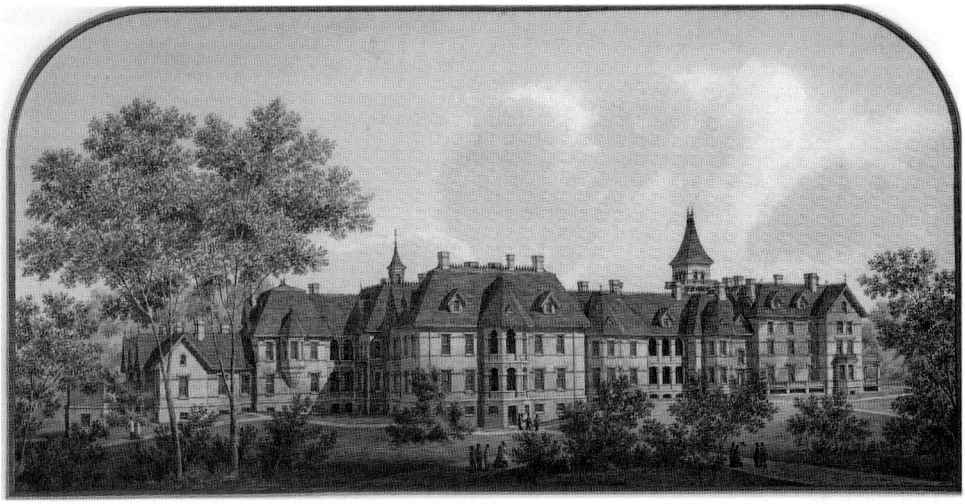

To meet a need that would otherwise be unmet…

Everything done for the comfort of the patient…

No patient to be confined below ground…

To carry forward and improve the ameliorated system of treatment of the insane, irrespective of expense…

If five persons were returned to health and reason, or even one, I would feel satisfied.

Moses Sheppard,
whose vision and generosity founded Sheppard Pratt in 1853

CONTENTS

Contributors xiii
Foreword xix
Richard J. Pollack
Introduction xxiii
Harsh K. Trivedi, M.D., M.B.A.
Steven S. Sharfstein, M.D., M.P.A.

1 History of Hospital Psychiatry 1
Jeffrey L. Geller, M.D., M.P.H.
Ashley J.B. MacLean, M.D.

PART 1
Inpatient Care

Units by Age Cohort

2 The Child Unit 47
Debra Heck, M.D.
Kathryn Burns, R.N., M.S.N.

3 The Adolescent Unit 67
Yasas Tanguturi, M.D., M.P.H.
Catharyn Turner II, M.D., M.Ed.

4 The Adult Crisis Stabilization Unit 87
Savitha Puttaiah, M.B.B.S., M.D.
Merle McCann, M.D.

5 The Geriatric Unit 113

Caitlin Lawrence, M.D.
Amy Halt, M.D., Ph.D.
Louis Marino, M.D.

Units by Diagnostic Cohort

6 The Developmental Disabilities Co-occurring Unit: Neuropsychiatry Across the Life Span 151

Scott R. Pekrul, M.D.
Robert W. Wisner-Carlson, M.D.
Thomas Flis, M.S.

7 The Eating Disorders Unit 183

Jennifer L. Goetz, M.D.
Steven F. Crawford, M.D.
Harry A. Brandt, M.D.

8 The Forensic Unit 211

Tobias D. Wasser, M.D.
Charles C. Dike, M.D., M.P.H., FRCPsych
Michael A. Norko, M.D., M.A.R.

9 The Psychotic Disorders Unit 229

Edward Zuzarte, M.D.
John J. Boronow, M.D.
Harsh K. Trivedi, M.D., M.B.A.

10 The Substance Use Disorders Co-occurring Unit 257

Sunil Khushalani, M.D., DFAPA, FASAM
George Kolodner, M.D., DLFAPA, FASAM

Specialty Settings

11 The State Hospital 291

Debra A. Pinals, M.D.
Brian M. Hepburn, M.D.
Ted Lutterman, B.A.

12 The Veterans Hospital 311

Anne Marie Stoline, M.D.
Marsden McGuire, M.D., M.B.A.

PART 2
The Continuum of Care

13 Community Mental Health and Hospital-Based Outpatient Services 341

Deepak Prabhakar, M.D., M.P.H.
Manan Shah, M.D.
Jason Addison, M.D.
Jeff Richardson, M.S.W., M.B.A.

14 Residential Treatment for Children and Adolescents 357

Virginia Susan Villani, M.D.

15 Residential Intensive Psychodynamic Psychotherapy for Adults 375

Eric M. Plakun, M.D.
Edward R. Shapiro, M.D.

16 Psychiatric Emergency Services and Interface With the General Hospital 399

Deepak Prabhakar, M.D., M.P.H.
Benedicto Borja, M.D.
Aaron Winkler, M.D.
Rachna Raisinghani, M.D.

PART 3
Hardwiring Excellence

17 Administration and Leadership 411

Gregory Gattman, FACHE
Kelly Savoca, CPA, M.B.A.
Harsh K. Trivedi, M.D., M.B.A.

18 Financing of Care 433

Paul Summergrad, M.D., FRCPsych (Hon)
Bruce J. Schwartz, M.D.
Peter Spyrou, M.D.

19 Quality, Measurement-Based Care, and Outcomes 447

Robert J. Schloesser, M.D.

20 Risk Management 463

Jerry Halverson, M.D.
Nathaniel Clark, M.D.
Terri Schultz, R.N., M.B.A.
Steven Hertig, B.A., CHPC

21 Preventing Conflict, Violence, and Use of Seclusion and Restraint 481

Kevin Ann Huckshorn, Ph.D., M.S.N., R.N., ICADC
Janice L. LeBel, Ph.D., ABPP

22 Lean and Operational Excellence 503

Sunil Khushalani, M.D., DFAPA, FASAM

23 Architecture and Thoughtful Design 517

Harsh K. Trivedi, M.D., M.B.A
Michelle S. Hooper, M.S.H., AIA
Antonio DePaolo, Ph.D.
Thomas D. Hess, M.B.A.
Roger Daub

PART 4
Workforce and Special Issues

24 Psychiatrists, Psychiatric Nurse Practitioners, and Psychologists 537

Todd Peters, M.D.
Kathleen Hilzendeger

25 Psychiatric Mental Health Nursing 547

Laura Lawson Webb, M.S.N., R.N., PMHN-BC

26 Social Work and Rehabilitation Therapies 557

Carrie Etheridge, LCSW-C
Vaune Kopeck, OTR/L
April Sobiech, LCSW-C

27 Working With Families 577

Lisa B. Dixon, M.D., M.P.H.
Thomas Jewell, Ph.D.
Sarah Piscitelli, M.A.

28 From Within: A Consumer Perspective on Psychiatric Hospitals 591

Howard D. Trachtman, B.S., CPS, CPRP, COAPS
Kenneth S. Duckworth, M.D.
Reverend Dr. Norma J. Heath
Ziona Rivera

PART 5
The Future of Hospital Psychiatry

29 Collaborative Care and Emerging Models 605

Ken C. Hopper, M.D., M.B.A.
Roger Kathol, M.D., CPE

30 The Future of Hospital Psychiatry 625

Harsh K. Trivedi, M.D., M.B.A.
Jennifer Weiss Wilkerson, M.H.S.A., FACHE
Thomas Glenn, M.S.F.

Index. 633

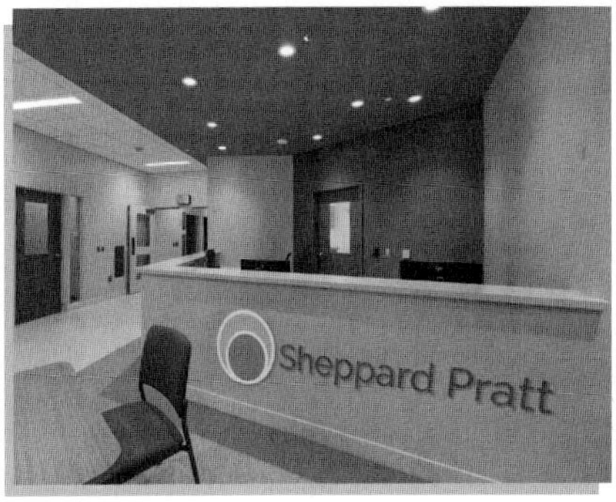

Contributors

Jason Addison, M.D.
Sheppard Pratt Health System, Baltimore, Maryland

Benedicto Borja, M.D.
Department of Psychiatry and Behavioral Sciences, George Washington University School of Medicine & Health Sciences, Washington, D.C.

John J. Boronow, M.D.
Sheppard Pratt Health System, Baltimore, Maryland

Harry A. Brandt, M.D.
University of Maryland School of Medicine; ERC Pathlight, Hunt Valley, Maryland

Kathryn Burns, R.N., M.S.N.
Sheppard Pratt Health System, Baltimore, Maryland

Nathaniel Clark, M.D.
Vanderbilt University School of Medicine, Nashville, Tennessee

Steven F. Crawford, M.D.
University of Maryland School of Medicine; ERC Pathlight, Hunt Valley, Maryland

Roger Daub
Hasta Advisors, LLC

Antonio DePaolo, Ph.D.
University of Maryland, Upper Chesapeake Health, Bel Air, Maryland

Charles C. Dike, M.D., M.P.H., FRCPsych
Yale University School of Medicine, New Haven, Connecticut; Connecticut Department of Mental Health and Addiction Services, Hartford, Connecticut

Lisa B. Dixon, M.D., M.P.H.
New York State Psychiatric Institute and Columbia University Vagelos College of Physicians and Surgeons, New York, New York

Kenneth S. Duckworth, M.D.
NAMI: National Alliance on Mental Illness

Carrie Etheridge, LCSW-C
Sheppard Pratt Health System, Baltimore, Maryland

Thomas Flis, M.S.
Sheppard Pratt Health System, Baltimore, Maryland

Gregory Gattman, FACHE
Sheppard Pratt Health System, Baltimore, Maryland

Jeffrey L. Geller, M.D., M.P.H.
University of Massachusetts Chan Medical School, Worcester, Massachusetts

Thomas Glenn, M.S.F.
Sheppard Pratt Health System, Baltimore, Maryland

Jennifer L. Goetz, M.D.
McLean Hospital/Harvard Medical School, Belmont, Massachusetts

Amy Halt, M.D., Ph.D.
Department of Psychiatry and Human Behavior, Brown University, Providence, Rhode Island

Jerry Halverson, M.D.
Rogers Behavioral Health

Reverend Dr. Norma J. Heath
NAMI Greater Boston Peer Support and Advocacy Network; AMRON International

Debra Heck, M.D.
Sheppard Pratt Health System, Baltimore, Maryland

Brian M. Hepburn, M.D.
National Association of State Mental Health Program Directors, Alexandria, Virginia

Steven Hertig, B.A., CHPC
Rogers Behavioral Health

Thomas D. Hess, M.B.A.
Sheppard Pratt Health System, Baltimore, Maryland

Kathleen Hilzendeger
Sheppard Pratt Health System, Baltimore, Maryland

Michelle S. Hooper, M.S.H., AIA
Marshall Craft Associates, Inc., Baltimore, Maryland

Ken C. Hopper, M.D., M.B.A.
TCU and UNTHSC School of Medicine, Fort Worth, Texas

Kevin Ann Huckshorn, Ph.D., R.N., M.S.N., ICADC
Recovery International, Inc.

Thomas Jewell, Ph.D.
New York State Psychiatric Institute and Columbia University, Department of Psychiatry, New York, New York

Roger Kathol, M.D, CPE
University of Minnesota, Minneapolis, Minnesota

Sunil Khushalani, M.D., DFAPA, FASAM
Kolmac Outpatient Recovery Centers; Department of Psychiatry, University of Maryland School of Medicine, Baltimore, Maryland

George Kolodner, M.D., DLFAPA, FASAM
Georgetown University School of Medicine, Washington, D.C.

Vaune Kopeck, OTR/L
Sheppard Pratt Health System, Baltimore, Maryland

Caitlin Lawrence, M.D.
Department of Psychiatry and Human Behavior, Brown University, Providence, Rhode Island

Janice L. LeBel, Ph.D., ABPP
Department of Mental Health, Commonwealth of Massachusetts

Ted Lutterman, B.A.
NRI, Falls Church, Virginia

Ashley J.B. MacLean, M.D.
University of Massachusetts Chan Medical School, Worcester, Massachusetts

Louis Marino, M.D.
Sheppard Pratt Health System, Baltimore, Maryland; Department of Psychiatry and Human Behavior, Brown University, Providence, Rhode Island

Merle McCann, M.D.
Sheppard Pratt Health System, Baltimore, Maryland

Marsden McGuire, M.D., M.B.A.
Department of Veterans Affairs, Washington, D.C.

Michael A. Norko, M.D., M.A.R.
Yale School of Medicine, New Haven, Connecticut; Connecticut Department of Mental Health and Addiction Services, Hartford, Connecticut

Scott R. Pekrul, M.D.
Sheppard Pratt Health System, Baltimore, Maryland

Todd Peters, M.D.
Sheppard Pratt Health System, Baltimore, Maryland

Debra A. Pinals, M.D.
University of Michigan Medical School, Ann Arbor, Michigan

Sarah Piscitelli, M.A.
New York State Psychiatric Institute, New York, New York

Eric M. Plakun, M.D.
Austen Riggs Center, Stockbridge, Massachusetts

Deepak Prabhakar, M.D., M.P.H.
Sheppard Pratt Health System, Baltimore, Maryland

Savitha Puttaiah, MB.B.S., M.D.
Baptist Behavioral Health, Jacksonville, Florida

Rachna Raisinghani, M.D.
Sheppard Pratt Health System, Baltimore, Maryland

Jeff Richardson, M.S.W., M.B.A.
Sheppard Pratt Health System, Baltimore, Maryland

Ziona Rivera
NAMI Greater Boston Peer Support and Advocacy Network; AMRON International

Kelly Savoca, CPA, M.B.A.
Sheppard Pratt Health System, Baltimore, Maryland

Robert J. Schloesser, M.D.
Sheppard Pratt Health System, Baltimore, Maryland

Terri Schultz, R.N., M.B.A.
Department of Compliance and Regulation, Rogers Memorial Hospital, Inc.

Bruce J. Schwartz, M.D.
Department of Psychiatry and Behavioral Sciences, Montefiore Medical Center and Albert Einstein College of Medicine, Bronx, New York

Manan Shah, M.D.
Sheppard Pratt Health System, Baltimore, Maryland

Edward R. Shapiro, M.D.
Austen Riggs Center, Stockbridge, Massachusetts; Clinical Professor of Psychiatry, Yale Medical School, New Haven, Connecticut

Steven S. Sharfstein, M.D., M.P.A.
Sheppard Pratt Health System, Baltimore, Maryland

April Sobiech, LCSW-C
Sheppard Pratt Health System, Baltimore, Maryland

Peter Spyrou, M.D.
Department of Psychiatry and Behavioral Sciences, Montefiore Medical Center and Albert Einstein College of Medicine, Bronx, New York

Anne Marie Stoline, M.D.
Perry Point VA Medical Center, Perry Point, Maryland

Paul Summergrad, M.D., FRCPsych (Hon)
Department of Psychiatry, Tufts University School of Medicine; Tufts Medical Center and Tufts Children's Hospital, Boston, Massachusetts; World Psychiatric Association

Yasas Tanguturi, M.D., M.P.H.
Vanderbilt Psychiatric Hospital; Vanderbilt University Medical Center, Nashville, Tennessee

Howard D. Trachtman, B.S., CPS, CPRP, COAPS
NAMI Greater Boston Peer Support and Advocacy Network

Harsh K. Trivedi, M.D., M.B.A.
Sheppard Pratt Health System, Baltimore, Maryland

Catharyn Turner II, M.D., M.Ed.
Children's Hospital of Philadelphia, Philadelphia, Pennsylvania

Virginia Susan Villani, M.D.
Sheppard Pratt Health System, Baltimore, Maryland

Tobias D. Wasser, M.D.
Yale School of Medicine, New Haven, Connecticut; Whiting Forensic Hospital, Middletown, Connecticut

Laura Lawson Webb, M.S.N., R.N., PMHN-BC
Sheppard Pratt Health System, Baltimore, Maryland

Jennifer Weiss Wilkerson, M.H.S.A., FACHE
Sheppard Pratt Health System, Baltimore, Maryland

Aaron Winkler, M.D.
University of Maryland/Sheppard Pratt, Baltimore, Maryland

Robert W. Wisner-Carlson, M.D.
Sheppard Pratt Health System, Baltimore, Maryland

Edward Zuzarte, M.D.
Sheppard Pratt Health System, Baltimore, Maryland

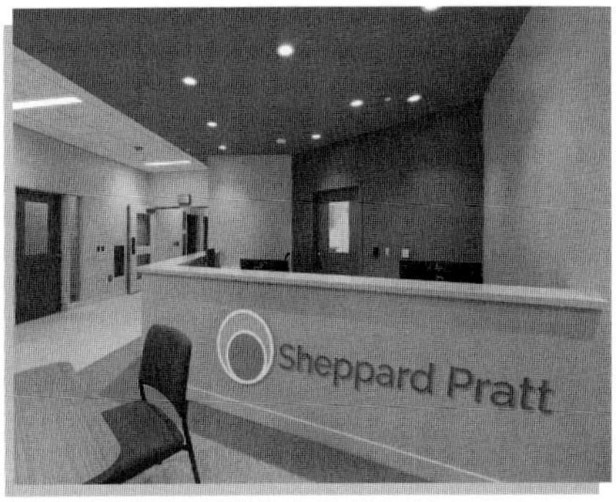

Foreword

With each passing day, the words of Dr. Brock Chisholm, the first director-general of the World Health Organization and a psychiatrist, become increasingly clear: "Without mental health there can be no true physical health." The American Hospital Association sees this link throughout our membership, which includes freestanding psychiatric hospitals, psychiatric units within general acute care facilities, and millions of individual clinicians. Even with improved access to community-based care, severely ill patients continue to need the intense and highly tailored medical treatments—for both mental and physical comorbidities—that are provided only in hospitals. As we continue to confront COVID-19, the world's greatest public health crisis in the past century, it is astounding how much has changed since the last published edition of this textbook . . . and how much remains the same.

Over the last decade, the field of hospital psychiatry has faced new clinical and policy challenges and opportunities. Spending by insurers for behavioral health treatments has increased significantly, and out-of-pocket spending for behavioral health treatments continues to rise. Accompanying this increase in spending is the nationwide explosion of the opioid crisis, which reminds us of the insidious entanglements of pain and addiction. Increasingly, patients seeking psychiatric care in hospitals suffer from a combination of behavioral and physical ailments, each exacerbating the others, resulting in highly sensitive and complex treatment regimens. As providers treat patients with complex conditions, they also must balance the growing regulatory demands, quality reporting programs, and progressively stricter survey and certification activities that have heaped numerous administrative requirements on hospitals. The ensuing environment of care is a constant juggling act of these pressures with efforts to advance evidence-based care protocols and quality improvement initiatives.

Even in the face of these obstacles, the field has expanded and treatment has evolved. Providers and policy-makers are increasingly aware of the importance of treating the whole person. Research demonstrates that integrating physical and behavioral health care improves outcomes and can reduce the total cost of care. Clinicians across specialties are adding behavioral health treatment into their regular courses of care, while psychiatric facilities and units address not only patients' physical ailments but also their postdischarge social needs, including housing, transportation, and nutrition. Many psychiatric facilities also are improving their health information technology capabilities to enhance care through the use of electronic medical records and telepsychiatry.

As the field has made progress in a number of areas, many age-old challenges remain. Inadequate reimbursement and insurance coverage for mental illnesses leave both patients and providers desperate for reform. Despite the passage of the Mental Health Parity and Addiction Equity Act in 2008, patients seeking mental health care are twice as likely to be denied coverage for services based on medical necessity as patients seeking physical health care, and behavioral health providers are still reimbursed less than those in other specialties. In addition, the long-standing workforce shortages are worsening, as practitioners in the baby boomer generation reach retirement age and their roles go unfilled by new graduates. The shortages are particularly severe in child, adolescent, and geriatric psychiatry.

These obstacles feed on and into pervasive undercurrents that have been present since the inception of hospital psychiatry. Disparities in access still leave people of color struggling to receive care at all, let alone culturally competent treatment. Individuals in the LGBTQ+ community are more likely to attempt or commit suicide, particularly during adolescence. The aging population is more likely than previous generations to live alone and without behavioral and social supports. And underscoring it all is the stigma associated with mental illness and substance use disorders. While it is encouraging that behavioral wellness has received some increased public attention, including from well-known personalities, unfortunately severe mental illnesses like schizophrenia and other psychotic disorders (the second most common diagnostic group treated in psychiatric hospitals) are associated with even higher levels of stigma than other behavioral health conditions.

Despite this intimidating environment, psychiatric hospitals are adapting and finding new ways of caring for severely ill patients. This textbook orients the practice of hospital psychiatry toward the future while seeking innovative solutions to these long-standing challenges. The forward-looking chapters focus on integrating physical and behavioral health care across specialty units, types of hospitals, and treatment settings. Authors at the vanguard of their field offer insights into modern delivery models that employ strategies such as telemedicine to extend the reach of the clinical workforce. Other chapters expound on the utility of collaborative care efforts, which incorporate professionals from various specialties, to address the full continuum of a patient's needs. Hospital and health system leaders extend guidance on the infrastructure capabilities necessary to balance the many, and often competing, clinical and administrative demands.

It is fitting that this new edition arrives following the tumultuous year of 2020. The COVID-19 pandemic, social and civil unrest, and the economic recession laid bare the critical and urgent need for behavioral health care. On the one hand, the events of that year have seriously affected the mental health of individuals across the nation, resulting in increases in depression, anxiety, drug overdoses, and self-harm. On the other, the surge in awareness of the importance of behavioral health care has hastened policy actions to enhance funding and ease regulatory burdens on psychiatric providers. This textbook will help the field take advantage of this historic and unprecedented opportunity to advance hospital psychiatry.

The American Hospital Association is proud to represent practitioners who face such a complex and challenging environment with integrity and compassion. As we strive to ensure a regulatory environment that reduces burden and supports innovation, clinicians work tirelessly to provide evidence-based, high-quality, and safe care to patients with acute conditions that are among the most difficult to treat. Together, and with the guidance of the experts featured in this textbook, we hope to continue to advance the practice of hospital psychiatry as we work to advance health in America.

Richard J. Pollack
President and Chief Executive Officer
American Hospital Association

of inpatient units, two major concepts exist: the existence or *availability* of psychiatric beds and the *accessibility* of those beds to all who need inpatient care.

Regarding availability of psychiatric beds, we have come a long way from the peak of public asylum psychiatry in 1955, when there were 559,000 individuals in psychiatric beds and length of stay was calculated in months or even years and lifetimes. State mental hospitals have been depopulated so that there are fewer than 40,000 beds in state hospitals, and these are largely forensic. In addition, there are 31,000 beds on psychiatric units in general hospitals, 25,000 beds in private psychiatric hospitals, 3,000 beds in Veterans Affairs hospitals, and 3,500 beds in other specialty mental health centers (Pinals and Fuller 2017). In the United States, we have 21 beds per 100,000 population according to the Organisation for Economic Co-operation and Development (OECD), as compared with an OECD average of 70 beds per 100,000. Only Chile, Italy, and Mexico have fewer.

In addition to availability of beds, it is important to note that access to psychiatric beds also remains a critical issue. With passage of legislation ensuring mental health parity, the substantial gains that were expected in access have not materialized because of lack of enforcement at the state level. Beyond the structure of the health benefits, insurers have attempted to change their internal definitions of what is covered and what is medically necessary. The landmark class action lawsuit *Wit v. United Behavioral Health* decision found that the insurer internally developed coverage determination guidelines and level of care guidelines more stringent than accepted standards to wrongfully deny care. A positive development in recent years has been the openness of younger generations in the United States and internationally about their mental health needs. They are actively demanding that their health insurance provide meaningful access to covered services, without the concerns for stigma that have prevented more of these issues from coming to light.

And while we cringe at the unscrupulous behavior of for-profit insurance companies, our largest federal payer of care for low-income individuals stands out for its own discriminatory practice. Indeed, the only section of "Medicaid law that prohibits federal payment for medically necessary care simply because of the type of illness being treated" (Treatment Advocacy Center 2016) is Medicaid's anachronistic institution for mental diseases, or IMD, exclusion. It restricts federal financial participation for individuals in the exclusion group and prevents access to inpatient psychiatric care for an entire population of people, particularly those with serious mental illness and those with comorbid substance use issues.

There is a significant role for psychiatric hospitals and psychiatric units in general hospitals in meeting mental health needs nationally. The impact of the COVID-19 pandemic on mental health and predicted increases in suicides and overdoses will only exacerbate availability and access issues for inpatient psychiatric beds.

We fundamentally believe that through the work of behavioral health integration, greater understanding of the impact of untreated and undertreated mental health on health outcomes, and the national need to better manage spiraling health care costs, psychiatric care will be thrust forward for the integral role it plays in overall health and as a driver of reducing the total cost of care. As these shifts occur, we are confident that a new national resource will emerge, the specialty psychiatric hospital—such as Sheppard Pratt. Throughout the nation, a handful of dedicated comprehensive specialty psychiatric hospitals will emerge—expert at managing all diagnoses, for all comers, with a comprehensive continuum of services, and able to manage the most complex cases in the nation. This comprehensive national resource will be a beacon of hope and a guiding force for best practice implementation, similar to the role of a specialty cancer hospital, a specialty orthopedic hospital, or a specialty cardiac hospital.

The Continuum of Care

The psychiatric hospital today, much like the rest of medicine, goes beyond the hospital walls and offers more than just an inpatient bed. This textbook is about the richness and diversity of levels of care, sites of care, and types of programs. While many communities experience a gap in the continuum of care, we are proud to share the broad system of care that Sheppard Pratt has created and refined over the course of decades. First starting most proximal to the inpatient unit, this portion of the textbook discusses hospital-based outpatient services. Residential treatment programs, day hospitals, intensive outpatient programs, specialty outpatient programs—all are part of the changing landscape of psychiatric treatment.

We end this part with a look at psychiatric emergency services, crisis stabilization, and the interface with the general hospital. The adolescent at risk for suicide and their family require a different approach than the aggressive geriatric patient admitted from a nursing home with dementia. Patients with co-occurring substance use and mental disorders, patients with eating disorders, and patients with co-occurring neurodevelopmental and mental disorders each require different approaches. The path forward is one in which we do not treat "mental illness" as a vanilla term that encompasses every DSM diagnosis and places people in general programs that try to treat every mental health issue within the same program. Rather, the path forward is more specific treatment based on the clinical needs of the patient, marked by the utilization of illness-specific treatment tracks and specialty programs for chronic disease management.

Hardwiring Excellence

As the field of psychiatry has progressed, so have the knowledge and expertise required to operate a high-quality, efficient, highly reliable, and fiscally sound hospital or health system. This portion of the textbook covers vital topics related to leadership, strategic planning, financial matters, and operational excellence. It delves into quality, safety, and risk management in hospital settings. It focuses on preventing conflict, violence, and use of seclusion and restraint. And, should you find yourself in the enviable role of getting to design a new space or remodel an existing space, it discusses the importance of design and architecture in creating a therapeutic space, engineering safety, and achieving optimal design for peak clinical and operational performance.

This newest version of the *Textbook of Hospital Psychiatry* was written to coincide with the unveiling of Sheppard Pratt's newest, state-of-the-art $150 million psychiatric hospital in the Baltimore-Washington corridor in July 2021. This hospital and its new 50-acre campus are a testament to the vision, strategic execution, and strong financial standing of Sheppard Pratt. This portion of the textbook defines the critical elements of why our path has been unique and unparalleled thus far in the field. The ability to build high-quality programs to scale and create the continuum of services to match the patient's journey is fundamental to good clinical care.

Workforce and Special Issues

Buildings are just buildings, but it is the people who infuse the care that breathes life and purpose to nurture hope and healing. This portion of the textbook covers the array of clinicians on a multidisciplinary care team and professional issues for each profession. It then expands to discuss working with families and presents a consumer perspective on psychiatric hospitals.

The Future of Hospital Psychiatry

The book ends with two impactful chapters. The substantial progress that will occur between now and the third edition of this textbook will be more seamless integration of behavioral health services across primary care and throughout medicine. The chapter on collaborative care and emerging models discusses a number of those efforts and ones that will indeed grow in the coming decade. The final chapter charts the path forward for the field of hospital psychiatry. It presents key disruptive forces as well as likely advances that will advance care in the years to come.

Final Thoughts

It is our hope that the knowledge provided in this textbook will help you to achieve meaningful advances in care in your programs and services. The images throughout the text reflect pictures of actual care settings. The descriptions of services are built and at scale. And they are provided with the aim of inspiring you and showing what is truly possible. We must each strive to implement meaningful change, to build new programs that create new access, and to advocate for appropriate funding of psychiatric care so that every individual can access lifesaving and life-changing care when they need it.

Acknowledgment

The editors would like to express their appreciation to Janet Bryan and Tamara Chumley for their help in the preparation of this manuscript. Their administrative skills in dealing with multiple authors, as well as the editors, during an unprecedented pandemic kept this work on track and (mostly) on time. Thank you.

Harsh K. Trivedi, M.D., M.B.A.
Steven S. Sharfstein, M.D., M.P.A.

References

Pinals DA, Fuller DA: Beyond Beds: The Vital Role of a Full Continuum of Psychiatric Care. Alexandria, VA, National Association of State Mental Health Program Directors, 2017. Available at: www.nasmhpd.org/sites/default/files/TAC.Paper_.1Beyond_Beds.pdf. Accessed December 12, 2020.

Sharfstein SS, Dickerson FB, Oldham JM (eds): Textbook of Hospital Psychiatry. Washington, DC, American Psychiatric Publishing, 2009

Treatment Advocacy Center: The Medicaid IMD Exclusion and Mental Illness Discrimination. Alexandria, VA, Treatment Advocacy Center, 2016. Available at: www.treatmentadvocacy-center.org/storage/documents/backgrounders/imd-exclusion-and-discrimination.pdf. Accessed January 19, 2021.

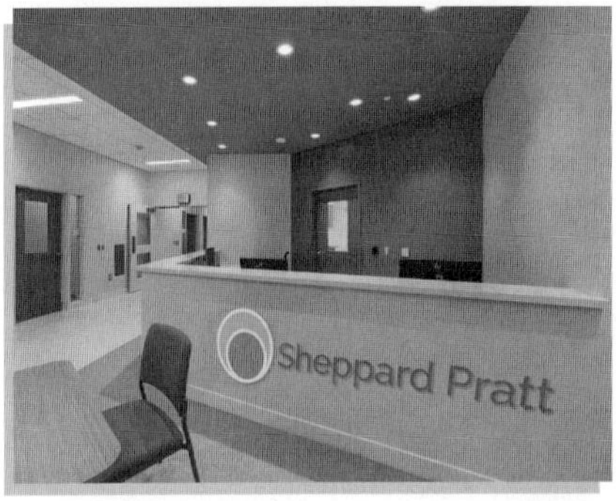

CHAPTER 1

History of Hospital Psychiatry

Jeffrey L. Geller, M.D., M.P.H.
Ashley J.B. MacLean, M.D.

The history of American psychiatry is fundamentally the history of inpatient psychiatry. Every generation in our nation's history has faced mental health as a significant societal challenge. While the methods of treatment have varied over time, what has been constant is the presence of stigma and the lack of full funding of adequate mental health services. Many original psychiatric hospitals have closed, and there has been a dramatic reduction in the availability of inpatient psychiatric beds in most communities nationally. Inadequate funding has led to an arbitrary pitting of various segments of care against one another. Examples include inpatient care versus community psychiatry and mental health versus substance use service funding. The separation of federal and local streams of funding for mental health, substance use disorders, developmental disorders, and social services has led to structural inabilities to provide comprehensive treatment planning and improved outcomes. Insurance, regulatory, and legislative barriers lead to suboptimal access to hospital-based psychiatry. Antiquated constructs of institutions for mental diseases (IMD) exclusion and discriminatory payment practices despite mental health parity remain barriers to effectuating the best outcome for the individual.

The architects of the American Psychiatric Association (APA) were founders of an association of medical superintendents, some from state hospitals, others from private

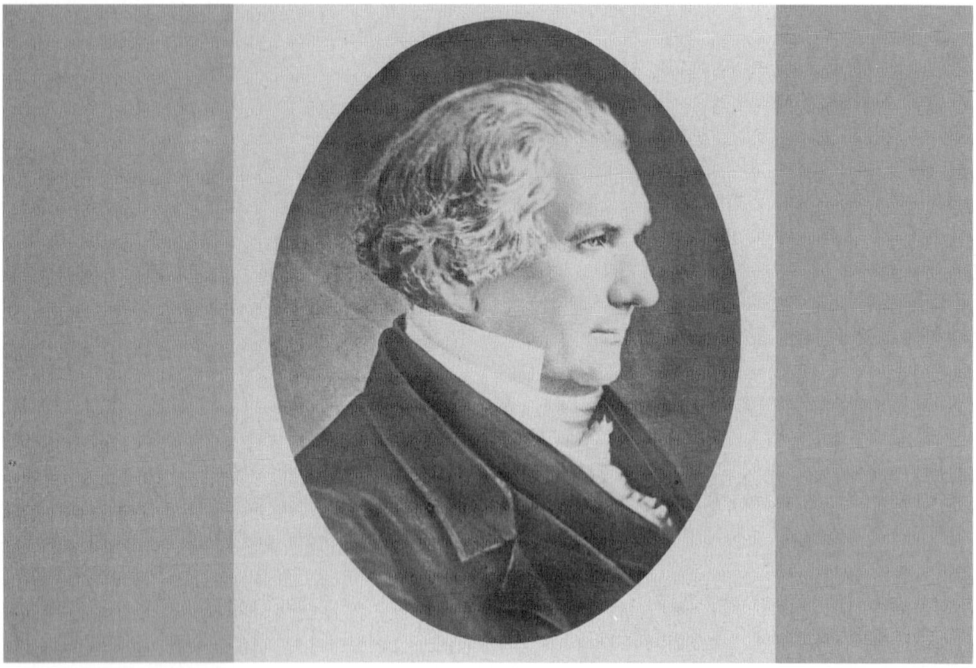

FIGURE 1–1. Samuel Bayard Woodward.
Source. John Curwen: *The Original Thirteen Members of the Association of Medical Superintendents of American Institutions for the Insane.* Courtesy of American Psychiatric Association Archives, Washington, D.C.

psychiatric hospitals. Nine of the original 13 members of the Association of Medical Superintendents of American Institutions for the Insane (AMSAII) had connections with private psychiatric hospitals. In 1844, they met in Philadelphia and established the first medical specialty organization in the United States. Thomas Story Kirkbride had trained at Friends Asylum and was superintendent of the Pennsylvania Hospital for the Insane. Samuel Bayard Woodward (Figure 1–1), Amariah Brigham, and John Butler had all been associated with the Hartford Retreat; Isaac Ray was connected with Butler Hospital; and Pliny Earle (Figure 1–2) had associations with both Friends and Bloomingdale Asylums. Two members, Nehemiah Cutter (Pepperell Private Asylum) and Samuel White (Hudson Lunatic Asylum), were founders of and ran proprietary psychiatric facilities, and Luther Vose Bell (Figure 1–3) headed McLean Asylum. These founders of American psychiatry, and the hospitals with which each was associated, set the course for hospital-based care and treatment.

The Early Years (The Beginning Through 1920)

Origins of Public Facilities

Public care of persons with insanity began concurrently at multiple levels of government. Prior to the nineteenth century, the care of insane persons was predominantly a local endeavor, took place largely in almshouses, and was generally custodial in na-

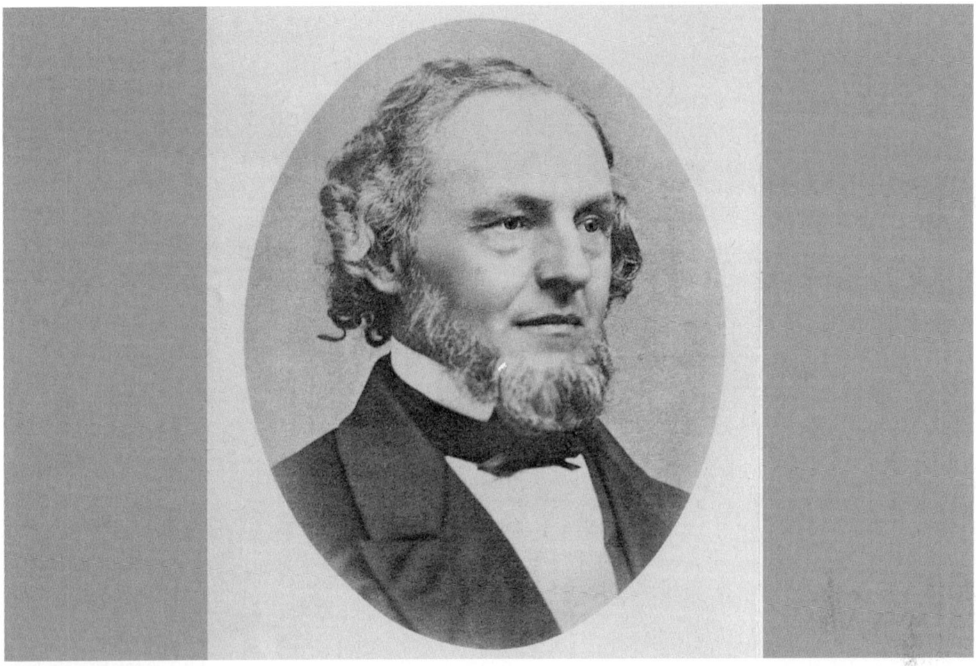

FIGURE 1–2. Pliny Earle.
Source. John Curwen: *The Original Thirteen Members of the Association of Medical Superintendents of American Institutions for the Insane.* Courtesy of American Psychiatric Association Archives, Washington, D.C.

ture (Hurd 1916–1917). When states took responsibility for insane paupers in this era, the state would auction these "confessedly undesirable persons" to the lowest bidder, because the state had to pay the private family to provide for the basic needs. If no family could be found, jails or strong pens under a relative's supervision were used (Deutsch 1949; Hurd 1916–1917).

In some states, care for the insane poor became organized at the county level. States created state boards of charity to inspect the county establishments that housed insane persons. This system was criticized because local variation was extreme and medical and nursing interventions were generally poor (Hurd 1916–1917).

At the outset, "state care" meant care received at a state institution that was established, built, and managed by the state but whose operation was funded by taxpayers and individuals. These were strictly speaking state-aided facilities. If the patient or family had resources, they paid for care; paupers were the responsibility of the county. Thus, the earliest public facilities—in Williamsburg, Virginia, and Columbia, South Carolina—were established pursuant to this model (Hurd 1916–1917).

State care in which the state was responsible for all insane persons and executed its responsibility through state-managed and funded hospitals began with Worcester State Hospital in 1833 (Hurd 1916–1917) (Figure 1–4). The development of state care progressed at quite different rates. New Hampshire, for example, did not have an act legalizing state care until 1913 (Hurd 1916–1917).

It was three decades after states began to take responsibility for their insane populations that states started to specifically consider the incurably insane. In 1865, New

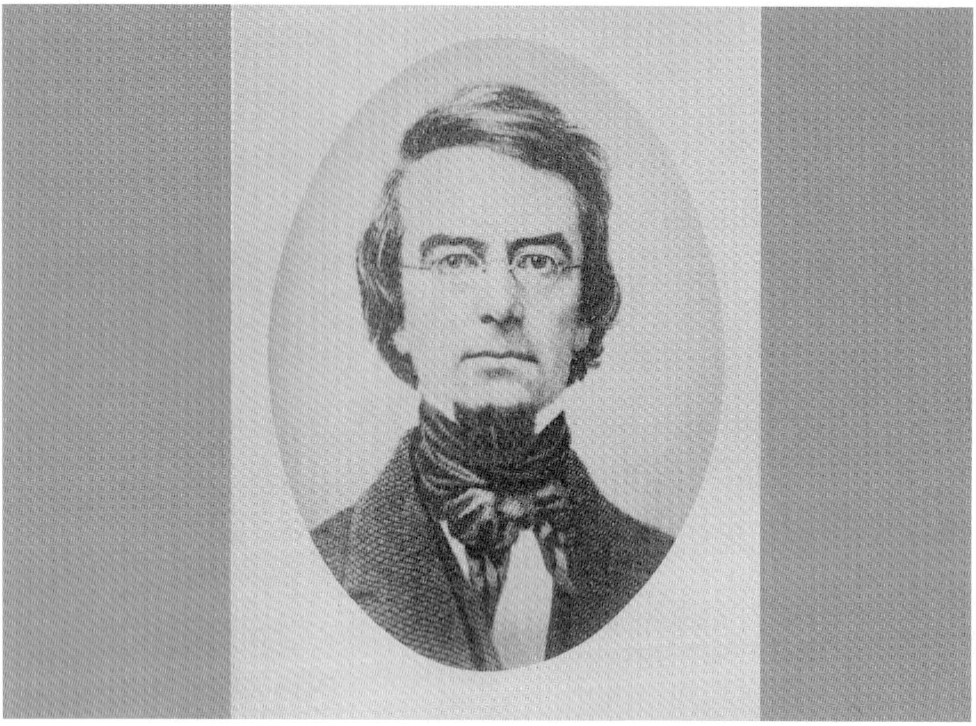

FIGURE 1–3. Luther Vose Bell.
Source. John Curwen: *The Original Thirteen Members of the Association of Medical Superintendents of American Institutions for the Insane.* Courtesy of American Psychiatric Association Archives, Washington, D.C.

York established the first asylum for persons with chronic insanity, the Willard Asylum for the Chronic Insane (Figure 1–5) (Deutsch 1949; Hurd 1916–1917). Not everyone was in favor of such institutions. Amariah Brigham (Figure 1–6), first superintendent of Utica State Hospital, in a letter to Dorothea Dix in 1866, indicated that he opposed "the establishment of hospitals solely for the incurable insane. They would, in my opinion, soon become objects of but little interest to any one, and where misrule, neglect, and all kinds of abuse would exist and exist without detection" (quoted in Deutsch 1949, p. 239).

At this same time, the members of the AMSAII articulated, at their annual meeting, what they believed the states' responsibilities were (Hurd 1916–1917):

1. The state should make ample and suitable provisions for all its insane.
2. No insane person should be treated in any county poorhouse or almshouse.
3. Proper classification is an indispensable element and can only be achieved in facilities specifically constructed for treatment.
4. Curable and incurable persons should not be in separate establishments.
5. States should have asylums placed so that individuals can get treatment near where they reside.
6. Hospitals should have enough wards to treat different classes of insane persons on different wards.
7. Hospitals could have up to 600 patients and properly care for the insane.

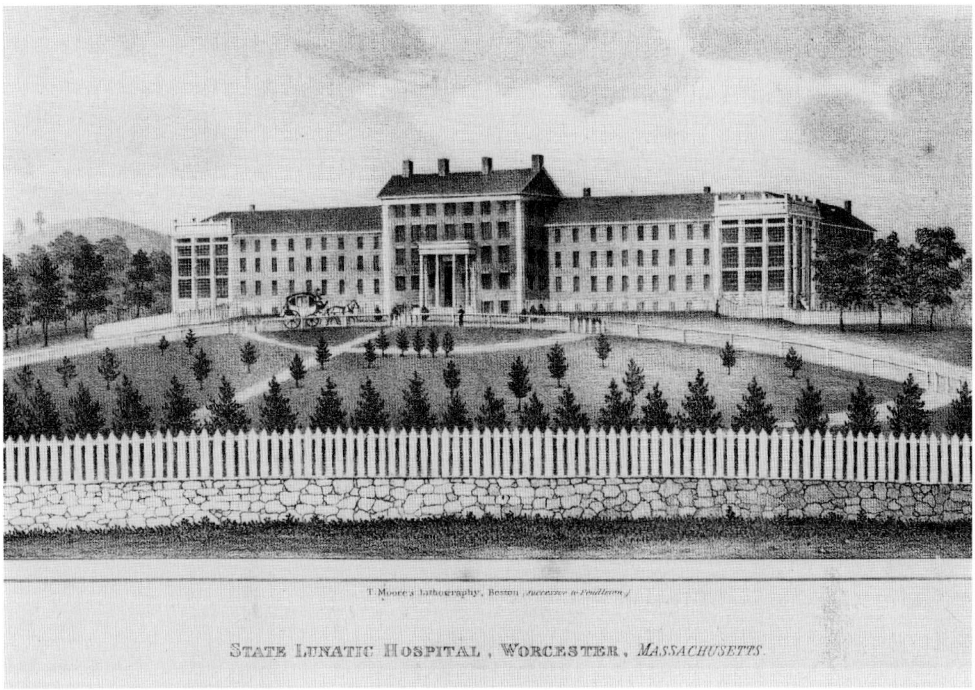

FIGURE 1–4. Worcester State Hospital.
Source. Courtesy of National Library of Medicine, Bethesda, Maryland.

In 1868, the AMSAII drafted suggested legislation concerning the admittance of patients (Hurd 1916–1917):

1. Insane persons may be placed in a hospital for the insane by their relatives, friends, or legal guardian, but never without the certificate of one or more reputable physicians, after a personal examination, made within 1 week.
2. Insane persons may be placed in a hospital by order of a magistrate who, after proper inquisition, finds that such persons are at large and dangerous to themselves or others or require hospital care and treatment; the fact of their insanity shall be certified as specified in the preceding section.
3. Insane persons may be placed in a hospital, by order of any high judicial officer, if, on statement in writing of any respectable individual that a certain person is insane, and that the welfare of himself or others requires his restraint, a duly appointed commission finds the person is a suitable case for confinement.

Origins of Private Psychiatric Hospitals

Three facilities began as parts of general medical hospitals. The Institute of the Pennsylvania Hospital started in the general hospital proposed by Benjamin Franklin, with insane persons scattered throughout the hospital, mostly in cellars. A separate wing of the general hospital was then completed, followed finally by a separate structure built in west Philadelphia, some distance from the general hospital, and funded by a colonial grant and subscriptions (Deutsch 1949; Kirkbride 1845).

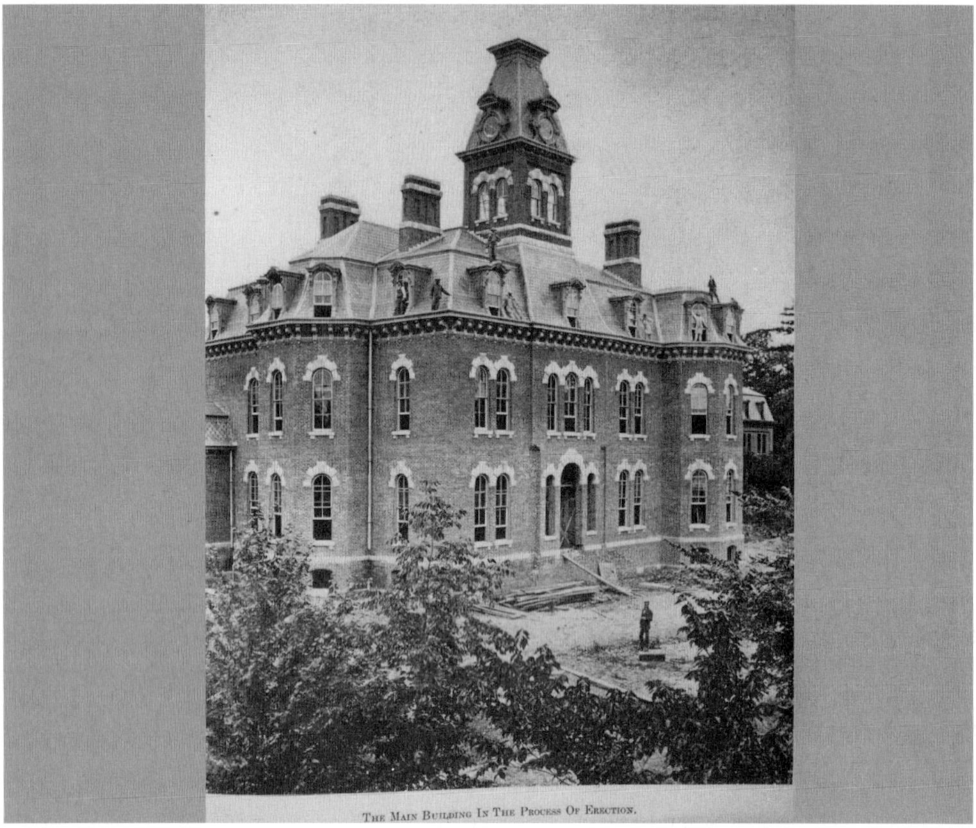

Figure 1–5. **Willard State Hospital (formerly Willard Asylum for the Chronic Insane).**
Source. Courtesy of American Psychiatric Association Archives, Washington, D.C.

The Bloomingdale Hospital in New York (Figure 1–7) began as a wing of a general hospital, funded by subscriptions from "philanthropic public spirited" citizens. The locus of care of the insane moved to a separate structure with a grant from the state (Deutsch 1949; Earle 1845).

McLean Hospital in Massachusetts started as part of a general hospital, but services for insane persons were provided in a separate facility from the outset. Initial funding was from bequests, subscriptions, and donations; 3 years after it opened, John McLean of Boston willed $100,000 to the asylum, and the asylum was renamed in his honor (Deutsch 1949; Massachusetts 1845).

Three private psychiatric hospitals began as freestanding institutions funded through different methods. Butler Hospital in Rhode Island (Figure 1–8) resulted from the legacy of a philanthropist, Nicholas Brown, and from a subscription campaign, with the major contributions coming from Cyrus Butler at the urging of Dorothea Dix (Deutsch 1949; Ray 1848). The Brattleboro Retreat, which began as the Vermont Asylum for the Insane, was funded through a bequest by the wife of a physician, with additional funds provided by the state (Deutsch 1949). The Hartford Retreat in Connecticut (subsequently named the Institute of Living) (Figure 1–9) resulted from a study by the Connecticut Medical Society that recommended the construction of a freestanding mental institu-

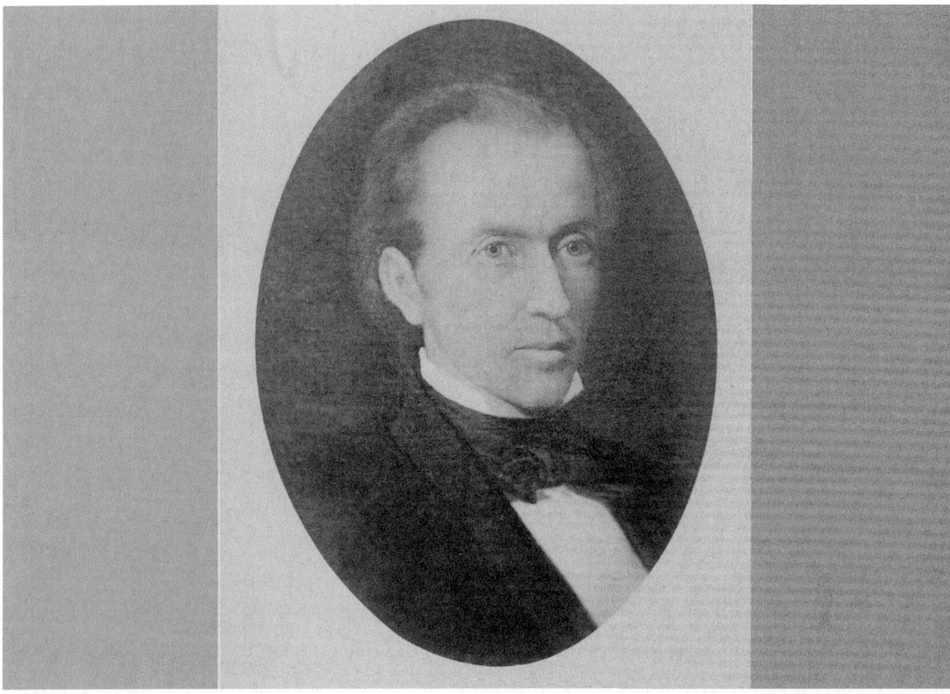

FIGURE 1–6. Amariah Brigham.
Source. John Curwen: *The Original Thirteen Members of the Association of Medical Superintendents of American Institutions for the Insane.* Courtesy of American Psychiatric Association Archives, Washington, D.C.

tion. The retreat was funded by a state grant, funds from the state medical society, private subscriptions, and a lottery (Connecticut 1845; Deutsch 1949). Two private hospitals were begun by religious organizations. The Friends Asylum in Pennsylvania was initiated by the Society of Friends. Modeled after the English Quakers' York Retreat, the Friends Asylum was funded by a subscription campaign and in-kind donations. The hospital was established to serve only members of the Society of Friends, but from 1834 to 1845 others were admitted. In 1845, admissions were limited to those connected with the Society of Friends and any others who were former patients (Deutsch 1949; Pennsylvania 1845).

Whereas all of these hospitals were formed under a for-profit model, the Mount Hope Institution in Maryland, which began as Mount Saint Vincent, was based on religious benevolence. Although a Catholic-affiliated institution, it accepted patients of all denominations.

The origins of many of the smaller facilities are much more obscure; many appear to have been set up as a form of private practice. Some that began in the early twentieth century, such as Chestnut Lodge and the Austen Riggs Center, were established as venues to practice certain types of psychiatry (Geller 2006). An interesting thesis for the founding of many nineteenth-century facilities is that physicians who had worked in the public sector needed income-producing ventures later in their careers because there was no public pension or retirement system (Gerald Grob, personal communication, November 2000). A few additional hospitals were created in a fashion similar to the earliest

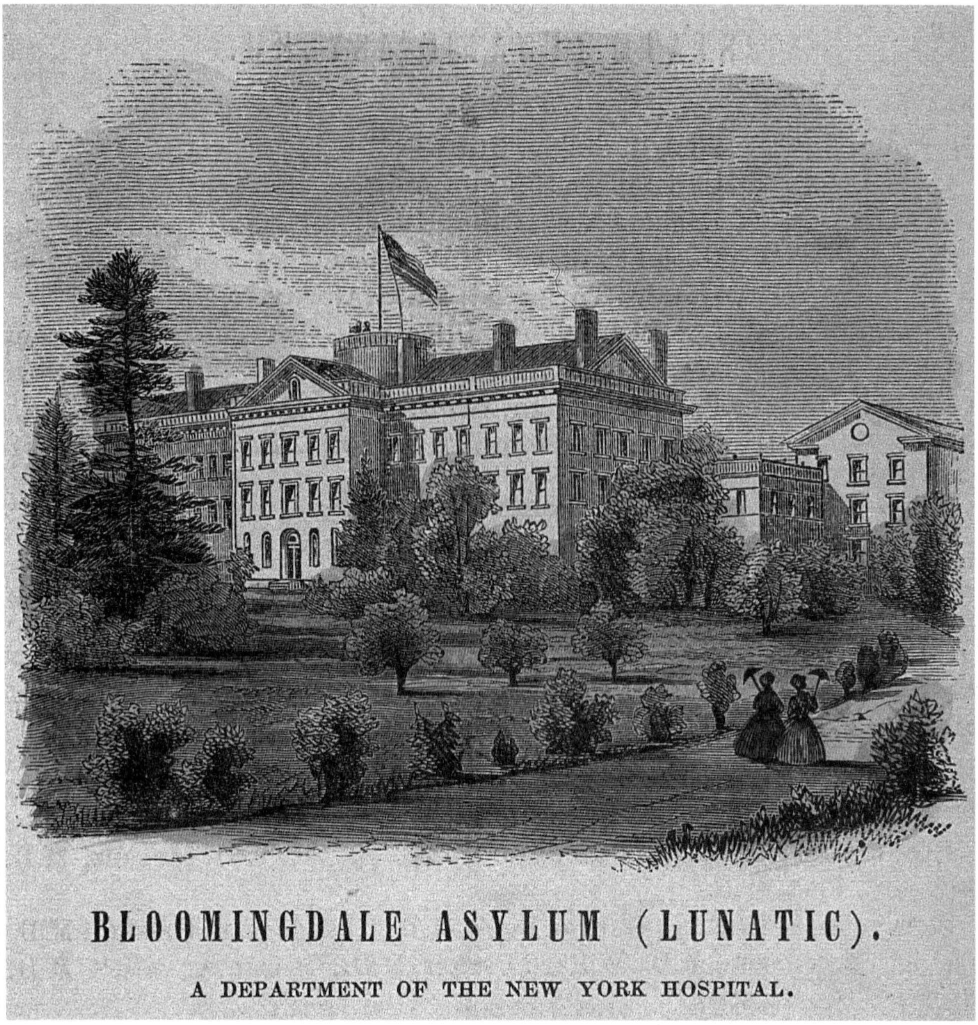

FIGURE 1–7. Bloomingdale Asylum (Bloomingdale Hospital), New York.
Source. Colored wood engraving. Courtesy of Wellcome Collection. Public Domain Mark.

asylums. Moses Sheppard planned for the establishment of a mental institution in Maryland and built a hospital that opened as the Sheppard Asylum (Figure 1–10). With a subsequent bequest from Enoch Pratt, the facility was renamed Sheppard and Enoch Pratt Hospital (Forbush 1971). Edward Jarvis, himself an operator of a private facility in Massachusetts, stated in 1860 that the role of the private facility was

> not to compete with the public institutions in matters of cheapness; but to provide liberally for all the proper wants of their inmates, and charge all for material, time, attention and responsibility, and receive a corresponding reward.
>
> Not to receive and treat the violent, the maniacal, the suicidal; but the mild, quiet, and manageable by personal influence.
>
> And principally to provide and offer to such patients as can properly enjoy and profit by them, an opportunity of using more of their faculties that are sane, a freer range of occupation and action, more of domestic and social life, more intercourse with the

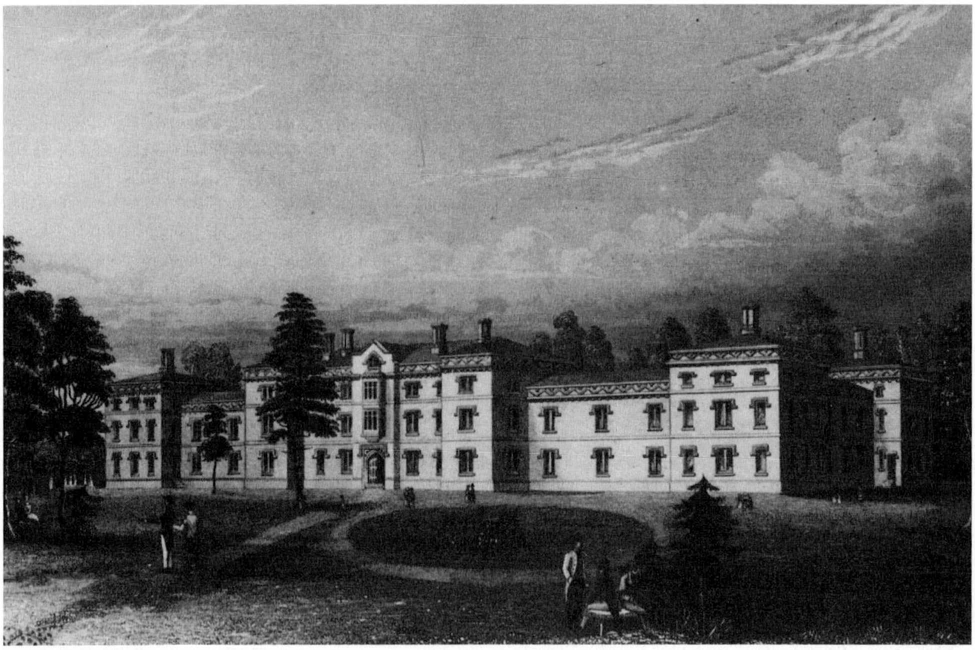

FIGURE 1–8. Butler Hospital, Providence, Rhode Island.
Source. *American Journal of Insanity*, Vol. 5, frontis. Courtesy of National Library of Medicine, Bethesda, Maryland.

> world, and a condition resembling more nearly that of their own homes than can be offered and enjoyed in the public hospitals. (Jarvis 1860, p. 31)

Private-Public Interface

Of the larger private facilities, all but one preceded the state's first public hospital, sometimes by more than 50 years. The private hospitals met a state's need for care of indigent insane persons by admitting "public" patients with varying methods of payment. This arrangement generally continued until the state determined it could provide for those insane who required public support more cost-effectively in state hospitals. Bloomingdale Asylum was aided by legislative appropriations for its first 30 years; this ended in 1849, and the facility then devoted itself to private patients only (New York 1872). William Rockwell, superintendent of the Vermont Asylum for the Insane (Brattleboro Retreat), proclaimed in 1867 that his hospital could accommodate all insane persons of Vermont who required hospital treatment (Vermont Asylum for the Insane 1868). The Hartford Retreat ended its relationship with the state of Connecticut after 30 years of "receiving such insane patients as were a public charge" (Connecticut 1871). Butler Hospital received an annual appropriation from the state that could be apportioned to specific patients at a fixed annual cap per patient (Butler Hospital for the Insane 1878). This continued even after Butler Hospital sent a large number of the indigent insane patients to the state facility at its opening. Pennsylvania Hospital (Figure 1–11) provided care to a limited number from the state, doing so "without charge of any kind" (Kirkbride 1845).

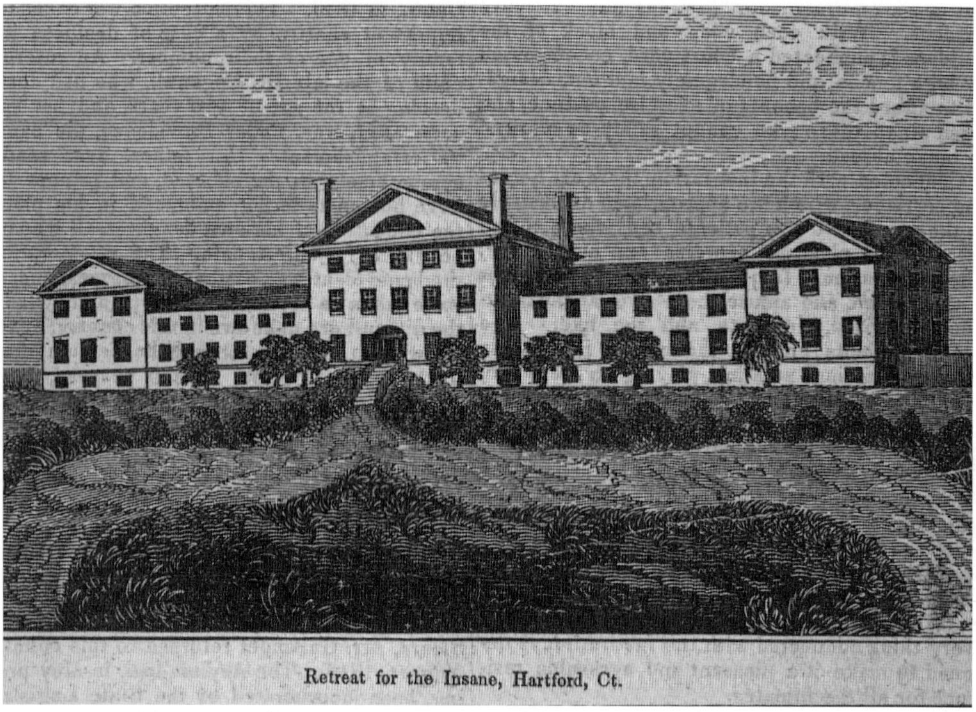

FIGURE 1–9. Hartford Retreat, Hartford, Connecticut.
Source. *American Journal of Insanity*, v. 5, frontis. Courtesy of National Library of Medicine, Bethesda, Maryland.

A social policy evolved in virtually every state that care of its insane citizens would predominantly be a public function. Despite the operation of many private facilities, these accounted for a small percentage of institutionalized persons by the early twentieth century. On January 1, 1920, there were 232,680 persons in institutions for mental disorders in the United States: 200,109 in state hospitals, 21,584 in county or city facilities, 1,040 in institutions for temporary care, 709 in Public Health Service hospitals, and 9,238 in private hospitals (Pollock and Forbush 1921). Thus, private facilities accounted for only 4% of persons in psychiatric facilities.

Comparison of Private and Public Facilities

It should come as no surprise that public and private facilities had some common features, because the establishment of many public asylums was directly influenced by the early private asylums. The Friends Asylum and Hartford Retreat influenced the erection and organization of Utica State Hospital (Figure 1–12); the Hartford Retreat affected the establishment of asylums in Worcester and Boston, Massachusetts; and the Brattleboro Retreat influenced the construction of the state asylum in New Hampshire (Hurd 1913).

At the turn of the twentieth century, the president of the New York State Commission in Lunacy argued that both public and private facilities should be able to admit patients for 48–72 hours on an emergency paper signed by a family physician. "Regular lunacy certification" would follow, and thus the use of jails and prisons for the reception

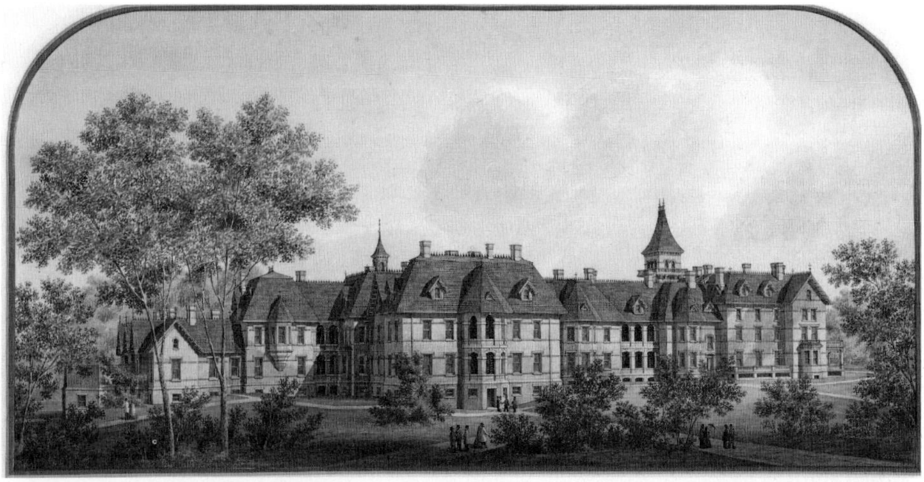

FIGURE 1–10. Sheppard Asylum.
Source. Courtesy of Sheppard and Enoch Pratt Hospital.

of persons "ill of brain disease" could be avoided (Peterson 1902). During the first two decades of the twentieth century, both public and private hospitals had open, unlocked wards, and both were striving to treat patients without the use of seclusion or restraint (Hurd 1916–1917; Page 1904).

Private facilities, like public ones, had issues with overcrowding ("Vermont" 1890), psychiatrists' violent deaths at the facility ("Death of Dr. George Cook" 1876), unwarranted admissions ("From the Report of the McLean Asylum" 1864), allegations of abuse (Stewart 1874), and stigma (Parsons 1881). Accounts decrying inappropriate admissions and ill treatment can be found from former patients of both public and private facilities (Geller and Harris 1994).

By the 1880s, most psychiatrists agreed that "insane patients can best be managed away from their own homes" (Parsons 1881, p. 586). Some psychiatrists postulated that "well-equipped and well-managed asylums for the insane are among the most important of the outgrowths of modern civilization and benevolence" (Parsons 1881, p. 567).

The private facilities were established for wealthier persons able to pay for more comfort, "suitable medical treatment," and "pursuits and diversions which are most congenial and desirable" ("Private Asylums" 1879, p. 243). Patients were such that when "you encounter persons variously occupied…you find yourself not infrequently quite at a loss to determine whether the persons met with are really the insane, or whether they may be visitors or officials in the establishment" (Wood 1853, p. 212). Private facilities allowed "more judicious social intercourse with the sane," greater personal freedom, more individuation of treatment, closer approximation to family life, greater ratios of physicians and attendants, and less use of "locked and bolted doors, and of barred windows" (Parsons 1881, p. 575). Public hospitals were entities of state, county, or municipal governments, and by mid-nineteenth century states had moved to centralize control and to decrease asylum superintendents' autonomy (Grob 1983). States' oversight over private facilities was extremely variable. By 1910, private

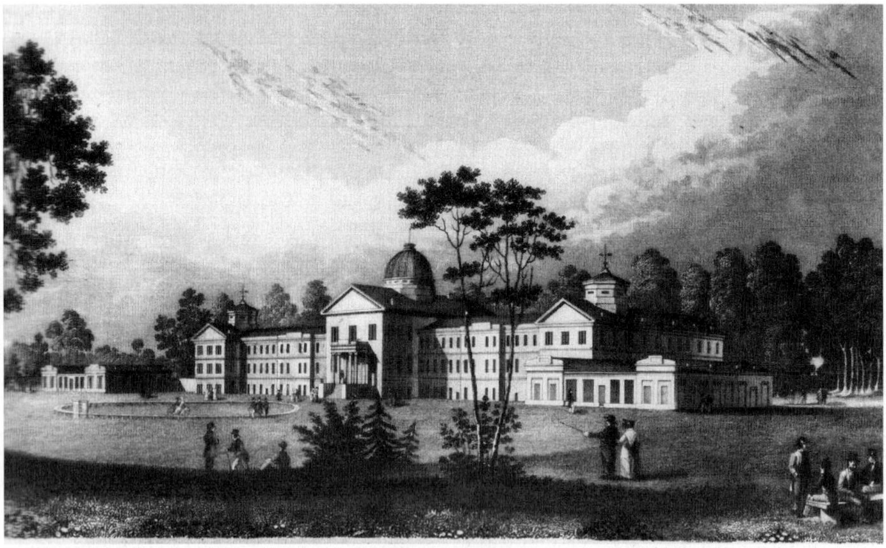

FIGURE 1–11. Kirkbride's Hospital (Institute of the Pennsylvania Hospital), Philadelphia, Pennsylvania.
Source. Courtesy of American Psychiatric Association Archives, Washington, D.C.

facilities came under the oversight of some form of a state board in 16 states. Three other states had alternative methods of oversight. In 11 states, private facilities were required to be licensed (Bureau of the Census 1914), but many were not.

Public institutions sought to lower their censuses even as state hospital populations grew and patients had progressively longer lengths of stay (Grob 1983); private facilities sought patients to maximize their occupancy rates. A fundamental criticism of private facilities was the inherent conflict of interest of the proprietor: "It is not for the interest of the proprietor of a private asylum to cure his patients, and hence they may not make an honest effort to promote their cure" (Parsons 1881, pp. 578–579). Private facilities advertised and were not infrequently endorsed in professional journal editorials ("Two Homes for the Nervous and Insane" 1880). Advertising by private facilities and by physicians was frequent enough that a code for professional advertising was proposed in 1894 ("Provision for Professional Advertising in the Code" 1894).

By the 1880s, some states (e.g., Connecticut, Indiana, Maryland, Massachusetts, New York, Pennsylvania, Rhode Island, Wisconsin) permitted the commitment of insane persons to private facilities (Board of State Commissioners of Public Charities of the State of Illinois 1885). As a way of relieving crowding at state hospitals, proposals were put forward to "furlough" patients from state hospitals to private facilities in an early version of contemporary "step-down procedures" ("Insane Hospital Annexes" 1880). Similar procedures were recently used in the state of Vermont, for example, for the same reason.

Private hospitals, in contrast to public hospitals, could become quite luxurious. Long Island House, in Amityville, New York, built a small cottage consisting of a sitting room, bedroom, bathroom, and clothespress for a single patient in 1900 ("Long Island House, Amityville, NY" 1900). Upham House, at McLean Asylum, included

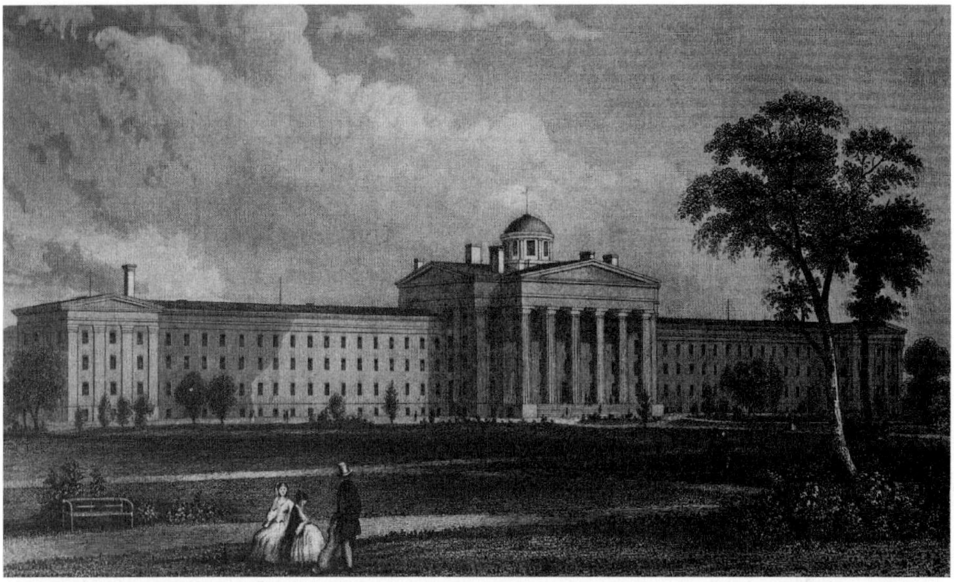

FIGURE 1–12. Utica State Hospital.
Source. Courtesy of American Psychiatric Association Archives, Washington, D.C./National Library of Medicine, Bethesda, Maryland.

nine suites, each containing a sitting room, bedroom, and bathroom; the house had two private halls, reception rooms, a dining room, a billiard room, and a Turkish bath ("The McLean Asylum for the Insane" 1893).

Greater resources led to remarkably favorable staffing ratios at private hospitals. In the 1850s, Friends Asylum had an attendant for every six patients ("The Asylum near Frankford, in Pennsylvania" 1851). Both Kirkbride (Pennsylvania Hospital for the Insane 1850) and Jarvis (Association of Medical Superintendents of American Institutions for the Insane 1853) described private attendants for every patient.

In 1851, John Butler (Figure 1–13), superintendent of the Hartford Retreat, noted both the importance of "mental occupations and amusements" and the fact that many asylums were lacking in the provision of these (Connecticut 1855). He repeated this theme 35 years later (Butler 1886). In this early period of inpatient psychiatry, the private facilities offered a remarkable array of activities for amusement and recreation, including baseball, boating, bowling, calisthenics and gymnasiums, concerts, cooking instruction, croquet, exhibitions, fishing, French lessons, golf, horseback riding, lantern slide shows, lectures, medicine ball, museums, pleasure grounds, reading rooms, skating, squash and tennis, stereoscopic views, tea parties, and wood carving ("At the Pennsylvania Hospital for the Insane" 1852; "Gymnasium for the Insane" 1897; Pennsylvania Hospital for the Insane 1854). Public hospitals did less well in providing amusements but had better developed work programs that were thought to be important to patients' recovery.

Despite their efforts, private hospitals suffered from the "premature removal of patients" (Butler Hospital for the Insane 1856; "Dr. Butler of the Hartford Retreat for the Insane" 1851; Pennsylvania Hospital for the Insane 1854; Sawyer 1879; Stokes 1851). In 1851, Butler expressed concerns about the outcomes for patients who left the asylum

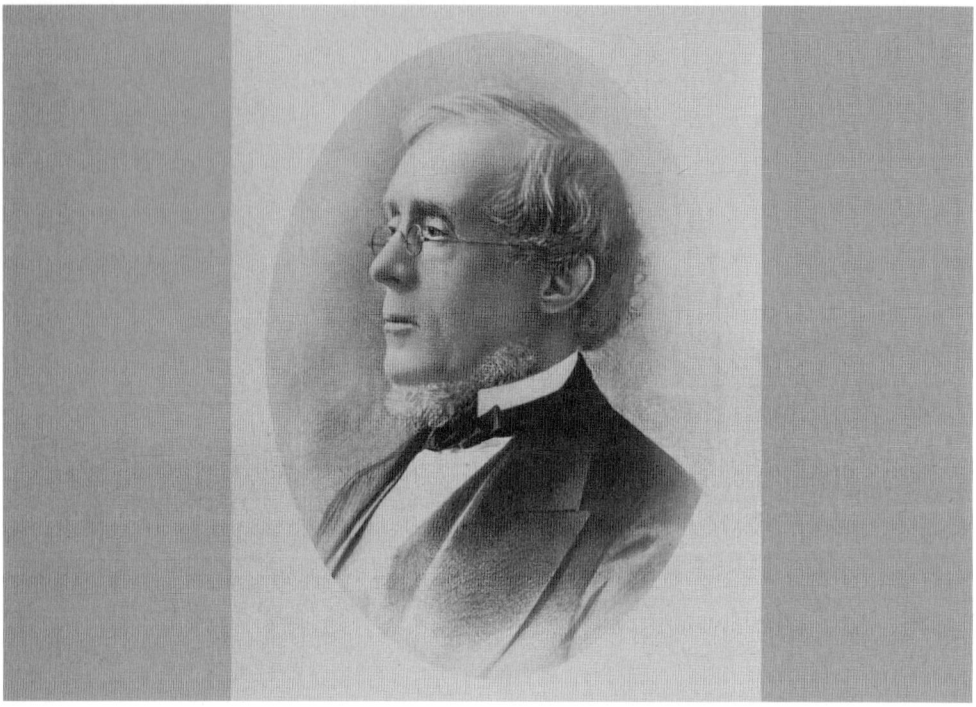

FIGURE 1–13. John S. Butler.
Source. John Curwen: *The Original Thirteen Members of the Association of Medical Superintendents of American Institutions for the Insane.* Courtesy of American Psychiatric Association Archives, Washington, D.C.

too soon: "Many have relapsed into an incurable state, while others remain half-crazed or nervous invalids, and will probably remain so for life" ("Dr. Butler of the Hartford Retreat for the Insane" 1851, p. 187). Isaac Ray of Butler Hospital (Figure 1–14) called the premature withdrawal of patients "a most disheartening experience of our calling" (Butler Hospital for the Insane 1856, p. 252). The superintendents of the private facilities during this era (unlike those of public facilities) did not have the authority to hold patients if family or friends insisted on their discharge (Stokes 1851). Some patients certainly left private facilities because of the inability to pay for further care (Butler Hospital for the Insane 1856; Stokes 1851). Ray, perhaps somewhat cavalierly, exclaimed, "We may indeed be shocked by this balancing of reason, God's greatest gift to man, with a paltry sum of money" (Butler Hospital for the Insane 1856, p. 282). Other patients were removed because family and friends were "impatient for the results" or unwilling to wait until "the disease is fully eradicated" (Stokes 1851, p. 211). Patients who were prematurely discharged from private facilities were not infrequently subsequently admitted to public facilities, because of the lack of an available bed, inadequate financial resources, or the patient's "unmanageable" behavior (Sawyer 1879). Others were concerned that patients discharged before they were medically ready could be a danger to the community from acts of violence (Sawyer 1879).

By the end of the 1880s, there was recognition that "the unparalleled progress in neurology, cerebral anatomy, physiology, pathology, and localization of function has enlarged the horizon of our knowledge of disease and of the action of causes" (Andrews

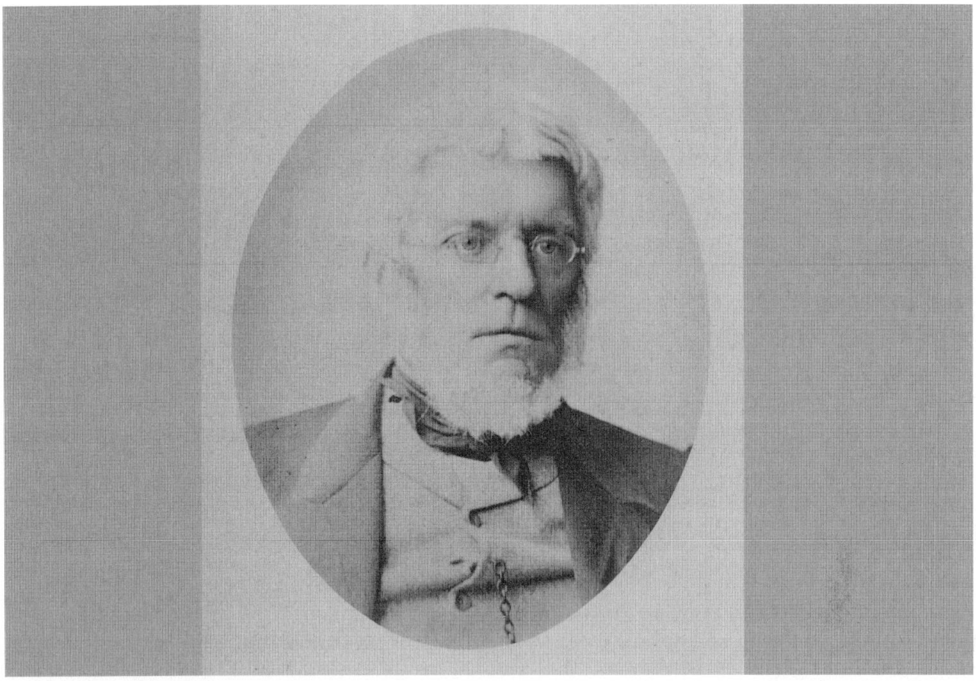

FIGURE 1–14. Isaac Ray.
Source. John Curwen: *The Original Thirteen Members of the Association of Medical Superintendents of American Institutions for the Insane.* Courtesy of American Psychiatric Association Archives, Washington, D.C.

1887, p. 199). This progress "furnished a scientific and positive basis for treatment in many cases of insanity which before was unattainable" (Andrews 1887, p. 199). Inpatient treatments near the end of the nineteenth century included electricity, massage, new medications and more rational prescribing, and oophorectomy (Andrews 1887); enforced rest (Sinkler 1892); hydrotherapy (Niles 1899); and physical training (Channing 1889). These approaches, although suspect in retrospect, represented significant advances for inpatient psychiatric treatment.

Hospitals devised new record-keeping systems to facilitate research ("McLean Hospital, Waverly" 1900); expanded clinical pathological laboratories ("Psychiatry at the Sheppard and Enoch Pratt Hospital" 1901); focused on such diseases as dementia praecox and syphilis ("Bloomingdale Hospital, White Plains" 1913); and hired physicians with research interests and expertise ("McLean Hospital, Waverly" 1900). The new focus on research is highlighted in a statement by Edward Brush, first superintendent of Sheppard and Enoch Pratt Hospital: "The most important function [of a hospital] is to study disease, its causes, progress, processes, termination and prevention" ("Psychiatry at the Sheppard and Enoch Pratt Hospital" 1901, p. 554).

In the end, however, it was Thomas Kirkbride (Figure 1–15) who made the most prophetic commentary for many of these hospitals: "So in regard to the support of hospitals for the insane, it will be a sad day for these institutions, and still sadder for the patients in them, when the rivalry of hospitals and their officers shall be, rather to discover for how little their inmates can be kept, than to secure what is best, and most thoroughly promotes the great objects for which they were established" (Kirkbride 1875, p. 99).

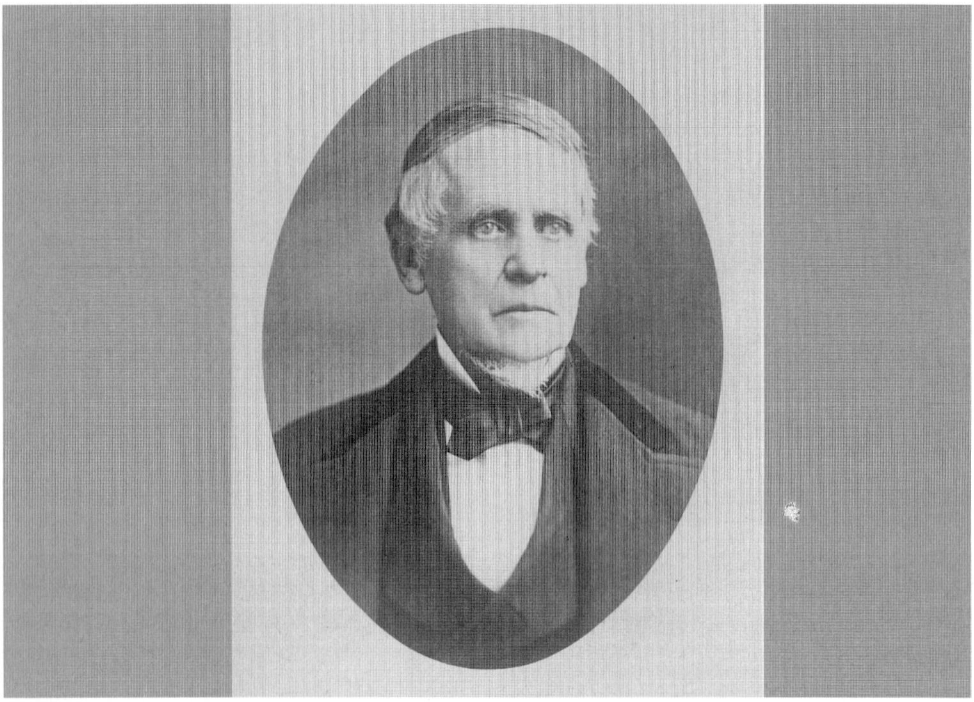

FIGURE 1–15. Thomas Kirkbride.
Source. John Curwen: *The Original Thirteen Members of the Association of Medical Superintendents of American Institutions for the Insane.* Courtesy of American Psychiatric Association Archives, Washington, D.C.

The Middle Period (1921–1970)

Changes in American psychiatry between 1921 and 1970 were dramatic and far-reaching. In terms of treatment modalities, psychoanalysis was introduced to the inpatient setting in the 1920s. The 1930s witnessed the introduction of the somatic treatments: insulin coma, metrazol shock, and electroshock therapy (Kalinowski and Hoch 1946). In the 1940s, attention was directed to establishing milieu therapy, in which "all aspects of the patient's life in the hospital were viewed as part of treatment" (Robbins 1966). In the 1950s, the introduction of the first antipsychotic medication, chlorpromazine, fundamentally altered inpatient psychiatry (Smith 1955). And in the 1960s, initial attempts to understand the mechanism of action of psychotropic drugs (Snyder et al. 1970) spurred efforts that to this day shape our pharmacological armamentarium.

Alternatives to psychiatric inpatient treatment, such as the day hospital, were initiated and promoted. Claims of being the "first day hospital in North America" were made by hospital staff in Boston, Montreal, and Topeka, Kansas. Psychiatric inpatient treatment based in general hospitals developed during this period (American Hospital Association 1970; Glasscote and Kanno 1965). Psychiatrists attempted to improve diagnostic validity and reliability (Jackson 1970) and to promulgate standards for inpatient psychiatric facilities (American Psychiatric Association 1969). New concepts, such as the rights of mental patients, emerged (Birnbaum 1960), and old, nineteenth-century ideas such as "recovery" reemerged (Menninger 1961). Insurances were developed or modified that began to cover the treatment of mental illness—both private and public.

Perhaps the most outstanding change between 1921 and 1970 was the beginning of the shift from hospital-based to non-hospital-based care and treatment of persons with mental illness, a movement retrospectively labeled "deinstitutionalization" but perhaps better characterized as "dehospitalization" (Geller 2000a). The peak year-end inpatient census for all psychiatric patients occurred in 1955.

The falling percentage of patients in public hospitals in the 1930s and 1940s was due to the creation and expansion of veterans hospitals and in the 1960s was due, in part, to the expanding role of the general hospitals. From the 1930s through the 1960s, the percentage of the total psychiatric inpatients accounted for by the private psychiatric hospitals was steady and small. The transfer of care from public inpatient setting to "the community" during the 1950s and 1960s contributed to the decline in utilization of state hospital beds.

1920s–1930s

In 1920, the National Committee for Mental Hygiene surveyed institutions for persons with mental diseases, mental deficits, epilepsy, alcoholism, and drug addiction and found 625 institutions in the United States, 388 public and 237 private. Thirty-two states had private institutions for mental patients, but their total census accounted for only 4% of the 232,680 persons with mental disorders actually in psychiatric hospitals (Pollock and Forbush 1921).

Institutions to treat persons with mental illness continued to open throughout the 1920s, whereas some private hospitals closed. In a 1923 report by the U.S. Census Bureau, there were 267,617 patients in 526 (55% public) hospitals. This rate of 242 resident patients per 100,000 general population was an increase from the 1880 rate of 82. This change was attributed to both an actual increase in the rate of mental diseases and a greater use of hospitals (Pollock 1925).

During the 1920s, psychoanalysis was introduced to hospitals. Occupational therapy, long used in public hospitals, became of greater interest to private hospitals. Dr. William Rush Dunton Jr., a psychiatrist and educator at Sheppard Pratt, published the first account of occupational therapy as a profession in 1917 and is acknowledged as the "father of occupational therapy." It was stressed that "therapeutic occupation" should be conducted off the wards in an "occupational building" (Haas 1924)—early "psychosocial rehabilitation malls."

In 1932, mental institutions represented 10% of the total number of all registered hospitals but accounted for nearly 50% of the patient population in hospitals ("Hospitals for Nervous and Mental Patients" 1933). Most patients were in public hospitals; private hospitals had just under 1% of all psychiatric inpatients ("Nineteen Hundred Thirty-Six Censuses of Mental Patients" 1938). Whereas public hospitals were struggling with limited resources for ever-expanding patient populations—420,553 nationwide in 1938—private hospitals had rather impressive staffing ratios, with 1 physician for every 17 patients ("Hospitals for Nervous and Mental Patients" 1933), 1 nurse for every 3 patients, and 1 attendant for every 4 patients (Grimes 1934).

Private sanatoriums, often located near large cities, were run for profit, emphasizing "comfort, hygiene, sanitation, beauty, and pleasure" (Grimes 1934). Public hospitals were generally constructed away from population centers and sometimes relocated if an urban center spread too close to the institution.

The sanatoriums were often owned by physicians, wholly or in part (Grimes 1934). The ratio of physicians to patients at sanatoriums was 1:17. The nurse-to-patient ratio was about the same, whereas the attendant-to-patient ratio was 1:3.5 ("Hospitals for Nervous and Mental Patients" 1933).

In the 1930s, somatic treatments moved from endocrine replacement therapy to narcosis, insulin convulsive therapy, metrazol shock, and electroshock therapy (Kalinowski and Hoch 1946). Other treatments included medication, hydrotherapy, psychotherapy, occupational therapy, physical therapy, and even surgery. Recreation was deemed important. Psychotherapy focused on extending patients' insight and available affective expression (Menninger 1936). Patients discharged as recovered or improved represented 65% of the total number of patients admitted (Grimes 1934).

There were also rest homes in the 1930s. These provided primarily custodial care for persons with some financial means who needed "mental medicine." Activities were limited, discharge of patients was slow, and many patients with chronic mental diseases lived their lives out in these rest homes (Grimes 1934).

New loci of treatment opened during the 1930s: the psychopathic hospital (Campbell 1930) and psychiatric ward in the general hospital (Heldt 1939). Although the presence of these psychiatric units was small (only 112 of 4,309 general hospitals had "departments for mental patients" in 1932), general hospitals were rapidly adding psychiatric units. Such units were not always welcomed by hospital medical staff, who were concerned that "noisy, destructive, violent or suicidal patients" would disrupt the general hospital (Young 1939).

The stigma of mental illness and of hospitalization were prominent no matter what the type of hospital. In 1936, the *American Journal of Psychiatry* commented on "the worry over the 'disgrace' of having been a patient in a mental hospital" ("The 'Stigma' of Mental Illness" 1936, p. 476). This editorial sadly opined that "psychosis as an illness to be considered and treated as a medical issue like other forms of disability" would do little to destigmatize the patient or the psychiatrist. Psychiatric patients organizing their own services and advocating for themselves has its modern roots in the 1930s (Friedman 1939).

1940s–1950s

The 1940s represent the nadir of America's public mental hospitals. Care of the mentally ill was described as substandard and a national disgrace. Deficiencies of state hospitals are well documented in the pages of professional journals such as *Mental Hygiene* (Klapman 1944). Exposés were available in books (Deutsch 1948), magazines (Maisel 1946), and fictionalized accounts (Ward 1946). In 1945, *The Modern Hospital* noted, "The sorriest spectacle in hospital service today is the treatment accorded the psychiatric patient" ("Modern Hospital Announces Prize Competition" 1945, p. 530). Private mental hospitals could not fill the need because they were just too costly. In 1945, the per capita annual expenditure in state, county, and city hospitals was $391 and $2,000 in private hospitals ("Costs of Long-Term Mental-Hospital Care" 1949). The middle class could simply not avail themselves of private inpatient treatment. This meant that those with moderate incomes had no choice but the public hospital (Sherman and Hoffman 1949).

Attempts were made to improve inpatient treatment through the promulgation of principles and standards, such as those put forward by the Division of Mental Hygiene of the U.S. Public Health Service, the National Committee for Mental Hygiene, and the APA's Committee on Psychiatric Standards and Policies, and through surveys (Liebman and French 1949). One such survey found that of inpatient facilities with fewer than 101 patients, 44 of 46 (96%) were private; of facilities with 101–1,000 patients, 10 of 40 (25%) were private; and of facilities with more than 1,000 patients, 0 of 99 were private (Liebman and French 1949). A 1947 survey of private mental institutions found that the total number of beds for mental illness (excluding mental retardation, epilepsy, and alcohol and drug abuse) in private sanatoriums, rest homes, and psychiatric units in general hospitals was 21,956. There were 10 states and territories with no beds in these categories of hospitals; 6 had fewer than 100, 26 had 100–999, and 6 had 1,000 or more beds. States in the last category were, in descending order of number of beds, New York, Pennsylvania, California, Illinois, Maryland, and Connecticut (Sherman and Hoffman 1949). Although there was relatively little hospital construction during the 1940s (Liebman and French 1949), the federal government became involved in the provision of inpatient psychiatric services in ways it had not been previously (Felix 1947). Much of the federal effort was directed to the public sector, but the Hill-Burton Act funded the construction of psychiatric units in general hospitals, and the National Mental Health Act supported research and training in private psychiatric facilities.

In the 1950s, attention turned to understanding the psychiatric hospital as a social system (Greenblatt et al. 1957). There was general agreement on the objective of any mental hospital (which sounds quite contemporary) "to effect maximum improvement of the individual patient as rapidly as possible. This should mean assisting him to return to the community as a contributing member of society" (Myers and Smith 1956, p. 6). If this objective could not be met, the hospital was to work out "the best adjustment possible for the patient within or without the hospital setting, with a persistent and continuous effort to improve the adjustment" (Myers and Smith 1956, p. 6).

Private hospitals accounted for less than 3% of the total mental hospital beds, but they accounted for 25%–40% of the annual admissions to all mental hospitals (Reed 1958). Rapid turnover of patients was accomplished through a four-decade trend of maintaining fewer "hard-core" patients, those hospitalized beyond 3 years' length of stay (Morris and Brunt 1957). Long-term patients were the responsibility of the state. Many psychiatrists running private psychiatric hospitals expressed concern about these hospitals' viability (Otis and Robinson 1951). The medical director of McLean Hospital stated at the 1950 APA Institute (in another quite modern-sounding refrain), "The time when you could run a private hospital as a hospital and make money has gone. Operating expenses have so increased that it is almost impossible to collect the cost from our patients" (Otis and Robinson 1951, p. 161).

Although some new private hospitals opened in the 1950s, other long-established, private mental hospitals went bankrupt, such as Norway Foundation in Indiana and Butler Hospital in Rhode Island (Reed 1958). (Butler Hospital reopened 1 year after it closed, in response in part to public support.) The demise of these two hospitals was attributed to expanding competition from general hospital psychiatric units (Dunn 1951), the inability to charge patients what they could afford and be able to meet expenses (Reed 1958), decaying physical plants, and staff dissatisfaction (Reed 1958).

Health insurance coverage that excluded mental disorders (Bennett 1959) made matters worse.

The absolute shortage of psychiatrists had a negative impact on all inpatient psychiatry. Despite an increase of 57% (from 5,534 psychiatrists in the United States to 8,713) between 1950 and 1956, there was "only one psychiatrist for every 19,200 citizens" in 1956 ("Care and Treatment" 1957). Between 1948 and 1957, during most of which the public hospital census was increasing, the state hospitals improved their psychiatrist-to-patient ratio from 1:259 to 1:161. This 37.6% improvement still left them far from the APA minimum standard of 1:30 (Tallman 1960). It was estimated at the end of the decade that an additional 12,000 psychiatrists would be needed (Squire 1961).

Innovations did emerge during this dark era for inpatient psychiatry, a period made worse by the burden World War II placed on these hospitals. Such innovations included the sending of follow-up questionnaires to discharged patients ("Post-Release Questionnaire" 1951), formation of ex-patient organizations ("Club Formed for Patients, Ex-patients, and Relatives" 1950), desegregation of psychiatric hospitals (Stevens 1952), evaluation of long-term intensive inpatient psychotherapy with psychotic patients, greater emphasis on rehabilitation ("Rehabilitation of the Mentally Ill" 1954), and development of day hospitals (Hayman 1957). Somatic treatments initiated prior to 1950 continued to be used during the decade: frontal lobotomy (Freeman 1957), insulin shock therapy (Brannon and Graham 1955), and electroshock therapy (Wolff 1955). The beginning of modern psychopharmacology was perhaps the greatest change in inpatient psychiatry in the 1950s. Treatment with chlorpromazine was reported from both public and private hospitals (Bennett et al. 1956; Kinross-Wright 1955). Research and development expanded during the later 1950s to include promethazine (Erwin 1957), thioridazine (Cohen 1958), and imipramine (Azima and Vispo 1958).

1960s

In the 1960s, opinions about private psychiatric hospitals varied from "I doubt if many private mental hospitals will survive the next ten years" (Barton 1962, p. 661) to "The private mental hospital will continue to be the central or primary resource supplying the psychiatric needs of the community" (Jones 1964, p. 336). One private hospital attending psychiatrist proclaimed, "It is the role of the private psychiatric hospital to be the leader, the pilot, on all fronts, in exploring new areas in the prevention and treatment of mental illness, in setting and maintaining standards, in fostering true multidisciplinary cooperation and activity, and in serving the community" (Barnard 1964, p. 22). Identified advantages of private hospitals included creating a microcosm of the community at large (Wayne 1961); providing patient-centered treatment (Barnard 1964; Wayne 1961); better integrating inpatient services into longitudinal treatment of the patient (Myers and Appel 1961); better serving first admissions (Barnard 1964; Wayne 1961); treating patients for shorter lengths of stay (Garber 1961); maintaining a better-trained staff with less administrative interference with clinical practice (Barnard 1964; Myers and Appel 1961); and providing treatment in a less stigmatizing environment (Garber 1961).

Inpatient psychiatric hospitalization outside of state hospitals became more available as health insurance for hospitalization expanded to include psychiatric treatment (Coordinating Committee on Professional Standards in Psychiatry 1961). Early efforts to include psychiatric treatment were made by the Federal Employees Health

Benefits Program in 1962 (Auster 1969), the United Auto Workers and the automobile industry in 1965 (Auster 1969), the Health Insurance Plan of Greater New York in 1965 (Goldensohn et al. 1969), Medicare in 1966 ("The Effect of Medicare on the Accreditation of Psychiatric Hospitals" 1966), and Blue Cross/Blue Shield nationally in 1969 (Auster 1969). Problems due to the perceived misuse of insurance for hospitalization for mental illness were already recognized in the 1960s. Interventions proposed to remedy these problems included peer review (Auster 1969), reimbursement for partial hospitalization and other alternatives to inpatient treatment (Felix 1965), and national health insurance (Gorman 1969). "Dumping" and "cost shifting" emerged as part of the everyday life of inpatient psychiatry. One public hospital superintendent lamented, "Most Blue Cross plans cover mental illness for only 21 days. So the patient goes to a private institution for three weeks. If he gets well, he goes home, saved from disgrace. If he fails to get well, he comes to us. Result: we get the failures, plus blame for having failures" (Davidson 1964, p. 280).

During the 1960s, the public sector became focused on psychotropic drugs' effects on state hospital utilization (Brill and Patton 1962) and the simultaneous use of two or more "tranquilizers," already referred to in the 1960s as "polypharmacy" (Merlis et al. 1970). University departments of psychiatry and private hospitals were examining the usefulness of the different phenothiazine derivatives (Casey et al. 1960), mechanisms of action of antidepressant medications (Schildkraut et al. 1971), and the merits of unilateral rather than bilateral electroconvulsive therapy (Whitehorn and Betz 1960). Hospitals, especially private ones, were interested in refining the roles of the psychiatrist (Whitehorn and Betz 1960), the nurse (Payne 1966), the social worker (Pinsky and Levy 1964), the psychiatric aide (Bernstein and Herzberg 1970), and the "multidisciplinary team" (Howard 1960). Psychiatrists grappled with understanding such concepts as therapeutic community (Gralnick and D'Elia 1969) and countertransference in milieu treatment (Wesselius 1968); improving intensive rehabilitation (Howard 1960); and understanding the effects of social competence on prognosis (Rosen et al. 1968).

Much happened in the 1960s that influences American inpatient psychiatry to this day: American presidents such as Kennedy (1964) and Johnson ("President Johnson Signs Comprehensive Health Planning Bill" 1967) showing a greater interest in mental health; members of the American bar advocating that committed psychiatric patients have a *right* to treatment (Bazelon 1969; Birnbaum 1965); new public funding streams for psychiatric treatment (Gibson 1967); and new standards for psychiatric facilities, including those defined by *Wyatt v. Stickney* (1971).

In 1965, the IMD exclusion was established in Section 1905(a)(B) of the Social Security Act. The IMD exclusion was created to contain cost of the newly formed Medicare program. There was a shifting of cost for the IMD exclusion group from federal to state budgets. As such, the IMD exclusion restricts federal financial participation (FFP) for individuals in the exclusion group. While the exclusion group definition was modified in 1972, 1988, 1990, and 2001 (DeLillo 2016), the IMD exclusion has, in effect, created substantial barriers to accessing hospital-based psychiatric care, particularly for those with serious mental illness.

In 1966, Lawrence Kubie forecast the necessary expansion of the private psychiatric hospital into a "treatment center" with "residential, vocational, educational and recreational" components; with "simple and natural" pathways in and out of the hospital; with intensive inpatient treatment, "night-care," and "day-care centers"; and with an expanded array of tasks and activities never previously thought to be functions of the private psychiatric hospital. Kubie (1968) doubted that the community could ever serve the needs of patients without psychiatric hospitals. Many of Kubie's thoughts echo those of his nineteenth-century predecessors.

The Modern Era (1971–2019)

It was in 1969–1970 that the Survey and Research Branch of the National Institute of Mental Health, and subsequently the Center for Mental Health Services, began to regularly collect data on all providers of mental health services. The National Association of Psychiatric Health Systems collects data annually on its membership. Other data sources include the American Hospital Association; the APA and the National Association for Mental Health conjointly as the Joint Information Service; the National Association of State Mental Health Program Directors.

When all sources of data are considered, it is clear that the total number of inpatients in the United States declined steadily from 1970 to 2000. The number of inpatient beds and percentage of the total that belonged to state hospitals declined steadily from 1970 to 1998; private hospitals showed an increase in both until a decline began after 1990; and general hospitals showed a generally steady increase in both. In 1970, the bed distribution was state hospitals, 78.7%; private hospitals, 2.7%; and general hospitals, 4.3%. By 1998, the percentages were 24.3%, 12%, and 20.7%, respectively.

The number of facilities and number of occupied beds show a similar pattern. In 1969, there were 310 state and county hospitals with 309,969 patients; private hospitals numbered 150, with a year-end census of 10,963; and the 604 general hospital psychiatric units had 17,808 beds. By 1998, the numbers had shifted: 229 state and county facilities had 56,955 patients; 348 private psychiatric hospitals had 21,478 patients; and 1,593 general hospitals had 37,002 patients. In 2000, for the first time in three decades, the number of facilities decreased in all three categories.

The total number of admissions increased progressively from 1969 through 1998, as did the percentage of admissions accounted for by private psychiatric hospitals. In the 1990s, private hospitals had small increases in the number of admissions; there were decreasing numbers of state hospital admissions, which were generally compensated for by increased admissions to general hospitals. From the 1960s through the 1990s, the private and general hospitals consistently had a greater percentage of admissions than they did percentage of beds, reflecting shorter lengths of stay than at state and county hospitals.

The work settings and caseloads for inpatient psychiatrists shifted substantially from 1976 to 1998. In 1976, there were 45 patients per psychiatrist in public facilities, 8 per psychiatrist in private hospitals, and 5 per psychiatrist in general hospitals. Over the two decades that followed, the burden on the public psychiatrist improved, that of the private hospital psychiatrist worsened, and that of the general hospital psychiatrist experienced little change. By 1998, psychiatrists' caseloads were 20 patients in public hospitals, 12 in private hospitals, and 4.5 in general hospitals.

Expenditures per civilian population between 1969 and 2000 decreased steadily for the public hospitals, peaked for the private hospitals in 1990, and increased for the general hospitals until 1994. These expenditures for the private hospitals were 345% higher in 1990 than in 1969 but were 23% lower in 1994, 55% lower in 1998, and 63% lower in 2000 than in 1990.

1970s

In the 1970s, states were contemplating phasing out state hospitals ("California Announces Plans to Close State Hospital" 1973; "Massachusetts Study Proposes Phase-Out of State Mental Hospitals" 1974), and general hospital psychiatric units were becoming more of a presence (Flamm 1979). In 1971, the average number of beds in a general hospital psychiatric unit was 35 (median 28), representing about 9% of the hospital's total beds; the average length of stay was 11 days (Greenhill 1979). The expanding role of general hospital psychiatry drew caution from some, who warned general hospital staff "to be on guard against some growing efforts to convert general hospital units into miniature state hospitals" (Flamm 1979, p. 191).

In the early 1970s, little attention was paid to improving the private sector's capacity for, and integrating the private sector into, the treatment of persons with the most debilitating psychiatric illnesses (Kanno 1971). However, private psychiatric hospitals began undergoing a fundamental change in the 1970s. In the 1960s, "long-term inpatient care was thought to be the best treatment money could buy" (Stone 2003) and hospitals provided psychoanalytically oriented treatment at a "leisurely pace that involved months or years of hospitalization" (Hirschowitz 1974, p. 730). Declining numbers of individuals willing or able to pay for such treatment and more readily available third-party coverage led to private hospitals admitting patients of different socioeconomic and ethnic backgrounds and keeping them for shorter lengths of stay. For some, this shift was not made easily (Hirschowitz 1974).

At the end of the 1970s, the president of Pennsylvania Hospital opined on the major problems facing psychiatrists in American hospitals: 1) rising health care costs; 2) planning and coordinating of health services for the good of all segments of the community; 3) "costly," "confusing," "onerous," "duplicative," and "counterproductive regulations"; 4) growing demand to collect data and provide survey information; and 5) questions about the best manner in which to govern hospitals (Cathcart 1979).

1980s

In 1982, an article published in *Hospital and Community Psychiatry* predicted that private hospitals would increasingly be owned by large corporations, whereas sole proprietorship and individual hospitals would decrease (Pottash et al. 1982). This became true, and more quickly than the authors might have imagined.

Expansion in the private sector in the 1980s was both remarkable and not distributed across the United States based on need. Distribution favored those states with the fewest regulations. By the end of the 1980s, states without "certificate of need" laws had an average of 33% more for-profit psychiatric beds than did regulated states (Sharkey 1994). About two-thirds of payments came from patients' fees in the 1980s, but Medicaid and state mental health agencies began to become more prominent payers as the 1980s progressed.

The 1980s presented a real opportunity for the growth of private psychiatric hospitals (Dorwart and Schlesinger 1988; Levenson 1982). Private corporations were ready to seize this opportunity to realize huge profits in the "psychiatric hospital industry" (Levenson 1982; Schlesinger and Dorwart 1984; Sharkey 1994). For-profit psychiatry, especially with its control of a large percentage of psychiatric beds, created its own set of problems. For-profit hospitals were the least likely to treat the most functionally disabled; would treat few, if any, patients who could not pay; usually had poorer staff-to-patient ratios than nonprofit hospitals; failed to provide education to students and professional trainees; failed to contribute adequately to research; provided a lower quality of care overall (Eisenberg 1984; Levenson 1982); were disengaged from the communities in which they were located (Dorwart et al. 1989); and hired away graduating residents from academic and public sector jobs with higher salaries (Brodie 1983). Evidence accumulated by mid-decade did not support the belief, much to the surprise of many, that for-profit hospitals were more efficient (Schlesinger and Dorwart 1984). Nonetheless, state governments began embracing privatization of state mental health services (Dorwart et al. 1989).

In 1979, there were seven psychiatric hospital chains (Levenson 1982). By 1982, most of the proprietary psychiatric beds were owned by chains, and the chains' power and influence rose. In 1983, there were 25 psychiatric hospital chains, and by 1984, there were 75 such chains. By 1983, the for-profit psychiatric chains were dominated by four corporations: Hospital Corporation of America in Nashville, Tennessee, with 3,162 beds; Charter Medical Corporation in Macon, Georgia, with 2,422 beds; National Medical Enterprises Inc., in Los Angeles, California, with 1,952 beds; and Community Psychiatric Centers in Pomona, California, with 1,838 beds. The growth and revenues of these for-profit psychiatric hospital chains throughout the 1980s can only be called astounding. By the mid-1980s, the four major providers of private psychiatric hospitals/beds controlled 85% of the market (Sharkey 1994).

Proponents of psychiatric chains claimed that they were poised to take on the public sector: "By the end of the decade, the private sector will have replaced most of the psychiatric services currently provided by federal, state and local governments" (Kuntz 1981, p. 90). Although this point was never reached, innovations that could affect private–public partnerships were explored and, in some instances, implemented (McNeill et al. 1980).

In the early 1980s, there was a debate throughout the United States as to which sectors of psychiatric inpatient treatment should be responsible for involuntary admissions and/or difficult-to-manage patients. In 1980, the Massachusetts Psychiatric Society disseminated a position paper on involuntary psychiatric admissions to general hospitals, asserting 1) there should be separate locked and unlocked units, 2) general hospitals should not be required to lock units, 3) involuntary patients should be staffed as though they required "psychiatric intensive care," 4) not all involuntary patients could be treated in a general hospital, 5) unresolved legal issues impeded implementation of involuntary treatment, 6) specially designed units would be required, 7) adequate reimbursement would have to be established, 8) the general hospital must be able to control its admissions and discharges, 9) partial hospitalization programs must be developed, and 10) there could not be "arbitrary governmental mandates" (McNeill et al. 1980).

Psychiatric hospitalization was becoming progressively more expensive, especially for the major payers: business and the federal government. Evidence emerged that private psychiatric hospitals were attempting to maximize the use of reimbursable days. A study of more than 120,000 persons ages 13–22 years showed that as days in hospital were approved at 7-day intervals, so too was there a pattern of peaks of discharge at 7-day intervals (Sharkey 1994). In a study of 32,240 discharges from private psychiatric hospitals, those discharges covered by Medicare showed a ratio of Medicare-covered days to total inpatient days near 1:1. To counteract escalating costs, employers began to adopt mechanisms to control psychiatric hospitalizations in the late 1980s (Sharkey 1994). Early efforts, such as prospective, concurrent, and retrospective utilization review, were quickly supplemented by prospective payment, capitation, insurance deductibles, copayments, and annual limits on inpatient days. Managed care companies specializing in psychiatric services management sprang up and almost as quickly consolidated to provide a range of "products" to control costs (Geller 1998). Some of these companies were accused of overly restricting access because at-risk contracts provided them a financial incentive to do so. Monitoring a patient's progress and refusing to pay once the patient could be taken out of the hospital to less expensive alternative care was not new to this era. Similar processes had been used by cities and towns when they bore the expenses for hospitalization of their residents at asylums in the nineteenth century (Grob 1983).

The 1980s did not lack for interest in what was occurring in psychiatric hospitals, such as who was being treated, by what methods they were treated, and what the staff's and patients' perceptions of treatment were. A study at High Point Hospital in New York showed that when comparing the 1980s with the 1960s, inpatients in the 1980s were younger (mean age dropped from 38 to 25 years), less likely to be diagnosed with a schizophrenic disorder and more likely to be diagnosed with an affective disorder; considerably more likely to have a substance use disorder (SUD), less likely to be referred by a physician (a drop from 90% to 50%), and likely to have a length of stay half as long (a drop from 2 years to 1 year) (Gralnick and Caton 1992).

Researchers at the Menninger Foundation conducted a study of staff perception of difficult inpatients. Their findings indicated "withdrawn psychoticism" was the variable most related to perceived difficulty. The next most related factor was character pathology. The "suicide–depressed" and "violence-aggression" factors were less related to perceived difficulty. The authors speculated that the false notion "violence looms large" in the perception of difficulty is secondary to administrative concerns and episodic concerns about violent patients (Colson et al. 1985). McLean Hospital staff studied patients' satisfaction with their hospital treatment 3 months after discharge. Rated as being associated with the greatest degree of satisfaction was the high quality of the staff (especially paraprofessionals and nurses); rated as lowest was the cost of treatment. Patients were also quite dissatisfied with the information they received regarding their treatment and progress (Eisen and Grob 1982).

In 1988, a major change occurred in the IMD exclusion as facilities with fewer than 16 beds were removed from the exclusionary group (DeLillo 2016). While there has been opposition to complete rollback of the IMD exclusion, this was seen as a way to provide reimbursement for care in smaller facilities or on smaller units. This change has had unintended consequences as well. There has been a proliferation of general 16-bed psychiatric units, often at the expense of specialty units for specific conditions such as psychosis or eating disorders. This led to a separate for-profit industry of inpatient management services operators. Because of a lack of progress in modernizing antiquated IMD exclusion language, there has also been the creation of multiple 16-bed facilities, all with separate licenses, on the same contiguous campus as a workaround to the 16-bed rule. A positive development at the end of the decade was removal of IMD exclusion of FFP for enrollees under age 21 (DeLillo 2016).

1990s

Throughout the 1990s, the total and average number of beds per private hospital decreased, as did the average length of stay (National Association of Private Psychiatric Hospitals 1991, 1992; National Association of Psychiatric Health Systems 1993, 1994, 1995, 1996, 1997, 1999, 2000, 2002, 2003b, 2003a). In the early 1990s, the practices the chain hospitals had used to fill beds were called into question, based in part on U.S. Department of Justice (DOJ) intelligence regarding fraud by private hospital chains (Sharkey 1994). Hospital chains began experiencing major losses, as high as $201.9 million in 1994. Assets were falling and lawsuits were flourishing, with settlements in the hundreds of millions of dollars ("NME to Provide $2.5 Million in Free Patient Care as Part of Settlement Agreement in Texas Lawsuit" 1992; Sharkey 1994; "Tenet Agrees to Pay Patients $100 Million in Malpractice Claims" 1997).

Several phenomena affected the fate of all psychiatric hospitals in the 1990s. First among these was managed care. By 1990, the provision of utilization management (i.e., preadmission certification, concurrent utilization review and case management) had become a major industry in and of itself. Although utilization management might have some beneficial effects, as Sharfstein (1990) pointed out, "the vast majority of utilization management…has as its objective cost containment pure and simple" (p. 965).

The loss of the psychiatrist's autonomy and treatment decision–making authority produced widespread consternation (Schlesinger et al. 1996; Sharfstein 1990; Wickizer et al. 1996). In a survey of 2,541 psychiatrists with active hospital affiliations, almost two-thirds reported needing prior approval from insurance companies for admission and more than three-quarters indicated some pressure from insurance companies to discharge patients earlier than they thought clinically appropriate (Schlesinger et al. 1996). Analysis of 2,265 utilization management cases revealed an overreliance on treatment protocols and evidence that almost all cases received prior approval for the same number of days despite a wide range of diagnoses (Wickizer et al. 1996).

The fact that cost benefits were examined from the perspective of the insurer but little account was taken of the hospitals' costs in executing repeated requests for extensions of stay was particularly burdensome for psychiatric hospitals (Sharfstein 1990; Wickizer et al. 1996). In the same analysis of the 2,265 cases just mentioned, investigators found that 70% of patients were approved for one or more treatment extensions and 40% of patients with extended stays had had three or more requests (Wickizer et al. 1996).

Managed care did decrease length of stay, and it appeared to do so progressively through the decade. Shorter lengths of stay meant increased pressure on private and general hospitals to keep beds filled and increased pressure on patients. One study found that close scrutiny by insurance companies became a major stressor to patients: insurance review became a focus of treatment; staff felt pushed into demanding improvement at a rate patients could not reasonably meet; and the more adversarial and irrational the review process, the more likely it was to feed into patients' and families' preexisting psychopathology (Gabbard et al. 1991).

Psychiatric hospital staff were generally dissatisfied with utilization management firms. In findings reported from a 1990 survey of 136 hospitals, 51% of hospitals indicated that patients left against medical advice after a reviewer said that treatment would not be covered, 49% reported that patients did not receive appropriate follow-up treatment because it was not covered, 47% said that preadmission review prevented patients' hospitalizations, 48% reported that utilization management firms lacked specific psychiatric criteria, 56% indicated difficulty making telephone contact with these firms, and 82% said that reviewers were unfamiliar with local resources ("Private Psychiatric Hospitals Report Wide Dissatisfaction With Managed Care Reviews" 1990). Hospitals were particularly concerned about these firms' lack of understanding of the relationship between psychiatric symptoms and social support systems. Hospital staff were taxed by spending an average of 63 hours per week on utilization management issues ("Managed Care Survey Finds Improvements, But Problems Remain" 1991).

By 1993, a survey of 141 private psychiatric hospitals showed improvements had been made. Reviewers were more often clinicians (70% of respondents), and these reviewers usually had experience in psychiatric or substance abuse treatment (65%). However, complaints remained about preadmission reviews preventing admissions (71%), reviews requiring discharges too early (89%), and discharges against medical advice when coverage was denied (51%) (National Association of Psychiatric Health Systems 1993).

The 1990s saw the privatization of public mental health services (Dorwart and Epstein 1993) in what could be considered a return to the early nineteenth-century utilization of private hospitals for public patients. Medicaid, Medicare, and state funds were directed to the private sector to greater degrees (Dorwart et al. 1991). States assisted freestanding private hospitals in obtaining waivers of the IMD rule (Geller 2000a) to become Medicaid eligible (Geller 1998) and developed public-sector managed care contracts, sometimes bypassing the state's department of mental health entirely (Geller 2000b).

Evidence emerged that the private psychiatric hospitals were not equally welcoming to all public sector patients. In national data sets (Dorwart et al. 1991; Olfson and Mechanic 1996), and in data from Maryland (Minkin et al. 1994) and Massachusetts (White et al. 1995), for example, consistent variables emerged that distinguished public from private admissions: behavioral history, diagnoses, and insurance. A greater reliance on the private system for those formerly treated in the public system precipitated many unintended consequences, including inpatient treatment farther from one's home community (Geller 1991), less continuity of inpatient treatment and associated longer lengths of stay (Geller et al. 1998), new loci and patterns of recidivism (Geller et al. 1998), and an ongoing debate about quality of care in private versus public settings (Dorwart et al. 1991). One measure of quality of care, staffing ratios (Dorwart et al. 1991), showed a narrowing of the difference between public and private facilities as the ratio of psychiatrists to patients improved in the public sector.

The concept of treatment in the "least restrictive alternative" affected all inpatient settings. An ill-defined concept, such treatment nonetheless was used to justify many alternatives to inpatient settings. The general and private hospitals were seen as less restrictive than the public hospitals for not entirely clear reasons (Geller 1991), but all manner of alternative service arrangements were seen as less restrictive than any hospital for acute or longer-term care and treatment (Geller 2000b; Sledge et al. 1996).

2000–2009

In 2007, the APA passed a position statement that was the most progressive step to altering the IMD exclusion put forth to that time:

> States should be offered the opportunity to receive a Federal exemption from the IMD Exclusion for State Hospitals and all Nonprofits over 16 beds, e.g., private hospitals, community residential programs, dual diagnosis residential treatment. To participate in the exemption a state must demonstrate a maintenance of effort (maintain its mental illness and substance abuse expenditures (excluding medication costs) from all sources, e.g., state's DMH, DPH, DMA, DMR, DOC, DSS, DYS, other) at a level no less than the state's average expenditure over the preceding five years. (American Psychiatric Association 2007)

This position addressed one of the major concerns of those who favored expansion for community-based services—namely, that weakening of the IMD exclusion would lead states to move funds from community programs back into public hospitals. The IMD exclusion became a focus of significant attention in the next decade.

States continued to close public psychiatric hospitals—Massachusetts, for example, closed a state hospital in 2003, bringing the number of its state hospitals to 3 from a peak of 12 in 1960. While often not increasing the number of state public psychiatric beds, states were constructing new state hospitals in this decade, indicating that states saw public inpatient treatment as an integral part of the public mental health system.

In 1955, there were 558,239 public psychiatric beds (state and county) available, or 340 psychiatric beds per 100,000 people. By 2005, this number decreased to 52,539 total public beds, or 17 beds per 100,000 people (Torrey et al. 2008).

The Mental Health Parity and Addiction Equity Act of 2008 (MHPAEA), passed on October 3, 2008, upheld and furthered the protections of the Mental Health Parity Act of 1996. MHPAEA is a federal law that requires that behavioral health benefits (for mental health and substance use disorders) be covered by most health insurance plans to be at par with medical and surgical benefits. This legislation impacted inpatient psychiatry by preventing employer groups offering behavioral health coverage from applying limits to the number of visits or days of inpatient coverage (Ettner et al. 2016).

2010–2019

The major change in hospital psychiatry in this decade was arguably the alterations in the IMD exclusion.

States were quite familiar with modifying IMD payment exclusions through the process of Section 1115 demonstration waivers. Although efforts in Congress to end the IMD exclusion had failed, the federal government offered states ways to apply the exclusions to expanding patient populations. The initial changes applied to SUDs. In July 2015, the Centers for Medicare & Medicaid Services (CMS) issued a State Medicaid Director letter that stated that under a Section 1115 waiver, states could receive FFP—the federal component of Medicaid—for short-term SUD treatment provided it was part of a transformed SUD treatment system in the state (Kunkel et al. 2018). Hospitals with a major focus on psychiatric disorders that were not SUDs became concerned that funds would be siphoned from them.

In 2016, by regulation 42 CFR 438.6(e), CMS indicated a state could make Medicaid payments to a managed care organization or a Prepaid Inpatient Health Plan for treatment in an IMD for up to 15 days per monthly capitation payment (Centers for Medicare and Medicaid Services 2016). A patient could actually stay longer than 15 days depending on when those hospital days fell within the months. This was a crack in the wall of the IMD exclusion as applied to mental illness. The 21st Century Cures Act, which incorporated the Helping Families in Mental Health Crisis Act, codified this change.

President Obama signed the $6 billion 21st Century Cures Act into law on December 13, 2016. The act authorized grants to maintain and expand assertive outpatient treatment (AOT) programs for adults in the hope that an effective AOT program could decrease the demand for inpatient psychiatric beds (U.S. Department of Health and Human Services 2018). This could be seen as a benefit to the state and a detriment to private psychiatric hospitals.

In August 2017, a State Medicaid Director letter gave states more flexibility under Section 1115 waivers for opioid and other SUD treatment (Kunkel et al. 2018). Again, mental health providers whose focus was on persons with serious mental illness were concerned about funds moving from this population to the SUD population. This concern was abated when on November 13, 2018, a State Medicaid Director letter permitted states to obtain Section 1115 waivers for the treatment of mental illness in IMDs (Centers for Medicare and Medicaid Services 2018).

As of November 2019, 26 states had a Section 1115 waiver to use Medicaid funds for IMD SUD services. Vermont was the only state with an IMD mental health waiver (Musumeci et al. 2019). Why are states holding back on applying for Section 1115 mental health waivers? The possibilities include the following: 1) the application process is very complex (see Centers for Medicare and Medicaid Services 2018); 2) the waiver is temporary, and states are reluctant to completely redo their inpatient and community delivery system as is expected by the waiver process; 3) states are wary because some states have had waivers pulled by CMS or waiver applications rejected, such as Massachusetts for a closed prescription drug formulary, Kansas for lifetime limits on Medicaid benefits, and Arizona for more frequent eligibility determinations (Hinton et al. 2019); 4) states are concerned that the DOJ will sue them if they put more patients into IMDs.

In the previous decade, DOJ had taken a rather formulaic approach to suing states under the Civil Rights of Institutionalized Persons Act (CRIPA) (Geller and Lee 2013). While CRIPA is about patients' rights in a public psychiatric hospital, DOJ used these suits as a way to get states to move patients out of hospitals, because a facility with inadequate staffing could improve its staff-to-patient ratio by keeping the staff the same and decreasing the hospital's census. In this decade, DOJ took a more direct approach, suing states under the provisions of *Olmstead v. L.C.* (1999).

Basing its decision on the Americans with Disabilities Act, the Supreme Court held, in a majority opinion written by Justice Ginsburg, that people with disabilities have a qualified right to receive state-funded supports and services in the community rather than in institutions when the following test is met:

> the person's treatment professionals determine community supports are appropriate; the person does not object to living in the community; and the provision of services in the community would be a reasonable accommodation when balanced with other similarly situated individuals with disabilities.

Apparently finding the Supreme Court's decision lacking, DOJ took it upon itself to expand upon *Olmsted*'s requirements by, for example, 1) proclaiming that a state over-relies on institutions, by comparing one state to national averages and ignoring morbidity, mortality, socioeconomic, and infrastructure data of the state; 2) holding a state at fault for building new public psychiatric beds, even while the state's overall inpatient census is decreasing; and 3) focusing on persons with mental illness not in institutions but in the community who are at risk of "unnecessary institutionalization" (i.e., being hospitalized). In the "unnecessary institutionalization" criteria, DOJ offers no evidence-based methodology it relies on to make such determinations (U.S. Department of Justice 2011). Perhaps the states are right in being wary of constructing new IMDs.

Nonetheless, states do continue to build new state hospitals, often closing and consolidating the functions of other public psychiatric hospitals. For example, when Massachusetts opened Worcester Recovery Center and Hospital in 2012, it actually was replacing the inpatient functions of three state hospitals and one community mental health center. States continue to make plans to replace antiquated state hospitals with new structures such as San Antonio State Hospital in Texas (Friedman 2019) and Central State Hospital in Virginia. The latter will have an increased capacity of 250 beds, just about doubling the size of the hospital (McCloskey 2019).

The private sector has been increasing its inpatient capacity in markets where it appears to be profitable to do so. For example, in this decade, in Massachusetts, four private psychiatric hospitals opened, with a total of 520 beds. Three of them are within 25 miles of one another. Most operate below capacity because they cannot find enough staff. There is no evidence these private psychiatric hospitals have impacted the major challenges facing state mental health systems, including emergency department boarding, persons with mental illness in jails and prisons, and the homeless who are mentally ill.

Hospital beds that might serve these patients outside of state hospitals are in general hospitals (Organisation for Economic Co-operation and Development 2019). Including private beds, among the 36 countries in the Organisation for Economic Co-operation and Development, the United States ranks low, at 32nd, in terms of the number of psychiatric beds, with 21 beds per 100,000 population compared with the average of 69 beds per 100,000 population as of 2016.

While these changes in the IMD exclusion were evolving, there were several other changes in existing practice and policy that also had an impact on inpatient psychiatry. In May 2013, DSM-5 (American Psychiatric Association 2013) was introduced, moving from a multiaxial system to a system with degrees of severity—the basis for a major change in clinical practice. DSM-5 did not seem to have a significant impact on inpatient psychiatry, nor was that its intention. There were concerns that DSM-5 might impact the allocation of scarce psychiatric resources (Blumenthal-Barby 2014). For a number of reasons, it took some states years to give up DSM-IV (American Psychiatric Association 1994) in favor of DSM-5.

Another significant change in this decade was MHPAEA, which took effect January 1, 2010. However, MHPAEA did not specify covered diagnoses, and initially there was no formal enforcement of its provisions. On February 2, 2010, the MHPAEA Interim Final Rule (IFR) was issued, requiring that states formally enforce compliance with MHPAEA provisions. The IFR made it clear that parity applied to nonquantitative treatment limits.

In November 2013, the MHPAEA Final Rule was issued, replacing the IFR. Looking at the impact of the parity rule on inpatient psychiatry, Mark et al. (2012) showed that prior to the parity law less than 10% of beneficiaries used over the maximum inpatient day limit. The California Health Benefits Review Program (2010) analysis found mixed results on the effect of parity on inpatient utilization, with results depending somewhat on diagnosis. It was hypothesized that the sickest patients would have a disproportionate benefit from the parity rule. Advocating for parity on the basis of equal civil rights for people with mental illnesses and SUDs runs the risk that when the standard insurance coverage is judged on the basis of comparability to medical-surgical coverage, insufficient coverage for the latter means insufficient behavioral health coverage under the parity standard (Frank 2018).

Ideally, the impact of MHPAEA on hospital psychiatry would be that people are getting more adequate outpatient services, leading to less demand on inpatient services. The problem was enforcement of compliance under MHPAEA.

According to the 2017 MHPAEA enforcement fact sheet (Employee Benefits Security Administration 2017), there were 187 health plan investigations in fiscal year 2017, with 92 violations for noncompliance. In 2018, a self-compliance tool was published by the Department of Labor to assist plan sponsors in determining whether their group health plans complied with MHPAEA (U.S. Department of Labor n.d.).

A study published in 2018 investigated the changes in copayments and coinsurance for SUD services before and after the implementation of MHPAEA. MHPAEA was associated with decreases in copayments for in-network inpatient detox services, improving the affordability of these services (Friedman et al. 2018). Davenport et al. (2019) examined disparities in the rate of use of out-of-network behavioral health services and out-of-network medical and surgical services in inpatient facilities. In 2017, out-of-network behavioral inpatient facilities were up to 5.2 times more likely to be used in comparison to out-of-network medical and surgical inpatient facilities, the difference having increased from 2.8 times more likely in 2013. Out-of-network SUD inpatient facilities were 10.1 times more likely to be used compared with out-of-network medical and surgical facilities, up from 4.7 times in 2013. This translates to greater access to beds.

To improve the parity in benefits for mental health and SUDs, the Behavioral Health Coverage Transparency Act was introduced in the House and Senate in May 2019 (Pellitt 2019). The bill mandated that health insurance companies disclose their practices around mental health and SUD benefits, with random audits of health plans to ensure enforcement. As of the end of 2021, the bill had not been passed.

In December 2020, Congress passed the Strengthening Behavioral Health Parity Act (SBHPA) provisions in the FY2021 Appropriations bill, to strengthen compliance with the Mental Health Parity and Addiction Equity Act (MHPAEA). The SBHPA requires the DOL to collect comparative analyses from group health plans and health insurance issuers about their compliance with the nonquantitative treatment limitation (NQTL) requirements of MHPAEA. NQTLs include prior authorization, provider network design, and reimbursement setting, among others. It requires DOL to step up MHPAEA compliance activity and increase the number of plans it evaluates every year.

Another major focus in the past decade was on The Joint Commission's efforts to reduce ligature risks in inpatient facilities. According to the Centers for Disease Control and Prevention, as of 2019, the 10th leading cause of death in the United States is suicide. Although the majority of suicides occur outside psychiatric facilities, suicides do occur in psychiatric hospitals and psychiatric units. To help hospitals reduce ligature risk, the Joint Commission started changing standards for hospitals. But surveyors had not reached agreements about what constitutes a ligature risk and about what mitigation strategies would be acceptable. To come up with a consensus, the Joint Commission created an expert panel; however, the panel's recommendations have not been universally accepted. The burden on hospitals to ameliorate ligature risks has been enormous. General hospitals are closing psychiatric beds because of lesser revenue compared with other specialties and higher costs due to structural modifications imposed by CMS through the Joint Commission for ligature risks (Beebe 2018; Wilusz 2019).

The Joint Commission also set out requirements for hospitals to have screening tools and procedures to prevent suicide, which became effective July 1, 2019. A hospital's recredentialing will involve consideration of how the hospital has designed and implemented methodologies of suicide prevention.

Conclusion

As we start the third decade of the twenty-first century, inpatient psychiatry appears to be weathering onslaught after onslaught against its role as an integral component of any system of care for persons with mental illness. In order for psychiatric hospitals to continue to function in their mixed roles of providing treatment, public safety, and asylum, all aspects of inpatient psychiatric treatment should be under frequent review; hence the impetus for the second edition of this book.

Psychiatric hospitals are shrinking, growing, being torn down, and being newly built all at the same time. Debates are ongoing as to the actual effects of the quest for parity, the misuse of jails and prisons as substitutes for psychiatric hospital beds (Banks et al. 2000; Domino et al. 2004), the misuse of psychiatric hospitals for persons with dementia or head trauma who have no resources, and the loss of beds for civil patients who are being displaced by forensic patients. No matter where one looks in the continuum of care, one finds patients waiting to be in another part of the continuum: emergency department boarding, patients in general hospital psychiatric units waiting for transfer to the state hospital, and patients in state hospitals waiting for community-based residential beds. In some states, patients in need of a psychiatric hospital bed have no place to wait but in jail.

Inpatient psychiatry started out with the best of intentions, awash in "magnificent beneficence" (President Franklin Pierce's description), with asylums reporting cure rates approaching 100%. All too soon the powerful scourge that insanity proved to be simply overwhelmed available resources. Take Danvers State Hospital in Massachusetts, for example. It opened in May 1878 amid public admiration that it was "light, airy, cheerful…with magnificent arrangements" ("Opening of the Hospital" 1878). The facilities were such that persons might not even know they were in an asylum, and hence the cutlery was stamped only "Danvers," not "Danvers Asylum" or "Danvers Hospital" ("Opening of the Hospital" 1878). At the turn of the twentieth century, the hospital's caliber of professional care and treatment was such that no restraint or seclusion was used (Page 1904). Yet the hospital's superintendent was soon lamenting, "It may be asserted that the lunatic hospital, per se, is not a remedy for insanity. In fact, as generally regarded by its inmates, it provokes inimical effects and in some cases aggravates the mental disease.... The physician may render some important service, but he is greatly in the dark as to the actual requirement" (Ramseur 2005, p. 103). By 1946, conditions were simply frightening. On September 13 of that year, there were nine staff persons to cover 13 wards with a census of 2,300 patients (Ramseur 2005).

In the years since World War II, attitudes have swung from a perspective that there was tremendous overreliance on inpatient beds to a conceptualization of inpatient hospitalization as a nefarious force of institutionalism, disempowerment, trauma, and deprivation of fundamental rights; to the current era where many wonder, where have all the beds gone?

As the future of hospital psychiatry evolves in this century, perhaps we would do well to keep in mind the sage advice Edward Jarvis gave to the AMSAII in the mid-nineteenth century:

> The wise manager of the insane carefully analyzes the condition of his patients, and ascertains what elements are diseased and what are sound. Having determined this, he cautiously respects and avoids all interference with every power and faculty, every principle, opinion, emotion, taste or desire, that is in good health, and applies his influence only to such as are not in good condition, and this he does in such a way as not to disturb the others. He therefore, so far as is consistent with the patient's recovery or best progress, applies no restraint, opposes no purpose, denies no indulgence, contradicts no opinions that are not disordered, and do not minister to the disease. Thus he sustains as great an amount of healthy mental and moral constitution as possible, by means of which he hopes to overcome the disturbance in those which are diseased. (Jarvis 1860, p. 28)

References

American Hospital Association: Mental Health Services and the General Hospital: A Guide to the Development and Implementation of Mental Health Service Plans. Chicago, IL, American Hospital Association, 1970

American Psychiatric Association: Standards for Psychiatric Facilities. Washington, DC, American Psychiatric Association, 1969

American Psychiatric Association: Diagnostic and Statistical Manual of Mental Disorders, 4th Edition. Washington, DC, American Psychiatric Association, 1994

American Psychiatric Association: Position statement on federal exemption from the Medicaid Institutions for Mental Diseases (IMD) exclusion. Washington, DC, American Psychiatric Association, 2007

American Psychiatric Association: Diagnostic and Statistical Manual of Mental Disorders, 5th Edition. Arlington, VA, American Psychiatric Association, 2013

Andrews JB: The distribution and care of the insane in the United States. Am J Insanity 44:192–211, 1887

Association of Medical Superintendents of American Institutions for the Insane: Proceedings of the Eighth Annual Meeting of the AMSAII. Second day—morning session. Am J Insanity 10:74–79, 1853

The asylum near Frankford, in Pennsylvania. Am J Insanity 8:179–181, 1851

At the Pennsylvania Hospital for the Insane. Am J Insanity 9:183–185, 1852

Auster SL: Insurance coverage for "mental and nervous conditions": developments and problems. Am J Psychiatry 126(5):698–705, 1969 5352624

Azima H, Vispo RH: Imipramine; a potent new anti-depressant compound. Am J Psychiatry 115(3):245–246, 1958 13571443
Banks SM, Stone JL, Pandiani JA, et al: Utilization of local jails and general hospitals by state psychiatric center patients. J Behav Health Serv Res 27(4):454–459, 2000 11070639
Barnard RI: The position of the private psychiatric hospital. Ment Hosp 15:19–22, 1964 14089082
Barton WE: Administration in Psychiatry. Springfield, IL, Charles C Thomas, 1962
Bazelon DL: The right to treatment: the court's role. Hosp Community Psychiatry 20(5):129–135, 1969 5786387
Beebe CE: Separating fact from fiction in ligature risk. Health Facilities Management, November 9, 2018. Available at: www.hfmmagazine.com/articles/3515-separating-fact-from-fiction-in-ligature-risk Retrieved December 8, 2019.
Behavioral Health Coverage Transparency Act. Available at: www.warren.senate.gov/imo/media/doc/Behavioral%20Health%20Coverage%20Transparency%20Act%20of%202019%20-%20one-pager.pdf. Accessed December 10, 2019.
Bennett AE: Problems in establishing and maintaining psychiatric units in general hospitals. Am J Psychiatry 115(11):974–979, 1959 13637271
Bennett AE, Ford FR, Turk RE: Clinical investigation of chlorpromazine and reserpine in private psychiatric practice. Am J Psychiatry 112(10):782–787, 1956 13302481
Bernstein S, Herzberg J: Small group experience with psychiatric aides. Ment Hyg 54:113–117, 1970
Birnbaum M: The right to treatment. Am Bar Assoc J 46:499–505, 1960
Birnbaum M: Some comments on "the right to treatment." Arch Gen Psychiatry 13:34–45, 1965 14306531
Bloomingdale Hospital, White Plains. Am J Insanity 70:536–537, 1913
Blumenthal-Barby JS: Psychiatry's new manual (DSM-5): ethical and conceptual dimensions. J Med Ethics 40(8):531–536, 2014, 24327374
Board of State Commissioners of Public Charities of the State of Illinois: Eighth Biennial Report of the Board of State Commissioners of Public Charities of the State of Illinois. Springfield, IL, HW Rokker, 1885
Brannon EP, Graham WL: Intensive insulin shock therapy: a five-year survey. Am J Psychiatry 111(9):659–663, 1955 14350085
Brill H, Patton RE: Clinical-statistical analysis of population changes in New York State mental hospitals since introduction of psychotropic drugs. Am J Psychiatry 119:20–35, 1962 13873092
Brodie HKH: Presidential address: psychiatry—its locus and its future. Am J Psychiatry 140(8):965–968, 1983 6135352
Bureau of the Census: Insane and Feeble-Minded in Institutions, 1910. Washington, DC, U.S. Government Printing Office, 1914
Butler JS: The individualized treatment of the insane. The Alienist and Neurologist 7:435–460, 1886
Butler Hospital for the Insane: Report of the trustees and superintendent of the Butler Hospital for the Insane. Am J Insanity 12:280–285, 1856
Butler Hospital for the Insane: Report of the Butler Hospital for the Insane, 1877. Am J Insanity 34:548, 1878
California announces plans to close state hospital. Hosp Community Psychiatry 24:249, 1973
California Health Benefits Review Program: Executive Summary: Analysis of Assembly Bill 1600: Mental Health Services. Report to California State Legislature. Oakland, California Health Benefits Review Program, 2010. Available at: http://analyses.chbrp.com/document/view.php?id=549. Accessed December 10, 2019.
Campbell CM: The work of the psychopathic hospital. Ment Hyg 14:883–900, 1930
Care and treatment. Ment Hyg 41:589, 1957
Casey JF, Lasky JJ, Klett CJ, Hollister LE: Treatment of schizophrenic reactions with phenothiazine derivatives: a comparative study of chlorpromazine, triflupromazine, mepazine, prochlorperazine, perphenazine, and phenobarbital. Am J Psychiatry 117:97–105, 1960 13808146

Cathcart HR: Issues facing American hospitals. Hosp Community Psychiatry 30(3):193–194, 1979 761858
Centers for Medicare and Medicaid Services: Special contract provisions related to payment. Electronic Code of Federal Regulations, 42 CFR 438.6 (e), 2016. Available at: www.law.cornell.edu/cfr/text/42/438.6. Accessed December 7, 2019.
Centers for Medicare and Medicaid Services: Opportunities to design innovative service delivery systems for adults with a serious mental illness or children with a serious emotional disturbance (SMD #18–001). Letter to State Medicaid Director, November 13, 2018. Available at: https://www.medicaid.gov/federal-policy-guidance/downloads/smd18011.pdf. Accessed December 7, 2019.
Channing W: Physical training of the insane. Am J Insanity 46:166–175, 1889
Club formed for patients, ex-patients, and relatives. APA Mental Hospital Services Bulletin 1:6, 1950
Cohen S: TP-21, a new phenothiazine. Am J Psychiatry 115(4):358, 1958 13583228
Colson DB, Allen JG, Coyne L, et al: Patterns of staff perception of difficult patients in a long-term psychiatric hospital. Hosp Community Psychiatry 36(2):168–172, 1985 3972342
Connecticut: Retreat for the Insane. Am J Insanity 2:66–68, 1845
Connecticut: Thirtieth annual report of the officers of the Retreat for the Insane at Hartford, Connecticut. April 1, 1854. Am J Insanity 11:257–261, 1855
Connecticut: Forty-fifth and forty-sixty annual reports of the officers of the Retreat for the Insane at Hartford, Conn: 1869 and 1870. Am J Insanity 27:326, 1871
Coordinating Committee on Professional Standards in Psychiatry: Report of the Coordinating Committee on Professional Standards in Psychiatry. Am J Psychiatry 117:757–760, 1961
Costs of long-term mental-hospital care. Ment Hyg 33:155–156, 1949
Davenport S, Gray TJ, Melek SP: Addiction and mental health vs. physical health: widening disparities in network use and provider reimbursement. Milliman Research Report, November 19, 2019. Available at: http://assets.milliman.com/ektron/Addiction_and_mental_health_vs_physical_health_Widening_disparities_in_network_use_and_provider_reimbursement.pdf. Accessed December 10, 2019.
Davidson HA: The snake pits hiss back: a letter to the APA from a hospital superintendent. Am J Psychiatry 121:279–280, 1964
Death of Dr. George Cook. Am J Insanity 33:132–135, 1876
DeLillo M: Institution for Mental Disease (IMD) as an "in lieu of" service. Milliman White Paper, 2016
Deutsch A: The Shame of the States. New York, Harcourt Brace, 1948
Deutsch A: The Mentally Ill in America. New York, Columbia University Press, 1949
Domino ME, Norton EC, Morrissey JP, Thakur N: Cost shifting to jails after a change to managed mental health care. Health Serv Res 39(5):1379–1401, 2004 15333114
Dorwart RA, Epstein SS: Privatization and Mental Health Care: A Fragile Balance. Westport, CT, Auburn House, 1993
Dorwart RA, Schlesinger M: Privatization of psychiatric services. Am J Psychiatry 145(5):543–553, 1988 3282448
Dorwart RA, Schlesinger M, Horgan C, et al: The privatization of mental health care and directions for mental health services research, in The Future of Mental Health Services Research (DHHS Publ No ADM-89-1600). Edited by Taube CA, Mechanic D, Hohmann AA. Washington, DC, U.S. Government Printing Office, 1989, pp 139–154
Dorwart RA, Schlesinger M, Davidson H, et al: A national study of psychiatric hospital care. Am J Psychiatry 148(2):204–210, 1991 1987819
Dr. Butler of the Hartford Retreat for the Insane. Am J Insanity 8:187–188, 1851
Dunn WH: Mental-health opportunities in the general hospital. Ment Hyg 35(2):190–198, 1951 14842783
Earle P: Historical and descriptive account of the Bloomingdale Asylum for the Insane. Am J Insanity 2:1–12, 1845
The effect of Medicare on the accreditation of psychiatric hospitals. Hosp Community Psychiatry 17:18–19, 1966

Eisen SV, Grob MC: Measuring discharged patients' satisfaction with care at a private psychiatric hospital. Hosp Community Psychiatry 33(3):227–228, 1982 7061060

Eisenberg L: The case against for-profit hospitals. Hosp Community Psychiatry 35(10):1009–1013, 1984 6386650

Employee Benefits Security Administration: Fact Sheet: FY 2017 MHPAEA Enforcement. Washington, DC, U.S. Department of Labor, 2017. Available at: www.dol.gov/sites/dolgov/files/ebsa/about-ebsa/our-activities/resource-center/fact-sheets/mhpaea-enforcement-2017.pdf. Accessed December 4, 2019.

Erwin HJ: Clinical observations on the use of promethazine hydrochloride in psychiatric disorders. Am J Psychiatry 113(9):783–787, 1957 13402966

Ettner SL, Harwood MJ, Thalmayer A, et al: The Mental Health Parity and Addiction Equity Act evaluation study: impact on specialty behavioral health utilization and expenditures among "carve-out" enrollees. J Health Econ 50:131–143, 2016

Felix RH: The National Mental Health Act: how it can operate to meet a national problem. Ment Hyg 31(3):363–374, 1947 20256577

Felix RH: Improving health insurance coverage for psychiatric illness. Am J Psychiatry 121:731–735, 1965 14267583

Flamm GH: The expanding roles of general-hospital psychiatry. Hosp Community Psychiatry 30(3):190–192, 1979 761857

Forbush B: The Sheppard and Enoch Pratt Hospital, 1853–1970: A History. Philadelphia, PA, JB Lippincott, 1971

Frank RG: Reflections on the Mental Health Parity and Addiction Equity Act after 10 years. Milbank Q 96(4):615–618, 2018 30280415

Freeman W: Frontal lobotomy 1936–1956: a follow-up study of 3000 patients from one to twenty years. Am J Psychiatry 113(10):877–886, 1957 13402981

Friedman C: Plans in place to replace San Antonio State Hospital to better serve patients' needs. KSAT 12 News, February 26, 2019. Available at: www.ksat.com/news/2019/02/27/plans-in-place-to-replace-san-antonio-state-hospital-to-better-serve-patients-needs. Accessed December 8, 2019.

Friedman JH: An organization of ex-patients of a psychiatric hospital. Ment Hyg 23:414–420, 1939

Friedman SA, Azocar F, Xu H, Ettner SL: The Mental Health Parity and Addiction Equity Act (MHPAEA) evaluation study: did parity differentially affect substance use disorder and mental health benefits offered by behavioral healthcare carve-out and carve-in plans? Drug Alcohol Depend 190:151–158, 2018 30032052

From the report of the McLean Asylum. Am J Insanity 21:235–238, 1864

Gabbard GO, Takahashi T, Davidson J, et al: A psychodynamic perspective on the clinical impact of insurance review. Am J Psychiatry 148(3):318–323, 1991 1992833

Garber RS: The private hospital's responsibility for leadership. Ment Hosp 12:16–17, 1961 13703465

Geller JL: "Anyplace but the state hospital": examining assumptions about the benefits of admission diversion. Hosp Community Psychiatry 42(2):145–152, 1991 1997363

Geller JL: Mental health services for the future: managed care, unmanaged care, mismanaged care, in Humane Managed Care? Edited by Schamess G, Lightburn A. Washington, DC, National Association of Social Workers, 1998, pp 36–50

Geller JL: Excluding institutions for mental diseases from federal reimbursement for services: strategy or tragedy? Psychiatr Serv 51(11):1397–1403, 2000a 11058186

Geller JL: The last half-century of psychiatric services as reflected in psychiatric services. Psychiatr Serv 51(1):41–67, 2000b 10647135

Geller JL: Avoiding extinction: successful private psychiatric hospitals in the opening decade of the twenty-first century. Psychiatr Q 77(2):189–201, 2006 16779684

Geller JL, Harris M: Women of the Asylum. New York, Anchor Books, 1994

Geller JL, Fisher WH, McDermeit M, Brown JM: The effects of public managed care on patterns of intensive use of inpatient psychiatric services. Psychiatr Serv 49(3):327–332, 1998 9525791

Geller J, Lee L: United States Department of Justice findings letters in psychiatric hospital CRIPA cases: an aid or a distraction? J Am Acad Psychiatry Law 41(2):174–190, 2013 23771930
Gibson RW: Title XIX: psychiatric provisions and limitations. Hosp Community Psychiatry 18(3):88–91, 1967 6041248
Glasscote RM, Kanno CK: General Hospital Psychiatric Units: A National Survey. Washington, DC, American Psychiatric Association and National Association for Mental Health, 1965
Goldensohn SS, Fink R, Shapiro S: Referral, utilization, and staffing patterns of a mental health service in a prepaid group practice program in New York. Am J Psychiatry 126(5):689–697, 1969 5352623
Gorman M: National health insurance: an idea whose time has come. Am J Psychiatry 126(5):708–711, 1969 5352626
Gralnick A, Caton CLM: Long-term hospital treatment: a 25-year study. Psychiatr Q 63(2):199–208, 1992 1488462
Gralnick A, D'Elia F: A psychoanalytic hospital becomes a therapeutic community. Hosp Community Psychiatry 20(5):144–146, 1969 5786390
Greenblatt M, Levinson DJ, Williams RH: The Patient and the Mental Hospital. Glencoe, IL, Free Press, 1957
Greenhill MH: Psychiatric units in general hospitals: 1979. Hosp Community Psychiatry 30(3):169–182, 1979 367914
Grimes JM: Institutional Care of Mental Patients in the United States. Chicago, IL, JM Grimes, 1934
Grob GN: Mental Illness and American Society, 1875–1940. Princeton, NJ, Princeton University Press, 1983
Gymnasium for the insane. Am J Insanity 53:626–627, 1897
Haas LJ: The backbone of an occupational building for mental and nervous patients. Ment Hyg 8:737–752, 1924
Hayman M: A unique day therapy center for psychiatric patients. Ment Hyg 41(2):245–249, 1957 13418333
Heldt TJ: Psychiatric services in general hospitals. Am J Psychiatry 95:865–871, 1939
Hinton E, Musumeci MB, Rudowitz R, et al: Section 1115 Medicaid demonstration waivers: the current landscape of approved and pending waivers. San Francisco, CA, Henry J. Kaiser Family Foundation, February 2019. Available at: https://collections.nlm.nih.gov/master/borndig/101740359/Issue-Brief-Section-1115-Medicaid-Demonstration-Waivers-The-Current-Landscape-of-Approved-and-Pending-Waivers.pdf. Accessed December 7, 2019.
Hirschowitz RG: Two psychiatric hospitals in transition; studies in staff behavior. Hosp Community Psychiatry 25(11):730–733, 1974 4416759
Hospitals for nervous and mental patients. JAMA 100:895–897, 901–910, 1933
Howard BF: An optimistic report on total rehabilitative potential of chronic schizophrenics. Arch Gen Psychiatry 3:345–356, 1960 13716205
Hurd HM: Three-quarters of a century of institutional care of the insane in the United States. Am J Insanity 69:469–481, 1913
Hurd HM (ed): The Institutional Care of the Insane in the United States and Canada. Baltimore, MD, Johns Hopkins Press, 1916–1917
Insane hospital annexes. The Alienist and Neurologist 1:558, 1880
Jackson B: The revised Diagnostic and Statistical Manual of the American Psychiatric Association. Am J Psychiatry 127:65–73, 1970
Jarvis E: On the proper functions of private institutions or homes for the insane. Am J Insanity 17:19–31, 1860
Jones CH: Discussion. Ment Hosp 15:336, 1964
Kalinowski LB, Hoch PH: Shock Treatments and Other Somatic Procedures in Psychiatry. New York, Grune & Stratton, 1946
Kanno CK: Eleven Indices: An Aid in Reviewing State and Local Mental Health and Hospital Programs. Washington, DC, Joint Information Service, 1971
Kennedy JF: Message from the President of the United States relative to mental illness and mental retardation. Am J Psychiatry 120:729–737, 1964 14115463

Kinross-Wright V: Chlorpromazine treatment of mental disorders. Am J Psychiatry 111(12):907–912, 1955 14376659
Kirkbride TS: A sketch of the history, building, and organization of the Pennsylvania Hospital for the Insane. Am J Insanity 2:97–114, 1845
Kirkbride TS: Pennsylvania: report of the Pennsylvania Hospital for the Insane, 1874. Am J Insanity 32:95–99, 1875
Klapman JW: Public relationships of the mental hospital. Ment Hyg 28:381–396, 1944
Kubie L: The future of the private psychiatric hospital. Int J Psychiatry 6(6):419–433, 1968 5701995
Kunkel C, Lewis CE, Savage J: Medicaid's winding path through Institutions of Mental Disease. Milliman White Paper, December 2018
Kuntz E: Multihospital system survey: hospital chains grab psychiatric business from government facilities. Mod Healthc 11(4):90–91, 1981
Levenson AI: The growth of investor-owned psychiatric hospitals. Am J Psychiatry 139(7):902–907, 1982 7091408
Liebman S, French RL: Patient population distribution in mental hospitals in the United States. Am J Psychiatry 105(7):489–493, 1949 18102426
Long Island House, Amityville, NY. Am J Insanity 57:403, 1900
Maisel AQ: Bedlam 1946. Life 20:102–118, 1946
Managed care survey finds improvements, but problems remain. Hosp Community Psychiatry 42:964–965, 1991
Mark TL, Vandivort-Warren R, Miller K: Mental health spending by private insurance: implications for the Mental Health Parity and Addiction Equity Act. Psychiatr Serv 63(4):313–318, 2012
Massachusetts: McLean Asylum for the Insane. Am J Insanity 2:55–58, 1845
Massachusetts study proposes phase-out of state mental hospitals. Hosp Community Psychiatry 25:492–493, 1974
McCloskey S: In-depth look at Central State Hospital and how plans to rebuild will help with treatment. ABC 8 News, April 18, 2019. Available at: www.wric.com/news/politics/capitol-connection/in-depth-look-at-central-state-hospital-and-how-plans-to-rebuild-will-help-with-treatment. Accessed December 8, 2019.
The McLean Asylum for the Insane. The Alienist and Neurologist 14:142, 1893
McLean Hospital, Waverly. Am J Insanity 57:397–399, 1900
McNeill DN, Stevenson J, Longabaugh RH: Short-term inpatient care and readmission rates: the CMHC approach versus the private approach. Hosp Community Psychiatry 31(11):751–755, 1980 6253384
Menninger K: The course of illness. Bull Menninger Clin 25:225–240, 1961 13769471
Menninger WC: Psychiatric hospital therapy designed to meet unconscious needs. Am J Psychiatry 93:347–360, 1936
Merlis S, Sheppard C, Collins L, Fiorentino D: Polypharmacy in psychiatry: patterns of differential treatment. Am J Psychiatry 126(11):1647–1651, 1970 5420467
Minkin EB, Stoline AM, Sharfstein SS: An analysis of the two-class system of care in public and private psychiatric hospitals. Hosp Community Psychiatry 45(10):975–977, 1994 7829051
Modern Hospital announces prize competition. Ment Hygiene 29:530–531, 1945
Morris HH Jr, Brunt MY Jr: Disposition of first admissions to a private psychiatric hospital, 1920–1951. Am J Psychiatry 113(11):1024–1029, 1957 13411285
Musumeci MB, Chidambaram P, Orgera K: State options for Medicaid coverage of inpatient behavioral health services. San Francisco, CA, Henry J. Kaiser Family Foundation, November 6, 2019. Available at: www.kff.org/report-section/state-options-for-medicaid-coverage-of-inpatient-behavioral-health-services-report. Accessed December 7, 2019.
Myers JM, Appel KE: Open staffs in psychiatric hospitals and services: experiences at the Institute of the Pennsylvania Hospital. Ment Hosp 12:39–43, 1961 14477682
Myers JM, Smith LH: The organization of a mental hospital. Ment Hosp 7(6):6–10, 1956
National Association of Private Psychiatric Hospitals: 1990 Annual Survey: Final Report. Washington, DC, National Association of Private Psychiatric Hospitals, 1991

National Association of Private Psychiatric Hospitals: 1991 Annual Survey: Final Report. Washington, DC, National Association of Private Psychiatric Hospitals, 1992
National Association of Psychiatric Health Systems: 1992 Annual Survey: Final Report. Washington, DC, National Association of Psychiatric Health Systems, 1993
National Association of Psychiatric Health Systems: 1993 Annual Survey: Final Report. Washington, DC, National Association of Psychiatric Health Systems, 1994
National Association of Psychiatric Health Systems: 1995 Annual Survey Report. Washington, DC, National Association of Psychiatric Health Systems, 1995
National Association of Psychiatric Health Systems: Trends in Psychiatric Health Systems: A Benchmarking Report. National Association of Psychiatric Health Systems 1996 Annual Survey Report. Washington, DC, National Association of Psychiatric Health Systems, 1996
National Association of Psychiatric Health Systems: Trends in Behavioral Healthcare Systems: A Benchmarking Report. National Association of Psychiatric Health Systems 1997 Annual Survey Report. Washington, DC, National Association of Psychiatric Health Systems, 1997
National Association of Psychiatric Health Systems: Trends in Behavioral Healthcare Systems: A Benchmarking Report. National Association of Psychiatric Health Systems 1998 Annual Survey Report. Washington, DC, National Association of Psychiatric Health Systems, 1999
National Association of Psychiatric Health Systems: Trends in Behavioral Healthcare Systems: A Benchmarking Report. National Association of Psychiatric Health Systems 2000 Annual Survey Report. Washington, DC, National Association of Psychiatric Health Systems, 2000
National Association of Psychiatric Health Systems: Trends in Behavioral Healthcare Systems: A Benchmarking Report. National Association of Psychiatric Health Systems 2001 Annual Survey Report. Washington, DC, National Association of Psychiatric Health Systems, 2002
National Association of Psychiatric Health Systems: Challenges Facing Behavioral Health Care: The Pressures on Essential Behavioral Healthcare Services. Washington, DC, National Association of Psychiatric Health Systems, 2003a
National Association of Psychiatric Health Systems: Trends in Behavioral Healthcare Systems: A Benchmarking Report. National Association of Psychiatric Health Systems 2002 Annual Survey Report. Washington, DC, National Association of Psychiatric Health Systems, 2003b
New York: Report of the Bloomingdale Asylum, 1871. Am J Insanity 28:549, 1872
Niles HR: Hydrotherapy in the treatment of mental diseases. Am J Insanity 55:443–447, 1899
Nineteen hundred thirty-six censuses of mental patients. Ment Hyg 22:340, 1938
NME to provide $2.5 million in free patient care as part of settlement agreement in Texas lawsuit. Hosp Community Psychiatry 43:852–853, 1992
Olfson M, Mechanic D: Mental disorders in public, private nonprofit, and proprietary general hospitals. Am J Psychiatry 153(12):1613–1619, 1996 8942459
Olmstead v L.C., 527 U.S. 581 (1999)
Opening of the hospital. Danvers Mirror, May 18, 1878
Organisation for Economic Co-operation and Development: Hospital beds (indicator). 2019. Available at: https://data.oecd.org/healtheqt/hospital-beds.htm. Accessed December 17, 2019.
Otis WJ, Robinson GW: Private hospitals, in Mental Hospitals 1950. Edited by Overholser W. Washington, DC, American Psychiatric Association, 1951, pp 159–171
Page CW: Mechanical restraint and seclusion of insane persons. Boston Med Surg J 151:590–595, 1904
Parsons RL: On the private care of the insane. The Alienist and Neurologist 2:564–588, 1881
Payne SM: The evolution of therapeutic care and clinical specialization in psychiatric nursing. Perspect Psychiatr Care 4(3):12–19, 1966 5177289
Pellitt S: Sen. Warren, Rep. Kennedy reintroduce bill to strengthen parity. Capitol Connector, May 23, 2019. Available at: http://thenationalcouncil.org/capitol-connector/2019/05/sen-warren-rep-kennedy-reintroduce-bill-to-strengthen-parity. Accessed December 4, 2019.
Pennsylvania: Asylum for the relief of persons deprived of the use of their reason. Am J Insanity 2:147–151, 1845

Pennsylvania Hospital for the Insane: Report of the Pennsylvania Hospital for the Insane for the year 1849. Am J Insanity 6:322–329, 1850
Pennsylvania Hospital for the Insane: Report of the Pennsylvania Hospital for the Insane for the year 1853. Am J Insanity 11:186–188, 1854
Peterson F: Twentieth century methods of provision for the insane. Am J Insanity 58:405–415, 1902
Pinsky S, Levy ES: Social group work in a private hospital. Ment Hosp 15:516–524, 1964 14172965
Pollock HM: Book Review: Report of Census of Institutions for Mental Disease. Washington, DC, U.S. Census Bureau, 1925
Pollock HM, Forbush EM: Patients with mental disease, mental defect, epilepsy, alcoholism and drug addiction in institutions in the United States, January 1, 1920. Ment Hyg 5:139–169, 1921
Post-release questionnaire. APA Mental Hospital Services Bulletin 2:5, 1951
Pottash ALC, Gold MS, Bloodworth R, Extein I: The future of private psychiatric hospitals. Hosp Community Psychiatry 33(9):735–739, 1982 7129389
President Johnson signs comprehensive health planning bill. Hosp Community Psychiatry 18(1):59, 1967
Private asylums. Boston Med Surg J 101:243, 1879
Private psychiatric hospitals report wide dissatisfaction with managed care reviews. Hosp Community Psychiatry 41:938–941, 1990
Provision for professional advertising in the Code. The Alienist and Neurologist 15:135–137, 1894
Psychiatry at the Sheppard and Enoch Pratt Hospital. Am J Insanity 57:553–558, 1901
Ramseur M: Haunted Palace: Danvers Asylum as Art and History. South Harwich, MA, ARTSHIP Publishing, 2005
Ray I: The Butler Hospital for the Insane. Am J Insanity 5:1–24, 1848
Reed PB: The role of the private psychiatric hospital. Ment Hosp 9:34–35, 1958
Rehabilitation of the mentally ill. Ment Hyg 38:692–693, 1954
Robbins LL: Reflections 1940–1966. Bull Menninger Clin 30(4):190–206, 1966 5938349
Rosen B, Klein DF, Levenstein S, Shanian SP: Social competence and posthospital outcome. Arch Gen Psychiatry 19(2):165–170, 1968 5664347
Sawyer JW: Rhode Island: report of the Butler Hospital for the Insane: 1878. Am J Insanity 35:584–586, 1879
Schildkraut JJ, Winokur A, Draskóczy PR, Hensle JH: Changes in norepinephrine turnover in rat brain during chronic administration of imipramine and protriptyline: a possible explanation for the delay in onset of clinical antidepressant effects. Am J Psychiatry 127(8):1032–1039, 1971 5541194
Schlesinger M, Dorwart R: Ownership and mental-health services: a reappraisal of the shift toward privately owned facilities. N Engl J Med 311(15):959–965, 1984 6472422
Schlesinger M, Dorwart RA, Epstein SS: Managed care constraints on psychiatrists' hospital practices: bargaining power and professional autonomy. Am J Psychiatry 153(2):256–260, 1996 8561208
Sharfstein SS: Utilization management: managed or mangled psychiatric care? Am J Psychiatry 147(8):965–966, 1990 2375463
Sharkey J: Bedlam, Greed, Profiteering, and Fraud in a Mental Health System Gone Crazy. New York, St Martin's, 1994
Sherman IC, Hoffman HR: Facilities in private mental institutions in the United States and territories. Am J Psychiatry 106(4):268–269, 1949 18148483
Sinkler W: Diseases and conditions to which the rest treatment is adapted. J Nerv Ment Dis 17:321–338, 1892
Sledge WH, Tebes J, Wolff N, Helminiak TW: Day hospital/crisis respite care versus inpatient care, Part II: service utilization and costs. Am J Psychiatry 153(8):1074–1083, 1996 8678177
Smith K: Chlorpromazine and Mental Health. Philadelphia, PA, Lea & Febiger, 1955
Snyder SH, Taylor KM, Coyle JT, Meyerhoff JL: The role of brain dopamine in behavioral regulation and the actions of psychotropic drugs. Am J Psychiatry 127(2):199–207, 1970 4319649

Squire MB: Open-staff policy opens the door to improved psychiatric therapy. Hospitals 35:64–67, 1961 13915981
Stevens RB: Interracial practices in mental hospitals. Ment Hyg 36(1):56–65, 1952 14899370
Stewart WF: Maryland: forty-third report of the Maryland Hospital for the Insane: 1872–1873. Am J Insanity 31:101–102, 1874
The "stigma" of mental illness. Am J Psychiatry 93:476–478, 1936
Stokes WH: Eighth annual report of the Mount Hope Institution, near Baltimore, for 1850. Am J Insanity 8:209–212, 1851
Stone AA: Reel life: Girl Interrupted. Clinical Psychiatric News, August 2003, pp 61–62
Tallman FF: The state mental hospital in transition. Am J Psychiatry 116:818–824, 1960 13836744
Tenet agrees to pay patients $100 million in malpractice claims. Psychiatr Serv 48:1216–1217, 1997
Torrey EF, Entsminger K, Geller J, et al: The Shortage of Public Beds for Mentally Ill Persons: A Report of the Treatment Advocacy Center. Arlington, VA, Treatment Advocacy Center, 2008. Available at: https://mentalillnesspolicy.org/imd/the-shortage-of-public-hospital-beds-for-mentally-ill-persons-pdf.html. Accessed December 17, 2019.
Two homes for the nervous and insane. The Alienist and Neurologist 1:391, 1880
U.S. Department of Health and Human Services: Testimony from Elinore F. McCance-Katz, M.D., Ph.D. on 21st Century Cure Implementation: Examining Mental Health Initiatives Before Committee on Energy and Commerce. Thursday, July 26, 2018 (18:45). Available at: www.hhs.gov/about/agencies/asl/testimony/2018–07/21st-century-cure-implementation-examining-mental-health-initiative.html. Accessed December 12, 2019.
U.S. Department of Justice: United States' investigation of the state of Mississippi's service system for persons with mental illness and developmental disabilities. Letter to the Honorable Haley R. Barbour, Governor, State of Mississippi, December 22, 2011. Available at: www.justice.gov/sites/default/files/crt/legacy/2012/01/26/miss_findletter_12-22-11.pdf. Accessed December 7, 2019.
U.S. Department of Labor: Self-Compliance Tool for the Mental Health Parity and Addiction Equity Act (MHPAEA), n.d. Available at: www.dol.gov/sites/dolgov/files/ebsa/about-ebsa/our-activities/resource-center/publications/compliance-assistance-guide-appendix-a-mhpaea.pdf. Accessed December 10, 2019.
Vermont. Am J Insanity 46:434, 1890
Vermont Asylum for the Insane: Thirty-first annual report of the officers of the Vermont Asylum for the Insane. Am J Insanity 24:420, 1868
Ward MJ: The Snake Pit. New York, Random House, 1946
Wayne GJ: The case for the psychiatric hospital. Ment Hosp 12(3):5–10, 1961
Wesselius LF: Countertransference in milieu treatment. Arch Gen Psychiatry 18(1):47–52, 1968 5634690
White CL, Bateman A, Fisher WH, Geller JL: Factors associated with admission to public and private hospitals from a psychiatric emergency screening site. Psychiatr Serv 46(5):467–472, 1995 7627670
Whitehorn JC, Betz BJ: Further studies of the doctor as a crucial variable in the outcome of treatment with schizophrenic patients. Am J Psychiatry 117:215–223, 1960 13855368
Wickizer TM, Lessler D, Travis KM: Controlling inpatient psychiatric utilization through managed care. Am J Psychiatry 153(3):339–345, 1996 8610820
Wilusz L: Rush closes mental health units after state finds potential risks to patients. Chicago Sun Times, May 31, 2019. Available at: https://chicago.suntimes.com/2019/5/31/18647800/rush-university-medical-center-mental-health-units-ligature-risks-patient-safety-concerns. Accessed December 8, 2019.
Wolff GE: Electric shock treatment: a "must" for chronic patients in mental hospitals. Am J Psychiatry 111(10):748–750, 1955 14361758
Wood GB: History of the Pennsylvania Hospital for the Insane. Am J Insanity 9:209–213, 1853
Wyatt v Stickney, 325 F. Supp. 781, 784 (M.D. Ala. 1971)
Young GA: Experiences with psychiatric departments in the general hospitals of Omaha. Am J Psychiatry 96:69–75, 1939

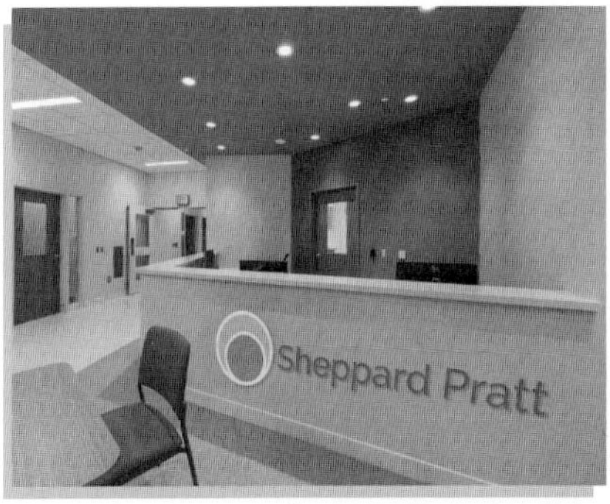

PART 1

Inpatient Care

Units by Age Cohort

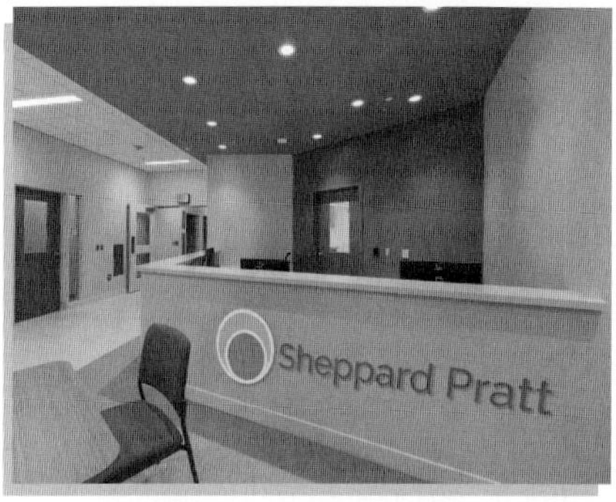

CHAPTER 2

The Child Unit

Debra Heck, M.D.
Kathryn Burns, R.N., M.S.N.

The chance to change a child's life for the better is an incredible opportunity that comes with tremendous responsibility. Careful diagnosis and consideration of psychosocial/environmental stressors are paramount in helping a child. There are many settings where this can happen: school, pediatrician's office, family environment, outpatient treatment. Inpatient hospitalization is the most restrictive setting and can be both lifesaving and life-changing for children who need help. There is no better way to observe a child than 24 hours a day in a clinically controlled setting with on-site family meetings and group therapy to help with diagnosis and treatment planning. Sometimes a complicated diagnosis with contradictory symptoms becomes clear because of the power of observation on an inpatient unit. Multidisciplinary teams can then create a treatment plan working with the family and at times the school system that will help the child be successful postdischarge. Inpatient hospitalization can allow the crystallizing moment that brings the adults in a child's life together to identify goals and a treatment plan. A child's life can be changed forever.

Reasons a Child Would Require Hospitalization

The American Academy of Child and Adolescent Psychiatry's Guidelines for Treatment Resources, Quality Assurance, Peer Review and Reimbursement offer the following requirements that justify inpatient admission (American Academy of Child and Adolescent Psychiatry 1989):

- The psychiatric disorder must be of such severity as to cause significant impairment of daily functioning in at least two important areas of the child and adolescent's life[,] such as school performance, social interactions, or family relationships.
- The treatment proposed must be relevant to the problems diagnosed and adjudged likely to benefit the patient.
- Other[,] less restrictive treatment resources must have been considered and determined to be not available or not appropriate to the patient's needs or have been attempted and proven unsuccessful. Examples of less restrictive treatment resources would include, but not be limited to, residential treatment, day treatment, or intensive outpatient care.

Safety issues such as suicidal thoughts or attempts, self-injurious behaviors, homicidal thoughts and aggression toward others, running away from home or school, and poor reality testing could all be considered dangerous behaviors and meet criteria for inpatient admission.

Also, a decreased level of functioning such as severe anxiety, obsessive-compulsive disorder (OCD), eating disorders, severe depression that causes decreased eating and sleeping, sudden unclear changes in mental status, conversion disorder, pseudoseizures, or other unclear diagnoses may be best addressed on the inpatient unit if the patient is failing to respond to other, less intensive levels of care.

As mentioned above, criteria for inpatient treatment typically involve a situation in which the child is a danger to themself or others. While depression, anxiety, and ADHD are often addressed in the outpatient setting, children being treated in the inpatient setting have complicating factors or a level of severity that requires a more restrictive setting for safety.

Evaluating a Child on an Inpatient Unit

Every child is different. To try to match symptoms of the child with the menu of symptoms in DSM-5 (American Psychiatric Association 2013) for diagnosis is simply not enough. Each child is a mosaic of their genetic makeup, life experiences, their culture, their successes and failures, their losses, their socioeconomic environment, their family role and family stressors, their self-perception, parental perception and parenting style, friendships, hopes, and dreams. Also important in a child's life is their social role and success in the school setting. Bullying and trauma in school are ever-present stressors in many children's lives. Sometimes their parents are not even aware because the child has not disclosed this to any adult out of fear or shame. Some children may have an undiagnosed learning disability or language disability that interferes with their ability to be successful no matter how hard they try. Some children may be with a peer group that pressures them to make poor decisions. Overall the need to belong and feel successful is a powerful force in a child's life and needs to be considered when seeking to understand a child's behaviors. All of this information is paramount in correct diagnosis and treatment and comes at a time when there is more pressure than ever to quickly make a diagnosis and treat the child. In what follows we offer suggestions to consider as part of an appropriate and thorough inpatient evaluation that is best done by a multidisciplinary treatment team.

Identifying the major concern that brought the child to treatment is very important in a crisis stabilization setting. There may be many issues or problems occurring at the same time, but focus must be maintained on the problem that put the patient in danger or made them dangerous to someone else. Most often this presents as aggression toward others or self in the form of suicidal thoughts or self-injurious behaviors. Questions include the following: When did the behavior start or worsen? Are there triggers or certain situations or people that exacerbate symptoms? What has been tried and has it been successful? Are there patterns as in the time of day that symptoms occur or the context where they occur, such as in school only? Was there a loss or change in the life of the child, such as the death of a family member, divorce, or move?

> Sally is a 9-year-old girl who was admitted with chronic suicidal thoughts and self-injurious behavior in the form of pulling out her hair and scratching herself with her fingernails. Several antidepressants had been tried that seemed to make her worse or cause side effects. She could not identify any triggers. It started last summer, according to her mother. "She became very sad, isolative, did not participate in sports like she used to." She did not want to go to activities and only wanted to stay at home with her mother. Her mother took a leave of absence from her job so she could spend more time with Sally and allowed her daughter to stay home from school to be with her, which was the only time Sally seemed happy. On interview, Sally denied any stressors, said she did not know why she became depressed, but she felt guilty because "I am afraid I am making my mom sad too."
>
> Careful review of the psychosocial history obtained by the social worker revealed that Sally's symptoms started when her mother became engaged and worsened when she got married and they moved in with her stepfather and stepsisters. Neither Sally nor her mother realized that her symptoms correlated with her mother's engagement and marriage. Helping Sally talk to her mother about her worries that she would lose her mother's attention allowed her mood to improve and for her to have hope. Sally and her mother planned activities they could do together that would help preserve their relationship.

Other changes that could contribute to increased dangerous behaviors would include medication noncompliance, or a recent change in medication. Collateral information from the outpatient treatment team and pharmacy can be valuable.

Questions about the child's overall health are important as well. How is the child eating and sleeping? What is their energy level, and how is their ability to focus and concentrate? Routine labs are typically done on the inpatient unit, evaluating a child's medical status and looking for any nutritional or biological contributors to mood lability, depressed mood, and anxiety. Vital signs and physical examination are also completed on admission and followed if abnormal. Staff do a routine skin assessment on admission to document any injuries that may be present. These are investigated if warranted. Children are also given brief standardized assessments such as a suicide-1 rating scale and questions about gender identity (assignment at birth and gender identification).

Family history of psychiatric disorders is important, as we learn more and more about how some mental illness can be hereditary. Also, family composition and home environment are important to ask about. Has the child had a chaotic household that could be a stressor for the child? Is there violence in the home or neighborhood that may be traumatizing for the child? Have they been exposed to inappropriate subject matter in person or seen it on media? Are they imitating behavior of a role model? It is important also to consider the child's culture when making a diagnosis.

Isabella is an 8-year-old girl who revealed to the school counselor that she was seeing "dead people." Isabella was a good student and a kind child, and staff were very concerned about her complaints of hallucinations. On interview, Isabella explained that she was seeing her great-grandmother and her great-aunt, dressed in the white lace wedding gowns that they were buried in, and that they would come to her most nights before she fell asleep to offer comfort and guidance. Isabella explained that "all the women in my family have the gift of communicating with the dead." Isabella's mother confirmed this was true and that she, like Isabella, also had this gift.

Also important to consider is how the child presents in different situations. It is not uncommon for a child to do well at school but not at home. This suggests there may be environmental stressors or conflicts with family members that exacerbate symptoms. Sometimes a child does well at home but has problems at school with aggression, elopement, and severe disruptive behaviors. These problems could be due to an undiagnosed learning disability, bullying in school, or peer or teacher conflicts.

Evaluating the Young Child

Research shows that the rate of psychiatric disorders in children ages 2–5 is similar to the rate in older children. These disorders interfere with functioning and are predictive of impairment in later childhood (Egger and Angold 2006). Especially important in the evaluation of young children is their developmental status and environmental stressors. Children should demonstrate healthy social and emotional development and be able to learn appropriately and function safely in home and school settings.

Very young children, age 4 or 5, typically present for inpatient treatment because of severe aggression related to prolonged tantrums. These tantrums sometimes appear unrelated to a trigger and occur quickly and without warning. For these children, a developmental history is especially important. Information about developmental milestones, in utero exposure to drugs or alcohol, patterns of play, and early peer relationships can be important and indicate the need for ruling out autism or other developmental disorders such as intellectual disability, speech and language disturbances, or fetal alcohol syndrome or the need for genetic testing. Identifying these issues early will allow for early intervention that can have a profound impact on a child's future development. Following is a discussion of typical diagnoses and how they present on an inpatient child unit.

Complicated ADHD in the Acute Care Setting

A 2016 survey by Danielson et al. (2018) found that 6.1% of children are diagnosed with ADHD, and of those, 64% of those have a second diagnosis: behavior or conduct problem, 52%; depression, 17%; or anxiety, 33% (cited in Centers for Disease Control and Prevention 2016). If a child with ADHD is admitted to the inpatient unit, it is because they have symptoms that are making them a danger to themself or others.

Trey is a 6-year-old kindergartner referred to inpatient care for severe aggression at school. Trey's mother states that Trey was never aggressive at home. In school, he would be disruptive and then have a tantrum when redirected. He was often "carried" out of the classroom and taken to a different room, where he would hit and kick staff and tantrum until his mother was called to come and get him. This happened on a daily basis. Despite a reported full-scale IQ of 133, Trey was in danger of repeating kindergarten and being placed in a self-contained classroom at school.

On observation, Trey was noticeably hyperactive and unable or unwilling to focus on group leaders, ran about the room, and engaged in disruptive behaviors such as yelling out random words like "Ow!" and then smiling and looking around at staff, waiting for a response. He would have a severe tantrum at about the same time every day (midday), when it was time to switch from a "fun" activity to a work activity. He was escorted to the quiet room at that time, and staff's efforts to help him calm down were unsuccessful. He would often cry out, "I want to go home!" and "I want my mommy!" He was unable to return to the group room for the rest of the day.

Focalin XR 5 mg was started for the patient, who responded well by being able to stay in his seat and engage appropriately in group activities. He continued to have the tantrum midday. Staff took a different approach with Trey by walking him to the quiet room and telling him to "calm yourself down before we can talk." Staff then ignored his tantrum. Trey's tantrums became much shorter in duration and less intense and were eliminated after 2 days.

Complicated ADHD may not respond to a typical regimen, or the child may not be able to take typical treatments because of side effects or medical concerns (e.g., seizures, tics). Children with complicated ADHD typically also have a comorbid illness such as mood disorder, anxiety, or trauma. If a child has a comorbid illness, then it is important to first treat ADHD effectively and then reevaluate other symptoms of the comorbid illness. The following strategies are outlined in the Texas algorithm (Pliszka et al. 2006). Treating ADHD effectively can be complicated. No medicine works for all children. Just as we are all different genetically, our receptors are different, and so response to medications may be varied. If there is a positive family response to a medication, then that medication should be tried first. There are four main types of stimulants: methylphenidate preparations (Ritalin, Metadate CD, Concerta, Daytrana, Quillivant), dexmethylphenidate preparations (Focalin, Focalin XR), amphetamine and dextroamphetamine mixed salts (Adderall, Adderall XR, Vyvanse), and dextroamphetamine (Dextrostat, Dexedrine, ProCentra). If a methylphenidate preparation does not work, then a different medication should be tried, such as dexmethylphenidate, and vice versa. If neither is helpful, an amphetamine and dextroamphetamine mixed salt such as Adderall should be tried. Finally, if none of the previously mentioned medications is helpful, a trial of a dextroamphetamine should be done. This is not necessarily the order in which medications should be tried. What is important is that a child's response to one medication may be superior to their response to the others. Often parents will say, "My child can't take a stimulant, because it makes him agitated" or "It does not work." Careful questioning often reveals that only one or two stimulants, or two preparations of the same stimulant (such as Adderall and Vyvanse, which are both composed of amphetamine and dextroamphetamine), have been tried. If a child is taking a high dose of medication and it is "not working," that is a sign that they are on the wrong stimulant. If a child "looks like a zombie," then they are on the wrong stimulant or the dose is too high.

Side effects can be medication related, dose related, or preparation related. For instance, a child may do very well when taking two doses of short-acting Adderall (morning and noon) but may not be able to sleep at night when they take one dose of Adderall

XR in the morning. A child may be dysphoric with Adderall but not with Focalin (or Concerta), or vice versa.

Appetite suppression is a common side effect of all stimulants. Often parents complain that their child while taking a stimulant won't eat all day but will then "wake up in the middle of the night and raid the kitchen!" This is because the stimulant has worn off by nighttime and the child is ravenous because they have not eaten all day. As with all medication and treatments, the benefits must outweigh the risk. If a stimulant is important to help a child be successful and safe, then there are strategies to help the child gain or maintain weight. Care must be given to provide the child with a nutritious, calorie-dense breakfast, eaten before the stimulant has had a chance to start working. A child may not want to eat much at lunch or dinner, however, and parents can save the child's dinner, to be eaten prior to bedtime when the child's appetite is returning. Also, parents can provide nutritious, calorie-dense foods as a bedtime snack to make up for missed calories during the day. Some parents and providers agree to give the child a break from stimulants on non-school days, including weekends, summer, and winter breaks, to allow the child to catch up on calories that are decreased on school days.

Children with ADHD often have difficulty falling asleep, even when they do not take a stimulant. It is important to not give stimulants later than the after-school dose needed for homework, as they may interfere with the child's ability to stay asleep or fall asleep. Short-acting stimulants are best in the afternoon. Some children respond well to a bedtime routine such as a bath and a bedtime story. Access to electronics can be stimulating and should be avoided. Some children require melatonin or clonidine for sleep.

The relationship between tics and stimulants is controversial. Based on clinical observation, a stimulant can exacerbate a tic. This exacerbation is often medication-specific and can also be preparation specific.

> James is an intelligent 8-year-old boy with severe ADHD. He had been tried on many different stimulants, but the only ones that worked for him were methylphenidate products. Unfortunately, he had a vocal and motor tic when he took Ritalin that made him embarrassed, and the tics were disruptive in the classroom. James was tried on Concerta and Daytrana at different times and with different dosing combinations of short-acting methylphenidate, but the tics persisted. James did not have a tic when he did not take the medications. His parents felt that James could not be successful without taking methylphenidate, so he did on school days. Finally, James tried Metadate CD, and it was effective without causing any tics.

Clonidine or guanfacine (Tenex, Intuniv) is often used with stimulants to target impulsivity, hyperactivity, and aggression. They should be tried before a neuroleptic or mood stabilizer is considered, because of their favorable side-effect profile.

Children with a seizure disorder may not be able to take stimulants because these medications can lower the seizure threshold. Nortriptyline can be used carefully for these patients. Typically it is given at bedtime because of sedation, and weight-based dosing is used because of potential cardiac side effects.

It is hard to describe the dramatic change in a patient with severe ADHD when they are taking the right stimulant. The youngster who was unable to stay in class suddenly becomes an A student and their life is transformed. Untreated or undertreated ADHD puts children at risk of conduct disorder because they are not successful in the classroom and are drawn to different peer groups in their school where they can feel successful. Early childhood is when one's self-image and self-worth are established, or not. Although ADHD is typically not thought of as a potentially life-threatening diagnosis, its impact on the life of the child can be profound. In a recent study, children with ADHD had nearly a fourfold higher risk of suicidal ideation compared with children who did not have ADHD (Chen et al. 2019). Untreated or undertreated ADHD can send a child down the wrong path in life.

Successfully treated ADHD can transform a child's life forever. Inpatient units are the ideal place to diagnose and treat complicated ADHD, for many reasons. Children can be observed in different settings, including group work, which simulates classroom settings and recreational settings. Different staff observe the patient at different times of the day and document behaviors and symptoms, including poor focus and inattention. Because stimulants are typically fast-acting, it only takes a day or two to discover if the medication being tried has the potential to be helpful. Careful observation for side effects is also more easily done in the inpatient setting than at home and school, where there may be confounders or conflicting information. If a medication is not working, it is easily discontinued, and a new medication can be tried the next day. If a medication is working but is causing side effects, this is best, and most quickly, addressed on the inpatient unit, where changes in dosing and timing can be ordered and results evaluated the next day.

ADHD and Depression

> Charles is a 10-year-old boy admitted after telling the school counselor he wanted to kill himself. Charles has also said this at home when he has gotten "in trouble" for something he said or did. Charles has ADHD and is impulsive and disruptive at home and at school. He has poor social skills. He does not listen or follow directions. He is silly at times, standing on chairs, running about the room, singing a funny song in an effort to gain attention or make others laugh. Often Charles does not understand what he has done wrong or why others are frustrated with him. He is depressed and suicidal at times because of his perception that he is not well liked. He has poor self-esteem and does not feel like he is good at anything. He internalizes his anger and sadness and becomes depressed, feeling that he is not wanted and should not be alive and that "everyone would be better off without me." Charles is started on a stimulant and does better at home and at school. He has more friends, and the adults in his life appreciate his efforts and praise him. Charles' self-esteem improves and his mood lifts. He is no longer suicidal. He continues to work on social skills in a group setting.

Depression is common in children with ADHD. In one study, 9%–38% of children with ADHD were found to have depression (Biederman et al. 1991). Of children that had a diagnosis of depression, ADHD was the most common comorbidity (34%). Aggression in children with ADHD can indicate depression (Turgay and Ansari 2006).

In children with ADHD and depression, the ADHD should be treated first per the Texas algorithm. If needed, a selective serotonin reuptake inhibitor (SSRI) can be added to target depressive symptoms after treatment for ADHD has been optimized.

ADHD and Trauma

> Allison is an 11-year-old girl who was referred for treatment because of bizarre behavior and aggression. Allison was placed in foster care after early and severe abuse and neglect. She urinated on the floor in her room. She complained of being always hungry and hoarded food and trash in her room (but did not eat the food). She stole items from

her foster mother and from staff at school. She was in constant motion, disorganized, and impulsive, and ran away from home and out of school multiple times. She was aggressive toward adults at home and at school who attempted to block her from eloping. She said she felt "more safe" when on the run than at home or at school. She was treated with stimulants and clonidine but still remained in a constant state of hyperarousal and overactivity. Low-dose quetiapine was added to her regimen. Her mood improved, and she was less impulsive. She was better able to sleep, and her compulsions (stealing, hoarding) improved. It was discovered that she and her younger brother had been locked in a room for long periods of time without access to food, water, or a bathroom by impaired (birth) parents. Her urinating on the floor happened when she was angry or felt she had been treated unfairly. Allison was referred to outpatient therapy to work on her feelings of sadness and rage.

In this case, the ADHD was addressed, but the patient also required treatment for symptoms related to her trauma history that put her in danger.

ADHD and Anxiety

Thirty-three percent of children with ADHD will also have anxiety (Centers for Disease Control and Prevention 2016). For some children, treating ADHD will decrease anxiety. It is also possible some children will have increased anxiety with stimulants. The ADHD should be treated first as recommended in the Texas Algorithm, with different stimulants tried if one increases anxiety. If the child still has anxiety after optimal treatment of ADHD, then using an SSRI and/or α_2-receptor agonist such as clonidine may help. Diphenhydramine or hydroxyzine may be helpful short term on an as-needed basis for anxiety while waiting for the SSRI to take effect. Cognitive-behavioral therapy is also recommended for anxiety, occurring mostly on an outpatient basis after discharge.

ADHD and Bipolar Disorder (Disruptive Mood Dysregulation Disorder)

A common concern of many parents is "Does my child have bipolar disorder?" In the recent past, many children were diagnosed with bipolar disorder. Whether or not the diagnosis was accurate is controversial. What is clear is that true childhood mania with cycling is rare and that some children have a persistent, severe irritability that affects their ability to function successfully in life. The newer diagnosis of disruptive mood dysregulation disorder is more commonly used than bipolar disorder in children. For the purpose of discussion in this chapter, both diagnoses will be included under the umbrella term *mood disorder*.

ADHD is one of the most common comorbid conditions in children diagnosed with mood disorders. It is found in 70%–90% of prepubertal children with bipolar disorder (Kowatch et al. 2005). Many children admitted to the inpatient unit seem to have symptoms of both ADHD and a mood disorder. ADHD and mood disorders may have overlap in symptoms. Also, to make matters more confusing, a child may have both ADHD and a mood disorder. Aggression or other dangerous behaviors may be present in children with ADHD.

It can be difficult to decide if a child has ADHD, a mood disorder, or both. Ultimately, it is necessary to address the child's unsafe behaviors, but because the medications used for ADHD and mood disorders are different, a clear diagnosis is important.

Mood stabilizers are not effective for ADHD, and medications for ADHD are not effective mood stabilizers, with the exception of clonidine or guanfacine, which can be used to target impulsivity and aggression in either diagnosis. If ADHD is suspected, it should be treated first and then the child should be reevaluated for a mood disorder (Pliszka et al. 2006). Because stimulants work fairly quickly, this is a good strategy on the inpatient unit, where time may be limited.

There are other things to consider when trying to decide if a child has ADHD, a mood disorder, or both. A child with ADHD will not have psychotic symptoms such as disorganized thoughts, tangential or loose thought process, or perceptual disturbances such as paranoia or sadistic impulses. The one exception is medication-induced psychosis from a stimulant. This is a rare side effect, and the correlation of the onset of psychotic symptoms and initiation of the stimulant should be apparent. Children with ADHD may break things because of carelessness or aimless exploring, but they do not break things out of anger. A child with a mood disorder may have severe temper tantrums with psychotic disorganization and may break things out of anger. These tantrums will often last over 30 minutes. The child may have a poor or absent memory of the tantrum. The child with a mood disorder will have irritability typically in the morning and may also have trouble waking up. A child with ADHD typically wakes up easily and often early. A child with ADHD is more likely to have learning disorders, language disorders, and problems with reading. Children with a mood disorder are often gifted verbally and artistically. Children with ADHD may be socially awkward, clumsy, and oblivious to danger. Children with a mood disorder seek and enjoy power struggles, seek danger, exhibit grandiosity, and seek recognition. They may like to climb to dangerous heights or play with fire. Children with ADHD will have an onset of hyperactivity and poor attention in early childhood, and these are persistent and chronic in most settings throughout their childhood. Children with a mood disorder may have a later onset with increased severity of mood swings as they get older. There may be a cyclical nature to their symptoms. Finally, a strong family history of either ADHD or mood disorder may help the treatment team discern the correct diagnosis.

Other Diagnoses on the Inpatient Unit

Trauma

The most common presentation of a child with trauma on the inpatient unit involves a child who presents with new-onset crying, sleep disturbance, enuresis, encopresis, and/or separation anxiety, or a child who has new onset of aggression or sexualized behaviors. Often the trauma is not recognized or known by the family on admission. A detailed history from the parents and the child is needed, looking for any changes in routines or people around the time of the symptom onset. Sometimes the child is too fragile to talk about the trauma but may be able to "act it out" in play therapy or draw about it in art therapy. Sometimes the trauma is not identified while the child is hospitalized. Some children are confused and ambivalent about the abuse and may seek to protect their abusers. Knowing about the trauma helps guide therapy and treatment decisions.

Trauma is common. More than two-thirds of children in the United States report having experienced at least one traumatic event by the age of 16 years (Copeland et al. 2007). Identification and treatment of childhood stress disorders such as PTSD and acute stress disorder is important for many reasons. First and foremost, the process of identification and treatment relieves the suffering of the child and allows them to return to normal functioning as soon as possible, to aid in their resilience, and allows them to be the most successful student and have the best childhood they can. But also, research shows that the more adverse childhood experiences (ACEs) a child has, the greater is the likelihood of negative health and life outcomes such as heart disease, stroke, diabetes, asthma, depression, alcohol and substance use, poor academic achievement, and unemployment (Hughes et al. 2017). The ACEs included in this study were physical, sexual, or emotional abuse; neglect; household violence; substance abuse; mental illness; parent divorce; and incarceration of a family member.

Because all children are different, what may be traumatizing for one child might not be traumatizing for another. Other things that can be traumatizing to some children include natural disasters, school violence, life-threatening illness in themselves or a family member, medical procedures, loss or death of a pet, neglect, death or incarceration of a family member or loved one, parental divorce, witnessing domestic violence, humiliation in a public place, and worries about parents or siblings being harmed or humiliated. Witnessing parents being treated violently can be traumatizing as well. Birth of a new sibling can also be stressful. Trauma and stressor-related symptoms include persistent, frightening thoughts and memories or flashbacks of a traumatic event or events. Other symptoms include jumpiness, sleep problems, problems in school, avoidance of certain places or situations, depression, headaches, and stomach pains. Children may also have regressed behavior (e.g., thumb-sucking, talking in baby talk, enuresis, and encopresis) after being successfully toilet trained. Some children may worry about dying at a young age. Some children may lose touch with reality or dissociate.

> Mathew is a 7-year-old boy who was "completely normal" according to school staff but who one day appeared to be confused and locked in his own world. He appeared to go into a trance and moved his arms as if he were folding laundry. He seemed unaware of his surroundings and did not respond when others talked to him. School staff and his mother worried that Mathew might have lost touch with reality, and he appeared psychotic. His school filed a petition for emergency evaluation. On admission, Mathew continued to act this way most of the day, every day. He said some words that appeared to be out of context and did not communicate with others in a meaningful way. Mathew was unable to explain what he was thinking or experiencing. Careful, detailed interviews of school staff and the patient's mother revealed the following details: Mathew's mother had recently left Mathew's dad for another man. She and the children moved into her boyfriend's trailer, where there were no doors on the rooms. Mathew and his siblings witnessed his mother having sexual relations with her boyfriend. This was traumatizing for Mathew. Mathew's mother was given support and education. Mathew was treated with fluoxetine. Mathew was not able to talk about what he was going through, but his dissociation decreased, and he was able to resume normal activities.

Unfortunately, there is no perfect medicine to treat trauma. Medication strategies should help bring relief and target anxiety, mood, and overall adrenergic tone. An SSRI can help with the depression and anxiety that a child may be experiencing. Clonidine can also help decrease adrenergic tone, helping to decrease the increased vigilance, exaggerated startle response, overreactivity, impulsivity, and subjective sense of fear. Medications such as diphenhydramine or hydroxyzine can also be used on an as-needed basis to help the child feel calm. An atypical neuroleptic may be needed for severe symptoms, such as trauma-related nightmares, self-injurious behavior, and dissociation (Donnelly 2003).

> Shane is a 7-year-old boy who was admitted for having "fits" whenever he was asked to use the bathroom at his foster home. Shane had been placed in foster care after being removed from his mother's care because of abuse and neglect. He did not want to take showers or baths or use the toilet. He had long screaming tantrums and would sometimes hit or kick when approached by his foster parents. Shane was unable to explain why he was afraid of the bathroom, other than saying, "There is a man looking through the window." Shane would say this even though the curtains were drawn. He was started on sertraline; however, Shane needed more immediate help. Low-dose olanzapine was added, and Shane was then able to use the bathroom at his home.

A child may need help in blocking intrusive thoughts that are interfering with their ability to function, such as eating, sleeping, going to school, playing sports, and participating in the normal activities of childhood. If a child is old enough to understand abstract thought, then the following exercise may be helpful for them.

Ask the child to create their own box and decorate it however they want. This can be real, drawn, or imaginary. Then ask them to put the box on a shelf in their mind. Then ask them to take all the painful memories and thoughts and place them in the box and put a lid on the box. These memories and thoughts are now contained and put away until it is time to work on them with a therapist, when they are ready.

While it is not unusual for a child with a history of trauma to dissociate in certain situations, dissociative identity disorder (DID) is a very rare sequelae of severe, early trauma. Its existence is controversial, and the occurrence rate is unknown.

> Sam is an 8-year-old boy living in foster care after being removed from his mother's care for abuse and neglect. Sam was admitted several times over 6 months because of increased aggression at the foster home. Sam had a good relationship with his foster mother, and his biological sister was also in the home. Sam's first admission was for setting a fire in the kitchen. He took paper and put it on the gas stove while it was turned on. Initially Sam admitted he wanted to kill his foster mother and sister and burn the house down. He was unable to explain why. Oddly, Sam later denied this, crying and saying he loved his sister and foster mother. Sam appeared inconsistent in other ways. Some days he spoke with a gruff voice, his hair and clothing were disheveled, and he appeared elevated, laughing, saying loudly that his "sister deserved to get killed!" and bragging on how he was able to "beat her up." Other days he was well groomed and quiet and appeared internally preoccupied. He stared off, seeming to daydream. Some days Sam did not know how to read. He appeared confused at times, asking what was for lunch after he had just eaten. He appeared to lose time, not knowing whether it was morning or evening. Sometimes he would say things that did not make sense and laugh when asked about them. He drew a picture in art therapy (Figure 2–1).
>
> The art therapist noted an unusual finding in Sam's picture:
>
>> In an art therapy session, patient made artwork that seemed to suggest symptoms of dissociation. Patient shared his artwork at the end of group, saying it was a "police officer and an animal." Patient drew a portrait of a person in a police uniform clearly and skillfully. The animal he drew looked like it was drawn by a much younger person. When asked what type of animal it was, he reported, "A zebra." Patient also made spirals, a number 5, letters, and doodle-like marks. When asked what it said or meant, he appeared confused and said, "I don't know." Patient's artwork seemed to reflect a complex and disorienting inner experience. His artwork shows perspectives of artwork from varying stages of development. It seemed to reflect aspects of how patient has coped with aspects of his history of trauma in a kind of dissociated dreamlike/trance state.

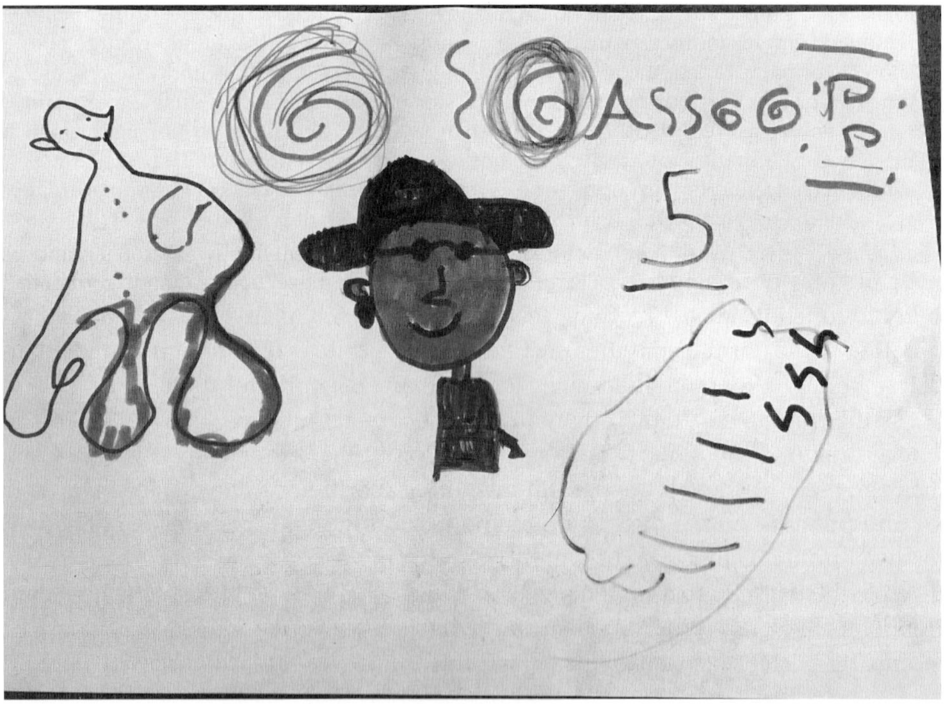

FIGURE 2–1. **Picture drawn by Sam, an 8-year-old boy living in foster care after being removed from his mother's care for abuse and neglect.**
To view this figure in color, see Plate 1 in Color Gallery.

Doodling can be a way to make marks in a soothing way and a way to mentally disconnect. With people who dissociate, shifting from different states of consciousness, these repetitive marks can be a way to function and cope. These types of marks occur with a higher frequency in children with severe dissociation, as was noted by Cohen and Thayer Cox (1995) in their research. This example does not prove or disprove the existence of DID, but it demonstrates how reality can be fractured for some children with a severe history of trauma.

Depression and Self-Injurious Behaviors

Typically, children with depression admitted to the inpatient unit have suicidal ideation or self-injurious behaviors. Children with depression can also present as aggressive and irritable. Collateral information is needed from the family regarding neurovegetative symptoms that might confirm a diagnosis of depression, such as decreased energy, decreased focus, sleep and appetite disturbance, anhedonia, decreased ability to manage activities of daily living, and poor grooming. Children are better than adults at brightening situationally, but often children with depression will appear sad and isolative on the unit and spend their time on the periphery of the milieu. Typically an SSRI is started; however, these medications do not work immediately. That is why it is important, when possible, to identify a stressor or loss that can be addressed while the child is inpatient to hopefully give the child relief and their family a better understanding of the patient. The team can work on strategies to help the families provide support and reassurance, identify warning signs with a safety plan, and give the child and their family hope that things will get better. Families may need referrals to organizations that offer grief counseling. A school consult may be needed to help advise parents on their rights and on protocols if their child is being bullied in school. Some children are overwhelmed in school and need evaluations for learning disabilities. Misunderstandings between family members that contribute to depression can be addressed in a family meeting.

> Aaron is an 11-year-old boy who lived with his paternal grandparents, having been abandoned by his birth mother at an early age. His father was in jail and told Aaron that when he gets out of jail they can be together again like a "real family." Aaron's grandparents were upset and worried and told Aaron, "That will never happen" and "Your dad is a criminal and a drug addict and you will never live with him." Aaron started cutting his arms and abdomen with a knife. Aaron denied this was an attempt to kill himself but said only, "I cut myself because that keeps me from hurting other people." After some time he revealed that he was angry at his grandparents for speaking badly about his father. During a family meeting, this was explained to his grandparents, and they apologized to Aaron. They agreed to not talk that way about his father anymore, and Aaron was less sad and angry and no longer felt the need to cut himself.

As in the example above, suicidal thoughts or self-injurious behaviors can be driven by anger, misunderstandings, and an inability to express one's feelings in a healthy and direct way.

Anxiety

Anxiety is common and underdiagnosed in young children. The most common presentation of anxiety on the inpatient unit is school refusal. A typical presentation is that a child will refuse to go to school and then become aggressive if parents or school staff attempt to force the child to enter the school building or stay in the school building. Reasons for school refusal are diverse and complex. Separation anxiety is a common reason. School issues such as bullying or trauma at the school can also be reasons for school refusal. Again, SSRIs with a combination of clonidine or hydroxyzine prn may be helpful. A neuroleptic may be needed temporarily for severe aggression.

Obsessive-Compulsive Disorder

OCD is rarely seen on the inpatient unit. To meet criteria for inpatient admission, the OCD must be severe enough to warrant a restrictive setting for safety. OCD symptoms can endanger a child's health or ability to attend school, or the child may become aggressive if their ritual is interrupted or if they are forced to "hurry up." Typically SSRIs are used for anxiety and obsessive thoughts. Neuroleptics may be helpful temporarily to decrease obsessive thoughts and decrease the intensity of the need to act on a compulsion. OCD is best treated over time with a combination of medication and therapy once patients are safe and have been stabilized.

Gender Dysphoria

Gender dysphoria is becoming more recognized. It is a risk factor for depression and anxiety. Children with gender dysphoria may be targeted for bullying. They may have family members who do not understand or accept them. Crisis intervention and stabilization on the inpatient unit can help children who are feeling depressed, anxious, or even suicidal. Staff can provide the family with support and education and referrals to community support groups and resources.

Psychotic Disorders

It is surprisingly common to have a child admitted because they reported they are "hearing voices" or "seeing things." Typically the child does not appear psychotic in other ways; for instance, they are not paranoid, delusional, or disorganized. They have good grooming, good sleep, and good appetite. They do not appear distressed by these experiences, and "hearing voices" seems to happen most often when they are "in trouble" and "the voices told me to do this." In fact, childhood schizophrenia is very rare. If a child does truly appear to be psychotic, treatment with a neuroleptic is appropriate. If the child has an underlying mood disorder or anxiety/trauma disorder, this should also be treated with an appropriate medication such as a mood stabilizer or an SSRI for anxiety and depression.

Typical presentations of hallucinations that are not psychotic in nature are in the context of grief (when a child reports seeing, typically at bedtime, a loved one who passed away) or being upset after watching graphic or violent media. If a child is asked to describe the voices, hearing the voices "outside" of their head is more likely reported for true psychotic hallucinations. Voices heard "inside" the head tend to be more ruminations or perseverating and may even be heard by the child as their own voice. Asking the child to describe what they are seeing or hearing can be helpful. If it is self-deprecating and mood-congruent, then it is more likely due to depression. If the hallucinations are related to trauma, then it is most likely PTSD. Sometimes a child will describe what sounds like a violent movie plot. If so, it is worthwhile to ask if the child has ever viewed a movie or materials similar to what they described. This type of investigation is not meant to prove or disprove if the hallucinations are "real." The hallucinations are experienced as "real" to the child and serve some purpose. These questions can help clarify the best course of treatment and avoid exposure to medications that may not be needed and avoid potential side effects.

Role of Family in Treatment

As mentioned at the beginning of this chapter, every child is different. The role of their environment cannot be underestimated. Collateral information is integral for correct diagnosis and treatment planning. A careful psychosocial evaluation needs to be done on admission to gather information about stressors in the family, the child's perceived role in the family, and the effect the child's illness is having on the family. This type of meeting also helps to identify treatment goals and build an alliance with the family. The plan can be set in motion prior to discharge.

A child's success after discharge depends on the family understanding and supporting the child and having realistic expectations and a plan for how to keep the child safe. Also important is to review the warning signs of worsening symptoms and the procedure for readmission if needed.

Role of Interface With School

Collateral information from the school is very important. The school is the primary setting for the child as far as competence, peer relationships, relationships with staff, ability to do work, and the ability to get along with others are concerned. No psychiatric evaluation is complete without information about how the child is doing in school. Also, sometimes the parent or the school will ask the treatment team to make recommendations to help the child be successful in the school setting. This can be very important and can change the child's chances of success in school going forward. Protocols regarding bullying should be discussed with the parents, along with their rights for pursuing a free appropriate public education, or FAPE, for their child. Staff may suggest testing for learning disabilities or speech and language disorders. Parents may need guidance regarding advocating for their child in the school system.

Role of Interface With Government Agencies

The inpatient treatment team ideally works hand in hand with government agencies such as the Department of Social Services (DSS) and Child Protective Services (CPS) to provide information about the child and recommendations for treatment or placement. DSS workers participate in evaluations of the children by providing history and consent for treatment when needed. They are also involved with advocating for the children, protecting the children, and setting goals for the children.

The inpatient treatment team members are mandated reporters and provide information to DSS/CPS if there is any cause for concern.

Role of Interface With Outpatient Providers

It is very important to collaborate with the outpatient provider regarding treatment history and planning. Often, they can provide information about the patient and the family, previous medication trials, and compliance with treatment. There may be information that is discovered or revealed while the child is on the inpatient unit that would be important for the outpatient treatment team to know. Also, information on prescriptions dispensed and recommendations made to the school is important for the outpatient treatment team to have for their records.

Milieu Therapy/Structure on the Inpatient Unit

The majority of children do best with structure. Ideally the inpatient unit has a schedule that is followed daily. Children have a combination of group therapies, art therapy, occupational therapy, recreational time, and quiet time. Meals and groups are at the same time every day. Bedtime is at the same time every day. Activities are planned to allow intervals of play in between groups. Efforts are made daily to take the children outside to play. The goal is to create a safe, therapeutic environment that will help the children get back to baseline as soon as possible. Safe behavior is encouraged by a reward-based system.

Reward-Based System

For managing the milieu, reward systems can be used to help provide structure and motivation for children to have safe behaviors. Reward systems are best when worked into the programming of the milieu such that by following directions, keeping hands and feet safe, and participating, a child knows they are meeting the criteria of the reward system. A good reward system is simple. Simplicity is especially important within an inpatient setting with short length of stay. There are two types of rewards on the unit, one that allows for instant gratification and one that has a larger but delayed reward.

The unit allows for patients to visit a store that is on the unit. This "point" store has items such as coloring books, modeling clay (e.g., Play-Doh), stuffed animals, fidget toys, tablet time, help-hand-out-snack cards, and pick-the-game-during-gym cards. If a patient is green for the day—"green" meaning that the patient has kept hands and feet to self, not postured or verbally threatened—they are able to visit the store. Each item within the store has points assigned to it. Rewards such as tablet time or helping to hand out snack cost 25 points, while Play-Doh might cost 15. A patient is able to earn points throughout the day.

Instant Reward

Many of the children on an inpatient unit struggle with patience, impulse control, and self-regulation. A child might have been listening and have heard that at the end of the group there would be a reward. However, for patients struggling with regulation waiting 30 minutes for a group to end to receive that reward is too long. The child for several reasons will have already forgotten what was going to happen in 30 minutes. The child could have become distracted and be now playing in their seat instead of sitting in it, or the child could have become upset with a peer.

The instant reward system used currently is one in which a child can be rewarded by staff immediately when the safe behavior is seen. Staff can do this by writing their initials or giving a stamp on a card that each patient carries with them. One staff initial or stamp equals one point. To the child who is becoming distracted staff might say, "Good job for sitting back down in your seat and keeping your feet on the ground; let me give you a stamp," or the child who is becoming upset with a peer might be told, "Good job for moving away from your peer when you were becoming upset; let me write my initials." In both cases, staff were able to give positive praise and reinforce good behavior in the moment. Staff can also give out points when they see acts of kindness such as a child holding the door open for a peer or a child helping a peer spell a word for an activity.

Delayed Reward

There is an expectation that all children will attend and participate in groups. Most likely this might look different for each child. Participation from a 6-year-old is going to be different than that from a 10-year-old. The overall group is structured to support every child. Staff will start the group by explaining how to earn points. A group leader might say, "If you raise your hand before speaking and listen to others, you will get one point at the end of group." Not only will the group leader verbally explain how to earn points, they will also remind the group by writing it on the group room board. Now a child has motivation for attending an entire group.

Changes and Failures

There have been many adjustments made to the process of points. At one time, the milieu was running with only instant reward and no reward for attending groups. Not surprisingly, children were coming and going to group with no motivation to stay. An attempt was then made to remove the cards children were carrying with them for instant points and to just have points be earned by attending groups. This again failed. For one, children who had just arrived on the unit were not yet stable enough to be expected to stay for an entire group. Many children when they first arrive need frequent breaks of taking space and playing in their bedroom or resource room. The new children were not earning any points and having tantrums when they saw other children attending the point store. For another, staff struggled with how to reward children in the moment and could only say "Good job," which quickly became empty words to many children.

Overall, the reward system should get the child to complete the unit goals. The reward system encourages group participation, and it encourages physical and emotional safety. Many of the children seeking inpatient treatment have difficulty thinking about the consequences that might happen later and tend to need more instant rewards rather than delayed rewards to stay motivated. However, as the child starts to stabilize, the program should also move toward setting delayed rewards such as having the child wait for the end of shift to attend the point store.

Groups, Coping Skills, and Taking Space

The number of staff assigned to the inpatient unit may vary depending on acuity and census. The number of groups may be increased to create a smaller number of children per group if needed for the particular patient population that day (e.g., younger children or older children might be better served if in their own group for the day). Groups are designed to help children identify and express their feelings appropriately and to work on communication and coping skills. Another goal is to help children feel successful and to improve their self-esteem. Children are encouraged to identify when they are getting angry or frustrated and to ask to "take space" by going to their room. While in their room they have access to their "calming box" to help themselves calm down. The calming box contains safe objects that they like that can help them calm down. Some examples might be a favorite stuffed animal, plastic bricks (e.g., Legos), crayons and paper, a favorite book or magazine, and Play-Doh. The hope is that all children will learn this technique and be able to use it at home and at school.

Another technique to help children identify goals and create a plan is a "social script." This document is created with the child's input and should use words or pictures that the child can understand. It is a written plan that is individualized and should be reviewed with the child at least twice a day. It is a physical reminder that should stay with the child, such as in their binder or notebook or taped to their desk. They can refer to it as needed, and staff can also remind the patient to refer to it. The following is an example of a social script, written by Jordan Segall, M.S., CCC-SLP:

School

School can be difficult and can cause me to feel stressed. Sometimes, I might not understand the work. Sometimes, I might think the work looks too hard. Other times, I just don't want to do it.

Students can make poor decisions when they are feeling stressed. Sometimes, I choose to run out of the classroom when I am feeling this way. This is not a safe choice. When I run out of the classroom, people worry about me. They wonder what's wrong and are afraid that I might get hurt.

> Talking to people when we feel stressed can help us think of safe ways to handle tough situations. When I'm feeling stressed, I will ask for help and/or tell staff how I am feeling before running out of the classroom.
>
> When I get stressed but don't feel like talking, I can take 5 minutes and use my strategies to help me feel better.
>
> - Take deep breaths
> - Draw or color a picture
> - Use positive self-talk (e.g., "I can do this.")
> - Squeeze a ball or a fidget
> - Think of something that makes me happy
> - Ask to take a quick walk
> - Ask to take a short break in a quiet space
>
> When I use these strategies, I will have more good days at school. My parents will be proud of me, my teachers will be proud of me, and I will feel proud of myself for staying calm and finding safe ways to handle my stress.

A constant challenge for staff is to set limits with the children in a way that allows them to save face and learn from the experience. Many children will push limits and seek conflict with staff. When a child is aggressive or threatening, they are asked to take space. They should go to their room as a respite, not as a punishment. As a last resort, if children are in danger of harming themselves or others, staff may be required to restrain the patient manually or walk them to the quiet room. Locked-door seclusion is always a last resort for a child who is harming others and cannot calm down with staff support and encouragement. Ideally, the unit staff should study the child and find what is effective for that specific child so that seclusion and restraint can be avoided as much as possible. It is important to determine the cause of aggression for each patient, and for staff to take on the role of creative problem-solving. If the child is acting out to seek attention, planned ignoring can be helpful. Perhaps there is an identifiable trigger, such as sharing or returning electronics when time is up. Once a strategy is identified, the strategy needs to be communicated to the rest of the treatment team. Ideally, it is also something that can be transferable to home and the school setting.

Team Members

An inpatient hospitalization can be helpful, even life-changing, for the child and their family. Time is often limited for a variety of reasons. It takes a dedicated team working together with the family to diagnose, treat, and create a plan that will help the child be safe and successful after discharge. Gathering the history and creating goals usually take place with the family, psychiatrist, social worker, and nursing staff. Collateral information can be obtained from the outpatient provider and (with parents' permission) the child's school. Often staff who work with the child in groups and in the milieu during play and recreational activities also pass along information that is very valuable about something the child did or said. Coming together as a team and talking about the child on a daily basis is crucial. Group notes and progress notes are also reviewed on a daily basis to crystallize the understanding of the child, and to steadily work toward reaching their goals for treatment. Consults may be required for psychological testing to clarify the diagnosis, to evaluate for autism, or even to test IQ if needed and if such testing has not been done recently. Art therapy and occupational therapy are important to help children on the unit and also to help staff gather information needed for diagnosis clarification and treatment planning. Discharge planning begins when the child is admitted to make sure the needed resources are in place at the time of discharge. A school consult is provided by a special education teacher on staff who is able to discuss school issues with the child, parent, and the school, to come up with a document that lists recommendations for the school to help the child be successful when they return. The child and their family are offered family therapy that is led by the social worker but may also include any member of the treatment team. The unit staff and structure are overseen by the unit manager for the unit, who works with staff to create and ensure standards and schedules are met and also helps problem-solve and work with families to achieve the best outcome for their child.

Future Directions

Standardized rating scales are becoming more popular in all settings of patient care. These scales may be computerized for quicker tracking and analysis. Prescribing practices are more closely tied to evidence-based treatment. Following recommended algorithms can improve results and speed up positive outcomes for patients. Parent education and support groups reduce the stigma of mental illness, provide information and resources for parents, and help raise the consciousness of communities. School systems and mental health systems must work together to identify children at risk and provide early intervention to reduce suffering and provide quicker results that can be life-changing for children and their families. Electronic access to medical records, while protecting a patient's privacy, will help with efficient and accurate diagnosing and strengthen outpatient connections to help the patient maintain stability after discharge. This will also allow better continuity of care, creating a safety net for children and their families. Individualized treatment plans can be transferable to home and schools and to the outpatient providers. As outpatient services become more readily available and better connected, the inpatient stay can be shortened. More children are receiving a diagnosis and being treated in less restrictive settings, such as day hospital or intensive outpatient programs, if their safety can be ensured in these settings.

References

American Academy of Child and Adolescent Psychiatry: Guidelines for Treatment Resources: Quality Assurance, Peer Review and Reimbursement. Washington, DC, American Academy of Child and Adolescent Psychiatry, 1989. Available at: www.aacap.org/AACAP/Policy_Statements/1989/Inpatient_Hospital_Treatment_of_Children_and_Adolescents.aspx. Accessed October 26, 2021.

American Psychiatric Association: Diagnostic and Statistical Manual of Mental Disorders, 5th Edition. Arlington, VA, American Psychiatric Association, 2013

Biederman J, Newcorn J, Sprich S: Comorbidity of attention deficit hyperactive disorder with conduct, depressive, anxiety, and other disorders. Am J Psychiatry 148(5):564–577, 1991

Centers for Disease Control and Prevention: Data and Statistics About ADHD. Atlanta, GA, Centers for Disease Control and Prevention, 2016. Available at: www.cdc.gov/ncbddd/adhd/data.html. Accessed November 11, 2019.

Chen Y-Y, Chen Y-L, Gau SS-F: Attention-deficit hyperactivity disorder and suicidality: the mediating effects of psychiatric comorbidities and family function. J Affect Disord 242:96–104, 2019 30173064

Cohen BM, Thayer Cox C: Telling Without Talking. Art as a Window Into the World of Multiple Personality. New York, WW Norton, 1995

Copeland WE, Keeler G, Angold A, Costello EJ: Traumatic events and posttraumatic stress in childhood. Arch Gen Psychiatry 64(5):577–584, 2007 17485609

Danielson ML, Bitsko RH, Ghandour RM, et al: Prevalence of parent-reported ADHD diagnosis and associated treatment among U.S. children and adolescents, 2016. J Clin Child Adolesc Psychol 47(2):199–212, 2018 29363986

Donnelly CL: Pharmacologic treatment approaches for children and adolescents with posttraumatic stress disorder. Child Adolesc Psychiatr Clin N Am 12(2):251–269, 2003 12725011

Egger HL, Angold A: Common emotional and behavioral disorders in preschool children: presentation, nosology, and epidemiology. J Child Psychol Psychiatry 47(3–4):313–337, 2006 16492262

Hughes K, Bellis MA, Hardcastle KA, et al: The effect of multiple adverse childhood experiences on health: a systematic review and meta-analysis. Lancet Public Health Aug; 2(8):e356–e366, 2017

Kowatch RA, Fristad M, Birmaher B, et al: Treatment guidelines for children and adolescents with bipolar disorder. J Am Acad Child Adolesc Psychiatry 44(3):213–235, 2005 15725966

Pliszka SR, Crismon ML, Hughes CW, et al: The Texas Children's Medication Algorithm Project: revision of the algorithm for pharmacotherapy of attention-deficit/hyperactivity disorder. J Am Acad Child Adolesc Psychiatry 45(6):642–657, 2006 16721314

Turgay A, Ansari R: Major depression with ADHD: in children and adolescents. Psychiatry (Edgmont) 3(4):20–32, 2006 21103168

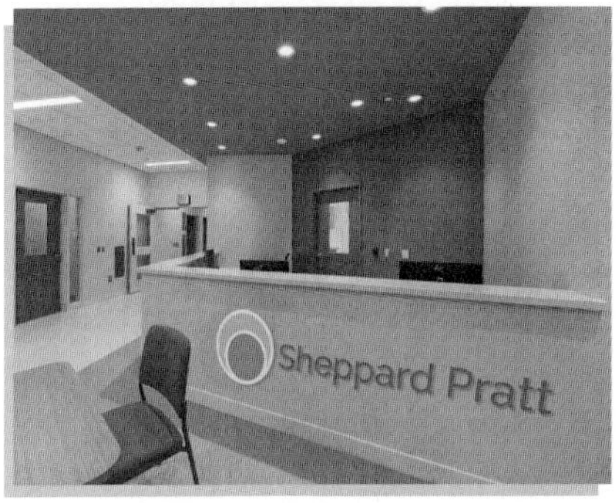

CHAPTER 3

The Adolescent Unit

Yasas Tanguturi, M.D., M.P.H.
Catharyn Turner II, M.D., M.Ed.

Adolescents with mental health needs require a spectrum of care that encompasses different types of treatment. Inpatient psychiatric units are at the highly intensive and most restrictive end of this spectrum. Inpatient psychiatry programs are the intensive care units of the mental health system. Adolescents who need inpatient services tend to be diagnostically complex and some of the most vulnerable members of the system (Geller and Biebel 2006a). Inpatient units are one component of a continuum of care that these adolescents should have access to. While the overall goal should be to provide treatment in the most normative and least restrictive setting, there is no denying the need and effectiveness of inpatient treatment (Geller and Biebel 2006a; Hayes et al. 2018; Winters et al. 2007). Hospital admission should not be a default substitute for absent or underdeveloped community-based mental health programs that could provide less restrictive care. However, availability of these services does not eliminate the need for inpatient treatment (Geller and Biebel 2006b). Inpatient units are meant to address the serious risks of and severe impairments caused by the most acute and complex forms of mental illness that cannot be managed effectively at any other level of care. They play a vital role in rapid clinical stabilization, diagnostic assessment, and identification of appropriate treatments and family engagement, with the goal of transition to a less intensive level of care (Sharfstein 2009).

Trends in Adolescent Inpatient Hospitalization

With the advent of managed care in the 1990s, adolescents have had increased rates of hospitalization, despite a decrease in number of beds and shorter lengths of stay (Meagher et al. 2013; Sharfstein 2009). An increase in admissions has also been accompanied by a rise in level of psychopathology and degree of acuity (Glick et al. 2011). In addition to managed care and a decrease in insurance reimbursements, other factors that have contributed to a shortening length of stay include availability of rapidly acting psychotropic medications, concerns around long hospitalizations, and adoption of a least restrictive systems of care philosophy (Vargas and Brambila 2005). Over the last decade and half, these trends have further intensified. Inpatient admissions for suicidal ideations, suicide attempts, and self-injury doubled between 2006 and 2011 for adolescents (Torio et al. 2015). There have been significant increases in the need for inpatient services (Teich et al. 2018) and emergency room visits for suicide and self-harm (Plemmons et al. 2018). These trends are also reflected in pediatric hospital settings, with an increase in children and adolescents with medical conditions and co-occurring psychiatric disorders (Zima et al. 2016). A reduction in the number of beds has unintended consequences for other elements of the system of care, including juvenile justice and child protective services (Geller and Biebel 2006b). Inpatient care is the clinical intervention with the weakest evidence base (Vargas and Brambila 2005). All these trends have created substantial demands on inpatient units to provide efficient and effective care (Geller and Biebel 2006a).

In this chapter we present an overview of the adolescent inpatient psychiatry unit through descriptions of admission criteria, assessment, treatment, management of aggressive and suicidal behaviors, and discharge planning. We also identify future directions and challenges for adolescent inpatient treatment.

Admission Criteria

Clinical criteria for admission must include significant signs and symptoms of active mental illness. Functional indicators for admission usually include a significant risk of harm to self or others, or an inability to meet basic self-care needs that jeopardizes the well-being of an adolescent. Commonly accepted criteria are listed in Table 3–1. The American Academy of Child and Adolescent Psychiatry (1989) guidelines stipulate that hospitalization should follow the least restrictive level of care principle and should involve clinical assessment by a qualified psychiatrist. The clinical heterogeneity in the child and adolescent population can complicate applying these criteria for admission. Decisions to hospitalize can also be dependent on systemic factors, including the nature and quality of available services within the community (Vargas and Brambila 2005). Admission criteria can also be used to help guide decisions around continued stay. Most insurances require a review of stay every few days.

In addition to generally accepted standards, each state has its own mental health statutes that identify legal requirements for voluntary or involuntary civil commitment (Vargas and Brambila 2005). Consent to admission is often required from parents and adolescents, especially for adolescents approaching the age of majority. Joint custody

TABLE 3–1. Admission criteria for adolescent inpatient unit

Dangerousness to self	Serious suicide attempt
	Suicidal ideations and intent
	Self-mutilation with severe injury
Dangerousness to others	Assaultive behavior or threatened violence
Inability to function	Delusions or hallucinations
	Manic episodes
	Bizarre or disorganized behavior
	Severe psychomotor agitation or retardation, catatonia
	Severe or life-threatening side effects of psychotropic medications

arrangements present a requirement that both custodial parents reach agreement about the admission decision. Due-process notifications related to legal rights and status must also be provided to patients and parents as part of the admission process. Practitioners should be thoroughly familiar with the specific state mental hygiene legal standards governing their location of inpatient practice.

Assessment

General Strategies and Methods

The principles and practices outlined in the "Practice Parameters for the Psychiatric Assessment of Children and Adolescents" are applicable to the inpatient assessment process (King and American Academy of Child and Adolescent Psychiatry 1997). The initial assessments on an inpatient unit should involve high-risk screening aimed at identifying and addressing potential sources of imminent harm. Screening covers past and current instances of significant physical illness, suicide, self-injury, violence as victim or perpetrator, fire setting, sexual abuse as victim or perpetrator, risky sexual behavior, and substance intoxication, abuse, or dependence. Clinical interventions necessary to establish and maintain patient safety are identified. Risk is subsequently reassessed prospectively over the course of hospitalization to maintain safety, evaluate intervention effectiveness, and gauge readiness for discharge. While admission assessments can be more narrowly focused on safety and functioning, hospitalization also offers a setting for a complete clinical diagnostic assessment.

A thorough diagnostic assessment should involve multiple sources of information from collateral contacts such as outpatient clinicians, pediatricians, community service providers, and school personnel. Consents to contact collateral information sources are needed at the outset of the admission. Adolescence spans the end of late childhood to the start of the young adult years. This period is characterized by a range of developmental phenomena with wide variation in social functioning and physical development. Providers need a good understanding of typical milestones and what can be considered normative. A determination of the concordance or discrepancy among the domains of physical, emotional, social, behavioral, cognitive, and adaptive functioning is particularly salient in assessing the impact of severe mental illness on developmental status. Failure to attain expected or loss of attained developmental milestones requires that a developmental disorder or neurodegenerative process be ruled out. A good developmental history should include medical history, cognitive and social functioning, peer and family relationships, physical and emotional development, and temperament (Geller and Biebel 2006b).

Assessments should utilize the diagnostic frame provided by DSM-5 (American Psychiatric Association 2013). Difficulties should be sufficiently persistent, functionally impairing, and distressing enough to warrant clinical attention. Inpatient assessment includes input from multiple other disciplines, including nursing, milieu therapy, social work, education, physical and occupational therapy, expressive therapy, psychology, and pediatrics (King and American Academy of Child and Adolescent Psychiatry 1997; Vargas and Brambila 2005). Co-occurring disorders tend to be underdiagnosed during adolescence (Geller and Biebel 2006b). Adolescence is the period in which psychotic and bipolar spectrum illnesses have their onset. Recent trends have demonstrated an increasing diagnosis of mood disorders and use of antipsychotic medications in hospitalized adolescents (Meagher et al. 2013). There is a high degree of comorbidity for substance use disorders as well, with significant increases in cannabis use (Wu et al. 2011). Screening should focus on symptoms of intoxication, dependence, and withdrawal. A comprehensive treatment plan to address multiple symptoms, diagnoses, and comorbidities should be developed. Assessments should also be informed by cultural sensitivity and the cultural context; the meaning and function of symptoms should also be considered.

The clinical interview remains the cornerstone of psychiatric assessment and diagnosis. It is where clinician and patient meet, rapport is established, the patient gains voice, cooperation is fostered, mental status is examined, the history is obtained, and the therapeutic relationship takes shape. Interviews are performed with the patient individually, with the parents separate from the patient, and with the patient and parents together. Interviews with adolescent and parents have the dual goals of gathering information and building rapport (Geller and Biebel 2006b). Treatment alliance is important with adolescents, and the team should be careful not to undermine it. Adolescents may commonly feel comfortable sharing information without the presence of a parent. Confidentiality involves a delicate balance of an adolescent's privacy interests with a parent's right to know about assessment findings and treatment planning, especially in matters pertaining to reproductive health and substance abuse. Reproductive health services are a core component of adolescent medicine practice. Services to address matters related to sexuality, pregnancy, sexually transmitted diseases, and sexual assaults should be available. This entails close coordination with emergency and child protective services to ensure timely collection of physical evidence, antiviral prophylaxis, and emergency pregnancy prevention. LGBTQ+ adolescents are particularly at risk for suicide and self-harm (Liu and Mustanski 2012). Careful analysis of the unique aspects of each case must be done to determine what constitutes a necessary disclosure to prevent harm and what adverse effects might result from a confidentiality breach. It is here that clinical, ethical, and legal analyses should pull together. The clinical interview also helps the provider assess modes and effectiveness of family communication and provides an opportunity for family engagement and for provider communication of findings and recommendations to family.

In addition to the clinical interview, structured instruments for symptom inventory allow for accurate, reliable, and efficient gathering of data. These tools can help with a comprehensive assessment but should not be used as a primary diagnostic modality (King and American Academy of Child and Adolescent Psychiatry 1997). Scales and instruments help rate illness severity and functional impairments and enhance the reliability of treatment monitoring during the hospital course. Questionnaires are useful in collecting and organizing relevant clinical data from parents and teachers. Recent research has also focused on measurement of outcomes of inpatient hospitalization within the domains of functioning, relationships, and symptom severity related to depression, anxiety, psychosis, and mania, as well as risk factors (Hayes et al. 2018). A list of structured instruments and outcome measures is included in Table 3–2. Psychological consultation and testing can also aid the diagnostic process. These may not be indicated in every case. Given the limited availability of provider resources, such consultation should be accessed judiciously based on the specific demonstrated individualized needs of each patient. Psychological consultation can also help inform behavioral planning during the stay. Care should be taken to not conflate findings and results during a crisis with normal baseline functioning. Providers should also seek to obtain the results of previous testing, including testing that informed development of the school Individualized Education Program (IEP), to aid with diagnosis.

Diagnostic Workup

Diagnostic assessment should include a careful medical history and thorough physical examination along with laboratory testing and imaging when indicated. Child and adolescent psychiatrists must maintain their knowledge of appropriate health screening and examination skills to meet national standards of practice for the physical evaluation of adolescents. Medical evaluation should not be shortchanged because of the presentation of the patient with acute behavioral and emotional issues. In the case of adolescents presenting with symptoms of psychosis or catatonia, careful assessment of likely medical causes should be performed (Merritt et al. 2020). Significant physical illness comorbidity rates have been noted in adolescent populations receiving psychiatric services (Warner 2006). A body map of injuries should be completed on admission and can provide documentation for child protective issues and in tracking of patterns of self-injury that might happen over the course of treatment. The medical clearance of overdoses usually requires a period of preadmission prospective monitoring of blood levels and clinical status to verify physical stability. Nutritional status should be screened routinely. Risk for cardiovascular and metabolic complications related to obesity must be identified and managed. BMI should be monitored in the context of an eating disorder or another severe neurovegetative disturbance. Immunization status and tuberculosis exposure and screening history must be checked and updated.

Laboratory tests may have limited screening utility in those presenting from emergency rooms (Donofrio et al. 2014); however, laboratory testing is indicated for baseline assessment, prior to initiation of psychotropic medications, and for monitoring for side effects, especially for second-generation antipsychotics (McLaren et al. 2017). Medical workup is also useful for monitoring adolescents with eating disorders (Lock et al. 2016). Brain imaging or electroencephalography in the absence of focal neurological findings is low yield in clinical populations with primary psychiatric disorders.

TABLE 3–2. Rating scales and outcome measures for use on the adolescent inpatient unit

Global functioning or descriptive symptom profile	Brief Psychiatric Rating Scale, Child Version (Hughes et al. 2001)
	Clinical Global Impression (CGI; Guy 1976)
	Children's Global Assessment Scale (CGA; Shaffer et al. 1983)
	Global Assessment of Functioning (GAF; Hayes et al. 2018)
Target symptom monitoring	Children's Depression Inventory (Kovacs 1985) (depression)
	Children's Yale-Brown Obsessive Compulsive Scale (Goodman et al. 1991) (obsessions and compulsions)
	Screen for Child Anxiety Related Emotional Disorders (SCARED; Birmaher et al. 1999) (anxiety)
	Conners' Rating Scales—Revised (Conners et al. 1998) (attention, hyperactivity)
	Young Mania Rating Scale (Young et al. 1978) (mania)
Risk and safety assessment	Overt Aggression Scale—Modified (Kay et al. 1988) (aggression)
	Columbia-Suicide Severity Rating Scale (CSSRS; Hill et al. 2017) (suicidality)
Side-effect measures	Abnormal Involuntary Movement Scale (AIMS; Guy 1976)

However, severe psychopathology in the severe mood symptoms, head trauma, neurological symptoms, or first-episode psychosis (Skikic and Arriola 2020) can provide reasons to pursue additional laboratory testing, electroencephalography, or brain imaging. Common laboratory tests and their rationale are listed in Table 3–3.

Treatment

Biopsychosocial Formulation and Treatment Planning

Assessment data are incorporated into a biopsychosocial formulation of the factors contributing most directly to the need for admission. An ideal treatment plan should use this biopsychosocial model and include contributions from the multidisciplinary team, utilizing different modalities such as medication, psychotherapy, educational services, activity therapy, therapeutic recreation, case management, and discharge planning (Vargas and Brambila 2005). A tailored treatment plan should utilize patient and family strengths and seek realistic attainable goals toward crisis stabilization. Treatment planning should also include collaboration with patients, families, and community-based providers. Patients can benefit from the continuity of care and clinical contact that occur when existing community-based providers are able to participate as members of the treatment team.

Psychotropic Medication

Medication treatment is one component of a balanced multimodal intervention plan informed by a formulation of the biological, psychological, and social factors. The main

TABLE 3–3. Rationales for use of laboratory tests during adolescent psychiatric inpatient hospitalization

Test	Monitoring rationale
Serum electrolytes	Baseline health measure; elevated bicarbonate level associated with vomiting
Blood urea nitrogen	Renal function measure, hydration status
Serum creatinine	Renal function measure, drug elimination
Serum phosphate	Indicator of nutritional status; critical shifts in refeeding syndrome
Complete blood count	Baseline health measure, medication side effects
Liver function tests	Baseline health measure, medication side effects
Pregnancy test	Baseline health measure relevant to multiple aspects of care
Serum prolactin	Hypothalamic-pituitary function baseline, neuroleptic effects
Urine toxicology screening	Detection of illicit drug ingestion
Urinalysis	Baseline health measure, renal function, hydration status
Serum drug levels	Therapeutic monitoring, management of overdose
Glucose, triglycerides, and serum lipids	Metabolic syndrome risk, medication side effects
Electrocardiography	Cardiac baseline, medication side effects

Note. Specific laboratory testing is governed by the clinical circumstances of each case.

foci of inpatient medication interventions are to select or adjust appropriate agents, establish dose tolerability to treatment initiation or change, and coordinate with outpatient providers to maintain continuity of clinical management through discharge. Psychopharmacology is symptom based and directed to address the most severe and impairing dimensions of active psychopathology. In the inpatient setting, clinical presentations are complex and multiple disorders frequently overlap. Providers should develop a medication plan based on the best available evidence and use the simplest effective medication strategy when treating multiple disorders (Walkup and Work Group on Quality Issues 2009). A clear rationale for using medication combinations should be identified.

Over the last few decades, the evidence base for the use of medications has expanded. The proportion of adolescents who are taking medications upon both admission and discharge has increased with significant increases in use of mood stabilizers and antipsychotics (Meagher et al. 2013). Bostic and Rho (2006) posited a model for dimensional treatment and symptom targeting that is well suited to the inpatient setting. Shaw and DeMaso (2010) also provided an example of target symptom prescribing that is concordant with these principles. Table 3–4 identifies different symptom domains and the class of medications for each.

Medication decision-making and consent procedures on an adolescent unit are triangulated between patient, parents or guardians, and clinician. Parental consent and patient assent are always required for medication treatment unless there are emergency exceptions, or a legal basis exists for treatment over objection. Emergency conditions for medication treatment entail an acute risk of harm if immediate treatment is not provided to address physiological compromise such as acute dystonic reactions or in-

TABLE 3–4. Target symptom approach to medication selection

Target symptom	Medication considerations
Aggression—chronic	Selective serotonin reuptake inhibitor
	Selective norepinephrine reuptake inhibitor
	Atypical or typical antipsychotic
	Mood stabilizer
	Alpha-agonist
	Beta-blocker
	Stimulant
Aggression—acute	Antihistamine (diphenhydramine, hydroxyzine)
	Benzodiazepine
	Atypical or typical antipsychotic
Agitation	Antihistamine (diphenhydramine, hydroxyzine)
	Benzodiazepine
	Atypical or typical antipsychotic
Anxiety	Selective serotonin reuptake inhibitor
	Antihistamine
	Benzodiazepine
	Alpha-agonist
	Buspirone
	Gabapentin
Depression	Selective serotonin reuptake inhibitor
	First-ever treatment should be fluoxetine or escitalopram (paroxetine should not be used in adolescents)
	Serotonin-norepinephrine reuptake inhibitor
Inattention/Hyperactivity	Stimulant
	Alpha-agonist
	Atomoxetine
	Bupropion
Insomnia	Melatonin
	Hydroxyzine
	Diphenhydramine
	Benzodiazepine
	Trazodone
	Hypnotic (e.g., zolpidem, zaleplon)
	Amitriptyline
	Mirtazapine
Mania	Atypical or typical antipsychotic
	Mood stabilizer
	Lithium
	Antiepileptic
Psychosis	Atypical or typical antipsychotic
	Benzodiazepine

TABLE 3–4. Target symptom approach to medication selection *(continued)*

Target symptom	Medication considerations
Withdrawal	Clonidine Benzodiazepine Gabapentin

Source. Adapted from Shaw and DeMaso 2010.

tolerable distress that is unresponsive to nonmedication interventions. The underlying cause for agitation should be identified and treatment should be targeted toward it. Patient autonomy should be respected, and adolescents should be given the option of taking oral medications first. Classes of medication that are used for acute agitation in adolescents include antihistamines, benzodiazepines, and antipsychotics (Sonnier and Barzman 2011). The emergency conditions and the rationale for such emergency medication use in such situations should be well documented, side effects should be anticipated, and the parent/guardian should be informed of the situation in a timely manner.

A detailed discussion around the risks and benefits of treatment, including side effects, should be shared with adolescents. This helps strengthen the provider-patient relationship and makes it more likely that the adolescent will adhere to treatment (Walkup and Work Group on Quality Issues 2009). Adolescents can be exquisitely sensitive to side effects, including changes in bodily appearance or function that are perceived to be related to illness or treatment. Weight gain is common with mood stabilizers and antipsychotics, and changes in weight can also occur with antidepressants and psychostimulants. Sexual side effects are also common with use of selective serotonin reuptake inhibitors. There should be a close working relationship with pharmacy services to evaluate potential drug interactions and gather relevant drug information to inform treatment decisions. Providers should be aware of the FDA regulation requiring that all antidepressants carry a black box warning about possible increased risk for suicide when they are used to treat depression in children and adolescents. Better research into this relationship has demonstrated an extremely favorable risk-benefit ratio for antidepressants, with significant lowering of suicide rates with their use (Birmaher et al. 2007).

Because the time frames of inpatient care are often shorter than the known dose-response effects of many medications, coordination with referring and follow-up providers to plan in-hospital adjustments and to map postdischarge monitoring of treatment is necessary to complete drug trials. The handoff of inpatient care should include communicating a clear monitoring plan to the receiving clinician because treatment effects and side effects can emerge weeks to months after changes are made.

Psychotherapy

Inpatient psychotherapy programs incorporate individual, group, and family therapy modalities to identify and support existing adaptive strengths of an adolescent and family as they attempt to come to terms with and manage the signs and symptoms of an acute mental illness. The psychotherapeutic frame of inpatient work is decidedly short term, with an emphasis on establishing and maintaining continuity in previous and future therapies. The inpatient unit provides an opportunity for consultation when there is already ongoing psychotherapeutic work in the community. Adolescents enter inpatient treatment with diverse needs and capacities for therapeutic engagement. Such settings require an adaptable psychotherapy program with individual, family, and group components that can be adjusted to meet the unique requirements of each clinical situation. The specific therapeutic techniques and orientations available on a unit will tap into the psychotherapy training and skills of the staff.

The evidence base for effective psychotherapeutic treatments for adolescents has increased. Multiple evidence-based treatments now exist for conditions such as attention and hyperactivity, autism, depression, disruptive behavior, eating issues, substance use, and traumatic stress (Chorpita et al. 2011). The evidence is strongest for family therapy, cognitive-behavioral therapy (CBT), dialectical behavior therapy (DBT), interpersonal therapy, motivational interviewing, parent management training, multisystemic therapy, exposure and response prevention, modeling, and psychoeducation, with lesser evidence for play therapy and psychodynamic approaches (Chorpita et al. 2011; Higa-McMillan et al. 2016). Many of these psychotherapies can be utilized and modified for the inpatient setting. Very little research has been published on inpatient unit–specific therapies in the last 20 years; however, recent studies have shown the benefit of empirically supported, brief, suicide-focused, CBT-based treatment modules on outcomes (Wolff et al. 2018). Expressive therapy modalities such as music (Shuman et al. 2016), art, movement, and drama can also provide adjunctive support in the therapeutic milieu. Table 3–5 provides a list of treatments of various clinical symptoms or syndromes.

Therapeutic alliances between clinicians, adolescents, and families are needed to support and sustain the clinical work to be done during the hospital admission. Alliance formation is fostered when a patient's and family's concerns are heard, appreciated, and addressed in the clinical work. Motivation to join in the therapeutic work will vary substantially among adolescents and their families. Motivational interviewing techniques are evolving as potentially useful tools to help adolescents participate as active agents in their health care decision-making (Erickson et al. 2005). Every effort is needed to have the work proceed in a collaborative spirit that is free from coercion. This is a challenging task to accomplish in situations involving involuntary commitment or in the presence of significant disagreements among treatment participants. A reframing of treatment orientation in terms of health and safety priorities can help to build consensus in such difficult situations. Navigation of these delicate scenarios requires thoughtful integration and compassionate application of clinical, ethical, and legal perspectives.

Individual Therapy

Individual therapy provides a partially sheltered psychotherapeutic venue for the adolescent. The scope of confidentiality for the individual therapy process must be explicitly delimited at the outset of treatment. Individual psychotherapy emphasizes therapeutic elements of relaxation training, stress reduction, anger management, self-monitoring, safety planning, communication building, symptom management, treatment planning, development of coping skills, and patient education. In the inpatient setting, therapy often is supportive in nature and limited given the time constraints, scope, and objectives of acute inpatient treatment. New skills or approaches can be

TABLE 3–5. Psychosocial treatment modality selection based on clinical indication

Clinical indication	Treatment modality
Depression	Cognitive-behavioral therapy
	Interpersonal therapy
	Psychodynamic psychotherapy
	Family therapy
Bipolar disorder	Cognitive-behavioral therapy
	Family-focused treatment
Emotional dysregulation	Cognitive-behavioral therapy
	Dialectical behavior therapy
Stress and trauma	Cognitive-behavioral therapy
	Trauma systems interventions
	Psychodynamic psychotherapy
	Dialectical behavior therapy
Psychosis	Social skills training
	Supportive psychotherapy
	Family therapy
Anxiety	Cognitive-behavioral therapy
	Exposure
	Modeling
	Habit reversal therapy
	Family therapy
Eating disorders	Family therapy
	Multidisciplinary team collaboration
	Motivational interviewing
Disruptive behavior	Behavioral systemic therapy
	Multisystemic therapy
	Cognitive-behavioral therapy
	Functional family therapy
Substance abuse	Motivational interviewing

introduced that might be practiced during the hospital stay. This therapy is by necessity brief and not intended to address long-term or ongoing issues that can and should be addressed in community settings.

Group Therapy

Types of group-based treatment, including group therapy, activity groups, and psychoeducation groups, have been shown to be components of effective inpatient treatment for adolescents (Hayes et al. 2018). Inpatient group therapy is an effective treatment for adults with mood disorders, trauma, and even psychosis (Kösters et al. 2006); however, it is unclear what components of the treatment are effective in adolescents (Hayes et al. 2018). Therapy groups can focus on specific therapeutic areas and skills such as anger management, relaxation training, social skills, hygiene, and grooming. They might have a health education orientation that focuses on matters of reproductive health, substance abuse, smoking cessation, or medication treatment. Single-gender girls' or boys' groups can be used to address issues related to identity formation and gender-based developmental issues. There are also task-oriented groups such as community meetings and goals groups. Group tasks can be supported by individual work that helps patients to prepare goals and agenda items for presentation in goals groups and community meetings. Goals are prepared daily, and during the morning goals group, someone should present a goal for the day that maintains relevance to his or her individual treatment goals. Closure groups are commonly conducted in the evening to follow up on the work that was done toward goals throughout the day.

Group therapy sessions offer significant exposure, desensitization, and practice opportunities for kids who are having difficulties joining and participating in social situations. Trained staff can also help identify adolescents at risk of disruptive behavior and assess whether they can be helped to prepare for the group or whether they require more individualized programming away from the group setting. Groups are excellent settings to make naturalistic observations pertinent to clinical and functional assessment. Multifamily groups can be welcome sources of support in which families learn about the treatment process, acquire parenting skills, identify community resources, or just find time to get together and share constructive diversion in a game or leisure activity. Many units hold parents' nights or family nights for this purpose.

Group therapy modalities draw on interpersonal dynamics, perspective sharing, collective support, and consensus building as therapeutic processes. Group formats should accommodate for the frequent shifting of membership and the possibility that patients might only be present for a single session. The changing membership of the group is addressed by having clear instructions and a consistent set of rules and expectations for participation available at the start of the group (Malekoff 2015). Therapists must continuously keep the process moving in a constructive direction. The tone and the atmosphere of groups must be calm, orderly, and respectful. Adolescent group members can provide powerful and enlightening feedback to peers.

Family Therapy and Psychoeducation

Multiple family therapy models have been utilized in adolescents. Family therapy for eating disorders has a strong evidence base for specialized inpatient practice. Other modalities identified in the literature that can be useful in an inpatient setting include brief strategic family therapy, family-focused CBT for anxiety and depression, psychoeducation in first-episode psychosis, attachment-based family therapy, and DBT for self-harm (Carr 2016). Inpatient family therapy should identify and support existing family strengths, enhance effective communication, resolve conflicts, negotiate consensus, establish safety, provide information, and formulate plans for the transition to the next setting of care. Shapiro (2015) defined five types of parent work: assessment and monitoring of change, help for parents in understanding their child, parent training, parent guidance, and parent counseling. Family therapy also seeks to build consensus on the aims of inpatient treatment. In addition, the family work provides a venue to present findings and recommendations related to assessment and treatment.

Psychoeducation is a core component of inpatient work. Family members usually need various forms of support to help them cope with the anxieties and uncertainties surrounding the adolescent's admission. Existing sources of support can be accessed within the family's relationships, cultural practices, spiritual beliefs, and community. Family empowerment is strongly rooted in the teaching and learning that occur between family members and the treatment team. It is a mutual learning process in which the treatment team gains knowledge about how to best help the family and the family learns the information needed to make informed decisions and be fully engaged in the care. Materials and information to support psychoeducation are designed to target adolescent health risks, medication information, diagnosis-specific information, parenting skills, and developmental topics. Resources such as AACAP's family website (American Academy of Child and Adolescent Psychiatry 2019) are particularly useful.

Milieu-Based Treatment Modalities

The unit milieu is a safe 24-hour treatment setting with patient-centered programming built from therapeutic and social components. All milieu interactions between unit staff and clients carry therapeutic potential. A values-based milieu approach should guide staff with well-defined written unit rules available on the unit. All persons participating on the unit should commit to the values of safety, health, human rights, mutual respect, nonviolence, fairness, and personal integrity. Training staff in trauma-informed care is essential. A safe environment and the interpersonal support, therapy, and psychoeducation they receive there are factors that adolescents identify as helpful experiences, while a lack of treatment responsiveness and anxiety-provoking experiences can be nonsupportive (Moses 2011).

The daily routine on the unit should convey a sense of predictability, planning, and order, with changes announced in a timely fashion. Patients' spiritual needs continue when they are admitted to the hospital. Availability of chaplaincy for various faiths should be maintained to support patients and families if they wish to maintain religious and spiritual observance (Moncher and Josephson 2004). An inpatient milieu is supported by the collaborative work of a multidisciplinary team involving all staff on the unit. Unit staffing should meet individual clinical needs while maintaining cohesive program functioning. Role definition and function of team members are defined by credentialing, experience, training, and areas of competence. Local workforce availability and hospital accreditation standards are also important.

Ideally, every unit should have a classroom program with a teacher who provides instruction and coordinates educational planning with local schools to identify potential learning needs and help patients maintain continuity of academic work and credit status between the community and hospital settings. With the shortening length of hospital stays, it may not be feasible for all units. A classroom-type setting can help the treatment team observe a patient's functional status in a naturalistic setting and identify issues with learning, concentration, and following directions, thus further informing treatment plans.

Rehabilitative emphasis is placed on the practice of activities of daily living, personal hygiene, symptom management, or development of social skills. Physical therapy might be indicated when motor or musculoskeletal deficits are noted. Occupational therapy might be needed to address sensory integration deficits. Speech and language specialists should be available to participate in the care of persons with sensory deficits or communication disorders. Hospitalized teenagers often require nutritional interventions. Patients with eating disorders will need specialized meal programs and nutritional restoration plans. Weight loss or gain due to appetite disturbance secondary to physical illness or medication side effects might need to be addressed through meal plan adjustments.

Well-delineated levels of supervision help in monitoring for safety. Level systems on short-stay units must be simple and quick to learn, motivate participation, and leave no unsupervised time. Control of the environment also requires surveillance for potentially harmful objects and substances, with interventions such as belongings checks. Well-trained staff are also able to utilize behavioral interventions to help alter reinforcement patterns and affect regulation and effect cognitive restructuring (Delaney 2006). Structured behavioral interventions can be applied in postdischarge settings and aid families with challenges at home. Patients requiring a high level of direct individual care can have broad impact on a milieu by diverting staff from performance of more general milieu management functions. Staff ratios should increase with patient care needs to ensure that patient safety and care quality can be maintained. The environmental design and management of the unit must guard against excessive visual, auditory, or tactile stimulation. Media access and content must also be closely monitored, and content should be consonant with values. There should be clinical awareness of media content as potential triggers for signs and symptoms of disorders. Leisure activities should be structured and well monitored in designated areas. Active involvement of patients by milieu staff in age-appropriate leisure activities that are enjoyable and interesting is more likely to keep patients constructively engaged.

Management of Aggressive and Suicidal Behaviors

Inpatient admissions for suicidal ideations, behavior, and self-harm and emergency room visits for impulse-control disorders have seen the greatest increases since 2006 (Torio et al. 2015). Maintaining patient safety during crisis is a key element of the inpatient process. A safe and effective crisis management approach continually aims to minimize the frequency, duration, and severity of behavioral crises to eliminate self-directed or interpersonal violence, and to implement the safest and least restrictive clinical interventions, ones that do not require the application of physical force. Familiarity with institutional guidelines and federal and state regulations is essential.

The process of identifying and managing risks of harm from aggression begins with admission. History regarding aggression and suicidality should be obtained on admission intake and should include triggers, warning signs, and prior history of such symptoms. Having specific information about the stay for both patients and parents can allay anxiety and prevent frustration that can further fuel emotional crises. The early identification of escalation triggers, fears, anxieties, frustrations, and concerns can help the clinical team and the patient work together on a plan to establish and maintain safety during the admission. A good diagnostic assessment can help identify potential vulnerabilities such as in those adolescents who have a history of trauma or processing difficulties, language-based learning disabilities, or sensory impairments. A strengths-based approach should be utilized in the development of a safety plan. The plan should include medication use to treat underlying psychopathology, which can help reduce distress, aid relaxation, and help a patient participate in the acquisition of cognitive, emotional, and behavioral skills. Trauma-informed therapeutic interactions, behavior-contingent strategies, availability of interpersonal space, and explicit and understandable communication are all helpful tools. Research in restraints and seclusion for children and adolescents continues to be lacking, with only a few multistrategy approaches, such as collaborative problem solving (Greene et al. 2006), showing good evidence for reduction (Valenkamp et al. 2014).

Levels of intervention for maintaining safety include nonrestrictive, restrictive, and most restrictive (Masters et al. 2002). Physical restraints (mechanical or chemical) and seclusion are interventions of last resort. They should be used only in cases of dangerousness to self or others and when other, less restrictive measures have failed. During restraints and seclusion, patient autonomy and dignity should be preserved. Staff involved must have specialized training and employ sound principles of physical management that minimize the opportunity for physical injury for both patients and staff. The Joint Commission (Crisis Prevention Institute 2009) guidelines stipulate that for children and adolescents between ages 9 and 17 years, orders for use of restraints can last only for 2 hours and need to be renewed. Patients should also be monitored continuously, especially to ensure there is no airway obstruction, and vitals should be checked every 15 minutes. Seclusion rooms for time-outs and early use of as-needed medication can be alternatives to physical restraints. Episodes should be documented meticulously in the medical record. Debriefings of the patient, parents, and staff for each restraint episode should be conducted. Any difficulties or lack of coordination should be identified and addressed through collaboration, practice, and training. Staff debriefings should be used as a place for analysis, problem solving, and support.

Effective suicide prevention requires work to develop the self-monitoring skills of the patient and the monitoring capacities of support network members. The therapeutic work will emphasize reduction of core symptoms contributing to suicide risk and the identification and practice of safe alternative coping strategies (Miller et al. 2006). A means reduction component might be needed as part of a safety plan to help family members to eliminate or limit access to dangerous objects and substances in the community setting. Imminently suicidal inpatients will likely need constant monitoring in a safe location of the unit until imminent risk of self-harm or suicide subsides. In self-injurious patients, injury patterns should be recorded at the time of admission and rechecked periodically at points during the admission to assess clinical progress.

The effectiveness of crisis management protocols requires ongoing evaluation to characterize and track event rates, intervention outcomes, and results of staff training. The use of structured instruments (see Table 3–2) can help with ratings of episode duration, severity, and behavioral specifics for quality improvement.

Discharge Planning

Patients are discharged "better," not well (Sharfstein 2009). With hospitalization focusing on acute stabilization, discharge planning begins at the time of admission. The goal of discharge planning is collaboration with patients and families, and the identification of services and resources that are available in the community. This identification entails active coordination and communication with aftercare service providers by discharge planners and utilization management personnel. The transition of care from the inpatient unit to the community has a number of challenges, including inadequate service coordination leading to gaps in treatment continuity (Winters et al. 2007). There should be minimal disruption in care and function for the benefit of patients and families. Shortages in appropriate services at lower levels of care, difficulties with transition from adolescent to adult systems, and lack of specialized services such as for substance use or for developmental disabilities are all common impediments. Step-down care might be needed in partial hospital or residential settings depending on the clinical needs. However, there are no guidelines or level-of-care criteria to determine aftercare. Ideally, services are chosen based on acuity and clinical needs. However, the type of services available might play a role. Further research to help inform evidence-based decision-making guidelines for discharge planning is necessary (Fontanella et al. 2008). Return to the educational environment will also need to be coordinated between hospital and school, often in the form of a school reentry meeting. Patients and parents often want guidance on how to discuss the inpatient admission with peers, family members, and school staff.

Discharge planning should also consider the risk of rehospitalization. Inpatient hospitalization is an expensive resource, and there is a significant elevated risk for readmission up to 3 months after discharge (James et al. 2010). There is equivocal evidence that posthospital discharge services are related to risk of readmission. The most consistent predictive factors are elevated acuity or risk (diagnosis, symptom severity, comorbidity, or suicidality) and negative familial factors (low engagement, satisfaction, adherence).

Future Directions

Inpatient psychiatry units will continue to provide the most intensive treatment role within an evolving system of adolescent mental health services. The essential inpatient work of rapid assessment, treatment planning, clinical stabilization, and effective transitioning of treatment to less intensive levels of care will remain in place. Several issues will impact adolescent psychiatric hospitalization in the foreseeable future.

Data on outcomes of hospitalization are limited (Vargas and Brambila 2005). Early research identified three broad groups of factors: patient, family, and treatment (Pfeiffer and Strzelecki 1990). Clinical meaningful outcomes can include change in symptoms and functioning, and the effectiveness of short-term interventions must be determined. Very little is also known about treatment planning and implementation and how they contribute to outcomes (Hayes et al. 2018). Rehospitalization can also be a target for quality improvement and can be used to measure effectiveness of treatment (James et al. 2010). Outcome measurement can help guide clinicians or families in advocating for needs and help with changes to public policy (Glick et al. 2011).

Recent literature has also shown promising results for specialized units for kids with autism spectrum disorder (Taylor et al. 2019). Units that target specific diagnoses such as eating disorders, substance use disorders, and autism spectrum disorder and other neurodevelopmental disorders may utilize the expertise of multidisciplinary teams and potentially improve outcomes. Adequate reimbursement is an important issue for adolescent units (Appelbaum 2003). While hospitalization is expensive, there are substantive health benefits (Green et al. 2007), and money invested in inpatient treatment can be recouped through other systems (Geller and Biebel 2006b). Further cost-effectiveness research is needed in adolescent systems of care. One other area that needs advocacy and attention is access to inpatient care for minorities (Vargas and Brambila 2005). There is also very little literature on how to carry out culturally responsive interventions in inpatient settings. Inpatient programs will need the advocacy of families, community providers, agencies, lawmakers, and professional organizations to ensure that the future for inpatient care is evidence based, ethically informed, human rights oriented, and delivered with compassion.

References

American Academy of Child and Adolescent Psychiatry: Inpatient hospital treatment of children and adolescents. Washington, DC, American Academy of Child and Adolescent Psychiatry, 1989. Available at: www.aacap.org/aacap/policy_statements/1989/Inpatient_Hospital_Treatment_of_Children_and_Adolescents.aspx. Accessed December 1, 2019.

American Academy of Child and Adolescent Psychiatry: Information for patients and their families. Washington, DC, American Academy of Child and Adolescent Psychiatry, 2019. Available at: www.aacap.org/AACAP/Resources_for_Primary_Care/Information_for_Patients_and_Their_Families/Home.aspx?hkey=bce12396-b276-4fed-8430-ca8628eb1a2b. Accessed December 8, 2019.

American Psychiatric Association: Diagnostic and Statistical Manual of Mental Disorders, 5th Edition. Arlington, VA, American Psychiatric Association, 2013

Appelbaum PS: The 'quiet' crisis in mental health services. Health Aff (Millwood) 22(5):110–116, 2003 14515886

Birmaher B, Brent DA, Chiappetta L, et al: Psychometric properties of the Screen for Child Anxiety Related Emotional Disorders (SCARED): a replication study. J Am Acad Child Adolesc Psychiatry 38(10):1230–1236, 1999 10517055

Birmaher B, Brent D, Bernet W, et al: Practice parameter for the assessment and treatment of children and adolescents with depressive disorders. J Am Acad Child Adolesc Psychiatry 46(11):1503–1526, 2007 18049300

Bostic JQ, Rho Y: Target-symptom psychopharmacology: between the forest and the trees. Child Adolesc Psychiatr Clin N Am 15(1):289–302, 2006 16321735

Carr A: Family therapy for adolescents: a research-informed perspective. Aust N Z J Fam Ther 37(4):467–479, 2016

Chorpita BF, Daleiden EL, Ebesutani C, et al: Evidence-based treatments for children and adolescents: an updated review of indicators of efficacy and effectiveness. Clinical Psychology: Science and Practice 18(2):154–172, 2011

Conners CK, Sitarenios G, Parker JD, Epstein JN: Revision and restandardization of the Conners Teacher Rating Scale (CTRS-R): factor structure, reliability, and criterion validity. J Abnorm Child Psychol 26(4):279–291, 1998 9700520

Crisis Prevention Institute: Joint Commission Standards on Restraint and Seclusion/Nonviolent Crisis Intervention Training Program. Milwaukee, WI, Crisis Prevention Institute, 2009. Available at: www.crisisprevention.com/CPI/media/Media/Resources/alignments/Joint-Commission-Restraint-Seclusion-Alignment-2011.pdf. Accessed December 1, 2019.

Delaney KR: Top 10 milieu interventions for inpatient child/adolescent treatment. J Child Adolesc Psychiatr Nurs 19(4):203–214, 2006 17118055

Donofrio JJ, Santillanes G, McCammack BD, et al: Clinical utility of screening laboratory tests in pediatric psychiatric patients presenting to the emergency department for medical clearance. Ann Emerg Med 63(6):666–675, 2014 24219903

Erickson SJ, Gerstle M, Feldstein SW: Brief interventions and motivational interviewing with children, adolescents, and their parents in pediatric health care settings: a review. Arch Pediatr Adolesc Med 159(12):1173–1180, 2005 16330743

Fontanella CA, Early TJ, Phillips G: Need or availability? Modeling aftercare decisions for psychiatrically hospitalized adolescents. Child Youth Serv Rev 30(7):758–773, 2008

Geller JL, Biebel K: The premature demise of public child and adolescent inpatient psychiatric beds, Part I: overview and current conditions. Psychiatr Q 77(3):251–271, 2006a 16912929

Geller JL, Biebel K: The premature demise of public child and adolescent inpatient psychiatric beds, Part II: challenges and implications. Psychiatr Q 77(4):273–291, 2006b 16927166

Glick ID, Sharfstein SS, Schwartz HI: Inpatient psychiatric care in the 21st century: the need for reform. Psychiatr Serv 62(2):206–209, 2011 21285100

Goodman W, Price L, Rasmussen S, et al: Children's Yale-Brown Obsessive Compulsive Scale (CY-BOCS). New Haven, CT, Yale University School of Medicine, 1991

Green J, Jacobs B, Beecham J, et al: Inpatient treatment in child and adolescent psychiatry—a prospective study of health gain and costs. J Child Psychol Psychiatry 48(12):1259–1267, 2007 18093032

Greene RW, Ablon JS, Hassuk B, et al: Innovations: child & adolescent psychiatry: use of collaborative problem solving to reduce seclusion and restraint in child and adolescent inpatient units. Psychiatr Serv 57(5):610–612, 2006 16675751

Guy W: ECDEU Assessment Manual for Psychopharmacology: Revised (DHEW Publ No ADM 76-338). Rockville, MD, U.S. Department of Health, Education and Welfare, Public Health Service, Alcohol, Drug Abuse and Mental Health Administration, NIMH Psychopharmacology Research Branch, Division of Extramural Research Programs, 1976, pp 534–537

Hayes C, Simmons M, Simons C, Hopwood M: Evaluating effectiveness in adolescent mental health inpatient units: a systematic review. Int J Ment Health Nurs 27(2):498–513, 2018 29194885

Higa-McMillan CK, Francis SE, Rith-Najarian L, Chorpita BF: Evidence base update: 50 years of research on treatment for child and adolescent anxiety. J Clin Child Adolesc Psychol 45(2):91–113, 2016 26087438

Hill RM, Hatkevich CE, Kazimi I, Sharp C: The Columbia-Suicide Severity Rating Scale: Associations between interrupted, aborted, and actual suicide attempts among adolescent inpatients. Psychiatry Res 255:338–340, 2017 28601718

Hughes CW, Rintelmann J, Emslie GJ, et al: A revised anchored version of the BPRS-C for childhood psychiatric disorders. J Child Adolesc Psychopharmacol 11(1):77–93, 2001 11322749

James S, Charlemagne SJ, Gilman AB, et al: Post-discharge services and psychiatric rehospitalization among children and youth. Adm Policy Ment Health 37(5):433–445, 2010 20063073

Kay SR, Wolkenfeld F, Murrill LM: Profiles of aggression among psychiatric patients, I: nature and prevalence. J Nerv Ment Dis 176(9):539–546, 1988 3418327

King RA, American Academy of Child and Adolescent Psychiatry: Practice parameters for the psychiatric assessment of children and adolescents. J Am Acad Child Adolesc Psychiatry 36(10 suppl):4S–20S, 1997 9606102

Kösters M, Burlingame GM, Nachtigall C, Strauss B: A meta-analytic review of the effectiveness of inpatient group psychotherapy. Group Dyn 10(2):146–163, 2006

Kovacs M: The Children's Depression Inventory (CDI). Psychopharmacol Bull 21(4):995–998, 1985 4089116

Liu RT, Mustanski B: Suicidal ideation and self-harm in lesbian, gay, bisexual, and transgender youth. Am J Prev Med 42(3):221–228, 2012 22341158

Lock J, La Via MC, American Academy of Child and Adolescent Psychiatry Committee on Quality Issues: Practice parameter for the assessment and treatment of children and adolescents with eating disorders. Focus (Am Psychiatr Publ) 14(1):75–89, 2016 31997944

Malekoff A: Group Work With Adolescents: Principles and Practice. New York, Guilford, 2015

Masters KJ, Bellonci C, Bernet W, et al: Practice parameter for the prevention and management of aggressive behavior in child and adolescent psychiatric institutions, with special reference to seclusion and restraint. J Am Acad Child Adolesc Psychiatry 41(2 suppl):4S–25S, 2002 11833634

McLaren JL, Brunette MF, McHugo GJ, et al: Monitoring of patients on second-generation antipsychotics: a national survey of child psychiatrists. Psychiatr Serv 68(9):958–961, 2017 28412899

Meagher SM, Rajan A, Wyshak G, Goldstein J: Changing trends in inpatient care for psychiatrically hospitalized youth: 1991–2008. Psychiatr Q 84(2):159–168, 2013 22855261

Merritt J, Tanguturi Y, Fuchs C, Cundiff AW: Medical etiologies of secondary psychosis in children and adolescents. Child Adolesc Psychiatr Clin N Am 29(1):29–42, 2020 31708051

Miller AL, Rathus JH, Linehan MM: Dialectical Behavior Therapy With Suicidal Adolescents. New York, Guilford, 2006

Moncher FJ, Josephson AM: Religious and spiritual aspects of family assessment. Child Adolesc Psychiatr Clin N Am 13(1):49–70, vi, 2004 14723300

Moses T: Adolescents' perspectives about brief psychiatric hospitalization: what is helpful and what is not? Psychiatr Q 82(2):121–137, 2011 20824339

Pfeiffer SI, Strzelecki SC: Inpatient psychiatric treatment of children and adolescents: a review of outcome studies. J Am Acad Child Adolesc Psychiatry 29(6):847–853, 1990 2273010

Plemmons G, Hall M, Doupnik S, et al: Hospitalization for suicide ideation or attempt: 2008–2015. Pediatrics 141(6):e20172426, 2018 29769243

Shaffer D, Gould MS, Brasic J, et al: A Children's Global Assessment Scale (CGAS). Arch Gen Psychiatry 40(11):1228–1231, 1983 6639293

Shapiro JP: Child and Adolescent Therapy: Science and Art. Hoboken, NJ, Wiley, 2015

Sharfstein SS: Goals of inpatient treatment for psychiatric disorders. Annu Rev Med 60:393–403, 2009 18729730

Shaw RJ, DeMaso DR: Textbook of Pediatric Psychosomatic Medicine. Washington, DC, American Psychiatric Publishing, 2010

Shuman J, Kennedy H, DeWitt P, et al: Group music therapy impacts mood states of adolescents in a psychiatric hospital setting. Arts Psychother 49:50–56, 2016

Skikic M, Arriola JA: First episode psychosis medical workup: evidence-informed recommendations and introduction to a clinically guided approach. Child Adolesc Psychiatr Clin N Am 29(1):15–28, 2020 31708044

Sonnier L, Barzman D: Pharmacologic management of acutely agitated pediatric patients. Paediatr Drugs 13(1):1–10, 2011 21162596

Taylor BJ, Sanders KB, Kyle M, et al: Inpatient psychiatric treatment of serious behavioral problems in children with autism spectrum disorder (ASD): specialized versus general inpatient units. J Autism Dev Disord 49(3):1242–1249, 2019 30465295

Teich JL, Mutter R, Gibbons B, et al: Use of inpatient behavioral health services by children and adolescents with private insurance coverage. Psychiatr Serv 69(9):1036–1039, 2018 29921189

Torio CM, Encinosa W, Berdahl T, et al: Annual report on health care for children and youth in the United States: national estimates of cost, utilization and expenditures for children with mental health conditions. Acad Pediatr 15(1):19–35, 2015 25444653

Valenkamp M, Delaney K, Verheij F: Reducing seclusion and restraint during child and adolescent inpatient treatment: still an underdeveloped area of research. J Child Adolesc Psychiatr Nurs 27(4):169–174, 2014 25100241

Vargas LA, Brambila ADD: Inpatient treatment models, in Handbook of Mental Health Services for Children, Adolescents, and Families. Edited by Steele RG, Roberts MC. New York, Springer, 2005, pp 133–149

Walkup J, Work Group on Quality Issues: Practice parameter on the use of psychotropic medication in children and adolescents. J Am Acad Child Adolesc Psychiatry 48(9):961–973, 2009 19692857

Warner LA: Medical problems among adolescents in U.S. mental health services: relationship to functional impairment. J Behav Health Serv Res 33(3):366–379, 2006 16752113

Winters NC, Pumariga A, Work Group on Community Child and Adolescent Psychiatry, Work Group on Quality Issues: Practice parameter on child and adolescent mental health care in community systems of care. J Am Acad Child Adolesc Psychiatry 46(2):284–299, 2007 17242631

Wolff JC, Frazier EA, Weatherall SL, et al: Piloting of COPES: an empirically informed psychosocial intervention on an adolescent psychiatric inpatient unit. J Child Adolesc Psychopharmacol 28(6):409–414, 2018 29648874

Wu L-T, Gersing K, Burchett B, et al: Substance use disorders and comorbid Axis I and II psychiatric disorders among young psychiatric patients: findings from a large electronic health records database. J Psychiatr Res 45(11):1453–1462, 2011 21742345
Young RC, Biggs JT, Ziegler VE, Meyer DA: A rating scale for mania: reliability, validity and sensitivity. Br J Psychiatry 133(5):429–435, 1978 728692
Zima BT, Rodean J, Hall M, et al: Psychiatric disorders and trends in resource use in pediatric hospitals. Pediatrics 138(5):e20160909, 2016 27940773

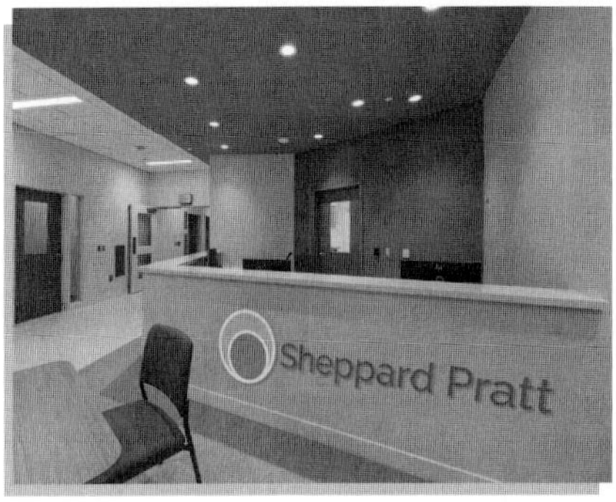

CHAPTER 4

The Adult Crisis Stabilization Unit

Savitha Puttaiah, M.B.B.S., M.D.
Merle McCann, M.D.

With the introduction of a range of effective psychopharmacological therapies in the 1950s, the function of psychiatric hospitalization changed from humane long-term care to active treatment. Whereas *short-term psychiatric hospitalization* in that era referred to hospital stays of less than 1 year, during the 1970s the average length of short-term psychiatric hospitalization decreased from 1 month to 2 weeks, and it has now been reduced to less than 1 week on average (Glick and Hargreaves 1979; Glick et al. 2003; National Association of Psychiatric Health Systems 2000; Sederer and Rothschild 1997). At the same time, the number of admissions has risen steadily, as has the severity of illness of the patients admitted to inpatient psychiatry units. Both patient turnover and the acuity of illness on the inpatient unit have increased significantly; this fact is supported by the greater severity of illness required to meet "medical necessity criteria" to "qualify" for hospitalization and the greater severity of illness at the time of discharge. These trends are not unique to the

We would like to sincerely thank the authors of the previous version of this chapter, Ira Glick, M.D., and Rajiv Tandon, M.D., for providing the framework for the current version of this chapter.

United States and are seen in countries across the world (Glick et al. 2003; Lelliot 2006; Ruud et al. 2006; Walsh 2006).

Settings in which acute inpatient psychiatric care may be provided vary substantially and include psychiatry units in a general hospital, specialized private or public psychiatry hospitals, crisis stabilization units that may or may not be attached to a hospital, and short-term residential treatment facilities (Geller 2006; Lipsitt 2003; Walsh 2006). With the number of state psychiatric beds rapidly disappearing, we are at an all-time low in the number of state hospital beds per capita in the United States since the 1850s (Torrey et al. 2016). Subsequently, there has been a significant increase in the population of the seriously mentally ill in the prison system. We are also seeing an alarming trend in reduction of the number of acute general psychiatric beds (Bastiampillai et al. 2016), and as a result, more unstable psychiatric patients are "boarding" in emergency departments (EDs) for days at a time. There are considerable differences in the staffing and scope of services that can be provided at each of the types of psychiatric hospital settings, and the licensing and other regulatory elements vary as well. Although each of these settings currently faces a different set of fiscal and competitive pressures, the settings share several common attributes and challenges.

Inpatient treatment is both the most expensive and the most restrictive station of psychiatric care. The imperatives of treating patients in the least restrictive setting and of cost containment, particularly fueled by managed care, have led to a perception that admission to an inpatient psychiatric setting represents a failure of treatment and is best avoided. This perception is in sharp contrast to the traditional view of the inpatient psychiatry setting as an opportunity to provide necessary intensive diagnostic and/or therapeutic services that can dramatically improve the trajectory of an individual's mental illness. We believe that this latter perspective remains valid, although it needs to be specifically operationalized in view of current realities; this is the focus of our chapter.

Model of the Adult Inpatient Unit and Admission Criteria and Objectives of Hospitalization

The model presented in this chapter is predicated on the realities of inpatient practice in the United States in 2021. Hospital type and case mix, along with the presence of housing resources and a support system, are associated with variations in length of hospitalization (Lee et al. 2012). Average stays vary from 3–5 days to 1 month depending on the population served and funding available.

A patient can arrive on the inpatient unit via transfer from another unit or hospital, through referral by an outpatient provider, through transport by police, or via transfer from medical floors. The majority of patients with psychiatric problems report to the ED of a hospital, which provides psychiatric assistance around the clock and also has a psychiatric department (Ziegenbein et al. 2006).

Whereas general admission criteria are based on symptom acuity and safety considerations, specific admission criteria depend on the nature and location of the inpatient unit, available acute psychiatric care alternatives, and funding sources. Although specific admission criteria vary depending on payer and health care system factors, all admission criteria include an emphasis on dangerousness and the absence of less restrictive alternatives (Constantine et al. 2006; Warner 1995). Given the varying levels of acuity and complexity and the often rushed manner in which psychiatric patients are medically cleared in the ED, we cannot stress enough the importance of the admitting provider being aware of the current unit acuity and involving the nursing staff early in the admission process to improve collaboration among care team members and reduce risks to maintaining milieu safety (Benolkin et al. 2015).

We illustrate this point with the example of a young man who was severely agitated in the emergency room, requiring two rounds of intramuscular medications and restraints and seclusion. He had attacked nursing staff and had attempted to uproot and destroy the emergency room toilet. He was medically stable and required psychiatric care and stabilization and was accepted to the unit. There was immediate and extensive communication between the accepting physician on call and the charge nurse on the unit and the nursing shift coordinator, and we were able to determine the best room for this patient. The room was close to the nursing station, the bed was able to accommodate restraints if they were needed, and there was facilitation of more male staff, placement of the right observation level, and appropriate as-needed medications for agitation. The ED was also advised to get another set of vitals and offer oral medications prior to his transfer. The patient's transfer was a success, as he slept through the night and posed no problems and improved steadily.

In this chapter, we share our experiences from short-stay (5–10 days) general psychiatric units from across the country and review studies on inpatient psychiatric care. (As we move through the text and discuss the basic tenets of an acute inpatient psychiatric hospitalization, the reader is referred to the appendix to this chapter, which summarizes the broad concepts in an easily digestible format.) Evolving from an asylum model emphasizing containment in the absence of effective therapies, the current model is more akin to a modern medical-surgical intensive care unit (ICU), with rapid diagnosis and psychopharmacological intervention as its foundation. Although most patients will be acutely stabilized and discharged within 3–10 days of a hospital stay, there is a bimodal curve in length of stay in that approximately 20% of patients require longer lengths of stay (14–21 days) because of symptom acuity, treatment-resistant illnesses, or the lack of safe discharge options in the community.

We provide a framework and guidelines from the hospital's ED or a central receiving facility, or as an urgent "direct" admission from an outpatient clinical facility. The focus of intervention is always the acute patient. Having said that, we should make explicit that the role of the hospital for the chronic psychiatric patient, hospitalized for both psychiatric and nonpsychiatric reasons (usually varying amounts of suicidal ideation and/or behavior, homelessness, or substance abuse), is still unsettled and problematic. Management of such patients varies from state to state depending on bed availability and other community resources available. Regardless of setting or length of stay, the objectives of the hospital admission are to rapidly gather relevant history, to make goals focused on the presenting problem, and to promptly initiate appropriate treatment.

Whereas the ultimate goal for most patients is to change the long-term life trajectory in a positive direction, the proximate objective is to change the patient's condition in order to enable the patient to successfully return to their community or another less restrictive setting; however, the extent of funding for hospital treatment constrains what can be done. In most cases, the funding is controlled by managed care administrator-clinicians who are not directly involved in treatment and are governed by insurance companies. The dilemma is that the unit physician has the legal responsibility for the patient but is not the ultimate decision-maker about the length of stay for which reimbursement will be made.

The single guiding principle of inpatient psychiatric treatment is crisis stabilization, with *crisis* broadly defined to include issues such as dangerousness to self or others, acute decline in function, and a therapeutic impasse. It should be emphasized that the primary clinician must think this through with each patient and the patient's family (or the caseworker if no family is available) at each hospitalization. It is critical that the inpatient treatment episode be viewed as one important step in a continuum of care and not as the entirety of care that can completely "fix" the problem or illness.

Hospitalization for psychiatric disorders has evolved in a manner similar to that of hospitalization for other medical and surgical conditions: the hospital is a setting where patients are admitted when they are acutely ill so that the treatment team can make one, or at most two, interventions to change the trajectory of the illness or problem. An analogy to an ICU may be appropriate in that although the inpatient psychiatric intervention is crucial to the overall treatment, it is only one station in a continuum of care.

The Family as Partner on the Treatment Team

Given the acuity of the illness in the context of short hospital stays and the fact that persons admitted to a psychiatric unit are acutely sick, working with families of psychiatric inpatients becomes mandatory. If there is no family, a case manager is almost always a necessity. In our experience, almost every patient has some significant other; the critical task is to find that person, a process that may involve some extra work by social work staff.

To successfully treat the kinds of patients now being hospitalized, the treatment team must include not only the patient but also the patient's outside support system. The individuals in the support system not only serve as diagnostic informants but also provide a transition to the community for the patient and offer a means to integrate knowledge of the patient from outside and within the hospital setting. Coordination with families and psychoeducation have been found to assist with relapse prevention and promote recovery. Family involvement also helps to reduce isolation and gain relevant information and support (Petrakis and Laxton 2017).

Typically family meetings are held prior to discharge, in the second half of the hospitalization, but there have been instances when we have held family meetings to coax the paranoid and delusional patient to trust the treatment team more or to accept the long-acting injectable (LAI) that could stabilize the patient for longer periods of time.

Diagnostic Workup

It is critical that the specific objective or objectives of a particular inpatient episode be spelled out early in the course of hospitalization and that resources be principally directed toward addressing those objectives. The necessary focus of an inpatient episode is formulated by understanding the presenting complaint in the context of the psychiatric multiaxial diagnosis and life circumstances, including recent stressors.

The key element in defining these focal objectives and developing a useful treatment plan is answering the following question: Why is this patient here at this time? To answer this question, the clinician needs input from not only the patient but also the outpatient provider, the family or other caregiver, and the admitting source such as the psychiatric ED or consultation-liaison service. In conjunction with other stakeholders, the inpatient team formulates a specific strategy for addressing the focal problem.

How can one expeditiously define these individualized objectives? On the inpatient units with which we are most familiar, the tasks of defining individualized objectives and reallocating resources are explicitly prioritized in order to address this function. We accomplish this function by expanding the roles that the staff members play in liaison and coordination with outpatient settings and helping staff members develop specific expertise in managing behavioral emergencies, psychopharmacology, and discharge planning. We have also attempted to achieve an optimal balance between the seemingly conflicting objectives of defining the focal problem accurately and doing so expeditiously. Because time is at a premium, we require that the focal problem be formulated within 24 hours of hospitalization, even on weekends, and that a strategy for addressing the problem be developed at the same time. This process requires adequate staffing at all times; psychiatrists must be available to make diagnoses and treatment plans even during nights and weekends, just as in an ICU.

The patient's preadmission course of psychiatric illness and pattern of mental health service utilization can be instructive (Bowers 2005; Ionescu and Ruedrich 2006). Is this a first-time admission with or without a previous history of mental health treatment? If the person has previously received psychiatric treatment, has the treatment been discontinued or is it ongoing? Does the recent course of illness suggest progressive gradual decompensation or a rapid acute deterioration?

A specific initial task is to make as accurate a diagnosis as possible in a very short period of time. This task fits nicely with mandates from the Joint Commission and state regulatory agencies that require clinicians to expeditiously perform comprehensive assessments for inpatients. A comprehensive diagnosis in DSM-5 (American Psychiatric Association 2013) combines the previous Axes I–III into a nonaxial diagnosis:

1. A phenomenological primacy diagnosis of psychopathology based on DSM-5 (e.g., major depressive disorder, recurrent episode, with psychotic features AND severe.
2. Personality disorder diagnosis (if present). This could also include an assessment of maladaptive personality features or defense mechanisms that do not meet criteria for a personality disorder. Importantly, a "personality disorder" can be primary (i.e., lifelong and starting at a young age) or secondary to the primary disorder (e.g., a mood disorder).
3. Diagnosis of any somatic medical conditions that may be present.
4. A systems diagnosis focusing on the patient's support system. This encompasses psychosocial and environmental problems.

Another useful way of understanding the problem that the patient presents with is the four-perspectives approach developed by Paul McHugh and Phillip Slavney, from Johns Hopkins: disease, dimensional, behavior, and life story (Peters et al. 2012). For the disease perspective, the essential question to ask is "What disease does the patient have?" To address the dimensional perspective, the clinician attempts to understand the person by asking the question "How can I best guide my patient toward success based on the kind of person they are?" The behavior perspective demands that clinicians ask of certain patients, "How can my patient's distress be explained by what they do and how can I help them by changing what they do?" Finally, the life-story perspective uses the logic of narrative, a sequence of events within a particular setting that leads to a specific outcome, to understand a patient's psychiatric presentation. With the life-story perspective, the clinician must ask, "How can I best understand my patient's symptoms based on what they encounter?"

The first priorities for the clinician should be to determine the nature of the disorder(s) and how this relates to the presenting problem: Why is the patient here now? Next, the clinician needs to determine what kinds of resources the patient and support system have to support the treatment that needs to be delivered. It is also important to identify the immediate stressors that have upset the balance in the patient's life and precipitated the admission and try to alleviate them as feasible. Specific questions that clinicians should ask as part of the assessment include the following:

1. Why is this patient being admitted?
2. Is the admitting diagnosis correct?
3. Were the medications prescribed prior to admission correct for the patient's symptomatology (which may be different from the medications being correct for the diagnosis)? Were the medications prescribed in the correct dosage and of adequate duration? Were the medications being taken as prescribed?
4. Is the patient or immediate family member receiving some type of psychotherapy? What has been the course of the psychotherapy? Have there been any recent changes in the circumstances of the psychotherapy? For example, is the therapist currently on vacation?
5. Has the patient's social support system changed or failed? Does the patient, correctly or incorrectly, anticipate a change in their social system, which includes the outpatient psychiatric clinicians?

One critical element in the diagnostic process is to rule out delirium or another psychiatric disorder secondary to substance use or a general medical illness. This can often be done most efficiently while the patient is hospitalized, when laboratory testing, imaging, and consultants in other medical specialties are readily available. To be efficient and efficacious, specific clinical protocols must be individualized for the specific setting for each of the most common disorders treated. This is all the more important given the life-threatening nature of some of the medical disorders that can cause psychiatric symptoms (e.g., head injury or seizure disorder). If a patient has a psychiatric diagnosis, physicians are often too ready to attribute all of the patient's symptoms to that diagnosis, while they may minimize or not conduct a serious workup for medical conditions.

It is also now incumbent on psychiatric physicians to assume responsibility for some of the primary medical care during an inpatient stay, no matter how short the stay. In addition to a comprehensive physical examination (including BMI and extensive neurological evaluation), all patients must receive a basic laboratory workup that includes a complete blood count, basic renal and hepatic functions (blood urea nitrogen, creatinine, alanine transaminase, aspartate transaminase, bilirubin), hemoglobin A_{1c}, lipid profiles, and a toxicology screening. Additional laboratory and radiological evaluations may be required. Other medical consultations should be expeditiously obtained if necessary.

Many important aspects of inpatient psychiatric treatment are captured in the following points and can be gleaned from the case vignette that follows:

- If your patient presents as a puzzle and does not fit neatly into a diagnostic box, you may need to think outside the box.
- Diagnosis depends on more than a checklist of symptoms. You need to know your patient's life story and what has gotten them to the point of needing inpatient treatment at this point in their life.
- Never hesitate to obtain second-opinion consultations, if your patient is not responding to what appears to be reasonable treatment.
- Always review available labs and think what might be missing. Do not forget about the benefit of syphilis screening for your patients, even if their initial profiles do not raise concern.
- Always seek out the impressions of your patient's support system and enlist their help in the common goals of successful inpatient treatment in the hospital and transition back to outpatient care.

Case Vignette 1

A 49-year-old married male presented to our crisis walk-in center (CWIC) on two separate occasions with a chief complaint of increased anxiety. He stated that he had a recent physical examination that was normal. He had a history of treatment with bupropion and sertraline for depression, and he was taking fluoxetine and buspirone when first seen. An initial referral to an intensive outpatient program was unsuccessful, in that he felt too overwhelmed to attend and was unable to participate in groups. He was seen by his outpatient psychiatrist, during which his medication was changed to escitalopram. His condition deteriorated, and he began to plan to overdose on available medication at home. He returned to the CWIC 2 weeks later and was referred to our inpatient unit. The patient had a master's degree, lived with his wife of 20 years, and had been laid off from his full-time job 2 years previously.

During most of his admission, the patient worried about poor concentration and "losing" his memory. He was diagnosed with recurrent major depressive disorder and generalized anxiety disorder initially, after his care was discussed with his outpatient psychiatrist. Initial treatment was up-titration of escitalopram. He began to complain that he couldn't "spell anymore or remember things as well." He described increased agitation/racing thoughts and began to worry that he could hurt other people. Thoughts of overdosing on medication became stronger. Bipolar disorder and obsessive-compulsive disorder were considered diagnostically, and low-dose quetiapine and lorazepam were introduced.

Within a week, he revealed his clandestine homosexual lifestyle to his wife in a precipitous manner. He claimed to have seen 30–50 men over time in their home while his wife was working. His condition worsened, as he made predictions that he would lose his marriage and his home. Unfortunately, these predictions did come true.

The patient became argumentative with the staff, ruminated over his strong suicidal impulses, stopped bathing, and began to refuse to eat. His sleep patterns became more erratic. Quetiapine dosage was increased, and electroconvulsive therapy (ECT) was recommended. The patient made odd, paranoid statements (about, e.g., a concern that his wife would call the police to have him arrested for soliciting male prostitutes). He was very ambivalent about having ECT and ended up refusing further treatments after his first two.

He began to refuse medications episodically. On occasion, he would become verbally aggressive with the staff, and announced that he was "giving up." He confabulated a story to his wife about having killed her dog, in an effort to further drive her away from him. Medications were changed to duloxetine and olanzapine. His wife reported to the social worker that her husband had had a seizure in 2000 and spent 5 days in an ICU but that no clear cause was identified.

A second-opinion consult was obtained from neuropsychiatry, and subtle cognitive changes were described: perplexity about the interview, halting speech, memory problems, and paraphasic errors. An organic workup was requested, but the patient refused to have an electroencephalogram or head MRI done. His behavior became odd. Once, he chose to squat by his bedroom door in the hallway all night rather than have the safety search required by his suicide special observation (SO) status. On other occasions, he would stand still in the same spot in public areas for hours.

Because of his worsening condition and ongoing safety concerns, a forensic consult was requested. This senior consultant felt that this patient's "protean, ill-defined, and variegated symptoms bespeak more an organic process than a defined mental illness." Specific focus on his tendency to confabulate was noted. As time progressed, the patient complained of not being able to taste or even swallow his food or drink fluids. He became more withdrawn and refused to have visitors. He forgot the names of his treatment team members sometimes and began to have difficulty with the date. Sleep was poor, and he claimed not to have slept for an entire month (which was not true). He was seen talking "gibberish" to himself, and echolalia during interview attempts grew more common. Disorientation tended to fluctuate. Records from his earlier ICU stay were obtained and revealed a negative organic workup (head computed tomography and MRI, electroencephalography, and lumbar puncture [LP]). Medications were changed from olanzapine to aripiprazole, and duloxetine was up-titrated.

Additional labs were ordered since the patient had not responded to multiple reasonable medication trials. HIV testing was negative, Lyme screen was positive, but his syphilis serology indicated higher reactive values. Treatment with intramuscular penicillin was recommended by our department of medicine.

Nearly 2 months after his admission and on the third actual attempt, the patient agreed to have an MRI done. Anterior nonspecific white matter hyperintensities were prominent, suggesting that previous head trauma, postinfectious or inflammatory changes, or the sequelae of chronic microvascular ischemic events be considered. The possibility of neurosyphilis led the treatment team to pursue an LP, which was done after nearly 2 months in the hospital. His results were negative for Lyme disease, but they showed a white blood count of 30 cells/µL, 98% lymphocytes, and a positive VDRL test result. He was transferred to a medical hospital for treatment of neurosyphilis with a successful course of intravenous penicillin G.

The patient returned to our psychiatric unit for a further 2-week stay. His condition had changed remarkably. Sensorium was clear, he participated well in groups, personal hygiene was good, and he ate and slept well. His agitation and complaints about anxiety and his extreme focus on suicide were diminished. He cooperated with efforts at locating a group home placement, since his wife had begun a process of divorce upon discovery of his syphilitic infection and would not allow him to return home. Our social worker established the patient's mother as his chief contact person for outpatient support. Some lasting neurological symptoms from his disease course were noted (e.g., Montreal Cognitive Assessment [MoCA] scores were 17–18). He was discharged in an improved state and educated about the need for further LPs and periodic serum syphilis testing in follow-up medical care. Discharge medication were duloxetine, aripiprazole, and melatonin.

Because patients may have difficulty providing a coherent history, another important diagnostic task is to gather collateral information. The patient's account of the events leading up to admission must always be supplemented with accounts from family members, friends, and especially other providers. We recognize that family and other significant others may not be available because of alienation or schedule conflicts. However, given the illness acuity plus the short length of stay involved in most admissions, we believe it is mandatory that just as in intensive care, staff members make every effort to contact the patient's immediate family, doctor, and caseworker.

Hospitalization allows a variety of professionals with different perspectives, including physicians, nurses, occupational therapists, and psychologists, to observe and evaluate the patient. The inpatient unit traditionally has significant resources that are relevant to the diagnostic task. Given decreasing lengths of stay and a focus on acute stabilization, clinicians are often tempted to defer definitive diagnosis in favor of a "not otherwise specified" diagnosis. However, we believe that this does the patient a disservice because it can lead to effective treatment being deferred, and symptoms may be overlooked that need attention. Instead, a "most likely" diagnosis or set of diagnoses should be formulated, with necessary caveats, and appropriate treatment should be promptly initiated.

The legal status of the patient and their competence and ability to understand the nature of illness and treatment alternatives should be ascertained. Informed consent is the bedrock of treatment. If the patient is unable to fully participate in this process, this should be ascertained at the time of admission or prior to it if a scheduled admission. Appropriate steps should be taken to address the situation, such as approaching the court to seek authorization for necessary treatment, family involvement, and/or appointment of a guardian advocate. Delays in initiating appropriate treatment on account of the inability of the patient to provide valid informed consent should be minimized (details vary by state).

By the end of the evaluation, the treatment team should have determined the likely clinical diagnosis or diagnoses, identified the set of circumstances that necessitated the current hospitalization, elucidated the immediate stressors and current resources, and ascertained specific patient vulnerabilities and system factors that may affect treatment. A formalized treatment plan should be in effect by the third day of the patient's hospitalization.

The master treatment plan is developed by next answering the question "What needs to happen in order to solve this focal problem or problems?" (Harper 1989). It is most efficacious if the focal problem is one that the inpatient psychiatry unit can better address than another type of setting such as a medical unit. Is it possible to develop objectives that are specific to the needs of the patient and have some possibility of modifying the course of the illness and yet are modest enough to be attainable? Our broad strategy is designed to address the specific circumstances of the inpatient episode in the context of the functions that an inpatient unit performs best.

Case Vignette 2

A 19-year-old female student is admitted to an inpatient unit on account of a drug overdose that followed the breakup of a significant relationship. The patient has been in outpatient treatment and has received a diagnosis of recurrent major depressive disorder and borderline personality disorder. Her inpatient treatment must address safety needs and include a diagnostic reevaluation and possible changes in the therapeutic plan, as well as respite to allow resolution of the trauma of the breakup.

How this patient should be treated is discussed next, and we will return to this vignette later in the chapter.

Goals of Treatment

After diagnosis, the next task is to identify the goals of the treatment. One must always ask patients what their goals are for the hospital stay. It is important to ask patients what they would like to see happen for them in the course of this hospital stay. Equally important is to ask family members the same question. It must be recognized that the goals that patients, families, or even outpatient therapists express may be different from those identified by the inpatient team. Finally, treatment goals should be discussed among the inpatient team and with the outpatient treatment team.

Chances for good treatment outcome improve to the extent that a consensus on diverse objectives can be achieved. As noted earlier, the most important tasks include identifying and alleviating, if possible, the stresses that upset the patient's balance and interfere with their ability to live outside the hospital; decreasing symptoms; changing the posthospital life trajectory from the prehospital downward course; and beginning the process of educating the patient and family.

Specific Treatment Interventions

Detoxification From Substances

Substance use disorders are highly comorbid with other psychiatric diagnoses, and problems related to substance abuse frequently precipitate or substantially contribute to the admission. Rapid detoxification is among the tasks that can best be accomplished in the hospital. Although some general psychiatry inpatient units still perform this function, specialized substance abuse detoxification units perform this function in many settings.

Family Intervention

It is very important to evaluate the patient's support system. Even during a very short stay, it is virtually mandatory to have at least one session with the people who are most important to the patient. This allows the clinical team to gather information, provide education about the patient's illness and its treatment, and undertake other interventions specific to the situation. The importance of education in leading to a better outcome is under-recognized (Glick et al. 1994). As noted earlier, the involvement of the family is also invaluable in obtaining the needed consent for both information gathering and treatment.

Individual Psychotherapy

Given the short length of stay now predominant, hospital staff often forget to talk to the patient. Regardless of how long the patient stays in the hospital, basic principles of individual therapy should be followed. These include establishing an alliance; providing support, hope, and education; and even, on occasion, making an interpretation, if it will advance the aims of the hospitalization. In fact, a 2007 study documented the effectiveness of adding both brief and intensive psychotherapy to pharmacotherapy for depressed inpatients (Schramm et al. 2007).

Group Psychotherapy

The role of recreational and leisure activities ("activity therapy") during an acute psychiatric hospitalization is very important. Although there has been a reduction in the use of such activities in the context of cost containment, very short hospital stays, and the changing role of a short-term psychiatric unit in a continuum of care, we highly recommend a dedicated recreational therapist whose sole responsibility is running of therapeutic groups for the patients. Such a therapist also provides valuable feedback on patients' performance to the treatment teams, shaping the diagnosis and treatment of the individual. The use of focused patient therapy groups, such as dialectical behavior therapy or cognitive-behavioral therapy, or art therapy or exercise and meditation, depends on the specific setting, the resources of the inpatient unit, and the population that it serves. Referral to consumer groups such as NAMI (National Alliance on Mental Illness) and the Depression and Bipolar Support Alliance is usually very helpful over the long run. Brief group mindfulness therapy interventions are well received and tolerated by acutely hospitalized psychiatric inpatients, including those with acute psychosis (Nikolitch et al. 2016).

Initiation or Modification of Psychopharmacological Treatment

Medication management is usually central to the treatment regimen (Glick et al. 1991; Kingsbury et al. 2001; Tandon et al. 2006). The crucial first step is to make an accurate diagnosis and identify target symptoms. An early decision point is whether to continue outpatient medications. To make this decision rationally, the clinician needs to undertake a significant amount of investigation in order to gather a medication history that includes dosages, duration, rationale for use, and, most important, prior therapeutic response and side effects. This labor-intensive task is essential in effectively and quickly developing an appropriate treatment plan. Taking a patient off medications is often as helpful an intervention as starting new medications, particularly given the issues related to drug interactions and potent clinical effects of treatment discontinuation.

In our inpatient units we tend to take a twofold approach. First, we select a primary medication for the patient's psychiatric illness (e.g., an antipsychotic or a mood stabilizer, or an antidepressant) and titrate it as tolerated to a therapeutic dosage. Because antipsychotics, mood stabilizers, and antidepressants all take days or weeks or months to achieve their full effectiveness, we treat symptoms such as agitation and anxiety with as-needed medication, to provide patients with some short-term relief. One of the most common, although understandable, mistakes is to attempt to speed up response by giving higher doses of the primary medication when what is mostly needed is an understanding of the normal course of response and patience on the part of the clinician. Such a mistake is often made based on the unrealistic hope that the patient will be asymptomatic at the time of discharge, whereas it is more realistic to expect that the patient's symptoms will be sufficiently reduced to allow continuation, and fine-tuning, of treatment in another setting. We very commonly use the day hospital programs and collaborate closely with family and outpatient providers to continue close monitoring of patients, especially as they await a full therapeutic trial of a medication, which is a full dose of the medication, for at least 8–12 weeks.

We also recommend making only one change in medication at a time, if possible. This strategy is often difficult given short lengths of stay, but our practice after making a diagnosis is to determine what is the most effective medication with which to start and its initial target dosage. Ideally, this is carried out concurrently with tapering of the patient's previous medications that, by history, seemed to be ineffective or inappropriate for the diagnosis. The hospital psychiatrist must identify the benefits versus the costs of each medication. By *cost*, we mean not just financial cost but more importantly the costs in terms of side effects and medication interactions. The pros and cons of discontinuing a previous medication must also be carefully considered and discussed with the prescribing outpatient provider. Although pharmacotherapy must be individualized, evidence-based guidelines can provide useful guidance (Tandon et al. 2006). We recommend American Psychiatric Association practice guidelines and the U.K.'s National Institute for Health and Care Excellence guidelines, along with the Texas Medication Algorithm Project for antipsychotic use. UpTodate is a very useful evidence-based clinical resource for ongoing patient care that can identify drug interactions, provide patient and family handouts on medications, and offer the latest recommendations and medication information.

It is important not to undermedicate the patient. Finding the best possible dosage in 3–10 days is a very difficult objective to achieve. Although there is considerable heterogeneity among patients with regard to the optimal dosage, we recommend rapidly achieving the average target dosage for the situation and making short-term adjustments only if absolutely necessary. Dosage selection needs to factor in diagnosis, age, stage of illness, prior response, and concurrent medical conditions as much as possible.

As a rule of thumb, we recommend using fewer rather than more medications. It is important not to get fixed in the practice of prescribing what may be described as the "usual cocktail" (e.g., an antipsychotic plus a mood stabilizer, an antidepressant plus a benzodiazepine plus a sleeping pill) (Kingsbury et al. 2001). It is important to remember that once a patient is discharged from an inpatient facility, the outpatient clinician is likely to continue this treatment regimen indefinitely, because the clinician may fear that changing the regimen may lead to worsening symptoms or a downward course.

Although we advocate using the minimum number of medications, we also recommend not temporizing when considering adding a medication because of an acute situation such as escalating agitation. The usual mistake is to delay until an adverse event occurs, such as the patient's becoming acutely agitated or assaultive. This situation arises more often when treating patients with schizophrenia or bipolar disorder mania, but it also occasionally occurs in treating patients with major depressive disorder or even severe personality disorder associated with substance abuse. The usual approach is to use a short-acting benzodiazepine (e.g., lorazepam) or diphenhydramine or increase the dosage of a sedating antipsychotic.

Nonadherence to medication treatment is a major problem that often leads to repeated hospitalizations. To improve patient adherence to treatment, we suggest working with significant others during the hospital stay, striving to minimize adverse effects, and focusing on patient and family education. If the treatment team is in doubt about a patient's willingness to take medication, team members should not hesitate to consider and prescribe a LAI, if an appropriate medication is available, to ensure compliance. LAIs are recommended when adherence is inadequate (American Psychiatric Association 2021; Moore et al. 2007; National Collaborating Centre for Mental Health 2010). The LAIs deal efficiently with covert nonadherence (Barnes and Curson 1994), relieve patients from the burden of daily dosing, and ease family burden because care providers are more aware of nonadherence (Barnes and Schizophrenia Consensus Group of British Association for Psychopharmacology 2011; Kane and Garcia-Ribera 2009). LAIs however remain underutilized (Fayek et al. 2003). Given the high nonadherence rate and readmission rates to the inpatient unit, it is important to consider the LAIs whenever possible with patients and to have an open discussion.

It is also important to remember that clozapine remains a highly effective treatment for treatment-resistant schizophrenia, with response rates between 30% and 60%. It has also been shown to significantly reduce incidents of self-harm and aggression in patients with severe borderline personality disorder. The level of coordination and monitoring that is often required during clozapine initiation is best accomplished in an inpatient setting. One other medication that needs to be considered in the inpatient setting is lithium: apart from its mood-stabilizing actions, lithium has antiaggressive and antisuicidal actions.

With regard to discharge medications, we recommend not making downward dosage adjustments immediately prior to discharge because lowering the dosage at this point may lead to an exacerbation of symptoms just at the time the patient must leave the hospital. Instead, it is better to have the outpatient physician regulate the dosage. Close coordination with the outpatient team is crucial; this entails ensuring a smooth handoff to the aftercare clinic or other setting where the patient will continue in treatment. Timely transmission of necessary clinical information to the outpatient team to facilitate an effective transfer of care is a very high priority. This builds on coordination of care with the outpatient team from the time of admission throughout the course of inpatient treatment. Time constraints can make such coordination challenging (Boyer et al. 2000), but it is one of the most important elements in ensuring good outcomes. It is usually necessary both to make verbal contact with the outpatient team and to actually transmit written documents, including the treatment goals and medications. We start filling out discharge summary templates right from day 1 of the patient's admission and continue to fill them out as we go along during the admission, and over time, we have been able to achieve sending out of discharge summaries within 24 hours of patient discharge.

We have found rating scales to be extremely useful in measuring the response of defined target symptoms to prescribed psychopharmacological treatment. Although administration of a lengthy battery of instruments is not desirable and may be cumbersome, the use of simple and reliable scales as individually appropriate is strongly recommended. The MoCA and the Brief Psychiatric Rating Scale are useful instruments to track cognitive impairment, especially if the patient is receiving ECT or has significant psychopathology, respectively (Tandon et al. 2006).

Lastly, we would like to highlight the importance of an often-overlooked modality of nonmedication treatment: ECT. ECT is a fast, safe, and highly effective treatment for treatment-resistant and agitated depression with a high degree of suicidality, especially in the elderly (Geduldig and Kellner 2016) and in refractory schizophrenia. We recall one interesting patient in particular for whom ECT was the only treatment that was effective in controlling a rare case of unremitting mania that had gone on for at least 3 months, with almost full recovery from the manic state by the end of 12 bilateral ECT treatments.

Having a standard protocol on the unit of going about ECT treatments by providing handouts, offering patient educational videos, seeking medical consultation for clearance for ECT, obtaining a signed consent for the treatments, and maintaining close liaison with families eases a patient's mind and makes them more amenable to the treatments. Contrary to the popular opinion, time and time again, we have seen, and a robust data set confirms, that ECT does not lead to longer-lasting cognitive deficits (Ziegelmayer et al. 2017). As patients start noticing improvements by the third to fifth ECT treatment, we often consider a step-down to the partial hospitalization program setting to complete the remainder of the index course of ECT and have a discussion of maintenance ECT with the outpatient provider, depending on the response and the patient's preference.

To summarize, here are some basic guidelines:

- Do NOT diagnose patients with "NOS" (not otherwise specified); make a working diagnosis as is done in the rest of medicine.
- Do initiate treatment promptly.
- Do NOT practice polypharmacy; less is more.
- Do NOT underdose; prescribe no more or less than needed.
- Do select treatment based on a comprehensive history of previous treatment response.
- Do NOT repeat a failed treatment; if it did not work the first time, it usually will not work the second.
- Do NOT assume that patients have no significant others (broadly defined); almost everyone has some significant other, even the homeless.
- Do NOT delay initiating treatment, but do not overmedicate either.
- Do track response with the use of reliable rating scales.
- Do consider ECT and offer to all patients where indicated.

Milieu Management

The structure and setting of the inpatient unit are central to its function, and the unit milieu is of critical therapeutic importance. The locations of patient rooms, group activity rooms, the nursing station, the meal room, and other elements of unit geography significantly affect the ability of the treatment team to effectively carry out unit functions. An explicit stable daily routine, along with a clear set of unit procedures and rules that are consistently implemented, facilitates a predictable and safe environment. We provide a welcome folder to all new patients that includes a printed schedule of all the unit activities for the week, along with a small journal that helps them capture the essence of their hospitalization as they go along. The schedule is also posted in a few key areas of the unit, acting as a useful reminder and helping patients orient to the unit.

We also practice daily morning team meetings with all available staff—and some hospitals practice an afternoon wrap-up meeting too—to briefly review the milieu and update observation levels, and provide consistent care with effective communication between all the disciplines.

Such an environment provides the context for effective therapy. Given the higher level of illness acuity in inpatient settings, the inherent design of the unit also helps. Ulrich et al. (2018) provide an overview of characteristics of an inpatient unit that, based on our experience, are helpful. Nursing professionals play the key role in the creation and maintenance of such a unit milieu. With the changing nature of the patient population on an inpatient psychiatry unit, the function of acute inpatient psychiatric nursing has continued to evolve (Bowers 2005; Deacon et al. 2006; Lamb and Weinberger 2005). Nursing personnel maintain safety on the unit and manage the unit environment, collect and communicate information about patients, provide personal care, manage disturbed behavior, and give and monitor treatment. Nursing personnel also may lead a variety of therapeutic groups, such as psychoeducational groups focusing on compliance and medication management.

From a staffing perspective, one needs to evaluate how resources can be best utilized within local constraints to address the objectives of the program. New educational programs for staff are usually necessary to adequately train clinicians of all disciplines. The organization of the inpatient treatment team needs careful attention. Different team members have defined and differentiated roles that must be effectively coordinated. The unit psychiatrist or service chief plays a key role as the team leader. It is important to emphasize that treatment is shaped not only by how much a psychiatrist knows but also by their attitudes and knowledge about the model of inpatient treatment.

Management of Suicidal and Aggressive Behavior

One basic role of the inpatient unit is to keep patients safe. On our units, about 30%–50% of patients are admitted involuntarily—that is, they are judged to be a danger to maintaining safety until the risk of harm is reduced, with the hospitalization actively reducing the risk of such harm. Specific expertise to perform these functions includes effective court liaison, violence and suicide management, and the ability to perform thorough risk assessments.

A careful history and evaluation to assess the risk of suicidal behavior are essential components of the initial clinical workup. In managing acutely suicidal patients, we concur with Jayaram et al. (2010) in recommending the use of one-to-one observation or observation by skilled nursing staff when a patient must be within an arm's reach of the observer and not 15-minute checks. Ensuring adequate staff training and maintaining systematic reports from each shift and observer are crucial for maintenance of quality of care.

Individualized assessment of risk and of the precipitants of aggressive behavior should also be performed at the time of admission (Serper et al. 2005). Staff members should be trained in appropriate techniques to manage aggressive behavior (Morrison 2003). Although seclusion and restraint should be utilized infrequently, if at all, staff members need to be trained in their safe and appropriate use (Sailas and Wahlbeck 2005). The risk of inpatient violence remains high at 30%–50% (Fisher 2016). The best predictor of violence remains a past history of severe attempts. It is important to understand the origin of violence—from psychosis or impulsivity or predatory characteristics—and accordingly address it (Fisher 2016).

Case Vignette 3

Ashley, a 29-year-old woman with a history of autistic disorder, ADHD, moderately severe learning disabilities, and schizophrenia was admitted from her group home for escalating violence toward staff and head-banging behavior.

Since she was a former patient on the unit, a treatment plan, detailed below, was initiated at the time of admission, after a careful assessment and good dialogue between all the disciplines:

Treatment Plan

Patient's Goal(s)
To get discharged from the hospital and return home with staff

Behaviors
Behaviors to Increase
Asking for assistance when dealing with distress

Behaviors to Decrease
1. Head banging
2. Suicidal actions and gestures (e.g., wrapping items around her neck)
3. Homicidal actions and gestures (e.g., hitting and charging after staff)
4. Crying/yelling

Contingencies/Staff Response
What Staff Can Do to Increase Behavior
1. Time on the patio: If patient goes 1 hour with no behavior (15-minute time limit)
2. Watch favorite DVD (at the end of the shift): If patient does not engage in behavior for the duration of the shift
3. Remain helmet-free: If no behavior occurs for 2 days and patient is off SO level

What Staff Can Do to Decrease Behavior
1. With sufficient staff, block the behavior. Limit attention yet keep patient in your sights.
2. Remind patient, "This is not helpful to you. What alternative coping skill can we use?"; ignore negative comments, and reinforce all positive comments immediately.

Each morning, staff will go over with Ashley what are the expectations of her behavior and what are the possible consequences if she does not follow her plan. An incentive plan will be in place that rewards Ashley when she makes positive choices and practices her alternative coping strategies. Ashley is to engage in three relaxation techniques and three sensory activities per day. To reduce satiation, staff offers Ashley opportunities to pick from each list to practice.

Sensory
- Lie with weighted blanket
- Play with Thera-Putty (check with OT [occupational therapy] for location of item)
- Play with fidgets (check with OT for location of item)
- Listen to soothing music
- Take a walk around the unit

Alternative Relaxation Skills
- Guided meditation
- Deep breaths
- Squeezing stress balls
- Self-massage
- Dance to music (Ashley loves country music)

Ashley's acting out may function as manipulation rather than a response to internal stimuli. If Ashley thinks something should be happening or happening faster than reality, or is told "no," she may react in dramatic ways:

- Become physically aggressive with staff
- Destroy property
- Become self-injurious (i.e., head banging, biting self, hitting self in the mouth)

Make sure Ashley's helmet is on and withdraw commenting by restricting attention to them as much as possible while still keeping her and others safe. If Ashley is engaging in behavior, remove the reinforcing behavior and attempt to refocus Ashley by offering alternative coping skills. If Ashley cannot recall alternatives, suggest to her what is on the list. If in the milieu Ashley is overstimulated, return to her room and offer choices again. If escalation persists, follow policy for ensuring patient safety.

The above detailed, well-thought-out treatment plan broke it down for everybody, including Ashley, and helped her speedy recovery and return to the group home.

Another important clinical issue is the situation in which a patient on an inpatient unit attacks or threatens to kill the treating psychiatrist or other staff members. The most appropriate response is to take the threatening behavior at face value, as though it could happen, rather than simply interpreting or ignoring it. One should assume that the behavior is part of the patient's acute symptomatology. A second step is to attempt to determine from referral sources if there is a history of threats or of actual violence. As a third step, it is prudent to reevaluate the medication regimen and consider increasing the dosage of medication for that particular illness. It may also be advisable to transfer the patient to another physician or another unit, especially if the treating staff are uncomfortable working with such a patient.

Discharge Planning

Given the briefer hospitalizations, discharge planning should start on day 1 of the patient's hospitalization. We have particularly found that having a dedicated discharge coordinator who exclusively handles discharge is highly effective. We always link the patient to an outpatient prescriber and a therapist; typically, an outpatient appointment is scheduled for the patient within 1 week of hospital discharge. Patients may also need help with other services such as case management and housing. Effectiveness of inpatient/outpatient handoffs is a primary index of high-quality inpatient psychiatric treatment (Joint Commission 2008). It is not uncommon that we hear that outpatient providers no longer feel equipped to manage patients with complex needs and, unfortunately, choose hospitalization as the time to make this change. Assisting the patient in obtaining higher level of care such as mobile treatment services or long-term psychiatric rehabilitation care can be life-changing for the patient.

Patients and family need help to change the posthospital trajectory, because the patient is usually on a downward slope during the acute illness. The objective is to make one or at most two interventions to change life for both the patient and the family after the hospital stay, targeting the types of psychosocial and environmental problems. This strategy can be the most important part of a hospitalization and has the potential to significantly change the course of a patient's illness. Inpatient education programs focused on surviving outside the protected hospital setting are helpful; these may include multiple structured small-group meetings focusing on education about the illness and coping strategies.

We also routinely recommend referral to appropriate consumer organizations such as NAMI and Alcoholics Anonymous in order to improve posthospital outcome (Glick and Dixon 2002).

At discharge, patients who smoke (roughly about 50% of the adult inpatients) should be offered nicotine replacement therapy and a referral to the state quit line, which can help them to stay nicotine-free even outside the hospital.

The flowchart in Figure 4–1 helps one understand a patient's tobacco use and level of interest in quitting assessed at the time of admission and interventions during the hospital stay, at discharge, and on follow-up. Quit line (1-800-QUIT-NOW) is an evidence-based telephone service that offers tobacco-cessation counseling and is available in all 50 states (Fiore et al. 2012).

Let us revisit the inpatient stay of the 19-year-old female student who was admitted to our inpatient unit on account of a drug overdose that followed the breakup of a significant relationship.

Case Vignette 2 (*continued*)

As previously noted, the patient has been in outpatient treatment and has received a diagnosis of recurrent depressive disorder and borderline personality disorder. After initial detoxification and life-supportive monitoring and therapy, the treatment team develops an individualized safety plan with the patient, and she learns coping skills in an individual and unit group setting. In view of nonresponse to an adequate trial of the current antidepressant, the agent is switched and a low dosage of a sedating antipsychotic is added to address symptoms of paranoia and insomnia. Three friends who reside in the same college dormitory as the patient and constitute her immediate support system (they accompanied the patient to the ED from which she was admitted to the inpatient unit) participate in two meetings with the patient and her inpatient social worker. Following discussion with the outpatient therapist, the patient is referred to a dialectical behavior therapy program.

Conclusion

Inpatient hospitalization for adults in crisis involves the following steps: defining the focal problem, making a diagnosis, formulating specific goals for the admission, determining which treatments to prescribe, reinforcing or rebuilding the patient's support system, and establishing outpatient care. The role of the family and significant others is central. Key tasks to be performed by the inpatient unit include liaison and coordination with multiple groups (e.g., outpatient team, psychiatry emergency services, the court system, family members, other caregivers, community mental health agencies, various social and governmental agencies), rapid comprehensive assessment (e.g., descriptive and diagnostic, medical, personality, system), maintenance of patient safety and a therapeutic environment (Boyer et al. 2000), and smooth and expeditious transfer to another residential and treatment system.

The approach to inpatient psychiatry we propose focuses on creating patient-specific objectives that are congruent with the functions that inpatient psychiatry units can best perform. The highlights of this approach include making an accurate diagnosis, delivering effective medication, involving the patient's support system, and coordinating care with outpatient providers. These are all things that can be accomplished or

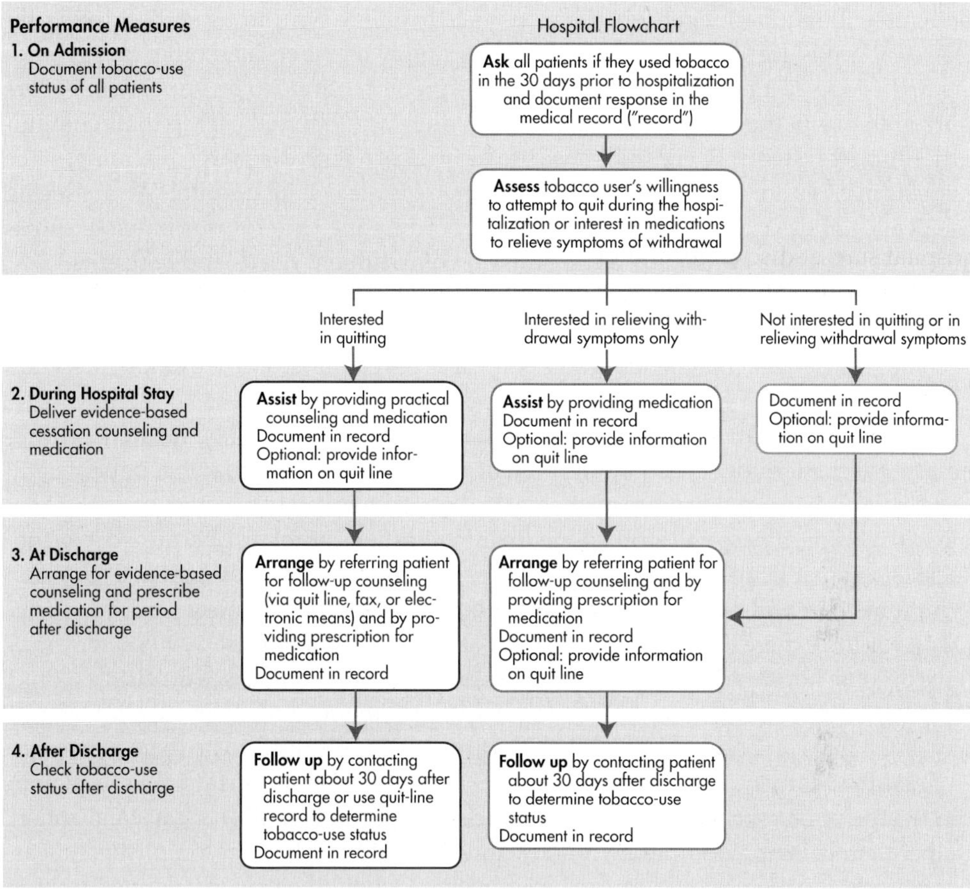

FIGURE 4–1. Assessment of a patient's tobacco use and level of interest in quitting at the time of admission and interventions during the hospital stay, at discharge, and on follow-up.

at least started during a relatively short hospital stay. It should be emphasized that the inpatient unit is only one station in a continuum of care and plays a specific role in this continuum. Because it is the most expensive component on this continuum, optimal and efficient utilization of this resource is essential.

More severely ill patients are coming into the hospital. Specialty units offer expertise in dealing with serious psychiatric conditions that may not be as available in general units; this specialization should be encouraged. Our patients are presenting with more medical problems, and incorporating care for the mind and the body will become even more essential to our mission. Even as we assess outpatient treatment needs for psychiatric aftercare, we should ensure that our patients have appropriate medical care available. In some respects, inpatient psychiatry has taken on a primary care responsibility, diagnosing and treating new medical problems and making sure that this treatment can be passed on to community providers.

We will be seeing greater collaboration between psychiatrists and other medical specialists and will view our patients more holistically. We need to be aware of all available lower level of care options (e.g., partial hospital program, intensive outpatient program, psychiatric rehabilitation programs, outpatient treatment teams) to decrease time in the more restrictive inpatient setting. But we need to realize that some of our patients will require longer lengths of stays to stabilize symptoms and address psychosocial needs. Keeping outpatient clinicians, family members, and other care providers in the loop as inpatient treatment progresses will continue to be important. We are only with our patients for a short time before they are "handed off" to their community support systems. Everybody needs to be on board with discharge planning, since patients in crisis are often more vulnerable when they leave the hospital. We are seeing the benefit of electronic medical records in coordinating care for our patients across all levels of care by aiding rapid transmission of treatment needs and concerns.

Psychiatric treatment is expanding in exciting directions. As options evolve, other treatments will probably become as commonplace in inpatient psychiatry as ECT has become. Transcranial magnetic stimulation, nasal esketamine, and Brexanolone should be made available in crisis stabilization programs.

Inpatient psychiatric clinicians can rest assured that there will be future job availability. No matter how broad an outpatient treatment network may be, patients will need a hospital to provide more intensive treatment when safety becomes an issue. People with chronic illness will stop taking their medications or relapse because of psychosocial stressors. People with no prior history of psychiatric treatment will develop symptoms that will put them at risk and require inpatient diagnosis and treatment. Our job is to be there for our patients, especially during times of stress, when they may have become hopeless and are sharing their deepest fears, sometimes for the first time. We have been handed a sacred duty to help our patients and their support system navigate what can be a foreboding health care system. We need to be their advocates.

The inpatient psychiatry system still has an extremely important role to play in the treatment of psychiatric illness. Its principal function is that of crisis stabilization. Rather than being preoccupied with how much could have been accomplished in earlier periods, inpatient providers can be enthusiastic about their clearly defined tasks in this new era of treatment. In addition, payers and utilization reviewers can be assured of meaningful and efficient inpatient stays from which patients are likely to benefit maximally. Finally, it is important to maintain a mechanism for assessing how well a particular inpatient unit or system is accomplishing its objectives over time. This assessment should include both objective measures of assessing treatment outcome (measured against admission goals) and the commonly used patient and family satisfaction measures.

References

American Psychiatric Association: Diagnostic and Statistical Manual of Mental Disorders, 5th Edition. Arlington, VA, American Psychiatric Association, 2013

American Psychiatric Association: The American Psychiatric Association Practice Guideline for the Treatment of Patients With Schizophrenia, 3rd Edition. Washington, DC, American Psychiatric Association, 2021

Barnes TR, Curson DA: Long-term depot antipsychotics: a risk-benefit assessment. Drug Saf 10(6):464–479, 1994 7917075

Barnes TR; Schizophrenia Consensus Group of British Association for Psychopharmacology: Evidence-based guidelines for the pharmacological treatment of schizophrenia: recommendations from the British Association for Psychopharmacology. J Psychopharmacol 25(5):567–620, 2011 21292923

Bastiampillai T, Sharfstein SS, Allison S: Increase in US suicide rates and the critical decline in psychiatric beds. JAMA 316(24):2591–2592, 2016 27812693
Benolkin L, Kinstler D, Delaney KR: Improving awareness of an acute psychiatric unit's capacity for admission. J Psychosoc Nurs Ment Health Serv 53(8):30–35, 2015 26268479
Bowers L: Reasons for admission and their implications for the nature of acute inpatient psychiatric nursing. J Psychiatr Ment Health Nurs 12(2):231–236, 2005 15788042
Boyer CA, McAlpine DD, Pottick KJ, et al: Identifying risk factors and key strategies in linkage to outpatient psychiatric care. Am J Psychiatry 157(10):1592–1598, 2000 11007712
Constantine R, Kershaw M, Robinson P: Florida's Mental Health Acute Care/Crisis Services: Background and Strategies for Reform. Tampa, University of South Florida, 2006
Deacon M, Warne T, McAndrew S: Closeness, chaos and crisis: the attractions of working in acute mental health care. J Psychiatr Ment Health Nurs 13(6):750–757, 2006 17087679
Fayek M, Flowers C, Signorelli D, Simpson G: Psychopharmacology: underuse of evidence-based treatments in psychiatry. Psychiatr Serv 54(11):1453–1454, 1456, 2003 14600298
Fiore MC, Goplerud E, Schroeder SA: The Joint Commission's new tobacco-cessation measures—will hospitals do the right thing? N Engl J Med 366(13):1172–1174, 2012 22417200
Fisher K: Inpatient violence. Psychiatr Clin North Am 39(4):567–577, 2016 27836152
Geduldig ET, Kellner CH: Electroconvulsive therapy in the elderly: new findings in geriatric depression. Curr Psychiatry Rep 18(4):40, 2016 26909702
Geller JL: A history of private psychiatric hospitals in the USA: from start to almost finished. Psychiatr Q 77(1):1–41, 2006 16397753
Glick ID, Hargreaves WA: Psychiatric Hospital Treatment for the 1980s: A Controlled Study of Short Versus Long Hospitalization. Lexington, MA, Lexington Press, 1979
Glick ID, Dixon L: Patient and family support organization services should be included as part of treatment for the severely mentally ill. J Psychiatr Pract 8(2):63–69, 2002 15985859
Glick ID, Burti L, Suzuki K, Sacks M: Effectiveness in psychiatric care, I: a cross-national study of the process of treatment and outcomes of major depressive disorder. J Nerv Ment Dis 179(2):55–63, 1991 1990072
Glick ID, Burti L, Okonogi K, Sacks M: Effectiveness in psychiatric care, III: psychoeducation and outcome for patients with major affective disorder and their families. Br J Psychiatry 164(1):104–106, 1994 8137088
Glick ID, Carter WG, Tandon R: A paradigm for treatment of inpatient psychiatric disorders: from asylum to intensive care. J Psychiatr Pract 9(5):395–402, 2003 15985960
Harper G: Focal inpatient treatment planning. J Am Acad Child Adolesc Psychiatry 28(1):31–37, 1989 2914833
Ionescu D, Ruedrich S: Inpatient treatment planning: consider six preadmission patterns. Curr Psychiatr 5:23–31, 2006
Jayaram G, Sporney H, Perticone P: The utility and effectiveness of 15-minute checks in inpatient settings. Psychiatry (Edgmont) 7(8):46–49, 2010 20877534
Joint Commission: Performance measurement initiatives: hospital-based, and patient psychiatric services. Candidate commercial. February 15, 2008. Available at: www.jointcommission.org/measurement/measures/hospital-based-inpatient-psychiatric. Accessed March 21, 2022.
Kane JM, Garcia-Ribera C: Clinical guideline recommendations for antipsychotic long-acting injections. Br J Psychiatry Suppl 52:S63–S67, 2009 19880920
Kingsbury SJ, Yi D, Simpson GM: Psychopharmacology: rational and irrational polypharmacy. Psychiatr Serv 52(8):1033–1036, 2001 11474046
Lamb HR, Weinberger LE: The shift of psychiatric inpatient care from hospitals to jails and prisons. J Am Acad Psychiatry Law 33(4):529–534, 2005 16394231
Lee S, Rothbard AB, Noll EL: Length of inpatient stay of persons with serious mental illness: effects of hospital and regional characteristics. Psychiatr Serv 63(9):889–895, 2012 22751995
Lelliot P: Acute inpatient psychiatry in England: an old problem and a new priority. Epidemiol Psichiatr Soc 15(2):91–94, 2006 16865927
Lipsitt DR: Psychiatry and the general hospital in an age of uncertainty. World Psychiatry 2:87–92, 2003

Moore TA, Buchanan RW, Buckley PF, et al: The Texas Medication Algorithm Project antipsychotic algorithm for schizophrenia: 2006 update. J Clin Psychiatry 68(11):1751–1762, 2007 18052569

Morrison EF: An evaluation of four programs for the management of aggression in psychiatric settings. Arch Psychiatr Nurs 17(4):146–155, 2003 14508770

National Association of Psychiatric Health Systems: Annual Survey Report: Trends in Behavioral Healthcare Systems. A Benchmarking Report: Length of Stay Declines as Patient Numbers Rise. Washington, DC, National Association of Psychiatric Health Systems, 2000

National Collaborating Centre for Mental Health: Schizophrenia: Core Interventions in the Treatment and Management of Schizophrenia in Adults in Primary and Secondary Care, Updated Edition. Leicester, UK, The British Psychological Society/Royal College of Psychiatrists, 2010

Nikolitch K, Laliberté V, Yu C, et al: Tolerability and suitability of brief group mindfulness-oriented interventions in psychiatric inpatients: a pilot study. Int J Psychiatry Clin Pract 20(3):170–174, 2016 27334931

Peters ME, Taylor J, Lyketsos CG, et al: Beyond the DSM: the perspectives of psychiatry approach to patients. Prim Care Companion CNS Disord 14(1):PCC.11m01233, 2012 22690367

Petrakis M, Laxton S: Intervening early with family members during first-episode psychosis: an evaluation of mental health nursing psychoeducation within an inpatient unit. Arch Psychiatr Nurs 31(1):48–54, 2017 28104058

Ruud T, Lindefors N, Lindhardt A: Current issues in Scandinavian acute psychiatric wards. Epidemiol Psichiatr Soc 15(2):99–103, 2006 16865929

Sailas E, Wahlbeck K: Restraint and seclusion in psychiatric inpatient wards. Curr Opin Psychiatry 18(5):555–559, 2005 16639118

Schramm E, van Calker D, Dykierek P, et al: An intensive treatment program of interpersonal psychotherapy plus pharmacotherapy for depressed inpatients: acute and long-term results. Am J Psychiatry 164(5):768–777, 2007 17475736

Sederer LI, Rothschild AJ: Acute Care Psychiatry: Diagnosis and Treatment. Baltimore, MD, Williams & Wilkins, 1997

Serper MR, Goldberg PR, Herman KG, et al: Predictors of aggression on the psychiatric patient service. Compr Psychiatry 46(2):121–127, 2005 15723029

Tandon R, Targum SD, Nasrallah HA, Ross R; Treatment Effectiveness in Schizophrenia Consortium: Strategies for maximizing clinical effectiveness in the treatment of schizophrenia. J Psychiatr Pract 12(6):348–363, 2006 17122696

Torrey EF, Bruce RD, Lamb HR, et al: Raising Cain: The Role of Serious Mental Illness in Family Homicides. Treatment Advocacy Center Reports, June 2016. Available at: www.treatmentadvocacycenter.org/storage/documents/raising-cain.pdf. Accessed September 11, 2021.

Ulrich RS, Bogren L, Gardiner SK, Lundin S: Psychiatric ward design can reduce aggressive behavior. J Environ Psychol 57:53–66, 2018

Walsh D: Coming in from the cold: from psychiatric to general hospital. The Irish experience. Epidemiol Psichiatr Soc 15(2):95–98, 2006 16865928

Warner R (ed): Alternatives to the Hospital for Acute Psychiatric Treatment. Washington, DC, American Psychiatric Press, 1995

Ziegelmayer C, Hajak G, Bauer A, et al: Cognitive performance under electroconvulsive therapy (ECT) in ECT-naive treatment-resistant patients with major depressive disorder. J ECT 33(2):104–110, 2017 28169947

Ziegenbein M, Anreis C, Brüggen B, et al: Possible criteria for inpatient psychiatric admissions: which patients are transferred from emergency services to inpatient psychiatric treatment? BMC Health Serv Res 6:150, 2006 17121672

Appendix: Approximate Timeline for an Acute Inpatient Psychiatric Hospitalization

	Day 1—Assessment and crisis management	Day 2—Completion of assessment and initiation of focused treatment	Day 3—Continuation of focused treatment	Day 4—Assessment of safety and discharge readiness	Day 5—Discharge with smooth handoff
Assessment	Physician: take history, conduct examination, make formulation, order laboratory tests, consultations Nursing: assess safety and other needs Social work: contact outpatient team/ collateral informants, determine legal status and resources BEGIN TO DEFINE THE FOCAL PROBLEM: *Why admission here, now?*	Finalize presumptive diagnosis, evaluate laboratory results Define mental/physical health needs, reevaluate safety Monitor safety, vital signs, sleep, nutrition, self-care Complete assessment of legal issues, living and financial needs CLEARLY DEFINE THE FOCAL PROBLEM	Assess physical health and psychopathology Monitor safety, vital signs, self-care, sleep Review progress toward defined target outcomes	Assess patient safety and physical/mental health Assess adequacy of self-care and support needs Evaluate response of target symptoms and needs Assess extent to which focal problem has been addressed	Carefully assess patient safety Repeat physical and mental examination Repeat structured assessments, including rating scales

	Day 1—Assessment and crisis management	Day 2—Completion of assessment and initiation of focused treatment	Day 3—Continuation of focused treatment	Day 4—Assessment of safety and discharge readiness	Day 5—Discharge with smooth handoff
Treatment	**Establish safety and plan for focused intervention** Continue outpatient medications as appropriate Implement safety precautions/monitoring as indicated Plan family/network interventions as appropriate Orient patient to the unit Plan individual therapy as feasible and indicated	Initiate new medication treatment and taper off prior medication as appropriate Use as-needed medications for specific target symptoms as appropriate Implement individual and group therapeutic interventions as appropriate Implement family and other network interventions Implement individualized safety and behavioral/cognitive plan	Continue to implement medication plan Continue group therapy Evaluate effectiveness of and response to interventions Continue family and other network interventions as required Implement medication and other patient education	Complete implementation of medication plan Prepare discharge prescriptions Continue to assess response to various interventions Evaluate learned coping strategies Assess patient and family understanding	Review safety plan Review postdischarge plan with patient and family Continue various interventions as appropriate Dispense postdischarge medications with education
	Finalize and begin definitive interventions **Define aftercare needs and develop a plan to address them**	**Finalize and begin definitive interventions**	**Concretize postdischarge plan**		

	Day 1—Assessment and crisis management	Day 2—Completion of assessment and initiation of focused treatment	Day 3—Continuation of focused treatment	Day 4—Assessment of safety and discharge readiness	Day 5—Discharge with smooth handoff
Discharge planning	Assess follow-up and living arrangements Assess financial stability and need for assistance Assess employment or educational issues Conduct safety evaluation in likely postdischarge setting Assess other specific needs and issues	Address specific post-discharge needs: legal, living, care, fiscal Define approximate length of stay on inpatient unit	Begin to arrange outpatient appointments Identify likely discharge date Coordinate other postdischarge arrangements as necessary	Identify tentative return-to-work/school date and complete necessary paperwork Complete discharge paperwork Confirm appropriate postdischarge living and care arrangements	Reconfirm and document post-discharge follow-up arrangements Complete all aftercare arrangements Review follow-up plan and confirm patient and family understanding **DISCHARGE PATIENT**

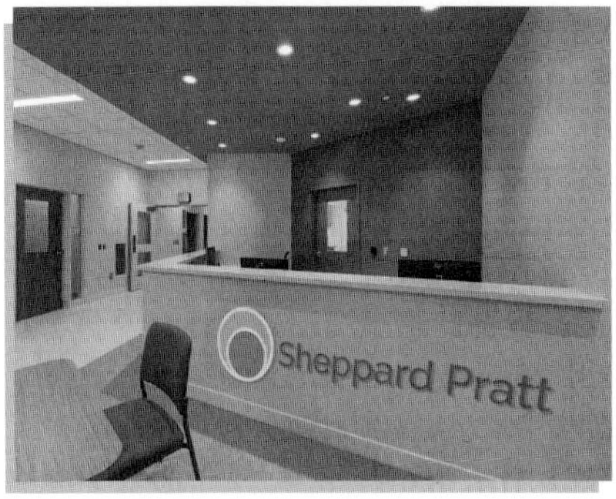

CHAPTER 5

The Geriatric Unit

Caitlin Lawrence, M.D.
Amy Halt, M.D., Ph.D.
Louis Marino, M.D.

Inpatient psychiatric treatment of the elderly requires a transdisciplinary approach for stabilization of this vulnerable and complex population. The most frequently treated psychiatric disturbances on the inpatient unit are depressive disorders and agitation related to dementia. Primary psychotic disorders, bipolar disorder, and delirium are also addressed on the inpatient unit, and personality disorders appear at a lesser frequency. The population served by each geriatric unit may vary according to unit culture and capabilities. Geriatric patients more commonly have complex medical problems that require careful preadmission screening and comanagement with consultative services that may include internal medicine, geriatrics, neurology, palliative care, speech therapy, occupational therapy, neuropsychology, and physical therapy. Use of psychopharmacology in the elderly population requires a tailored approach because of the changes in drug metabolism, higher rates of drug-drug interactions secondary to polypharmacy, and greater sensitivity to side effects. Suicidal ideation is of particular concern in the elderly, given the comparatively high lethality of suicide attempts made by elderly adults compared with younger adults. A particular challenge of inpatient geriatric psychiatry is the assessment and management of agitation in patients with dementia, given the morbidity and mortality related to antipsychotic use in this population. Integration of family into assessment and treatment planning and use of dedicated case management and social work services are essential for supporting patients with extensive aftercare needs. Innovations and reforms will help to improve delivery of effective community-based care to geriatric patients as this population grows.

Admission Criteria

Elderly patients are brought to the psychiatric hospital from a variety of settings, including their residence, assisted living facilities, and nursing homes, or as transfers from inpatient medical facilities. Elderly patients are often hospitalized in medical settings awaiting the availability of a psychiatric bed, and this places them at risk for restraint, drug interactions, and hospital-acquired infections.

Indications for the admission of the geriatric inpatient are similar to those for the admission of adult inpatients and include severe mood and psychotic disorders, with the goals of crisis stabilization, diagnosis, and initiation of treatment. An elderly patient with severe psychiatric symptoms may be particularly vulnerable to weight loss, severe malnourishment, and self-neglect. Elderly patients can be referred for admission for electroconvulsive therapy (ECT) after failed medication trials or intolerable drug-drug interactions or for treatment of severe depression with psychotic features.

The inpatient geriatric unit is uniquely suited for the treatment of neuropsychiatric symptoms of dementia, including psychosis, behavioral disturbance, and aggression. Patients exhibiting violent or uncontrollable behaviors are at risk for harming themselves, their caregivers, or other nursing home residents. Hospitalization may be indicated to increase the level of treatment and provide closer observation. Environmental, behavioral, and pharmacological interventions can be undertaken more intensively in the inpatient setting (American Psychiatric Association 2007). The hospitalization can be an opportunity for planning for discharge to a more supportive living arrangement (Sharfstein 2009).

Suicidal ideation and suicide attempts are strong indicators of the need for admission in the elderly patient. The risk of suicide in people older than 75 years is nearly 30%–40% higher than that in the general population, increases with age, and is most often related to firearm injuries (Kochanek et al. 2019). Suicide attempts in the elderly are significantly more lethal than those in younger adults, with estimates that one in every four attempts results in death (Fremouw et al. 1990). Suicide risk is increased by the presence of psychotic depression, alcoholism, sedative-hypnotic medication use, bereavement, and disability (Alexopoulos et al. 2001).

Some elderly patients are brought to the hospital for assessment of difficult behaviors that may not meet criteria for inpatient admission. If these behaviors do not pose a safety risk and are not interfering with necessary care, alternative strategies for outpatient management may be considered first, including options for caregiver support or enhanced services in the home. Geriatric inpatient psychiatry is a scarce resource. The average length of stay for a geriatric inpatient is over 2 weeks, and the stay is lengthened by receiving ECT, positive psychotic symptoms, falling, pharmacological complications, multiple prior hospitalizations, legal proceedings for treatment, and consultations (Blank et al. 2005).

Evaluation for Medical Stability

There is no universal protocol for medical clearance prior to psychiatric admission, though greater care should be taken with the geriatric patient. Older adults are vulnerable to medical complications; have higher exposure to hospital-acquired infections; have a greater burden from chronic medical illness and complications from polypharmacy; and may not be able to accurately report their symptoms. Medical illness can also present atypically in the elderly—for example, with a blunted or afebrile immune response to infections (Norman 2000), or acute cardiac events that manifest without chest pain (Brieger et al. 2004).

The extent of workup necessary for medical "clearance" of the psychiatric patient remains controversial, although there is a consensus that greater care is taken with the elderly. The goal of this workup is to identify medical illness masquerading as psychiatric symptoms and to identify acute medical issues in complex patients that cannot be appropriately treated on the inpatient psychiatric unit. The minimum medical evaluation should include a thorough medical history, physical examination, brief cognitive examination, and vital signs. Across age groups, a thorough history has a high sensitivity in identifying medical illness in psychiatric patients presenting to an emergency room and outperforms both vital signs and laboratory studies (Olshaker et al. 1997). American Association for Emergency Psychiatry task force consensus guidelines for the medical evaluation of psychiatric patients recommend further screening in patients with any of the following: new-onset psychiatric symptoms after age 45 years, age over 65 years, cognitive deficits or delirium, a positive review of systems indicative of a physical etiology, focal neurological findings or evidence of head injury, substance intoxication or withdrawal, a decreased level of awareness, or other abnormalities in the preliminary assessment (Wilson et al. 2017). Geriatric patients are likely to meet a number of these criteria. Targeted use of urinalysis, complete blood count, basic metabolic panel, liver function tests, urine drug screening, thyroid studies, and chest radiography aids in this medical evaluation, particularly when patients are unable to accurately report symptoms or provide a reliable history. In patients with complaints of pain, anatomical imaging may be indicated, especially in frail elderly patients with recent falls. Electrocardiography is prudent in patients with a cardiac history or cardiopulmonary symptoms or in those taking medications contributing to QT prolongation. Brain imaging may be helpful in patients with recent falls, loss of consciousness, localizing neurological symptoms, seizures, or an acute change in mental status. In complex cases in which a neurological disorder may be driving the psychiatric or behavioral disturbance, consultation with neurology, electroencephalography (EEG), or lumbar puncture may be indicated prior to admission.

Patients with acute mental status changes or a waxing and waning encephalopathy should be screened for delirium and the medical disturbance identified. The occurrence rate of delirium in hospitalized patients is 11%–42% (Siddiqi et al. 2006), although 60%–72% of cases of delirium in elderly patients are unrecognized by the primary treatment team (Collins et al. 2010; de la Cruz et al. 2015). In patients transferring from a general medical setting, acute medical illnesses should be treated and resolving and vital signs stable, and the receiving inpatient psychiatric unit must have the capabilities to continue treatment of any ongoing medical needs. Some geriatric psychiatric units may be better equipped for medical and psychiatric comanagement and can accommodate patients with greater medical needs.

Diagnostic Workup

Assessment of the geriatric inpatient includes attention to psychiatric symptoms, medical illness, cognition, functional status, and psychosocial support. First, a thorough history is taken, including a survey of the patient's history of psychiatric, neurological, and physical signs and symptoms. When patients are unable to provide a full, reliable history, family members and caregivers—ideally the person who is most familiar with the patient—are asked for additional history.

The psychiatric interview should include a mental status examination similar to that used in nonelderly adults, but often with a greater reliance on an assessment of physical appearance, rating scales, and cognitive assessments. Inappropriate attire and poor grooming may indicate poor functioning related to depression, thought disorder, or dementia. Behaviors such as anergia or apathy can be seen in both depression and dementia, while agitation and combativeness may stem from a thought disorder, delirium, or advanced dementia. Rating scales can be useful in identifying mood disturbance when the clinical interview is unclear (Poon 1986). The Geriatric Depression Scale (GDS; Yesavage et al. 1982–1983) is made up of yes-no questions and designed specifically for older adults, though the Hamilton Depression Rating Scale (HDRS; Berrios and Bulbena-Villarasa 1990) and Patient Health Questionnaire–9 (PHQ-9; Kroenke et al. 2001) are also easily utilized. All patients should be observed for responses to internal stimuli and asked about auditory hallucinations, visual hallucinations, and delusions. Perceptual disturbance can manifest not only in thought disorders but also in dementia and delirium and in patients experiencing sensory deprivation.

The medical history of the elderly patient is often complex, and recent medical illnesses may be contributing to a patient's presentation. A full list of prescribed medications, over-the-counter pills, and supplements is assessed for compliance, drug-drug interactions, and side effects, especially in the patient presenting with confusion or falls. Medication-induced causes of confusion, sedation, and mood disturbances are not uncommon. Opioid and benzodiazepine medications are used at greater frequency in the elderly than in younger patients (Han et al. 2017; Olfson et al. 2015). The Beers criteria medication list identifies opioids, sedative-hypnotics, antidepressants, and antiepileptic medications as contributors to falls, and anticholinergic medications as contributors to confusion, constipation, and other symptoms of anticholinergic toxicity (American Geriatrics Society Beers Criteria Update Expert Panel 2019).

Obtaining the patient's past psychiatric history is focused on determining early- versus late-onset mood and psychotic disorders and identifying both substance use and prior suicide attempts. A full family history takes into consideration psychiatric disorders, neurodegenerative illness, and suicide attempts. In patients undergoing workup for cognitive disorders, attention is paid to family members with prior diagnoses of dementia, elucidating early- versus late-onset symptoms, neuropsychiatric manifestations of the illness, and progression. The social history includes a targeted assessment of social network, family involvement, the extent of support in the living arrangements, financial issues, spirituality, and issues of loss and bereavement. With the help of a caregiver, the patient is assessed for their ability to participate in activities of daily living (ADLs) like grooming, toileting, and eating, and instrumental activities of daily living (IADLs) like driving, medication management, and financial management. The ADL assessment can include the use of standardized rating scales like the Lawton Instrumental Activities of Daily Living Scale (Lawton and Brody 1969).

Geriatric patients should have an objective assessment of cognition, especially when an undiagnosed cognitive disorder is being considered. The Mini-Mental State Examination (MMSE) and the Montreal Cognitive Assessment (MoCA; Nasreddine et al. 2005) are frequently used in geriatric psychiatry, although a variety of other methods can be utilized. The MMSE takes only 5–10 minutes to complete and examines registration, attention, calculation, recall, language, orientation, and ability to follow commands (Folstein et al. 1975). It is less sensitive to mild cognitive impairment and may not adequately measure visuospatial and executive function, and its results are impacted by demographics like age and education (Crum et al. 1993; Wind et al. 1997). The MoCA includes measures of short-term recall, visuospatial abilities, executive functions, attention, concentration, working memory, language, and orientation (Nasreddine et al. 2005). This test has a high sensitivity for detecting dementia, but also a high false positive rate (Davis et al. 2015). Some geriatric psychiatrists utilize the Clinical Dementia Rating (CDR) Scale, which uses patient and caregiver interviews to assess memory, orientation, judgment, problem solving, community affairs, home, hobbies, and personal care (Hughes et al. 1982). There are a number of other cognitive screening measures that may be used. Formal neuropsychology testing may aid in determining the presence, etiology, and severity of dementia when diagnostic clarification is needed and especially when deficits are mild or a rare cause of dementia is suspected. In patients with a known diagnosis of dementia, the etiology (e.g., Alzheimer's disease, vascular dementia, alcohol-related dementia, frontotemporal dementia, dementia with Lewy bodies), its clinical course, and treatment history are appraised.

Risk assessment of the geriatric patient exceeds that of a typical adult patient. Psychiatrists must fully assess suicidal and homicidal thoughts and recognize the higher rate of lethality of suicide attempts in the elderly. Additionally, there is careful consideration of the patient's ability to safely manage at home, considering the potential for accidents in daily activities like cooking, managing stairs, taking medications, and driving. Occupational therapy and physical therapy assessments are integral to this process.

If not completed during a preadmission workup, targeted diagnostic laboratory tests aid in the diagnosis of medical issues contributing to psychiatric symptoms. Chronic and acute medical illnesses are identified with a full medical history and physical examination, and laboratory abnormalities are scrutinized as potential contributors to psychiatric symptoms. Nutrition status is assessed, with attention to recent weight loss, anorexia, or difficulties with oral intake. A swallowing evaluation aids in diagnosis and dietary modifications in patients with dysphagia. Ambulatory status, postural vital signs, and fall risk are evaluated immediately. In patients undergoing a workup for cognitive impairment, labs may include a complete blood count, thyroid function tests, liver function tests, vitamin B_{12} level, antibody screens for HIV and syphilis (if risk factors are present), and in some cases, neuroimaging (American Academy of Neurology 2004). In patients with focal neurological symptoms, seizure-like episodes, or a rapidly progressive change in mental status, brain imaging, EEG, or lumbar puncture may be warranted, which can necessitate workup in a medical setting.

When the patient lacks capacity or willingness to engage in treatment and has a guardian or a power of attorney for medical decision-making, the surrogate is involved in the diagnostic workup and treatment planning.

Treatment Considerations

Beyond diagnostic evaluation and psychopharmacology, successful inpatient treatment of the elderly relies on environment design and integration of a transdisciplinary team into treatment planning. There are a number of resources available to meet the needs of the geriatric inpatient. Each geriatric unit will have its own milieu, goals, and culture for treatment, which will guide how ancillary treatment strategies and professionals are integrated into care, drawing from the resources most appropriate for each patient.

Environment Design

Ideally, a geriatric unit is designed to minimize fall risk, decrease overwhelming stimuli, promote engagement in daily activities, and enhance orientation. Units should be well lit to best support patients with visual impairment from cataracts, glaucoma, or macular degeneration. A calming, consistent color palette may decrease confusion and agitation. Patients are frequently oriented to their surroundings by staff, with the help of clocks, calendars, and exposure to daylight. Furniture should be arranged to decrease hazards for ambulatory patients. Efforts are made to encourage the use of communal areas for groups and meals. Patients receive assistance for grooming and hygiene, which may have been poorly attended to outside the hospital. Patients have access to appropriate devices to assist with ambulation and toileting, and furniture that can accommodate mobility issues.

Transdisciplinary Team

Assessment and treatment of the geriatric patient require collaboration between psychiatrists, nursing, physical therapy, occupational therapy, social work, and milieu therapists, who work together to identify solutions for each patient.

Elderly patients with social withdrawal or difficult behaviors benefit from supportive engagement from this transdisciplinary team. In dementia and late-life mood disorders, a patient may experience a reduction of activity levels and difficulty participating in ADLs, which can perpetuate confusion, weakness, depression, and agitation. Nonpharmacological approaches are recommended as the first-line treatment for managing behavioral symptoms in elderly patients with dementia and may reduce the use of polypharmacy for behavioral symptoms (Lyketsos et al. 2006). Patients may respond well to structure, reassurance, and distraction. Recreational activities such as music therapy, exercise, pet therapy, and simple cognitive exercises such as trivia or Bingo can help engage patients during inpatient treatment and facilitate appropriate involvement in a social setting (Grossberg and Desai 2003). Family members can aid in the identification of preferred activities, and recreational activities can be modified based on the capabilities of each patient. Cognitive stimulation and caregiver education can have lasting effectiveness for managing neuropsychiatric symptoms (Livingston et al. 2005). Although some professionals have questioned the ethics of the practice, providing dolls or plush toys to select patients living with dementia can improve engagement, enhance communication, and reduce distress (Mitchell and O'Donnell 2013).

Occupational therapy is an integral component of inpatient geriatric treatment. Occupational therapists often aid in the assessment of a patient's cognitive and functional skills and identify areas of concern that are pertinent for safe discharge planning. Occupational therapy interventions are designed to enhance the patient's remaining capabilities and to provide caregivers with skills to manage difficult situations (Miller and Butin 2000).

Patients may have weakness and muscle wasting as a result of sedentary behaviors. Physical therapists assess the ability of each patient to ambulate safely, taking into consideration physical limitations, confusion, and agitation. Physical therapists can recommend assistive devices, provide structured rehabilitation for regaining strength and mobility while on the unit, and recommend appropriate aftercare for continued rehabilitation. Physical therapists help identify when issues of agitation, confusion, and difficult behavior place patients at risk for falls or injury.

A growing number of elderly patients suffer from dysphagia related to cerebrovascular events or progressive dementia. Speech and language pathologists provide assessment of swallowing and recommendations for dietary modifications to reduce choking or aspiration risks. Nutritionists can assess each patient's nutritional needs and assist with strategies for optimizing the nutrition of vulnerable patients who have lost weight or are having difficulty eating.

Medical Consultation

Compared with younger adults, geriatric patients have a greater need for medical comanagement of underlying medical issues that complicate psychiatric treatment during an inpatient admission. Frailty, mobility issues, and use of psychotropic medications place patients at greater risk of falls and associated injuries. Elderly patients with complex medical histories are at high risk for polypharmacy, which may be contributing to difficulties with alertness, ambulation, or orientation. Sedentary patients may require specialized medical care, including considerations for anticoagulation. Aging patients with depression and comorbid medical illnesses can often present with recurrent somatic complaints (Drayer et al. 2005) that may be difficult to interpret and may benefit from a transdisciplinary approach. Some patients have changes in their mental status or character of unclear etiology, and benefit from a careful physical examination that may exceed the capabilities of a typical geriatric psychiatrist.

A dedicated team of physicians must coordinate their efforts to continue the balance of health within this delicate population. There are multiple models that can be utilized to provide integrated care, including comanagement on dual medical-psychiatric units and the utilization of medical consultants. Forming a treatment relationship with a team of internal medicine or geriatric medicine providers can facilitate timely recognition and treatment of evolving medical issues, aid in the treatment of delirium, help in the management of pain, and appraise or reduce polypharmacy. Palliative care consultation may also provide patients and families with assistance in determining goals of care and can be of particular importance in the assessment of patients with advanced dementia. Patients with advanced dementia have a high mortality rate in the months and years after psychiatric hospitalization (Chen et al. 2018) and may be admitted with behavioral symptoms related to terminal agitation. In these cases, coordination with palliative and hospice care can be of particular benefit for patients and families.

Caregiver Involvement

To the extent that is possible and helpful for each patient, visits from close supports are encouraged, which can improve a patient's orientation and adjustment to the unit. Caregivers are often needed to provide a history for each patient, identify areas of concern, and assist in the assessment of response to intervention, and are necessary contributors to discharge planning. There is a high prevalence of depression, anxiety, and burnout in caregivers, who may also have higher rates of physical illness (Schulz et al. 1995). The hospitalization can be an opportunity for providing families with education regarding diagnosis and treatment, and referrals for additional support. Well-designed caregiver support programs can increase caregiver knowledge and potentially reduce levels of caregiver burden and depression (Belle et al. 2003; Gitlin et al. 2003; Sörensen et al. 2002). There are significantly more resources tailored for supporting caregivers of patients with dementia compared with caregivers of those with late-life mood disorders or other psychiatric disturbance (Schulz et al. 2005).

Diagnosis and Treatment of Specific Disorders

Late-Life Depression

Major Depressive Disorder in Elderly Adults

DSM-5 diagnostic criteria for major depressive disorder in elderly adults do not differ from those in younger adults (American Psychiatric Association 2013), although the presentation of depression in the elderly can be more nuanced. Recognizing symptoms of geriatric depression can be challenging, given that older patients often underreport symptoms related to mood and depression (Gallo and Rabins 1999) and may focus instead on anhedonia or somatic complaints. Compared with younger adults with depression, geriatric patients frequently describe somatic complaints relating to poor sleep, low energy, poor appetite, and weight loss. There may be a tendency for providers and patients to overattribute these physical complaints to medical illness. Most patients do have physical symptoms that stem from medical illness, but their experiences are intensified by depression (Alexopoulos et al. 2002a). When it is difficult to establish the diagnosis of depression, better clarity can be reached by querying symptoms of anhedonia, social isolation, hopelessness, helplessness, worthlessness, guilt, psychomotor changes, and impaired decision-making and planning abilities (Alexopoulos et al. 2002b). In elderly depressed patients without dementia, there can be deficits in attention, processing speed, and executive function that may persist even after the remission of depression (Elderkin-Thompson et al. 2003; Kindermann et al. 2000; Lockwood et al. 2002). Psychotic features may be present in nearly one-half of geriatric inpatients with depression (Meyers 1995) but are often misdiagnosed or unrecognized (Rothschild et al. 2008). Psychotic features are most commonly delusions, particularly somatic, guilty, nihilistic, and persecutory (Alexopoulos et al. 2004).

It can be difficult to classify early versus late onset of depressive illness, and this classification may not be particularly useful for guiding treatment. There are additional syndromes of late-life depression that are not specifically included in the current DSM classification but have importance for treatment.

Depression With Reversible Dementia

A high proportion of geriatric patients with depression carry a risk of reversible dementia, which has sometimes been termed *pseudodementia.* For most patients, the cognitive impairment improves with remission of depression, although many patients continue to experience some level of dysfunction, and 40% will eventually develop an irreversible dementia within the next 3 years (Alexopoulos et al. 1993).

Vascular Depression

Cerebrovascular disease is viewed as a potential contributor to a particular phenotype of depression characterized by increased apathy, psychomotor retardation, poor insight, greater disability, and cognitive impairment (Alexopoulos et al. 1997a; Krishnan et al. 1997). These patients typically experience less guilt and agitation than depressed patients without cerebrovascular disease. Cognitive testing often shows impairments particularly in verbal fluency and object naming (Alexopoulos et al. 1997a). These patients may benefit from antidepressants that improve ischemic recovery through dopaminergic or noradrenergic properties (Alexopoulos et al. 1997b). Treatment of any underlying vascular disease and reduction of vascular risk are also of benefit.

Depression–Executive Dysfunction Syndrome

The depression–executive dysfunction syndrome is seen in a subset of patients with fronto-striatal-limbic system dysfunction. The syndrome is characterized by psychomotor retardation, decreased interest in activities, suspiciousness, and impairment in IADLs, but a relative sparing of neurovegetative symptoms. Patients with this syndrome do not respond as well to antidepressants as those with other subsets of depression (Alexopoulos et al. 2001, 2002b, 2005; Potter et al. 2004).

Depression can be more intimately related to health in late life and is frequently correlated with poor outcomes and disease-related complications. In older adults, depression is associated with weight loss (Morley and Kraenzle 1994), cardiovascular disease (Frasure-Smith et al. 1993), increased mortality after myocardial infarction (Romanelli et al. 2002), heart failure (Williams et al. 2002), poor self-rated health (Han 2002), and poor functional outcomes after stroke (Pohjasvaara et al. 2001). Depression is closely associated with functional impairment (Zeiss et al. 1996) and disability (Bruce 2001; Penninx et al. 1999). The transdisciplinary approach to treatment on the geriatric unit is well suited for identifying and managing these comorbidities.

Treatment of Major Depressive Disorder Without Psychotic Features

Geriatric inpatients with depression will often have moderate to severe illness, with or without psychotic features. First-line options for treatment of depression without psychotic features include pharmacotherapy alone and combination pharmacotherapy and psychotherapy. Elderly adults should be started with a trial of a single antidepressant. If there is partial response, augmentation strategies are tried. If there is no response to the first antidepressant, a trial of another antidepressant monotherapy should follow. Generally, if the first antidepressant trialed is inefficacious or only partially efficacious, conclusions about efficacy gained through the STAR*D study are likely applicable to the treatment of older adults; the mechanism of action of the subsequent antidepressant strategy may not preferentially affect response (Rush et al. 2006). Most antidepressants are similarly effective for treating major depression (Salzman et al. 2002). Attention to the side-effect profile and drug interactions of the medication may be of greater significance for selecting an appropriate antidepressant for each individual. Antidepressants are frequent inhibitors of cytochrome P450 isozymes, particularly 3A4, 2D6, 1A2, and 2C9.

Selective serotonin reuptake inhibitors (SSRIs) are preferred antidepressants in older adults when compared with tricyclic antidepressants (TCAs), given the former's more favorable side-effect profile (Mulsant et al. 2001a), relative safety in overdose, and lack of cardiovascular effects. There is also evidence for antidepressant use in vascular depression (Salloway et al. 2002). However, there are risks of SSRI use in the elderly. Daily SSRI use is associated with an increased risk of falls and double the risk of fragility fractures (Richards et al. 2007). The risk of suicide in elderly patients approaches a fivefold increase in the month after SSRI treatment is started (Juurlink et al. 2006), but at least part of this risk is postulated to be attributable to the underlying depressive illness. Patients should be monitored for suicidality closely in the first month of treatment. Citalopram, escitalopram, and sertraline may be preferred in some geriatric patients with a high burden of medical illness or polypharmacy, owing to the relatively lower potential for drug-drug interactions. Selective serotonin-norepinephrine reuptake inhibitors (SNRIs) are also regarded as first-line agents, although they require monitoring for elevation in blood pressure, which has been seen in both immediate- and extended-release formulations and is dose dependent (Staab and Evans 2000; Thase 1998). Elderly patients taking SSRIs or SNRIs are at risk for serotonin syndrome (Gillman 1999), gastrointestinal bleeding (de Abajo et al. 1999), and hyponatremia related to the syndrome of inappropriate secretion of antidiuretic hormone (SIADH) (Bouman et al. 1998). Bupropion, mirtazapine, and TCAs can also be used, though TCAs should be avoided in patients with cardiac conduction defects. Nortriptyline and desipramine are preferred over doxepin, imipramine, and amitriptyline because of their more favorable side-effect profiles. Patients taking TCAs benefit from monitoring of drug levels, postural vital signs, and electrocardiographic changes. Trazodone monotherapy for depression is generally avoided in the geriatric population.

ECT is an effective alternative treatment strategy in the elderly (Tew et al. 1999) and is considered safe in patients with comorbid medical conditions (Alexopoulos et al. 2004). ECT should be considered in patients who have had two adequate antidepressant trials that have failed, are at acute risk of suicide, and have medical comorbidities complicating antidepressant medication treatment. In the immediate phase, patients may experience deficits across neuropsychological domains, including language, processing speed, autobiographical memory, and cognitive flexibility (Lisanby et al. 2019). Though still in investigational stages, repetitive transcranial magnetic stimulation is also emerging as a possible safe and effective treatment in late-life depression, and elderly patients may have a more robust response compared to younger adults (Desbeaumes Jodoin et al. 2019; Iriarte and George 2018; McDonald 2016).

Treatment of Unipolar Major Depressive Disorder With Psychotic Features

Expert guidelines recommend treatment of major depression with psychotic features using either ECT or combination pharmacotherapy with an antidepressant and antipsychotic (American Psychiatric Association 2000; National Institute for Clinical Excellence 2004). Historically, there were inadequate data to support the use of combination therapy in elderly adults, because early studies using TCA and antipsychotic combination therapy did not show efficacy in the geriatric population (Mulsant et al. 2001b; Wijkstra et al. 2006). Newer trials have preferentially studied a second-generation antipsychotic with an SSRI or SNRI. The Study of the Pharmacotherapy of Psychotic Depression (STOP-PD) established the superiority of combined treatment with olanzapine and sertraline over antipsychotic monotherapy for remission of psychotic depression in both younger adults and older adults in the acute phase of treatment. Older adults also had less weight gain and lower increases in glucose levels than younger patients with this treatment (Meyers et al. 2009). There is evidence of benefit of combined treatment in the outpatient setting even after remission of symptoms in order to prevent relapse (Flint et al. 2019). Stabilization of depression with psychotic features can also improve cognitive dysfunction, especially in elderly patients under 70 years old (Victoria et al. 2017). Preferred antidepressants continue to be SSRIs and SNRIs for elderly patients with psychotic depression, and antipsychotics are considered based on side-effect profiles and drug interactions. Although guidelines differ on when to consider ECT in comparison to medication treatment given the relative lack of controlled trials (Rothschild 2013), ECT can be associated with a higher recovery rate in older patients with psychotic depression (Flint and Rifat 1998).

Bipolar Disorder

Bipolar Disorder in Elderly Adults

Elderly patients with bipolar disorder have a greater nonsuicide mortality rate and a higher likelihood of inpatient admission compared with elderly patients with unipolar depression (Bartels et al. 2000; Shulman et al. 1992). Compared with younger patients with bipolar disorder, older patients are less likely to have comorbid substance use disorders but have significantly greater functional impairment, cognitive impairment, confusion, and disorientation (Depp and Jeste 2004).

Generally, the prevalence of bipolar disorder decreases with age, and there are distinctions in early- versus late-onset bipolar illness. Consensus on defining late-onset bipolar disorder is mixed, though most investigators draw the distinction for late-onset illness anywhere between 40 and 65 years (Almeida and Fenner 2002; Schürhoff et al. 2000). In any geriatric patient presenting with late-onset manic symptoms, there should be a careful evaluation for secondary mania that may be caused by a general medical illness or medication effect. Antidepressants, sympathomimetics, dopaminergic medications for Parkinson's disease, corticosteroids, and benzodiazepines can all contribute to mania (Sajatovic et al. 2005). Patients with late-onset bipolar disorder are less likely to have a family history of bipolar disorder and more likely to have neurological disease, and have significantly greater vascular risk factors like hypertension, cerebrovascular accidents, coronary artery disease, atrial fibrillation, diabetes, and hyperlipidemia (Cassidy and Carroll 2002). Neuroimaging studies have shown a higher burden of frontal deep white matter changes in elderly patients with bipolar disorder and have suggested that a greater intensity of these changes may be associated with late-onset mania (de Asis et al. 2006), lending support to the hypothesis that vascular disease is a potential etiology or risk factor for late-onset bipolar disorder. Any patient with late-onset bipolar disorder should have a careful assessment of vascular risk, followed by well-managed treatment of hypertension, vascular disease, and diabetes.

Compared with patients with late-onset bipolar illness, elderly patients with early-onset manic symptoms are more likely to have a positive family history of bipolar disorder, a history of medication nonadherence, aggressive or threatening behavior, or a need for emergency petition for hospitalization (Lehmann and Rabins 2006).

Treatment of Bipolar Disorder in Older Adults

Until recently, treatment of late-life bipolar disorder was based primarily on uncontrolled trials. While lithium and divalproex were the most common agents studied, there were few evidence-based guidelines for dosing strategies or concentration targets.

The GERI-BD trial was the first randomized, double-blind controlled trial assessing the pharmacological treatment of mania in older patients with bipolar disorder and suggested that both lithium and divalproex monotherapy can be effective in treating elderly patients with mania, hypomania, or mixed episodes. Substantial response and remission rates were achieved with relatively lower serum concentrations (0.8–0.99 mEq/L for lithium, 80–99 µg/mL for valproex) compared with those used in younger adults, although there was a greater reduction in mania severity in patients treated with lithium. Rates of side effects (i.e., sedation, tremor, weight gain, nausea, vomiting) were similar between groups. Most patients were stabilized without the addition of an antipsychotic medication (Young et al. 2017). Lithium has traditionally been considered a preferred agent secondary to its possible neuroprotective effects (Kessing et al. 2008) and properties in reducing suicide rates (Cipriani et al. 2013). Use of lithium should be considered in the context of the patient's medical comorbidities and potential drug-drug interactions, particularly renal disease and use of antihypertensives, nonsteroidal anti-inflammatory drugs, and angiotensin converting enzyme inhibitors. Patients taking lithium will need long-term monitoring of drug levels, kidney function, thyroid function, and electrolytes.

Experts have also identified carbamazepine as a second-line treatment for bipolar mania, though this medication can be difficult to manage in the elderly, given the risks of neurological side effects (e.g., dizziness, vertigo, ataxia, cognitive impairment), cardiac conduction abnormalities, bradyarrhythmias, rashes, and blood dyscrasias; the high rate of drug-drug interactions; and the need for dose increases due to autoinduction (Aziz et al. 2006).

There is a significant gap in the evidence base for treatment of geriatric bipolar depression. The FDA-approved medications (i.e., quetiapine, lurasidone, and combination therapy with olanzapine and fluoxetine) have not been well studied in elderly adults. Generally, lithium monotherapy is preferred. Lamotrigine can be considered when added to lithium or divalproex (Robillard and Conn 2002). If necessary, an antidepressant can be added, though antidepressant monotherapy is not advised.

There are no current studies comparing ECT and pharmacotherapy in elderly patients with bipolar disorder. ECT can be considered in both depressive and manic phases of geriatric bipolar disorder and may be a preferred method in treating severely ill or rapidly deteriorating patients, for whom a rapid response is necessary; in patients who cannot tolerate the side effects of pharmacotherapy; or in patients in whom the relative risk from pharmacotherapy is greater than that from ECT (Young et al. 2004).

Schizophrenia

Schizophrenia in Elderly Adults

Schizophrenia is becoming increasingly common in the aging population, with adults over 55 representing nearly one-quarter of individuals with schizophrenia (Cohen et al. 2008). From a population perspective, health care systems are not prepared to support this growing population. Elderly adults with schizophrenia live in community settings, long-term hospitals, or nursing homes, but those in the latter two categories appear to have worse symptom control and cognitive deficits. While the DSM and ICD criteria do not currently make this distinction, the psychiatric community has often conceptualized distinctions in early-onset schizophrenia, late-onset schizophrenia, and very-late-onset schizophrenia-like psychosis (Howard et al. 2000). Although these distinctions certainly may not apply to each patient, older patients with early-onset schizophrenia have negative symptoms that can fluctuate over time and may have some stabilization of positive symptoms in later life. Late-onset schizophrenia resembles early-onset schizophrenia, with symptoms arising between age 40 and age 60, often with a female predominance, lower symptom severity, and less executive dysfunction. Very-late-onset schizophrenia-like psychosis is markedly more prevalent in women, and symptom onset occurs after age 60. There is a higher prevalence of persecutory and partition delusions and more frequent visual, tactile, and olfactory hallucinations. Negative symptoms are rare, and there is a paucity of other symptoms of thought disorder (Maglione et al. 2014). The diagnosis of late-onset schizophrenia is particularly challenging given the potential for other etiologies of psychosis in the aging population, including mood disorders, sensory dysfunction, medication effects, medical disorders, and dementia.

For any cases of new-onset schizophrenia in late life, other causes of psychosis should first be considered. For patients presenting with predominant hallucinations, providers should screen for visual impairment, hearing impairment, or localized brain lesions in centers affecting perception. Dementia with Lewy bodies may also be considered in patients with vivid visual hallucinations. Patients should routinely be assessed for cognitive impairment, because hallucinations, delusions, and other forms of psychosis occur with increasing frequency across dementia diagnoses. A severe mood disorder could also be entertained, given the higher incidence of psychotic features in elderly patients with depression compared with younger adults. Finally, an unrecognized delirium should be considered, especially when psychotic symptoms appear to be waxing and waning.

Elderly patients with schizophrenia have greater medical needs relative to age-matched peers, making integration of medical assessment into treatment of particular importance (Bartels 2004). An early diagnosis of schizophrenia confers a shortened life expectancy by over 20 years (Tiihonen et al. 2009), a two- to three-times increased risk of mortality, and a high prevalence of cardiovascular disease, diabetes, and metabolic syndrome. Medical needs are often unmet or undertreated because of medication nonadherence, lower health literacy, or potential bias within health care settings (Cohen et al. 2015).

Nearly half of patients with schizophrenia have symptoms that likely meet criteria for mild dementia (Evans et al. 1999). Even early-onset schizophrenia can cause marked cognitive impairment (Howard et al. 2000). Most cognitive deficits appear to date back to early in the disease course and can be worsened with age-related cognitive decline, although a small subset of patients in community samples have shown a rapid cognitive decline in later life (Thompson et al. 2013). There is interest in the potential use of biomarkers to help differentiate dementia from schizophrenia, especially in cases of late-onset or very-late-onset psychotic illness.

Treatment of Schizophrenia in Older Adults

Evidence-based research on pharmacological treatment of older adults with schizophrenia is limited (Cohen et al. 2015). The mainstay of treatment is the use of antipsychotic medications. All antipsychotic medications carry an increased risk of cardiovascular adverse events and noncardiovascular mortality when used in elderly patients, although cardiovascular adverse events appeared greatest in the first few months after initiation of antipsychotic treatment, and when these medications were used in elderly patients with dementia or preexisting cardiovascular disease (Sahlberg et al. 2015). When one is making the decision to start an antipsychotic medication, this risk must be weighed in consideration of the efficacy of antipsychotic medications for improving psychosis and quality of life in patients with schizophrenia. Because of a paucity of research, two recent Cochrane reviews were unable to identify enough evidence to guide treatment recommendations for the most appropriate drug to prescribe in elderly patients with schizophrenia (Marriott et al. 2006) or late-onset schizophrenia (Essali and Ali 2012), making expert opinion the best driver of treatment. Generally, older adults with schizophrenia require intermediate doses of antipsychotic medications compared with their younger counterparts. Consensus guidelines favor use of risperidone at 1.25–3.5 mg/day, followed by quetiapine 100–300 mg/day, olanzapine 7.5–15 mg/day, or aripiprazole 15–30 mg/day (Alexopoulos et al. 2004), although medication selection should be determined on the basis of the unique characteristics of each patient. Use of any medications, and especially antipsychotic medications, should be undertaken with extra care in the elderly, given the higher risk of drug-drug interactions and the physiological changes that alter the concentrations, clearance, and volume of distribution of medication (Pollock 1998). Patients who have developed renal failure, heart failure, arrhythmias, and movement disorders such as Parkinson's disease may be particularly vulnerable to side effects. Generally, the following guiding principles, outlined by Klimstra et al. (2009), can be applied:

1. The "start low and go slow" approach will apply differently for each patient. Elderly patients often are more sensitive to side effects even at lower concentrations. Consideration of a patient's age, comorbid illnesses, and general state of health will help guide initiation and titration.
2. Initiation of the medication and titration should be based on a patient's diagnosis and assessment of target dosing. Use of neuroleptics is diagnosis dependent. Elderly patients with schizophrenia will require lower target doses of neuroleptics than will younger adults, and patients with dementia-related psychosis will require even lower doses (Alexopoulos et al. 2004; Madhusoodanan et al. 2007).
3. Drug-drug and drug-disease interaction checkers should be routinely used before any addition of a new medication.

4. Routine use of as-needed medications should be reviewed often and minimized when possible. As-needed medications can lead to inappropriate accumulation of drug levels and can also cloud the treatment plan.

Older adults are more prone to side effects of antipsychotic medications than are younger adults and should be carefully screened for tardive dyskinesia, QTc prolongation, and metabolic side effects. Given that many patients do not achieve full remission of symptoms with medications alone, there is support for referral to cognitive remediation, social skills therapy, and cognitive-behavioral therapy when appropriate. All elderly patients with schizophrenia will require social services on discharge.

Dementia With Behavioral Disturbance

Neuropsychiatric Symptoms of Dementia

Nearly half of elderly patients older than age 85 have been diagnosed with dementia, most commonly dementia related to Alzheimer's disease, vascular dementia, or dementia with Lewy bodies (Rahkonen et al. 2003; Small et al. 1997). Noncognitive and neuropsychiatric symptoms of dementia occur in 60%–90% of patients and include agitation, aggression, delusions, hallucinations, yelling or vocalizations, and wandering. These symptoms more commonly occur in moderate to advanced disease and are associated with caregiver stress, depression, underemployment, and lost income (Borson and Raskind 1997; Clyburn et al. 2000; Coen et al. 1997; Nagaratnam et al. 1998). Neuropsychiatric symptoms can lead to nursing home placement and are estimated to directly contribute to 30% of the cost of caring for patients with Alzheimer's disease (Beeri et al. 2002). Still, there is no defined standard of care for treatment of neuropsychiatric symptoms of dementia.

Psychotic symptoms are very common across dementia diagnoses. In Alzheimer's disease, 41% of patients exhibit psychosis, commonly visual hallucinations and delusions, which are most often paranoid in nature, involving the misidentification of people and perception of theft. In Alzheimer's disease, psychosis seems to improve as the disease progresses, although it is unclear if this happens because patients lose the ability to communicate these symptoms. While 43% of patients with Parkinson's disease without dementia have psychosis, this grows to 89% in patients with dementia related to Parkinson's disease. Visual hallucinations in Parkinson's disease are usually stereotyped and nonfrightening, while delusions are less common but tend to be paranoid in nature. In dementia with Lewy bodies, well-formed and nonfrightening visual hallucinations start early in the disease course (Colijn et al. 2015).

Inpatient admission for patients with dementia is reserved for those whose behavior puts them at risk of harm to themselves or others or has contributed to a significant decline in functioning. There must be a careful review of potential contributors to the problematic behaviors. Common causes of agitation in patients with dementia include delirium, depression, psychosis, dysuria, dyspnea, discomfort related to constipation, and pruritus (Alexopoulos et al. 2004, 2005), although in some cases an etiology cannot be identified. For all patients, a careful physical examination, identification of an acute mental status decline, and standard laboratory evaluation including complete blood count, complete metabolic panel, urinalysis, and urine culture must be completed (Steinberg et al. 2012). When pain, delirium, or other medical etiologies of agitation are identified, their treatment becomes the obvious first step in care.

Treatment of Neuropsychiatric Symptoms of Dementia

Addressing neuropsychiatric symptoms of dementia remains a challenging part of inpatient psychiatric care. Medication treatments have only modest efficacy and carry a high risk of adverse effects and even death. Nonpharmacological behavioral interventions should be trialed first, and pharmacotherapy should be considered only after these have failed (Salzman et al. 2008). Environmental overstimulation or understimulation, space restriction, and caregiver behaviors are easily modifiable targets for intervention (Cohen-Mansfield 2001). Patients may improve when their hearing and vision are optimized, care is provided in more supportive tone, or alternative means of communication (i.e., nonverbal) are used (Klimstra et al. 2009). Structured social and recreational activities, music therapy, sensory stimulation, and caregiver/staff education can be helpful approaches. Unfortunately, only 5% of research studies utilizing nonpharmacological interventions used in a long-term-care setting showed statistically and clinically significant outcomes (Seitz et al. 2012), leading to concern that there are difficulties translating behavioral interventions into consistently meaningful real-world practice (Kales et al. 2014). Studies utilizing a person-centered approach have been most encouraging.

When depressive symptoms are present in the agitated patient, an antidepressant trial can be considered. SSRIs may not reliably improve acute agitation but can help prevent future episodes of agitation. In the Citalopram for Agitation in Alzheimer Disease Study (CitAD)—a randomized, placebo-controlled, double-blind trial—citalopram titrated to 30 mg/day outperformed placebo for reducing agitation in patients with Alzheimer dementia (Porsteinsson et al. 2014). These results may translate to other antidepressants. SSRIs are usually the preferred antidepressants given their tolerability and efficacy, although a person-centered approach to selecting an antidepressant is prudent. For example, there is mounting evidence that SNRIs and noradrenergic TCAs may have equal or better efficacy in treating patients with depression related to Parkinson's disease, although side effects must be carefully considered (Seppi et al. 2019).

Untreated, unreported pain is an easily modifiable contributor to reduced quality of life, dysphoria, isolation, and agitation in patients with dementia. Even in patients who are not reporting pain, regularly scheduled acetaminophen is a low-risk and effective intervention for improving social interaction and engagement (Chibnall et al. 2005).

Cognitive enhancers such as acetylcholinesterase inhibitors are not helpful for acute control of behavioral disturbance. However, in the long term, acetylcholinesterase inhibitors (Rösler 2002) and the NMDA receptor antagonist memantine (Wilcock et al. 2008) may improve behavioral and psychological symptoms of dementia and potentially reduce the need for psychotropic medications.

When agitation has not improved with environmental measures or other treatments, atypical antipsychotics can be considered and may be most efficacious in patients with psychosis. Atypical antipsychotics show a modest benefit for neuropsychiatric symptoms of dementia (Katz et al. 1999; Street et al. 2000; Streim et al. 2008). The Clinical Antipsychotic Trials of Intervention Effectiveness—Alzheimer's Disease (CATIE-AD) indicated that symptoms like anger, aggression, and paranoid ideas were likely to improve with the atypical antipsychotics studied (risperidone, olanzapine, quetiapine) when compared with placebo (Sultzer et al. 2008), and that risperidone and olanzapine outperformed placebo in an analysis of discontinuation due to lack of efficacy (Schneider et al. 2006b). Typical antipsychotics are considered to pose a greater safety risk and are not preferentially offered over atypical antipsychotics. In patients with dementia, side effects are minimized by starting at the lowest possible doses with a very slow titration, typically with target dose ranges of 0.25–1 mg of risperidone, 2.5–7.5 mg of olanzapine, 12.5–150 mg of quetiapine, and 5–10 mg of aripiprazole (Steinberg and Lyketsos 2012). Chemistry profile, lipid profile, fasting blood glucose or hemoglobin A_{1c}, and weight should be assessed at baseline, 3 months, 6 months, and then every 6 months after starting treatment. ECG monitoring for assessment of QTc prolongation may be necessary, especially in patients with a history of cardiovascular illness or QTc prolongation (Trifirò et al. 2009). In the inpatient setting, patients should be assessed frequently for response, and medication should be discontinued or switched if not efficacious within a target dose range.

Antipsychotics must be used cautiously because of the risks of metabolic side effects, increased cardiovascular events, and increased noncardiovascular mortality, particularly in elderly patients with dementia (Sahlberg et al. 2015). Antipsychotics carry a black box warning from the FDA for use in elderly patients with dementia because of a 1.5- to 1.7-times increased risk of mortality when used in patients with dementia (Schneider et al. 2005; Trifirò et al. 2009) and a 2- to 3-fold increased risk of cerebrovascular events (Schneider et al. 2006a). This warning was initially instituted by the FDA for atypical antipsychotics in 2005 and then extended to typical antipsychotics in 2008. When used in dementia, antipsychotics may also contribute to sedation, falls, confusion, extrapyramidal symptoms, and metabolic side effects. Still, consensus guidelines recommend that antipsychotics may be appropriate when trials of nonpharmacological approaches have been carried out and have failed, and when the potential benefits outweigh the risks, such as when behaviors put the patient and others at risk of harm (Rabins and Lyketsos 2005; Zuidema et al. 2015). Informed consent must include a discussion with the patient and surrogate decision-maker about the risks and benefits of treatment, including a discussion of the risks of cardiovascular events and mortality. Both patients and surrogates maintain the right to decline proposed treatment with an antipsychotic and to opt for treatment with a safer but less efficacious alternative.

Patients with Parkinson's disease and dementia with Lewy bodies are exquisitely sensitive to the extrapyramidal side effects of antipsychotic medications. Prior to initiation of antipsychotic therapy, the severity of psychotic symptoms should be reviewed, including an assessment of the distress experienced by the patient or caregivers. There is mixed evidence that a trial of an acetylcholinesterase inhibitor or memantine may improve psychosis in this population, and these may be more effective tools in dementia with Lewy bodies over Parkinson's disease (Edwards et al. 2007; Emre et al. 2010; Matsunaga et al. 2015; McKeith et al. 2000; van Laar et al. 2011; Weintraub and Hurtig 2007). If other strategies have been tried and antipsychotic medication appears necessary, atypical antipsychotics with the lowest risk of extrapyramidal side effects can be considered. Quetiapine is reasonably tolerated in this population, though clozapine is more efficacious for psychosis (Seppi et al. 2019), and the choice between these two medications may be tempered by the side-effect profile of clozapine and need for frequent monitoring for agranulocytosis. Pimavanserin is a new medication that acts as a serotonin 5-HT_{2A} receptor inverse agonist, is very well tolerated, and has no impact on motor symptoms; it has been FDA approved for treatment of psychosis in Parkinson's disease (Cummings et al. 2014; Meltzer et al. 2010).

Delirium on the Inpatient Unit

Geriatric inpatient units will accept patients for the care of delirium with variable frequency, depending on unit culture and capabilities. The geriatric unit can be an ideal place to manage delirium, given the transdisciplinary approach to care, a design that is sensitive to the sensory needs of elderly patients, and nursing staff who are attentive to the nuanced needs of patients with acute and chronic encephalopathies. Even in patients who are admitted to the inpatient unit for other indications, there remains a high incidence of comorbid delirium in geriatric inpatients. Patients of advanced age or with multiple medical comorbidities, recent illness, dementia, visual or hearing impairment, dehydration, sleep deprivation, and mobility impairment are at particularly higher risk. All patients on the inpatient unit should be screened for delirium, and treatment plans modified to address this condition.

By definition, delirium is an acute disorder of attention and cognition that often occurs after acute illness, surgery, or hospitalization and can drastically worsen morbidity and mortality. Diagnosis is made clinically; features of delirium recognized by DSM-5 include symptoms with acute onset, fluctuating course, inattention, impaired consciousness, and disorganization of thought (including disorientation, language impairment, and memory disturbance). Patients may also experience disruptions in sleep-wake cycle, hallucinations, delusions, emotional lability, or inappropriate behavior (Inouye et al. 1990). The latter symptoms are often more recognized in hyperactive delirium. Hypoactive delirium is often undiagnosed, has higher rates of mortality (Kim et al. 2015), and is more common among the elderly. Despite efforts to increase the diagnosis of delirium, the rate of delirium cases that go unrecognized by the treating physician in hospital settings remains at 60% (de la Cruz et al. 2015). An episode of delirium can trigger a rapid decline in functioning, leading to a loss of independence and often a transition to an institutionalized setting. In patients with dementia and a superimposed delirium, there is an accelerated rate of cognitive decline and there are longer hospital stays and higher rates of rehospitalization, institutionalization, and death (Fick et al. 2013; Gross et al. 2012; Morandi et al. 2014).

Before the diagnosis of delirium is made, a baseline mental status and the acuity of mental status changes must be established, with the expectation that symptoms of delirium will have developed over hours to days. Determining the acuity of the change will help differentiate a case of delirium from the chronic cognitive deficits that are seen in depression, dementia, or psychosis. Recognition of delirium has been advanced by the development of new, brief screening tools. Patients with acute changes should be given a brief cognitive screening test like the MMSE or Mini-Cog (Borson et al. 2000), and a validated delirium instrument such as the Confusion Assessment Method, 3-Minute Diagnostic Assessment, or 4A's Test (Oh et al. 2017).

When delirium is diagnosed, patients must have a full physical evaluation and targeted laboratory testing based on the clinical presentation that broadly assesses for precipitating factors such as infections, and metabolic derangements, medication-induced states, and poorly controlled pain. Lumbar puncture and cerebrospinal fluid analysis may be considered in patients with signs suggestive of meningitis or encephalitis, and neuroimaging may be useful in cases in which there is rapidly deteriorating mental status, focal neurological findings, or recent falls (Lai and Wong Tin Niam 2012). EEG is supported in patients with a history of seizures, findings suggestive of seizures, a history of brain trauma or stroke, or treatment with medications that lower the seizure threshold.

Management of Delirium on the Inpatient Unit

Primary prevention with multicomponent nonpharmacological approaches by a multidisciplinary team remains the most effective way to minimize the risk of delirium in hospitalized patients (Oh et al. 2017). The Hospital Elder Life Program (HELP) is a system of care delivery that has emerged as a leading model for treatment of hospitalized elderly patients. In this care plan, each patient's individual needs guide interventions such as daily visitors, therapeutic activities, early mobilization, nonpharmacological sleep interventions, feeding assistance, geriatric interdisciplinary care, provider education, and discharge assistance. The program has been effective in reducing the incidence of delirium and rate of falls (Hshieh et al. 2018). There is minimal evidence to support the use of medications for the prevention of delirium, including antipsychotics, acetylcholinesterase inhibitors, and melatonin or melatonin receptor agonists (Siddiqi et al. 2016).

Once delirium is diagnosed, treatment of the underlying contributing condition is the most effective intervention. Otherwise, strong evidence-based treatment options for management are limited. Oh et al. (2017) outline both nonpharmacological and pharmacological strategies for delirium management. Nonpharmacological strategies include adequate nutrition, access to eyeglasses and hearing aids, minimal interruptions in sleep time, and low-level lighting at night. Oh et al. also suggest efforts to prevent complications of delirium, such as aspiration, poor nutrition, skin breakdown, and deep venous thrombosis. Medications with deliriogenic potential (e.g., sedative-hypnotics, narcotics, anticholinergic medications, corticosteroids) should be reviewed and eliminated, depending on the clinical picture (Fong et al. 2009).

A comprehensive systematic review (Neufeld et al. 2016) concluded that the evidence does not support the use of antipsychotics for treatment of delirium in hospitalized older adults. In the 19 studies reviewed, use of oral risperidone, oral olanzapine, oral quetiapine, intramuscular ziprasidone, and intramuscular haloperidol showed no change in delirium incidence, duration, or severity; hospital length of stay; or mortality. Generally, antipsychotic medications are reserved for circumstances when delirium-associated agitation and hallucinations pose a safety risk to others or interrupt necessary care (Oh et al. 2017). Severe agitation may improve with low-dose antipsychotic medication such as quetiapine, olanzapine, risperidone, or haloperidol. Depending on the frequency of high-risk behaviors, a trial of an antipsychotic could be carried out on an as-needed or standing schedule, with an attempt to taper the antipsychotic after about 2 days if possible. Antipsychotics should be used at the lowest effective dose and for the shortest duration possible (Fong et al. 2009). Patients should be closely monitored for extrapyramidal symptoms, orthostasis, and QTc prolongation if antipsychotics are used.

There are limited studies that have examined other pharmacological approaches in the treatment of delirium. Because of a paucity of studies, there are inadequate data to support the use of acetylcholinesterase inhibitors (Overshott et al. 2008). Lorazepam and other sedative-hypnotics are generally avoided because of the risk of worsening cognition and orientation. Melatonin and melatonin receptor agonists have also been inadequately studied (Choy et al. 2018), but either appears to be a low-risk intervention for patients with dysregulated sleep cycles.

Special Considerations in the Treatment of Elderly Adults

Falls

Falls put geriatric patients at high risk of morbidity. Falls with injury increase morbidity and mortality, hospital length of stay, and the cost of care (Wong et al. 2011). Geriatric inpatients are at very high risk of falls because of multiple risk factors, including confusion, delirium, communication deficits, deconditioning, arthritis, cardiac comorbidities, sensitivity to medication side effects, and movement disorders. Physical frailty also increases an elderly patient's risk of injury with falls, and timely evaluation for traumatic injury is of critical importance in the elderly population. Fall prevention is a priority of hospital systems and regulatory agencies, and most hospitals have implemented a protocolized fall prevention program. One psychiatric unit reported a 9.5% fall rate across all unit patients admitted over the course of 3 years, with female gender, ECT, use of mood stabilizers, cardiac arrhythmias, parkinsonian syndrome, and dementias all associated with increased risk (de Carle and Kohn 2001). As discussed earlier in this chapter, effective unit design, a transdisciplinary approach, and physical therapy interventions can be helpful for reducing fall risk.

Suicidal Behaviors

Suicide attempts in the elderly are significantly more lethal than those in younger adults, with estimates that one in every four attempts results in death (Fremouw et al. 1990). Older age is associated with more determined and planned acts, less violent means, and fewer warnings of suicidal intent (Conwell et al. 1998). Elderly inpatients require immediate and ongoing assessment of the risk of suicide and self-injury. Assessment is similar to that of younger adults, and risk factors include a history of attempts, active suicidal ideation, lethal plans for suicide, and psychosis. Social isolation, bereavement, being a widow or widower, cognitive impairment, psychiatric illness, physical illness, and physical pain are all risk factors related to suicidal ideation and behavior in older adults (Conejero et al. 2018). Risk is greatest within the first week of admission and the first week of discharge from a hospital setting (Erlangsen et al. 2006). For high-risk patients, implementing one-to-one continuous observation and treating severe anxiety and agitation can be effective ways to minimize risk (Busch et al. 2003).

Aggressive Behaviors, Seclusion, and Restraint

Aggression related to dementia is addressed earlier in this chapter but remains a unique challenge in the context of managing the geriatric inpatient unit. When compared with younger patients, victims of patient assault are more likely to be fellow unit patients, rather than staff (Wystanski 2000). Patient-to-patient assaults can be particularly challenging, because of the obvious risk to other frail patients, and the barriers this creates for finding an appropriate aftercare arrangement. Attempts should be made to determine if there are any environmental triggers or diurnal trends to agitation, and environmental interventions should be developed to target this behavior. As described earlier, pharmacological management should be considered only after environmental interventions have been ineffective. Distraction and stimulation reduction can be particularly effective. Restraints should be avoided when possible because of the risk of injury to frail patients. For the impulsive patient, use of bed alarms and strategies like positioning the patient near the nursing station enhance monitoring and increase the likelihood of effective staff intervention before an adverse event. Each unit will have different patterns of use of seclusion and restraint, depending on the population served, the capabilities of the unit, and guidelines imposed by regulatory boards. Restraints may include bed rails, belts, and chair-tables. One study found that restraints occurred most often at the beginning of a hospitalization and were used most in patients with severe cognitive impairments and mobility impairments (Bredthauer et al. 2005).

Sexual Disinhibition

Sexual disinhibition in dementia is an ethically challenging dilemma that impacts patient safety, freedom, and autonomy and has legal implications (Cipriani et al. 2016). Sexual interest does not decline with aging (Mulligan and Siddiqi 2003), though a decline in cognition and judgment in dementia can result in inappropriate displays and potentially aggression. Sexual inhibition appears to happen in later stages of dementia and segregates into two subtypes—intimacy-seeking and disinhibited (de Medeiros et al. 2008). Disinhibition, however, can happen even in the early stages of frontotemporal dementia. When issues of sexuality arise on an inpatient unit, care teams are put in the position of considering a patient's ability to give consent, deciding how to manage sexual interactions between patients, and assessing whether to intervene when sexual behaviors are expressed in situations that are not traditionally considered appropriate. The moral and ethical complexity of managing these situations goes beyond the scope of this chapter. In general, when intervention is necessary, nonpharmacological treatments are preferred and include reducing precipitating factors, providing private opportunities to relieve sexual urges, enhancing other opportunities for nonsexual affection from family or pets, and distraction with other activities (Cipriani et al. 2016). There is a paucity of evidence-based research for management of sexual disinhibition in dementia and no FDA-approved medication for this indication. Reviews (De Giorgi and Series 2016; Guay 2008) suggest that when environmental interventions are ineffective, a trial of pharmacotherapy can be carried out, often starting with SSRIs given their safety profile and antilibidinal profile. Tricyclics, mirtazapine, trazodone, antiandrogens, gonadrotropin-releasing hormone agonists, estrogens, neuroleptics, and mood stabilizers have also been used, although evidence is limited, and a full discussion of the ethical implications is not included here.

Screaming

Shouting, yelling, screaming, and use of abusive language are common behaviors that can be a cause of concern in patients with dementia. In itself, this behavior is not an indication for a psychiatric inpatient admission, although it can be the source of significant caregiver strain and distress. Screaming is associated with cognitive impairment, depression, poor social networks, and severely impaired ADLs, and occurs more often when patients are alone during the evening hours (Cohen-Mansfield et al. 1990). Patients' yelling may be due to experiences of pain, discomfort, hallucinations, anxiety, boredom, difficulty communicating, or overstimulation. There is limited evidence to support a particular treatment for vocalizations, although environmental approaches are considered the mainstay of treatment (Barton et al. 2005). Making attempts at engagement and orientation and providing opportunities for socialization may help. Individual interventions are frequently inefficacious, and a multi-intervention approach is often recommended. In one study of nursing home residents, only 33% had objective reductions in vocalizations after a coordinated outreach program, which provided an average of 13–14 interventions for vocalizations (Draper et al. 2003). Identifying and treating underlying symptoms such as pain, depression, anxiety, or hallucinations with appropriate pharmacotherapy can be helpful. Taking these possible contributors into consideration, treatment planning should be tailored for the individual patient (McMinn and Draper 2005). In a few cases in which severe, persistent yelling did not respond to environmental interventions or pharmacotherapy, ECT was efficacious (Carlyle et al. 1991; Roccaforte et al. 2000) even in some nondepressed patients, although the mechanism is unclear, and this is not considered a standard of care.

Assessment of Capacity in Late Life

Inpatients are frequently required to make medical decisions of varying complexity. Capacity is often questioned when a patient makes a decision that puts their health, safety, or assets at risk and is not able or willing to accept help (Moye et al. 2013). Throughout the hospitalization, the health care professional is required to make formal and informal judgments about a patient's capacity to make decisions, defined here as a dichotomous clinical judgment about whether an individual can perform a specific task or make a specific decision (Moye and Marson 2007). Because there is variability between jurisdictions, physicians should consult with local professional organizations about standards for capacity, the role of the physician, and precedents for decision-making (Barbas and Wilde 2001). Capacity is distinguished from competency, which is the legal determination made by a judge about a person's abilities, although in practice there is not necessarily a strict delineation of these terms.

Dementia and late-life psychiatric disorders can lead to impairments in cognition that diminish a patient's ability across any domain of function, including the ability to live independently, manage finances, provide consent for medical treatment, drive a motor vehicle, participate in legal matters, or even provide consent for sexual activity. Impaired capacity in one domain does not imply impairment in another. While no disease should in itself be equated with incapacitation, there is a high rate of incapacitation in patients with dementia. Incapacitation is nearly universal in patients with severe dementia, and impairments in capacity are noted in over half of patients with mild to moderate dementia, with executive function and memory deficits being most predictive (Kim et al. 2002). Impairments in some domains of capacity are also common in patients with acute episodes of schizophrenia (Grisso and Appelbaum 1995) and bipolar disorder (Palmer et al. 2007), and less common in depression—with a lack of insight into illness being the strongest predictor of incapacitation (Cairns et al. 2005). No brief neuropsychology screening measure has consistently been able to identify patients at risk for impaired capacity, although the MMSE score has been shown to correlate with clinical judgments of incapacity (Raymont et al. 2004), with scores under 19 being highly likely to be associated with incapacity (Kim and Caine 2002).

The assessment of capacity for medical decision-making includes verifying that there has been an informed consent process, and conducting an assessment of a patient's ability to 1) communicate a choice, 2) understand the relevant information, 3) appreciate the situation and its consequences, and 4) reason about treatment options (Appelbaum 2007). In cases of impairment, the ethical principles of autonomy and beneficence are often at odds, and one must determine whether the impairment meets a threshold for incapacitation. Generally, a patient's autonomy is respected in indeterminate cases, although more stringent assessment and interpretation are used when the consequences of a patient's decisions are more serious. In cases that are particularly difficult or that may require a resolution in court, standardized instruments such as the MacArthur Competence Assessment Tool for Treatment (Grisso and Appelbaum 1998) may be used.

When a patient's ability to live independently is being evaluated, providers should pursue an assessment of all basic and instrumental ADLs through patient and family interview. Occupational therapy assessment, nursing report, and observation of the patient on the unit will provide useful feedback regarding a patient's capabilities. When patients maintain insight into deficits, education may be provided to the patient, family, and caregivers. In patients with mild to moderate impairments, modifications and adaptations may be made to reduce demands in their environment and promote prolonged independence. In patients who clearly do not have the capability to live safely with their current level of supervision, social work will help identify appropriate options for enhanced home care, assisted living, or treatment in a nursing home (Barbas and Wilde 2001).

When patients are identified as lacking capacity to make a decision about their treatment or living arrangement, the decision may be delayed if further treatment and education are likely to improve or restore a patient's ability to participate in the decision (Appelbaum 2007). In cases in which active psychiatric symptoms or delirium is contributing to the impairment, a period of treatment and intensive education may bolster understanding of the relevant information. The presence of family and other support may help the patient better process the information. In cases in which patients exhibit cognitive fluctuations, the assessment of capacity should occur at a point in time when the patient is in "good shape," and education provided using simple language, using visual aids if necessary, and with family or other support present (Trachsel et al. 2015).

When a patient is determined to lack capacity to make a decision, and efforts to restore capacity have not been successful or are not practical, a substitute decision-maker is identified. Ideally, a patient will have previously drafted advance directives, with a living will to provide preferences for medical treatment, and a durable power of attorney identifying a trusted person to make decisions about health care or finances when the patient is no longer able to. When patients do not have advance directives, a surrogate decision-maker must be identified according to local guidelines, which usually determine the order in which family members are approached. Making treatment decisions can have a negative emotional effect on up to one-third of surrogates (Wendler and Rid 2011). Surrogates may feel unsure of a patient's preferences, uncomfortable with the hospital environment, be in conflict with the treatment team, require more communication, or struggle with feelings of responsibility and guilt associated with the decision. Identifying and addressing these stressors can facilitate a more successful and less burdensome process of shared decision-making.

In practice, many of these affairs are resolved informally without an official declaration of incompetence or court involvement (Moye and Marson 2007); concerned caregivers slowly assume responsibility for helping manage finances, restrict driving, or become involved in managing medical affairs. In complex cases, including those involving disagreement among family members or the inability to identify a willing surrogate, a court may appoint a guardian to ensure that a patient's day-to-day needs are met. Obtaining guardianship is a lengthy and expensive process, often requiring court testimony and representation by an attorney, and will vary between states.

Discharge Planning

Psychotherapies

The role of psychotherapy in an acute inpatient psychiatric hospitalization is limited by the abbreviated nature of the hospitalization and the difficulties in implementing effective psychotherapy in patients with moderate to advanced dementia. Still, combination psychotherapy and psychopharmacology is the ideal treatment for geriatric depression. Referral to outpatient psychotherapy may be appropriate for some patients. There is evidence for cognitive-behavioral therapy (Thompson et al. 2001), problem-solving therapy (Alexopoulos et al. 2003), and psychodynamic psychotherapy as efficacious psychotherapies in geriatric major depression (Frazer et al. 2005). Adaptations to therapy have been made to address elderly patients with cognitive impairment. For example, interpersonal psychotherapy for cognitive impairment (IPT-CI) can address role conflicts and incorporate the needs of both the caregiver and patient into therapy (Miller and Reynolds 2007). A home-delivered problem adaptation therapy for cognitively impaired, disabled elderly (PATH) is an effective model that uses compensatory strategies and invites caregivers' participation when patients are unable to problem-solve alone (Kiosses et al. 2010).

Disposition Considerations

Arranging safe, effective, and appropriate aftercare is more complex in the elderly. For higher-functioning patients living in the community, referral to a partial hospital or intensive outpatient program may facilitate ongoing improvement, maintain stabilization, and reduce the risk of hospital readmission (Forster et al. 1999; Hoe et al. 2005; Mackenzie et al. 2006). Patients who are reliant on caregivers may be able to return to a supervised home environment, potentially with enhanced home health services or options for adult day care. Those without options for adequate in-home support may be transferred to an assisted living facility or nursing home, including options for locked-unit dementia care in either type of facility.

Patients with a deteriorating quality of life and difficulty managing physical symptoms may benefit from palliative care services on discharge. In the rare cases of terminal agitation or terminal delirium, a transition to hospice can be most appropriate. Cost coverage options and insurance eligibility are increasingly complicated. Given the complexity, early involvement of skilled case management services is an essential part of inpatient geriatric treatment. Patients who are treated on geriatric psychiatry units receive more appropriate referral to age-specific aftercare (Yazgan et al. 2004).

Caregiver Support

Family caregiver roles can vary significantly between patients. Family members may be uninvolved, provide a supportive role, act as surrogate decision-makers, or be the patient's primary caretaker on discharge. The care team can help educate family about the patient's disease, cognitive challenges, and issues related to mood and behavior. For family caregivers, the unit can provide teaching about effective behavioral strategies. Effective case management will also incorporate the needs of the caregiver and could include referral to psychotherapy, enhanced home services, options for caregiver respite, or liaison with local caregiver support groups. Enhancing caregiver strengths can improve quality of life for patients and caregivers and can delay institutionalization (Schulz et al. 2005). Caregivers may also need assistance with accessing legal resources for complex tasks such as obtaining guardianship or financing care.

Future Directions

There is an indisputable need for growth in psychiatric care for elderly adults both inside and outside the hospital setting. In the wake of the "silver tsunami," the estimated number of Americans over age 65 with mental health or substance use disorders will reach 10.1 to 14.4 million by 2030 (Institute of Medicine 2012). There remain significant challenges to developing an adequate workforce trained to manage the unique needs of this growing population (Juul et al. 2017). Until solutions to facilitate training and improve reimbursement are developed to support a growth in geriatric medicine and geriatric psychiatry, innovations are needed to continue to care effectively for elderly adults with mental health disorders.

The transdisciplinary team approach to care should become more pervasive across inpatient geropsychiatric units nationwide. Given the growing complexity of the aging population, development of innovative payment models should allow for the creative treatment of complex medical and behavioral health problems that is necessary for supporting this population.

Novel strategies for providing care in the community may broaden disposition options and reduce admission rates to the geriatric unit. Interventions like telepsychiatry and in-home monitoring will allow providers and families to more effectively support elders in their homes and allow for sustained independence and quality of life. While telepsychiatry has a growing presence in nursing homes and rural areas, systems for broadening the application of this model must be developed (Gentry et al. 2019). Enhancements and innovations in community care may provide more robust resources to patients and families outside a hospital setting, and a platform for trialing environmental interventions to manage neuropsychiatric symptoms of dementia before inpatient hospitalization is necessary. The rise of palliative care will broaden options for patients living with dementia and their caregivers, and potentially reduce the burden of neuropsychiatric symptoms by attending longitudinally to issues related to quality of life. With earlier introduction to palliative care, growth in hospice care, and more emphasis on end-of-life choices, referral rates to the inpatient geriatric unit for the neuropsychiatric effects of dementia may decrease.

We are hopeful that growing research into the diagnosis and treatment of memory disorders will allow for early and effective intervention in dementia. With the improved ability to anticipate dementia before the onset of symptoms and the development of disease-modifying agents, the morbidity of dementia may someday be reduced.

References

Alexopoulos GS, Meyers BS, Young RC, et al: The course of geriatric depression with "reversible dementia": a controlled study. Am J Psychiatry 150(11):1693–1699, 1993 8105707

Alexopoulos GS, Meyers BS, Young RC, et al: Clinically defined vascular depression. Am J Psychiatry 154(4):562–565, 1997a 9090349

Alexopoulos GS, Meyers BS, Young RC, et al: 'Vascular depression' hypothesis. Arch Gen Psychiatry 54(10):915–922, 1997b 9337771

Alexopoulos GS, Katz IR, Reynolds CF 3rd, et al: The Expert Consensus Guideline series: pharmacotherapy of depressive disorders in older patients. Postgrad Med Spec No Pharmacotherapy October, 1–86, 2001 17205639

Alexopoulos GS, Borson S, Cuthbert BN, et al: Assessment of late life depression. Biol Psychiatry 52(3):164–174, 2002a 12182923

Alexopoulos GS, Kiosses DN, Choi SJ, et al: Frontal white matter microstructure and treatment response of late-life depression: a preliminary study. Am J Psychiatry 159(11):1929–1932, 2002b 12411231

Alexopoulos GS, Raue P, Areán P: Problem-solving therapy versus supportive therapy in geriatric major depression with executive dysfunction. Am J Geriatr Psychiatry 11(1):46–52, 2003 12527539

Alexopoulos GS, Streim J, Carpenter D, et al: Using antipsychotic agents in older patients. J Clin Psychiatry 65 (suppl 2):5–99, discussion 100–102, quiz 103–104, 2004 14994733

Alexopoulos GS, Kiosses DN, Heo M, et al: Executive dysfunction and the course of geriatric depression. Biol Psychiatry 58(3):204–210, 2005 16018984

Almeida OP, Fenner S: Bipolar disorder: similarities and differences between patients with illness onset before and after 65 years of age. Int Psychogeriatr 14(3):311–322, 2002 12475092

American Academy of Neurology: Guideline Summary for Clinicians: Detection, Diagnosis, and Management of Dementia. Minneapolis, MN, American Academy of Neurology, 2004

American Geriatrics Society Beers Criteria Update Expert Panel: American Geriatrics Society 2019 updated AGS Beers criteria for potentially inappropriate medication use in older adults. J Am Geriatr Soc 67(4):674–694, 2019 30693946

American Psychiatric Association: Practice guideline for the treatment of patients with major depressive disorder (revision). Am J Psychiatry 157(4 suppl):1–45, 2000 10767867

American Psychiatric Association: Practice guideline for the treatment of patients with Alzheimer's disease and other dementias. Second edition. Am J Psychiatry 164(12 suppl):5–56, 2007

American Psychiatric Association: Diagnostic and Statistical Manual of Mental Disorders, 5th Edition. Arlington, VA, American Psychiatric Association, 2013

Appelbaum PS: Clinical practice: assessment of patients' competence to consent to treatment. N Engl J Med 357(18):1834–1840, 2007 17978292

Aziz R, Lorberg B, Tampi RR: Treatments for late-life bipolar disorder. Am J Geriatr Pharmacother 4(4):347–364, 2006 17296540

Barbas NR, Wilde EA: Competency issues in dementia: medical decision making, driving, and independent living. J Geriatr Psychiatry Neurol 14(4):199–212, 2001 11794448
Bartels SJ: Caring for the whole person: integrated health care for older adults with severe mental illness and medical comorbidity. J Am Geriatr Soc 52(12 suppl):S249–S257, 2004 15541165
Bartels SJ, Forester B, Miles KM, Joyce T: Mental health service use by elderly patients with bipolar disorder and unipolar major depression. Am J Geriatr Psychiatry 8(2):160–166, 2000 10804077
Barton S, Findlay D, Blake RA: The management of inappropriate vocalisation in dementia: a hierarchical approach. Int J Geriatr Psychiatry 20(12):1180–1186, 2005 16315148
Beeri MS, Werner P, Davidson M, Noy S: The cost of behavioral and psychological symptoms of dementia (BPSD) in community dwelling Alzheimer's disease patients. Int J Geriatr Psychiatry 17(5):403–408, 2002 11994927
Belle SH, Czaja SJ, Schulz R, et al: Using a new taxonomy to combine the uncombinable: integrating results across diverse interventions. Psychol Aging 18(3):396–405, 2003 14518803
Berrios GE, Bulbena-Villarasa A: The Hamilton Depression Scale and the numerical description of the symptoms of depression. Psychopharmacol Ser 9:80–92, 1990 2399249
Blank K, Hixon L, Gruman C, et al: Determinants of geropsychiatric inpatient length of stay. Psychiatr Q 76(2):195–212, 2005 15884745
Borson S, Raskind MA: Clinical features and pharmacologic treatment of behavioral symptoms of Alzheimer's disease. Neurology 48(5 suppl 6):S17–S24, 1997 9153156
Borson S, Scanlan J, Brush M, et al: The mini-cog: a cognitive 'vital signs' measure for dementia screening in multi-lingual elderly. Int J Geriatr Psychiatry 15(11):1021–1027, 2000 11113982
Bouman WP, Pinner G, Johnson H: Incidence of selective serotonin reuptake inhibitor (SSRI) induced hyponatraemia due to the syndrome of inappropriate antidiuretic hormone (SIADH) secretion in the elderly. Int J Geriatr Psychiatry 13(1):12–15, 1998 9489575
Bredthauer D, Becker C, Eichner B, et al: Factors relating to the use of physical restraints in psychogeriatric care: a paradigm for elder abuse. Z Gerontol Geriatr 38(1):10–18, 2005 15756482
Brieger D, Eagle KA, Goodman SG, et al: Acute coronary syndromes without chest pain, an underdiagnosed and undertreated high-risk group: insights from the Global Registry of Acute Coronary Events. Chest 126(2):461–469, 2004 15302732
Bruce ML: Depression and disability in late life: directions for future research. Am J Geriatr Psychiatry 9(2):102–112, 2001 11316615
Busch KA, Fawcett J, Jacobs DG: Clinical correlates of inpatient suicide. J Clin Psychiatry 64(1):14–19, 2003 12590618
Cairns R, Maddock C, Buchanan A, et al: Prevalence and predictors of mental incapacity in psychiatric in-patients. Br J Psychiatry 187:379–385, 2005 16199799
Carlyle W, Killick L, Ancill R: ECT: an effective treatment in the screaming demented patient (letter). J Am Geriatr Soc 39(6):637, 1991 2037760
Cassidy F, Carroll BJ: Vascular risk factors in late onset mania. Psychol Med 32(2):359–362, 2002 11866328
Chen R, Chien W, Chu H, et al: Mortality and risk factors in psychiatric inpatient with dementia: a 13-year long-term data analysis. Neuropsychiatry 8(3):930, 2018
Chibnall JT, Tait RC, Harman B, Luebbert RA: Effect of acetaminophen on behavior, well-being, and psychotropic medication use in nursing home residents with moderate-to-severe dementia. J Am Geriatr Soc 53(11):1921–1929, 2005 16274373
Cohen CI, Meesters PD, Zhao J: New perspectives on schizophrenia in later life: implications for treatment, policy, and research. Lancet Psychiatry 2(4):340–350, 2015 26360087
Choy SW, Yeoh AC, Lee ZZ, et al: Melatonin and the prevention and management of delirium: a scoping study. Front Med (Lausanne) 4:242, 2018 29376051
Cipriani A, Hawton K, Stockton S, Geddes JR: Lithium in the prevention of suicide in mood disorders: updated systematic review and meta-analysis. BMJ 346:f3646, 2013 23814104
Cipriani G, Ulivi M, Danti S, et al: Sexual disinhibition and dementia. Psychogeriatrics 16(2):145–153, 2016 26215977

Clyburn LD, Stones MJ, Hadjistavropoulos T, Tuokko H: Predicting caregiver burden and depression in Alzheimer's disease. J Gerontol B Psychol Sci Soc Sci 55(1):S2–S13, 2000 10728125
Coen RF, Swanwick GR, O'Boyle CA, Coakley D: Behaviour disturbance and other predictors of carer burden in Alzheimer's disease. Int J Geriatr Psychiatry 12(3):331–336, 1997 9152717
Cohen CI, Vahia I, Reyes P, et al: Focus on geriatric psychiatry: schizophrenia in later life: clinical symptoms and social well-being. Psychiatr Serv 59(3):232–234, 2008 18308900
Cohen-Mansfield J: Nonpharmacologic interventions for inappropriate behaviors in dementia: a review, summary, and critique. Am J Geriatr Psychiatry 9(4):361–381, 2001 11739063
Cohen-Mansfield J, Werner P, Marx MS: Screaming in nursing home residents. J Am Geriatr Soc 38(7):785–792, 1990 2370397
Colijn MA, Nitta BH, Grossberg GT: Psychosis in later life: a review and update. Harv Rev Psychiatry 23(5):354–367, 2015 26332218
Collins N, Blanchard MR, Tookman A, Sampson EL: Detection of delirium in the acute hospital. Age Ageing 39(1):131–135, 2010 19917632
Conejero I, Olié E, Courtet P, Calati R: Suicide in older adults: current perspectives. Clin Interv Aging 13:691–699, 2018 29719381
Conwell Y, Duberstein PR, Cox C, et al: Age differences in behaviors leading to completed suicide. Am J Geriatr Psychiatry 6(2):122–126, 1998 9581207
Crum RM, Anthony JC, Bassett SS, Folstein MF: Population-based norms for the Mini-Mental State Examination by age and educational level. JAMA 269(18):2386–2391, 1993 8479064
Cummings J, Isaacson S, Mills R, et al: Pimavanserin for patients with Parkinson's disease psychosis: a randomised, placebo-controlled phase 3 trial. Lancet 383(9916):533–540, 2014 24183563
Davis DH, Creavin ST, Yip JL, et al: Montreal Cognitive Assessment for the diagnosis of Alzheimer's disease and other dementias. Cochrane Database Syst Rev (10):CD010775, 2015 26513331
de Abajo FJ, Rodríguez LA, Montero D: Association between selective serotonin reuptake inhibitors and upper gastrointestinal bleeding: population based case-control study. BMJ 319(7217):1106–1109, 1999 10531103
de Asis JM, Greenwald BS, Alexopoulos GS, et al: Frontal signal hyperintensities in mania in old age. Am J Geriatr Psychiatry 14(7):598–604, 2006 16816013
de Carle AJ, Kohn R: Risk factors for falling in a psychogeriatric unit. Int J Geriatr Psychiatry 16(8):762–767, 2001 11536342
De Giorgi R, Series H: Treatment of inappropriate sexual behavior in dementia. Curr Treat Options Neurol 18(9):41, 2016 27511056
de la Cruz M, Fan J, Yennu S, et al: The frequency of missed delirium in patients referred to palliative care in a comprehensive cancer center. Support Care Cancer 23(8):2427–2433, 2015 25617070
de Medeiros K, Rosenberg PB, Baker AS, Onyike CU: Improper sexual behaviors in elders with dementia living in residential care. Dement Geriatr Cogn Disord 26(4):370–377, 2008 18931496
Depp CA, Jeste DV: Bipolar disorder in older adults: a critical review. Bipolar Disord 6(5):343–367, 2004 15383127
Desai AK, Grossberg GT: Recognition and management of behavioral disturbances in dementia. Prim Care Companion J Clin Psychiatry 3(3):93–109, 2001 15014607
Desbeaumes Jodoin V, Miron JP, Lespérance P: Safety and efficacy of accelerated repetitive transcranial magnetic stimulation protocol in elderly depressed unipolar and bipolar patients. Am J Geriatr Psychiatry 27(5):548–558, 2019 30527274
Draper B, Turner J, McMinn B, et al: Outcome of treatment of vocally disruptive behavior in nursing home residents. Aust J Ageing 22(2):80–84, 2003
Drayer RA, Mulsant BH, Lenze EJ, et al: Somatic symptoms of depression in elderly patients with medical comorbidities. Int J Geriatr Psychiatry 20(10):973–982, 2005 16163749
Edwards K, Royall D, Hershey L, et al: Efficacy and safety of galantamine in patients with dementia with Lewy bodies: a 24-week open-label study. Dement Geriatr Cogn Disord 23(6):401–405, 2007 17409748

Elderkin-Thompson V, Kumar A, Bilker WB, et al: Neuropsychological deficits among patients with late-onset minor and major depression. Arch Clin Neuropsychol 18(5):529–549, 2003 14591448

Emre M, Tsolaki M, Bonuccelli U, et al: Memantine for patients with Parkinson's disease dementia or dementia with Lewy bodies: a randomised, double-blind, placebo-controlled trial. Lancet Neurol 9(10):969–977, 2010 20729148

Erlangsen A, Zarit SH, Tu X, Conwell Y: Suicide among older psychiatric inpatients: an evidence-based study of a high-risk group. Am J Geriatr Psychiatry 14(9):734–741, 2006 16943170

Essali A, Ali G: Antipsychotic drug treatment for elderly people with late-onset schizophrenia. Cochrane Database Syst Rev (2):CD004162, 2012 22336800

Evans JD, Negron AE, Palmer BW, et al: Cognitive deficits and psychopathology in institutionalized versus community-dwelling elderly schizophrenia patients. J Geriatr Psychiatry Neurol 12(1):11–15, 1999 10447149

Fick DM, Steis MR, Waller JL, Inouye SK: Delirium superimposed on dementia is associated with prolonged length of stay and poor outcomes in hospitalized older adults. J Hosp Med 8(9):500–505, 2013 23955965

Flint AJ, Rifat SL: The treatment of psychotic depression in later life: a comparison of pharmacotherapy and ECT. Int J Geriatr Psychiatry 13(1):23–28, 1998 9489577

Flint AJ, Meyers BS, Rothschild AJ, et al: Effect of continuing olanzapine vs placebo on relapse among patients with psychotic depression in remission: the STOP-PD II randomized clinical trial. JAMA 322(7):622–631, 2019 31429896

Folstein MF, Folstein SE, McHugh PR: "Mini-mental state": a practical method for grading the cognitive state of patients for the clinician. J Psychiatr Res 12(3):189–198, 1975 1202204

Fong TG, Tulebaev SR, Inouye SK: Delirium in elderly adults: diagnosis, prevention and treatment. Nat Rev Neurol 5(4):210–220, 2009 19347026

Forster A, Young J, Langhorne P, et al: Systematic review of day hospital care for elderly people. BMJ 318(7187):837–841, 1999 10092260

Frasure-Smith N, Lespérance F, Talajic M: Depression following myocardial infarction: impact on 6-month survival. JAMA 270(15):1819–1825, 1993 8411525

Frazer CJ, Christensen H, Griffiths KM: Effectiveness of treatments for depression in older people. Med J Aust 182(12):627–632, 2005 15963019

Fremouw WJ, dePerczel M, Ellis TE: Suicide Risk: Assessment and Response Guidelines. New York, Pergamon, 1990

Gallo JJ, Rabins PV: Depression without sadness: alternative presentations of depression in late life. Am Fam Physician 60(3):820–826, 1999 10498109

Gentry MT, Lapid MI, Rummans TA: Geriatric telepsychiatry: systematic review and policy considerations. Am J Geriatr Psychiatry 27(2):109–127, 2019 30416025

Gillman PK: The serotonin syndrome and its treatment. J Psychopharmacol 13(1):100–109, 1999 10221364

Gitlin LN, Belle SH, Burgio LD, et al: Effect of multicomponent interventions on caregiver burden and depression: the REACH multisite initiative at 6-month follow-up. Psychol Aging 18(3):361–374, 2003 14518800

Grisso T, Appelbaum PS: The MacArthur Treatment Competence Study, III: abilities of patients to consent to psychiatric and medical treatments. Law Hum Behav 19(2):149–174, 1995 11660292

Grisso T, Appelbaum PS: MacArthur Competence Assessment Tool for Treatment (MacCAT-T). Sarasota, FL, Professional Resource Press, 1998.

Gross AL, Jones RN, Habtemariam DA, et al: Delirium and long-term cognitive trajectory among persons with dementia. Arch Intern Med 172(17):1324–1331, 2012 23403619

Grossberg GT, Desai AK: Management of Alzheimer's disease. J Gerontol A Biol Sci Med Sci 58(4):331–353, 2003 12663697

Guay DR: Inappropriate sexual behaviors in cognitively impaired older individuals. Am J Geriatr Pharmacother 6(5):269–288, 2008 19161930

Han B: Depressive symptoms and self-rated health in community-dwelling older adults: a longitudinal study. J Am Geriatr Soc 50(9):1549–1556, 2002 12383153

Han B, Compton WM, Blanco C, et al: Prescription opioid use, misuse, and use disorders in U.S. adults: 2015 National Survey on Drug Use and Health. Ann Intern Med 167(5):293–301, 2017 28761945

Hoe J, Ashaye K, Orrell M: Don't seize the day hospital! Recent research on the effectiveness of day hospitals for older people with mental health problems. Int J Geriatr Psychiatry 20(7):694–698, 2005 16021660

Howard R, Rabins PV, Seeman MV, et al: Late-onset schizophrenia and very-late-onset schizophrenia-like psychosis: an international consensus. Am J Psychiatry 157(2):172–178, 2000 10671383

Hshieh TT, Yang T, Gartaganis SL, et al: Hospital Elder Life Program: systematic review and meta-analysis of effectiveness. Am J Geriatr Psychiatry 26(10):1015–1033, 2018 30076080

Hughes CP, Berg L, Danziger WL, et al: A new clinical scale for the staging of dementia. Br J Psychiatry 140:566–572, 1982 7104545

Inouye SK, van Dyck CH, Alessi CA, et al: Clarifying confusion: the confusion assessment method: a new method for detection of delirium. Ann Intern Med 113(12):941–948, 1990 2240918

Institute of Medicine: The Mental Health and Substance Use Workforce for Older Adults: In Whose Hands? Washington, DC, National Academies Press, 2012

Iriarte IG, George MS: Transcranial magnetic stimulation (TMS) in the elderly. Curr Psychiatry Rep 20(1):6, 2018 29427050

Juul D, Colenda CC, Lyness JM, et al: Subspecialty training and certification in geriatric psychiatry: a 25-year overview. Am J Geriatr Psychiatry 25(5):445–453, 2017 28214074

Juurlink DN, Mamdani MM, Kopp A, Redelmeier DA: The risk of suicide with selective serotonin reuptake inhibitors in the elderly. Am J Psychiatry 163(5):813–821, 2006 16648321

Kales HC, Gitlin LN, Lyketsos CG, Detroit Expert Panel on Assessment and Management of Neuropsychiatric Symptoms of Dementia: Management of neuropsychiatric symptoms of dementia in clinical settings: recommendations from a multidisciplinary expert panel. J Am Geriatr Soc 62(4):762–769, 2014 24635665

Katz IR, Jeste DV, Mintzer JE, et al: Comparison of risperidone and placebo for psychosis and behavioral disturbances associated with dementia: a randomized, double-blind trial. J Clin Psychiatry 60(2):107–115, 1999 10084637

Kessing LV, Søndergård L, Forman JL, Andersen PK: Lithium treatment and risk of dementia. Arch Gen Psychiatry 65(11):1331–1335, 2008 18981345

Kim SY, Caine ED: Utility and limits of the Mini Mental State Examination in evaluating consent capacity in Alzheimer's disease. Psychiatr Serv 53(10):1322–1324, 2002 12364686

Kim SY, Karlawish JH, Caine ED: Current state of research on decision-making competence of cognitively impaired elderly persons. Am J Geriatr Psychiatry 10(2):151–165, 2002 11925276

Kim SY, Kim SW, Kim JM, et al: Differential associations between delirium and mortality according to delirium subtype and age: a prospective cohort study. Psychosom Med 77(8):903–910, 2015 26397939

Kindermann SS, Kalayam B, Brown GG, et al: Executive functions and P300 latency in elderly depressed patients and control subjects. Am J Geriatr Psychiatry 8(1):57–65, 2000 10648296

Kiosses DN, Arean PA, Teri L, Alexopoulos GS: Home-delivered problem adaptation therapy (PATH) for depressed, cognitively impaired, disabled elders: a preliminary study. Am J Geriatr Psychiatry 18(11):988–998, 2010 20808092

Klimstra SA, Latoussakis V, Kiosses DN, Alexopoulos GS: The geriatric unit, in Textbook of Hospital Psychiatry, 1st Edition. Washington, DC, American Psychiatric Publishing, 2009, pp 71–88

Kochanek KD, Murphy SL, Xu JQ, Arias E: Deaths: final data for 2017. Natl Vital Stat Rep 68(9):1–76, 2019

Krishnan KR, Hays JC, Blazer DG: MRI-defined vascular depression. Am J Psychiatry 154(4):497–501, 1997 9090336

Kroenke K, Spitzer RL, Williams JB: The PHQ-9: validity of a brief depression severity measure. J Gen Intern Med 16(9):606–613, 2001 11556941

Lai MM, Wong Tin Niam DM: Intracranial cause of delirium: computed tomography yield and predictive factors. Intern Med J 42(4):422–427, 2012 21118407

Lawton MP, Brody EM: Assessment of older people: self-maintaining and instrumental activities of daily living. Gerontologist 9(3):179–186, 1969 5349366

Lehmann SW, Rabins PV: Factors related to hospitalization in elderly manic patients with early and late-onset bipolar disorder. Int J Geriatr Psychiatry 21(11):1060–1064, 2006 16955445

Lisanby SH, McClintock SM, Alexopoulos G, et al: Neurocognitive effects of combined electroconvulsive therapy (ECT) and venlafaxine in geriatric depression: phase 1 of the PRIDE study. Am J Geriatr Psychiatry 28(3):304–316, 2019 31706638

Livingston G, Johnston K, Katona C, et al: Systematic review of psychological approaches to the management of neuropsychiatric symptoms of dementia. Am J Psychiatry 162(11):1996–2021, 2005 16263837

Lockwood KA, Alexopoulos GS, van Gorp WG: Executive dysfunction in geriatric depression. Am J Psychiatry 159(7):1119–1126, 2002 12091189

Lyketsos CG, Colenda CC, Beck C, et al: Position statement of the American Association for Geriatric Psychiatry regarding principles of care for patients with dementia resulting from Alzheimer disease. Am J Geriatr Psychiatry 14(7):561–572, 2006 16816009

Mackenzie CS, Rosenberg M, Major M: Evaluation of a psychiatric day hospital program for elderly patients with mood disorders. Int Psychogeriatr 18(4):631–641, 2006 16684397

Madhusoodanan S, Shah P, Brenner R, Gupta S: Pharmacological treatment of the psychosis of Alzheimer's disease: what is the best approach? CNS Drugs 21(2):101–115, 2007 17284093

Maglione JE, Thomas SE, Jeste DV: Late-onset schizophrenia: do recent studies support categorizing LOS as a subtype of schizophrenia? Curr Opin Psychiatry 27(3):173–178, 2014 24613985

Marriott RG, Neil W, Waddingham S: Antipsychotic medication for elderly people with schizophrenia. Cochrane Database Syst Rev (1):CD005580, 2006 16437531

Matsunaga S, Kishi T, Iwata N: Memantine for Lewy body disorders: systematic review and meta-analysis. Am J Geriatr Psychiatry 23(4):373–383, 2015 24406251

McDonald WM: Neuromodulation treatments for geriatric mood and cognitive disorders. Am J Geriatr Psychiatry 24(12):1130–1141, 2016 27889282

McKeith I, Del Ser T, Spano P, et al: Efficacy of rivastigmine in dementia with Lewy bodies: a randomised, double-blind, placebo-controlled international study. Lancet 356(9247):2031–2036, 2000 11145488

McMinn B, Draper B: Vocally disruptive behaviour in dementia: development of an evidence based practice guideline. Aging Ment Health 9(1):16–24, 2005 15841828

Meltzer HY, Mills R, Revell S, et al: Pimavanserin, a serotonin(2A) receptor inverse agonist, for the treatment of Parkinson's disease psychosis. Neuropsychopharmacology 35(4):881–892, 2010 19907417

Meyers BS: Late-life delusional depression: acute and long-term treatment. Int Psychogeriatr 7(suppl):113–124, 1995 8580387

Meyers BS, Flint AJ, Rothschild AJ, et al: A double-blind randomized controlled trial of olanzapine plus sertraline vs olanzapine plus placebo for psychotic depression: the Study of Pharmacotherapy of Psychotic Depression (STOP-PD). Arch Gen Psychiatry 66(8):838–847, 2009 19652123

Miller MD, Reynolds CF 3rd: Expanding the usefulness of interpersonal psychotherapy (IPT) for depressed elders with co-morbid cognitive impairment. Int J Geriatr Psychiatry 22(2):101–105, 2007 17096459

Miller PA, Butin D: The role of occupational therapy in dementia: C.O.P.E. (Caregiver options for practical experiences). Int J Geriatr Psychiatry 15(1):86–89, 2000 10637409

Mitchell G, O'Donnell H: The therapeutic use of doll therapy in dementia. Br J Nurs 22(6):329–334, 2013 23901451

Morandi A, Davis D, Fick DM, et al: Delirium superimposed on dementia strongly predicts worse outcomes in older rehabilitation inpatients. J Am Med Dir Assoc 15(5):349–354, 2014 24566447

Morley JE, Kraenzle D: Causes of weight loss in a community nursing home. J Am Geriatr Soc 42(6):583–585, 1994 8201141

Moye J, Marson DC: Assessment of decision-making capacity in older adults: an emerging area of practice and research. J Gerontol B Psychol Sci Soc Sci 62(1):P3–P11, 2007 17284555

Moye J, Marson DC, Edelstein B: Assessment of capacity in an aging society. Am Psychol 68(3):158–171, 2013 23586491

Mulligan T, Siddiqi W: Changes in male sexuality, in Geriatric Medicine: An Evidence Based Approach, 4th Edition. Edited by Cassel CK, Leipzig RM, Cohen HJ, et al. New York, Springer-Verlag, 2003, pp 719–726

Mulsant BH, Pollock BG, Nebes R, et al: A twelve-week, double-blind, randomized comparison of nortriptyline and paroxetine in older depressed inpatients and outpatients. Am J Geriatr Psychiatry 9(4):406–414, 2001a 11739067

Mulsant BH, Sweet RA, Rosen J, et al: A double-blind randomized comparison of nortriptyline plus perphenazine versus nortriptyline plus placebo in the treatment of psychotic depression in late life. J Clin Psychiatry 62(8):597–604, 2001b 11561930

Nagaratnam N, Lewis-Jones M, Scott D, Palazzi L: Behavioral and psychiatric manifestations in dementia patients in a community: caregiver burden and outcome. Alzheimer Dis Assoc Disord 12(4):330–334, 1998 9876961

Nasreddine ZS, Phillips NA, Bédirian V, et al: The Montreal Cognitive Assessment, MoCA: a brief screening tool for mild cognitive impairment. J Am Geriatr Soc 53(4):695–699, 2005 15817019 (Erratum in: J Am Geriatr Soc 67(9):1991, 2019)

National Institute for Clinical Excellence: Depression: Management of Depression in Primary and Secondary Care. NICE Clinical Guideline 23. London, National Institute for Clinical Excellence, 2004

Neufeld KJ, Yue J, Robinson TN, et al: Antipsychotic medication for prevention and treatment of delirium in hospitalized adults: a systematic review and meta-analysis. J Am Geriatr Soc 64(4):705–714, 2016 27004732

Norman DC: Fever in the elderly. Clin Infect Dis 31(1):148–151, 2000 10913413

Oh ES, Fong TG, Hshieh TT, Inouye SK: Delirium in older persons: advances in diagnosis and treatment. JAMA 318(12):1161–1174, 2017 28973626

Olfson M, King M, Schoenbaum M: Benzodiazepine use in the United States. JAMA Psychiatry 72(2):136–142, 2015 25517224

Olshaker JS, Browne B, Jerrard DA, et al: Medical clearance and screening of psychiatric patients in the emergency department. Acad Emerg Med 4(2):124–128, 1997 9043539

Overshott R, Karim S, Burns A: Cholinesterase inhibitors for delirium. Cochrane Database Syst Rev (1):CD005317, 2008 18254077

Palmer BW, Dunn LB, Depp CA, et al: Decisional capacity to consent to research among patients with bipolar disorder: comparison with schizophrenia patients and healthy subjects. J Clin Psychiatry 68(5):689–696, 2007 17503977

Penninx BW, Leveille S, Ferrucci L, et al: Exploring the effect of depression on physical disability: longitudinal evidence from the established populations for epidemiologic studies of the elderly. Am J Public Health 89(9):1346–1352, 1999 10474551

Pohjasvaara T, Vataja R, Leppävuori A, et al: Depression is an independent predictor of poor long-term functional outcome post-stroke. Eur J Neurol 8(4):315–319, 2001 11422427

Pollock BG: Psychotropic drugs and the aging patient. Geriatrics 53 (suppl 1):S20–S24, 1998 9745631

Poon LW: The use of rating depression scales in the elderly, in Handbook for Clinical Memory Assessment of Older Adults. Washington, DC, American Psychological Association, 1986

Porsteinsson AP, Drye LT, Pollock BG, et al: Effect of citalopram on agitation in Alzheimer disease: the CitAD randomized clinical trial. JAMA 311(7):682–691, 2014 24549548

Potter GG, Kittinger JD, Wagner HR, et al: Prefrontal neuropsychological predictors of treatment remission in late-life depression. Neuropsychopharmacology 29(12):2266–2271, 2004 15340392

Rabins PV, Lyketsos CG: Antipsychotic drugs in dementia: what should be made of the risks? JAMA 294(15):1963–1965, 2005 16234504

Rahkonen T, Eloniemi-Sulkava U, Rissanen S, et al: Dementia with Lewy bodies according to the consensus criteria in a general population aged 75 years or older. J Neurol Neurosurg Psychiatry 74(6):720–724, 2003 12754338

Raymont V, Bingley W, Buchanan A, et al: Prevalence of mental incapacity in medical inpatients and associated risk factors: cross-sectional study. Lancet 364(9443):1421–1427, 2004 15488217

Richards JB, Papaioannou A, Adachi JD, et al; Canadian Multicentre Osteoporosis Study Research Group: Effect of selective serotonin reuptake inhibitors on the risk of fracture. Arch Intern Med 167(2):188–194, 2007 17242321

Robillard M, Conn DK: Lamotrigine use in geriatric patients with bipolar depression. Can J Psychiatry 47(8):767–770, 2002 12420655

Roccaforte WH, Wengel SP, Burke WJ: ECT for screaming in dementia (letter). Am J Geriatr Psychiatry 8(2):177, 2000 10804080

Romanelli J, Fauerbach JA, Bush DE, Ziegelstein RC: The significance of depression in older patients after myocardial infarction. J Am Geriatr Soc 50(5):817–822, 2002 12028166

Rösler M: The efficacy of cholinesterase inhibitors in treating the behavioural symptoms of dementia. Int J Clin Pract Suppl (127):20–36, 2002 12139365

Rothschild AJ: Challenges in the treatment of major depressive disorder with psychotic features. Schizophr Bull 39(4):787–796, 2013 23599251

Rothschild AJ, Winer J, Flint AJ, et al; Study of Pharmacotherapy of Psychotic Depression (STOP-PD) Collaborative Study Group: Missed diagnosis of psychotic depression at 4 academic medical centers. J Clin Psychiatry 69(8):1293–1296, 2008 18384244

Rush AJ, Trivedi MH, Wisniewski SR, et al: Acute and longer-term outcomes in depressed outpatients requiring one or several treatment steps: a STAR*D report. Am J Psychiatry 163(11):1905–1917, 2006 17074942

Sahlberg M, Holm E, Gislason GH, et al: Association of selected antipsychotic agents with major adverse cardiovascular events and noncardiovascular mortality in elderly persons. J Am Heart Assoc 4(9):e001666, 2015 26330335

Sajatovic M, Madhusoodanan S, Coconcea N: Managing bipolar disorder in the elderly: defining the role of the newer agents. Drugs Aging 22(1):39–54, 2005 15663348

Salloway S, Boyle PA, Correia S, et al: The relationship of MRI subcortical hyperintensities to treatment response in a trial of sertraline in geriatric depressed outpatients. Am J Geriatr Psychiatry 10(1):107–111, 2002 11790641

Salzman C, Wong E, Wright BC: Drug and ECT treatment of depression in the elderly, 1996–2001: a literature review. Biol Psychiatry 52(3):265–284, 2002 12182932

Salzman C, Jeste DV, Meyer RE, et al: Elderly patients with dementia-related symptoms of severe agitation and aggression: consensus statement on treatment options, clinical trials methodology, and policy. J Clin Psychiatry 69(6):889–898, 2008 18494535

Schneider LS, Dagerman KS, Insel P: Risk of death with atypical antipsychotic drug treatment for dementia: meta-analysis of randomized placebo-controlled trials. JAMA 294(15):1934–1943, 2005 16234500

Schneider LS, Dagerman KS, Insel P: Efficacy and adverse effects of atypical antipsychotics for dementia: meta-analysis of randomized, placebo-controlled trials. Am J Geriatr Psychiatry 14(3):191–210, 2006a 16505124

Schneider LS, Tariot PN, Dagerman KS, et al: Effectiveness of atypical antipsychotic drugs in patients with Alzheimer's disease. N Engl J Med 355(15):1525–1538, 2006b 17035647

Schulz R, O'Brien AT, Bookwala J, Fleissner K: Psychiatric and physical morbidity effects of dementia caregiving: prevalence, correlates, and causes. Gerontologist 35(6):771–791, 1995 8557205

Schulz R, Martire LM, Klinger JN: Evidence-based caregiver interventions in geriatric psychiatry. Psychiatr Clin North Am 28(4):1007–1038, x, 2005 16325738

Schürhoff F, Bellivier F, Jouvent R, et al: Early and late onset bipolar disorders: two different forms of manic-depressive illness? J Affect Disord 58(3):215–221, 2000 10802130

Seitz DP, Brisbin S, Herrmann N, et al: Efficacy and feasibility of nonpharmacological interventions for neuropsychiatric symptoms of dementia in long term care: a systematic review. J Am Med Dir Assoc 13(6):503–506.e2, 2012 22342481

Seppi K, Ray Chaudhuri K, Coelho M, et al: Update on treatments for nonmotor symptoms of Parkinson's disease—an evidence-based medicine review. Mov Disord 34(2):180–198, 2019 30653247

Sharfstein SS: Goals of inpatient treatment for psychiatric disorders. Annu Rev Med 60(1):393–403, 2009 18729730

Shulman KI, Tohen M, Satlin A, et al: Mania compared with unipolar depression in old age. Am J Psychiatry 149(3):341–345, 1992 1536272

Siddiqi N, House AO, Holmes JD: Occurrence and outcome of delirium in medical inpatients: a systematic literature review. Age Ageing 35(4):350–364, 2006 16648149

Siddiqi N, Harrison JK, Clegg A, et al: Interventions for preventing delirium in hospitalised non-ICU patients. Cochrane Database Syst Rev 3:CD005563, 2016 26967259

Small GW, Rabins PV, Barry PP, et al: Diagnosis and treatment of Alzheimer disease and related disorders: consensus statement of the American Association for Geriatric Psychiatry, the Alzheimer's Association, and the American Geriatrics Society. JAMA 278(16):1363–1371, 1997 9343469

Sörensen S, Pinquart M, Duberstein P: How effective are interventions with caregivers? An updated meta-analysis. Gerontologist 42(3):356–372, 2002 12040138

Staab JP, Evans DL: Efficacy of venlafaxine in geriatric depression. Depress Anxiety 12 (suppl 1):63–68, 2000 11098416

Steinberg M, Lyketsos CG: Atypical antipsychotic use in patients with dementia: managing safety concerns. Am J Psychiatry 169(9):900–906, 2012 22952071

Street JS, Clark WS, Gannon KS, et al: Olanzapine treatment of psychotic and behavioral symptoms in patients with Alzheimer disease in nursing care facilities: a double-blind, randomized, placebo-controlled trial. Arch Gen Psychiatry 57(10):968–976, 2000 11015815

Streim JE, Porsteinsson AP, Breder CD, et al: A randomized, double-blind, placebo-controlled study of aripiprazole for the treatment of psychosis in nursing home patients with Alzheimer disease. Am J Geriatr Psychiatry 16(7):537–550, 2008 18591574

Sultzer DL, Davis SM, Tariot PN, et al: Clinical symptom responses to atypical antipsychotic medications in Alzheimer's disease: phase 1 outcomes from the CATIE-AD effectiveness trial. Am J Psychiatry 165(7):844–854, 2008 18519523

Tew JD Jr, Mulsant BH, Haskett RF, et al: Acute efficacy of ECT in the treatment of major depression in the old-old. Am J Psychiatry 156(12):1865–1870, 1999 10588398

Thase ME: Effects of venlafaxine on blood pressure: a meta-analysis of original data from 3744 depressed patients. J Clin Psychiatry 59(10):502–508, 1998 9818630

Thompson LW, Coon DW, Gallagher-Thompson D, et al: Comparison of desipramine and cognitive/behavioral therapy in the treatment of elderly outpatients with mild-to-moderate depression. Am J Geriatr Psychiatry 9(3):225–240, 2001 11481130

Thompson WK, Savla GN, Vahia IV, et al: Characterizing trajectories of cognitive functioning in older adults with schizophrenia: does method matter? Schizophr Res 143(1):90–96, 2013 23218560

Tiihonen J, Lönnqvist J, Wahlbeck K, et al: 11-year follow-up of mortality in patients with schizophrenia: a population-based cohort study (FIN11 study). Lancet 374(9690):620–627, 2009 19595447

Trachsel M, Hermann H, Biller-Andorno N: Cognitive fluctuations as a challenge for the assessment of decision-making capacity in patients with dementia. Am J Alzheimers Dis Other Demen 30(4):360–363, 2015 24946784

Trifirò G, Spina E, Gambassi G: Use of antipsychotics in elderly patients with dementia: do atypical and conventional agents have a similar safety profile? Pharmacol Res 59(1):1–12, 2009 18977443

van Laar T, De Deyn PP, Aarsland D, et al: Effects of cholinesterase inhibitors in Parkinson's disease dementia: a review of clinical data. CNS Neurosci Ther 17(5):428–441, 2011 21951368

Victoria LW, Whyte EM, Butters MA, et al: Improvement in depression is associated with improvement in cognition in late-life psychotic depression. Am J Geriatr Psychiatry 25(6):672–679, 2017 28285771

Weintraub D, Hurtig HI: Presentation and management of psychosis in Parkinson's disease and dementia with Lewy bodies. Am J Psychiatry 164(10):1491–1498, 2007 17898337

Wendler D, Rid A: Systematic review: the effect on surrogates of making treatment decisions for others. Ann Intern Med 154(5):336–346, 2011 21357911

Wijkstra J, Lijmer J, Balk FJ, et al: Pharmacological treatment for unipolar psychotic depression: systematic review and meta-analysis. Br J Psychiatry 188:410–415, 2006 16648526
Wilcock GK, Ballard CG, Cooper JA, Loft H: Memantine for agitation/aggression and psychosis in moderately severe to severe Alzheimer's disease: a pooled analysis of 3 studies. J Clin Psychiatry 69(3):341–348, 2008 18294023
Williams SA, Kasl SV, Heiat A, et al: Depression and risk of heart failure among the elderly: a prospective community-based study. Psychosom Med 64(1):6–12, 2002 11818580
Wilson MP, Nordstrom K, Anderson EL, et al: American Association for Emergency Psychiatry Task Force on Medical Clearance of Adult Psychiatric Patients, Part II: controversies over medical assessment, and consensus recommendations. West J Emerg Med 18(4):640–646, 2017 28611885
Wind AW, Schellevis FG, Van Staveren G, et al: Limitations of the Mini-Mental State Examination in diagnosing dementia in general practice. Int J Geriatr Psychiatry 12(1):101–108, 1997 9050431
Wong CA, Recktenwald AJ, Jones ML, et al: The cost of serious fall-related injuries at three Midwestern hospitals. Jt Comm J Qual Patient Saf 37(2):81–87, 2011 21939135
Wystanski M: Assaultive behaviour in psychiatrically hospitalized elderly: a response to psychosocial stimulation and changes in pharmacotherapy. Int J Geriatr Psychiatry 15(7):582–585, 2000 10918337
Yazgan IC, Greenwald BS, Kremen NJ, et al: Geriatric psychiatry versus general psychiatry inpatient treatment of the elderly. Am J Psychiatry 161(2):352–355, 2004 14754785
Yesavage JA, Brink TL, Rose TL, et al: Development and validation of a geriatric depression screening scale: a preliminary report. J Psychiatr Res 17(1):37–49, 1982–1983 7183759
Young RC, Gyulai L, Mulsant BH, et al: Pharmacotherapy of bipolar disorder in old age: review and recommendations. Am J Geriatr Psychiatry 12(4):342–357, 2004 15249272
Young RC, Mulsant BH, Sajatovic M, et al: GERI-BD: a randomized double-blind controlled trial of lithium and divalproex in the treatment of mania in older patients with bipolar disorder. Am J Psychiatry 174(11):1086–1093, 2017 29088928
Zeiss AM, Lewinsohn PM, Rohde P, Seeley JR: Relationship of physical disease and functional impairment to depression in older people. Psychol Aging 11(4):572–581, 1996 9000290
Zuidema SU, Johansson A, Selbaek G, et al: A consensus guideline for antipsychotic drug use for dementia in care homes: bridging the gap between scientific evidence and clinical practice. Int Psychogeriatr 27(11):1849–1859, 2015 26062126

Units by Diagnostic Cohort

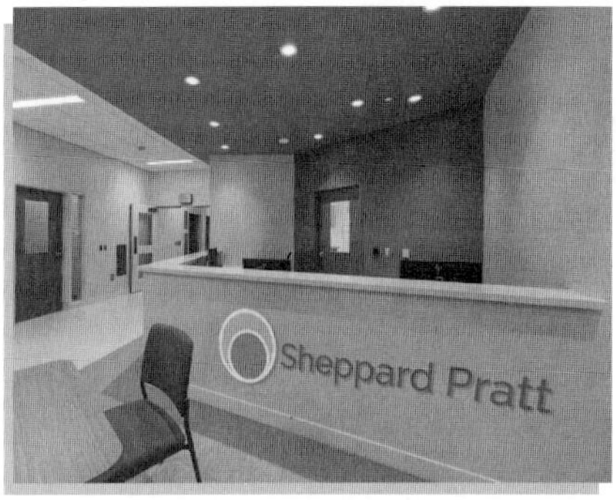

CHAPTER 6

The Developmental Disabilities Co-occurring Unit

Neuropsychiatry Across the Life Span

Scott R. Pekrul, M.D.
Robert W. Wisner-Carlson, M.D.
Thomas Flis, M.S.

Some would argue there is only neuropsychiatry. Certainly, in the early days of the asylum movement, institutions served people suffering from epilepsy, neurosyphilis, dementia, and encephalitis, as well as melancholia, manic-depressive illness, dementia praecox, and catatonia (Ovsiew and Jobe 1999; Shorter 1997). Neuropsychiatry arose as a discipline in this context during the mid-nineteenth century and fell from prominence in the twentieth century, only to reemerge as a specialty of psychiatry and neurology in the late twentieth century (Yudofsky and Hales 1989). Neuropsychiatry can be seen as an amalgam of neurology and psychiatry, a discipline dealing with the psychiatric aspects of neurological disorder and the borderland between clinical neurology and psychiatry (Lishman 1992; Ramirez-Bermudez et al. 2017) with a set of patients who have fallen between the cracks of the early-twentieth-century fracture between neurology and psychiatry (Trimble 2016). Conditions dealt with in neuropsychiatry include cognitive disorders such as dementias; psychiatric and behavioral concomitants of neurological disorders such as epilepsy, multiple sclerosis, and traumatic brain injury; and neurodevelopmental disorders such as intellectual disability (ID) and autism spectrum disorder (ASD) (Sachdev 2007). In this chapter we focus primarily on the inpatient neuropsychiatric treatment of psychiatric and behavioral conditions occurring in ID and ASD, referred to as a group as *intellectual and developmental disabilities*. We begin the chapter with a brief review of custodial or inpatient care of this patient population, followed by a description of the unique characteristics of the population of individuals with intellectual and developmental disabilities warranting a specialized neuropsychiatry inpatient unit. This will then inform our discussion of the unique needs and challenges in evaluating and treating this patient population.

History of the Hospitalization of Individuals With Intellectual and Developmental Disabilities and Other Neuropsychiatric Disorders

In the nineteenth century, education and reintegration into society were the goals for individuals with intellectual and developmental disabilities. As with individuals with mental illness who were given asylum from society for treatment and recovery, individuals with intellectual and developmental disabilities were committed to long-term public residential schools and centers with the goal of protection from society and habilitation (Lowrey 1944). However, in the late nineteenth and early twentieth centuries, the American eugenics movement emerged and portrayed people with ID as being a threat to society. This led to legislative support for long-term custodial and institutional care as a de facto form of incarceration. Between 1880 and 1900 the population of institutionalized individuals with intellectual and developmental disabilities rose from just more than 4,000 to 15,000. Over time, each state developed public institutions housing thousands of people with mental illness or intellectual and developmental disabilities, with the largest housing as many as 20,000 people. By the late 1960s, state institutions across the nation brimmed with an alarming 156,000 people with intellectual and developmental disabilities and 550,000 additional people experiencing mental illness (Lowrey 1944; Shorter 1997). This institutionalization movement led to the incarceration of individuals with intellectual and developmental disabilities regardless of dangerousness, maladaptive behaviors, or comorbid psychiatric illness (Day 1994; Lowrey 1944). By the 1960s and 1970s, in the setting of general social reform, institutions for individuals with intellectual and developmental disabilities and, also, the mentally ill came under scrutiny. It was recognized that vulnerable individuals were being housed in deplorable living conditions, and a push for deinstitutionalization emerged. Deinstitutionalization was accelerated by the passing of the Individuals with Disabilities Education Act (IDEA) in 1990. The end result was a massive decrease in the number of institutional settings for those with intellectual and developmental disabilities.

The deinstitutionalization of persons with intellectual and developmental disabilities came with the assumption that the behavioral and mental health problems of people with intellectual and developmental disabilities were a consequence of living in an institution. This turned out to be only partially correct. The goal had been to move services to large-scale community-based programs. However, over time, it became increasingly clear that individuals with ID and ASD had unique needs as well as higher rates of psychiatric disorders compared with the general population. The need for specialized services for this population was increasingly recognized from the 1980s to the 1990s (Moss et al. 1997). Several reasons have been identified for specialty services for this population, including the difficulties in making an accurate diagnosis, the need for modification of the services provided, and the development of staff competencies in handling this population (Day 2001).

The need for specialized neuropsychiatric units is large, and while most persons with neurodevelopmental disorders are admitted to general inpatient units, the number of specialized neuropsychiatric units has increased since the early 2000s. The most recent survey has identified nine pediatric neuropsychiatric units in the United States (Siegel et al. 2012). Prior to the age of 21, 11% of children and adolescents with ASD will be psychiatrically hospitalized in the United States (Croen et al. 2006; Mandell 2008) to either a general or a specialized unit. According to a survey completed by Siegel and colleagues (2012), pediatric neuropsychiatric units admit ASD patients at a higher rate, with ASD accounting for up to 76% of the admissions. In addition, 88% of patients had a full-scale IQ of less than 75. Further, the patients admitted had high rates of language impairment, with 27% classified as nonverbal (less than 10 words), 26% as limited verbal (primarily echolalia and scripting), and 45% as verbal (phrase speech) (Siegel et al. 2012). Individuals with ASD with this level of impairment are also at higher risk of medical comorbidities, including epilepsy. Analysis of patients with ID and/or ASD on a specialized neuropsychiatry unit showed improved outcomes, with significant decreases in aggression, self-injury, and tantrum behavior upon discharge that were sustained at 2 months postdischarge (Siegel and Gabriels 2014). The average length of stay was 45 days. A retrospective study (Gabriels et al. 2012) compared outcomes for ID and ASD pediatric patients with similar presentations admitted to either a general psychiatry unit or specialized units. The pediatric patients admitted to the specialized unit were found to have shorter average lengths of stay (26 vs. 45 days) and a lower 1-year readmission rate (12% vs. 33%).

Intellectual Disability and Autism Spectrum Disorder

ID and ASD are part of the broad category of intellectual and developmental disabilities. There can be considerable overlap in aspects of each category, particularly when ID and ASD are more severe and, likely, occurring together.

Intellectual Disability

ID is a developmental neurocognitive disorder characterized by deficits in general mental abilities and adaptive functioning (American Psychiatric Association 2013). In this context, *general mental abilities* refers to intelligence, a construct that can be complicated and even divisive. Generally, intelligence is considered a single trait, possibly supported by more specialized cognitive abilities. As well, intelligence has been conceptualized as a multidimensional construct (e.g., crystalized [knowledge and information] and fluid [abilities in reasoning and memory]) (Schalock et al. 2009). Thus, intelligence as a construct is complicated and beyond the scope of this chapter to explore fully.

ID is diagnosed by clinical assessment combined with standardized testing. General mental abilities or intelligence is tested with intelligence testing such as the Wechsler Adult Intelligence Scale or the Stanford-Binet Intelligence Scale. Adaptive functioning or adaptive behavior is "the collection of conceptual, social and practical skills that have been learned and are performed by people in their everyday lives" (Schalock et al. 2009, p. 43). Three domains of adaptive function are identified by DSM-5 as conceptual, social, and practical (American Psychiatric Association 2013). For ID to be diagnosed, reliable IQ testing scores must fall at least two standard deviations below the mean, and adaptive functioning, as measured with standardized testing such as the Vineland-II (Vineland Adaptive Behavior Scales, 2nd Edition), must be significantly impaired in at least one domain such that ongoing support is needed for adequate functioning. This latter testing must be confirmed by clinical assessment.

ID has an overall prevalence in the general population of 1%, with severe ID occurring in 6 per 1,000. By definition, the condition begins during the developmental period. It occurs more frequently in males, with a male-to-female ratio of 1.6:1 for mild ID and 1.2:1 for severe ID (American Psychiatric Association 2013). A multitude of genetic conditions, diseases, exposures, and so forth can cause ID. These can be divided into prenatal, perinatal, and postnatal causes, with risk factors in four realms: biomedical, social, behavioral, and educational (American Psychiatric Association 2013; Harris 2006; Schalock et al. 2009; Wehmeyer et al. 2017).

ID is an example of an impairment in the dimensional characteristic of intelligence present in all people. Individuals with ID are at risk for distress and behavioral disorder due to provocations overwhelming their cognitive abilities (McHugh and Slavney 1998). Psychiatric conditions and problem behaviors occur at a higher rate in individuals with ID (Cooper et al. 2007; Fletcher et al. 2017). Special considerations apply when diagnosing psychiatric and behavioral conditions in individuals with ID and other developmental disabilities, including ASD. Special diagnostic classification systems exist, including the *Diagnostic Manual—Intellectual Disability*, 2nd Edition (DM-ID 2; Fletcher et al. 2017), which is correlated with DSM-5 (American Psychiatric Association 2013), and the Diagnostic Criteria for Psychiatric Disorders for Use With Adults With Learning Disabilities/Mental Retardation (DC-LD) of the Royal College of Psychiatrists (Royal College of Psychiatrists 2001). Four phenomena need to be considered in evaluating individuals with intellectual and developmental disabilities: baseline exaggeration, intellectual distortion, psychosocial masking, and cognitive disintegration (Fletcher et al. 2017; Sovner and Hurley 1986). Baseline exaggeration and cognitive disintegration are considered later in the chapter.

Autism Spectrum Disorder

First described separately by Kanner in 1943 (Kanner 1943, 1968) and Asperger in 1944 (Asperger 1944, 1991), *Autism spectrum disorder* is defined as a complex, lifelong neurodevelopmental condition characterized by impairments in communication and social interaction combined with repetitive or rigid behaviors and restricted interests. The worldwide prevalence has been estimated to be 1%–2%. The most recent Centers for Disease Control and Prevention estimate of prevalence in the United States is 1 in 54, or 1.85%. ASD is about four times more common in boys than in girls (American Psychiatric Association 2013; Lai et al. 2014; Maenner et al. 2020). ASD is highly genetic, with a current heritability estimate of 83% (Folstein and Rutter 1977; Levy et al. 2009; Sandin et al. 2017; Yuen et al. 2019). Although syndromic autism is found in numerous genetic conditions (Benvenuto et al. 2009; Caglayan 2010), and genetic conditions that cause ID also commonly cause ASD (Coleman 2009), common genetic variation is thought to contribute the greatest portion of the risk (Gaugler et al. 2014). Individuals with ASD have an atypical cognitive profile with impairments in social cognition and executive function and atypical perceptual and information processing (Lai et al. 2014). Medical and psychiatric comorbidity is high (Davignon et al. 2018; Lai et al. 2019; Mosner et al. 2019; Rosen et al. 2018). Epilepsy is more common in ASD, present at a rate of 30%; ASD co-occurs in epilepsy also at a rate of 30% (Clarke et al. 2005; Tuchman and Rapin 2002; Tuchman et al. 2010). The epilepsy risk in ASD is a function of ID severity, female gender, and poorer verbal abilities (Amiet et al. 2008; Bolton et al. 2011; Mannion and Leader 2014).

Key Syndromes and Behavioral Phenotypes

ASD and ID are not uniform conditions and can manifest in different manners with varying characteristics. Part of this variation relates to the numerous causes as described above. Syndromal causes of ID and ASD, both genetic and environmental, are important to identify because of expected important findings and comorbid cognitive, behavioral, medical, and psychiatric conditions. Thus, the clinician on a neuropsychiatry inpatient unit should be familiar with a number of key syndromes for diagnosis, recognition of common comorbidities, and treatment planning.

An important concept in this regard is the *behavioral phenotype* associated with the syndrome. A behavioral phenotype is "a characteristic pattern of motor, cognitive, linguistic and social observations that is consistently associated with a biologic disorder" (O'Brien 2002, p. 2). Examples of behavioral phenotypes include self-injurious behavior in Lesch-Nyhan (Nyhan 1972, 1976) and Smith-Magenis (Elsea and Girirajan 2008) syndromes and hyperphagia in Prader-Willi syndrome (Whittington and Holland 2004) leading to morbid obesity.

Down syndrome is a well-recognized cause of ID, well known to the medical and lay community. First described in the nineteenth century by physician John Langdon Down, Down syndrome is the most common genetic cause of ID and was the first intellectual disability syndrome described. It is due to a trisomy of chromosome 21. Individuals with Down syndrome have characteristic physical characteristics, including facial features, short stature, and small hands with a palmar crease. ID in Down syndrome tends to fall in the moderate to severe range. Adults with Down syndrome have a significantly increased risk of dementia starting in middle to later adulthood (40 years and older) (McGlinchey et al. 2020). Though temperamentally described as good-natured, individuals with ID can have behavioral and psychiatric problems, including depression and anxiety. Though once felt to be rare in Down syndrome, ASD is now diagnosed in individuals with Down syndrome at a significantly higher frequency than in the general population (DiGuiseppi et al. 2010). Medical comorbidities such as hypothyroidism, obstructive sleep apnea, hearing loss, and cataracts may play a role in behavioral and psychiatric presentations that can lead to an inpatient admission.

Prader-Willi syndrome is a less common genetic syndrome but exemplifies the various issues that arise connected to syndromal neurodevelopmental disorders. It is the most common genetic cause of childhood and adult obesity. Prader-Willi syndrome is an example of genomic imprinting (i.e., the turning off of genes differentially in the maternally and paternally derived chromosomes). Deletion of the 15q11.2–q13 region in the father, maternal uniparental disomy (both copies of chromosome 15 are derived from the mother), or a defect in the imprinting center can cause this region to be nonfunctional and produce Prader-Willi syndrome. Individuals with Prader-Willi syndrome have learning disabilities, low normal intelligence, or mild ID. Autism occurs at a higher rate (Baker et al. 2018; Dykens et al. 2017; Veltman et al. 2005). Individuals with Prader-Willi syndrome are often stubborn and prone to temper tantrums, manipulation, compulsive behaviors, and problems with changes in routines. These traits can lead to challenging behaviors, agitation, aggression, and inpatient admission. Because of the lack of satiety in eating, individuals with Prader-Willi syndrome are very food focused and engage in various problematic behaviors around food, including overeating, food hoarding, secretive eating, agitation and aggression when deprived of food, and food bingeing to the point of gastric rupture (Stevenson et al. 2007). Psychosis is also increased in individuals with Prader-Willi syndrome, especially in the maternal uniparental subtype (Vogels et al. 2003; Whittington and Holland 2004). Bipolar disorder and cycloid psychosis predominate (Verhoeven et al. 2003). Thus, temperamental, psychiatric, and medical issues all can play a role in the psychiatric presentation of an individual with Prader-Willi syndrome.

Angelman syndrome, a genetic neurobehavioral condition and another example of imprinting, is characterized by developmental delay with severe ID and absent language; movement or balance disorders, especially ataxic gait; frequent laughing or happy demeanor; and epilepsy (Dan 2008, 2009). Angelman syndrome is estimated to occur at an incidence of 1 in 12,000 to 1 in 20,000. Genetically, it can be seen as the "mirror image" of Prader-Willi syndrome, with disruption of function of *UBE3A* mapping to the chromosome region 15q11.2–q13. This disruption occurs due to one of four genetic abnormalities: 1) deletion of the 15q11.2–q13 region maternally derived chromosome, 2) paternal uniparental disomy of chromosome 15 (both copies of chromosome 15 being derived from the father), 3) imprinting defects, or 4) *UBE3A* mutations (Williams and Dagli 2010). Problematic behaviors can derive from hyperactivity, poor attention, and noncompliance, sometimes leading to aggression (Pelc et al. 2008; Summers et al. 1995).

Alcohol is the greatest cause of ID. Fetal alcohol syndrome, the more severe manifestation of the broader fetal alcohol spectrum disorder (FASD), exemplifies an environmentally caused neurodevelopmental disorder. Prevalence estimates for fetal alcohol syndrome range from 0.2 to 1.5 per 1,000 (Centers for Disease Control and Prevention n.d.; Popova et al. 2017) and for FASD as high as 1%–5% (May et al. 2018). Prenatal alcohol exposure has both a dose and a timing effect, with higher doses earlier in gestation causing greatest harm. Genetic factors also play a role (Chudley and Longstaffe 2005; Eberhart and Parnell 2016; Ramsay 2010). With alcohol as the provocative factor, five permissive factors can be identified in enhancing the teratogenic prenatal effects: 1) peak maternal blood concentrations from alcohol bingeing; 2) timing of prenatal exposure; 3) socioeconomic status as an indicator of poor maternal nutrition and health, decreased access to prenatal care, and increased maternal distress; 4) polydrug use; and

5) genetic factors (Nulman et al. 2018). Features of FASD include characteristic facial features, including a flat philtrum with a thin upper lip and short palpebral fissure; evidence of pre- and postnatal growth retardation; neurocognitive deficits; and CNS dysfunction. Fetal alcohol exposure cannot always be confirmed, and diagnostic guidelines take this into account (Mukherjee et al. 2006). CNS abnormalities and functional abnormalities, including decreased IQ, learning disabilities, executive function deficits, motor functioning delays, attention and hyperactivity problems, and social skills problems, may be present (Bertrand et al. 2005). ADHD occurs frequently in individuals with FASD. Other reported psychiatric conditions include depression, anxiety disorder, PTSD, oppositional defiant disorder, reactive attachment disorder, bipolar disorder, and psychotic disorder. Co-occurring risk factors such as maternal smoking, poor maternal nutrition, genetic risks of mental illness, socioeconomic status, parenting issues, and foster care placements can contribute to the development of these psychiatric conditions beyond the teratogenic effects of prenatal alcohol exposure. Adverse childhood experiences (ACEs), including neglect, emotional abuse, and physical abuse, occur more frequently in FASD (Weyrauch et al. 2017) and may increase the risk of developing neurodevelopmental and psychiatric disorders in this population (Kambeitz et al. 2019). Thus, the individual with FASD may be multiply burdened by the teratogenic effects of prenatal alcohol exposure, the genetic propensity to psychiatric conditions, environmental risks (including ACEs), and cognitive and functional deficiencies in dealing with these burdens. In particular, individuals with FASD often have executive function problems, including difficulty in foreseeing consequences, problems learning from experience, poor abstract thinking, poor adaptability, impaired judgment, and emotional regulatory problems (Kodituwakku and Kodituwakku 2014; Koren et al. 2003).

22q11.2 deletion syndrome (velocardiofacial syndrome; 22q11DS) is the most common microdeletion syndrome in humans, with a prevalence of 1 per 3,000–6,000 live births. Learning difficulties or developmental disability, including nonverbal learning disability, is almost always present (in 70%–90% of individuals with the deletion) (McDonald-McGinn et al. 1999, 2015). Average IQ tends to be in the borderline range in the low 70s, though individuals can have normal intelligence (Harris 2006; Oskarsdóttir et al. 2005). IQ scores are lower in individuals with larger deletions (Zhao et al. 2018). 22q11DS is a single-gene cause of psychosis and one of the greatest risk factors for developing psychosis, with up to 41% of adults older than 25 years with 22q11DS developing psychosis (Schneider et al. 2014). Psychotic experiences emerge in early adolescence, correlating with anxiety and ADHD (Chawner et al. 2019). A cognitive decline may have preceded the development of psychosis (Gothelf et al. 2013; Pontillo et al. 2019; Vorstman et al. 2015). Psychiatric disorders in general are highly prevalent in 22q11DS (Tang et al. 2014). Individuals with 22q11DS may have characteristic facial features; a variety of medical conditions, including heart defects; abnormalities of the palate; immune system problems; and cognitive and learning disabilities. A variety of other medical problems can be present.

Fragile X syndrome is the most common inherited form of ID and ASD. It is due to a trinucleotide repeat (CGG) with >200 repeats silencing *FMR1*. The prevalence is estimated at 1 in 5,000 males and 1 in 4,000 to 1 in 8,000 females, though lower rates in females have also been reported (Hagerman et al. 2017). Individuals with fragile X syndrome have ID in the severe to moderate range (Harris 2006; Sansone et al. 2014).

ASD occurs in 50%–70% of individuals with fragile X syndrome (Kidd et al. 2020), though higher rates have been reported (Haebig et al. 2020). Other psychiatric and behavioral problems include ADHD, anxiety, impulsivity, unstable affect, self-injurious behavior, and aggression (Hagerman et al. 2017; Tranfaglia 2011).

Rett syndrome is the most common cause of profound ID in girls and women. It has a prevalence of 1 in 10,000 to 1 in 23,000 girls. A few male cases have been reported (Harris 2006; Kaur and Christodoulou 2001; Neul et al. 2019). The core clinical criteria of Rett syndrome are loss of hand skills, loss of spoken language, gait abnormality, stereotypic hand movements, and a period of regression followed by recovery or stabilization. Most cases result from a mutation on *MECP2*, which maps to Xq28 (Leonard et al. 2017). Seizures, scoliosis, foot deformities, gastrointestinal reflux, constipation, long QT syndrome, autonomic dysfunction, breathing problems, sleep problems, and crying and screaming spells can require clinical management (Schultz et al. 2018; Smeets and Schrander-Stumpel 2005). Although Rett syndrome is no longer classified as a pervasive development disorder or part of the autism spectrum, a behavioral phenotype with autistic symptoms has been described (Moss and Howlin 2009; Mount et al. 2002, 2003a, 2003b; Richards et al. 2015).

The discussion above highlights some of the special characteristics and needs of this patient population. Issues such as language and communication problems, concrete thinking with problems in abstracting, and difficulties with adaptive functioning and performance of activities of daily living (ADLs) are examples of special characteristics of this population requiring a special approach. Also, this patient population has a higher comorbidity of medical problems and, sometimes, special medical issues. The composition, expertise, and training of the inpatient treatment must reflect these needs.

The Inpatient Treatment Team

Because of the multiple needs of neuropsychiatric patients on an inpatient unit, a multidisciplinary treatment team is required, covering a range of expertise and professions. Team members include a psychiatrist, psychiatric nurses, an internist/pediatrician, a social worker, a behavioral therapist, a psychologist, a speech and language pathologist (SLP), an occupational therapist (OT), and educators.

Psychiatrist

As leader of the treatment team, the psychiatrist performs a psychiatric evaluation to assess the patient and devises the treatment plan in coordination with other disciplines. The psychiatrist must be knowledgeable about the varieties of psychiatric presentations of individuals with ID, ASD, and various genetic and other syndromes as described above. Familiarity with medical comorbidities is crucial to ruling out medical causes or contributors to behavioral problems in this population. Education of the treatment team about these issues is important. The psychiatrist needs to know about ASD and ID in general, but also about genetic and other neurodevelopmental syndromes as described above and in Table 6–1. In some situations, the psychiatrist will coordinate the medical care, consulting with outpatient specialists including geneticists and neurologists and confirming that emergency department (ED) physicians, internists, and pediatricians have done their due diligence in evaluating the patient. There are more than 7,000 rare diseases (Haendel et al. 2019), and one cannot know all of them. Many rare diseases have neuropsychiatric manifestations (Lauterbach et al. 2016), and the psychiatrist must self-educate and educate the treatment team appropriately. Though *Smith's Recognizable Patterns of Human Malformations* (Jones et al. 2013) has been the standard reference text, numerous internet-based resources are now available and recommendable, including GeneReviews at the NCBI Bookshelf (www.ncbi.nlm.nih.gov/books/NBK1116); the NORD (National Organization for Rare Disorders) website (https://rarediseases.org); the Genetic and Rare Diseases Information Center (https://rarediseases.info.nih.gov) of the NIH National Center for Advancing Translational Services; the Genetics reference page of the U.S. National Library of Medicine (https://ghr.nlm.nih.gov); UpToDate (www.uptodate.com); and MedLink Neurology (www.medlink.com).

Psychiatric Nurse

The role of the psychiatric nurse is multifaceted, involving compassionate, patient-centered care in the context of teamwork and collaboration, underpinned by respect and open communication. The psychiatric nurse is responsible for the psychiatric nursing assessment, which involves an analysis of the patient's problems and a nursing plan with interventions to address those problems (Halter 2018; Manaka et al. 2018). The nurse is also responsible for enacting much of the general treatment plan, including physical and biologic interventions, such as administering medications; physical assessment and care; working with families; behavioral interventions; and safety/risk management (Taua et al. 2012). Both children and adults with ID and ASD may need significant assistance with ADL, sometimes requiring full care. Other aspects of the patient population need to be recognized and accommodated in the nursing process, such as language issues and difficulties with abstract reasoning. For example, one must ask questions and give directions with simple language and vocabulary. Some individuals with ASD may have minimal spoken language but use other communication devices. It is important to ascertain the best way to communicate with the patient from parents and/or caregivers (Evans et al. 2016). More emphasis on observation of behaviors and nonverbal communication may be needed. Overall, the unique qualities and needs of individuals with ID and ASD determine the skills that are required by the nursing staff. Individuals with ASD and ID often have behaviors, particular interests, hypersensitivities, and special triggers that need to be known to the staff to appropriately manage the person while a patient is on the unit. Nurses or their supervisees also collect data both formally and informally. Because of the patient's deficits in language and self-reflection, behavioral observations are paramount in determining the success of the treatment plan or to guide the adjustments that need to be made to it. The nurse is responsible for the overall functioning of the milieu, including the safety of the patients and staff. Other duties include psychoeducation, including medication education, for the patient and family.

Internist/Pediatrician

Because of the higher burden of comorbid medical problems in this population, the internist or pediatrician must be available for initial medical assessment and ongoing

TABLE 6–1. Genetic and other neurodevelopmental syndromes

Syndrome	Incidence	Cause	Characteristics	Intellectual / Cognitive	Language	Behavioral phenotype	Psychiatric comorbidities	Medical comorbidities	References
Down syndrome	1/800 to 1/700 live births Most common genetic cause of ID	Trisomy 21	Characteristic facial, palmar, and other features	Moderate to severe ID	Receptive language better than expressive	Friendly and affable Can be quite obstinate	Dementia in adults (50% by age 50 years) (McGlinchey et al. 2020) Anxiety Depression	Hypothyroidism Structural cardiac abnormalities Cataracts Hearing loss Obstructive sleep apnea (Startin et al. 2020)	Esbensen and MacLean 2017; Harris 2006
Prader-Willi syndrome	1/10,000 to 1/30,000 live births	Absence of paternally expressed imprinted genes at 15q11.2-q13	Characteristic facial features; strabismus; short stature; obesity starting in childhood	Low normal IQ to mild ID Learning disabilities	Delayed Verbal abilities generally a relative strength	Temper tantrums, stubbornness, manipulative and compulsive behaviors Skin picking	Psychosis OCD Autism	Hypogonadism Obesity Scoliosis Sleep disturbance Type II diabetes Central adrenal insufficiency Hypothalamic dysfunction	Whittington and Holland 2004
Angelman syndrome	1/12,000 to 1/20,000	Disruption of function of *UBE3A*	Developmental delay Severe ID	Severe ID	Absent language	Exuberant behavior Happy demeanor Prominent smiling Disrupted sleep Fascination with water	ASD	Epilepsy	Dan 2008, 2009; Moss and Howlin 2009; Moss et al. 2013; Pelc et al. 2008; Richards et al. 2015; Williams and Dagli 2010

TABLE 6–1. Genetic and other neurodevelopmental syndromes *(continued)*

Syndrome	Incidence	Cause	Characteristics	Intellectual / Cognitive	Language	Behavioral phenotype	Psychiatric comorbidities	Medical comorbidities	References
Fetalalcohol syndrome	14.6 per 10,000	Fetal alcohol exposure	Characteristic facial features Prenatal and postnatal growth deficiency Neurocognitive deficits	Reduced IQ Mild to moderate ID		Attentional problems Conduct problems	ADHD And others	Cardiac abnormalities Ophthalmologic conditions Hearing loss Middle ear disease	Chudley and Longstaffe 2005; Harris 2006; Popova et al. 2017
22q11.2 deletion syndrome	1 in 3,000 to 1 in 6,000	Microdeletion 22q11.2	Characteristic facial features and hypernasal speech due to palatal abnormalities Congenital Cardiac abnormalities	Usually normal to mild ID Learning disabilities NVLD	Relative strength	Shy, socially withdrawn with poor social skills Impulsive, disinhibited, and prone to temper tantrums	Psychosis Anxiety ADHD Autism Mood disorders	Palatal abnormalities Congenital Heart defect Immunodeficiency Hypocalcemia	Harris 2006; McDonald-McGinn et al. 2010, 2015; Sandini et al. 2020; Tang et al. 2014
Fragile X syndrome	1 in 5,000 males 1 in 4,000–8,000 females	Trinucleotide repeat (CGG) > 200 on X chromosome silencing *FMR1*	Elongated face Large protruding ears Hyperflexible joints Macroorchidism Gaze aversion	Moderate to severe ID	Receptive better than expressive	Anxiety Gaze aversion Hyperactivity Sensory hyperarousal Impulsivity Tantrums Aggression	ASD ADHD Anxiety	Seizures Recurrent otitis media Later parkinsonism	Hagerman 2010; Hagerman et al. 2017; Harris 2006

Note. ASD=autism spectrum disorder; NVLD=nonverbal learning disorder; OCD=obsessive-compulsive disorder.

assessment and management of medical conditions. As with other disciplines, the consultant must be knowledgeable about the medical comorbidities that are common in these disorders and help the treatment team in ruling these out as causes or contributors to the presenting behavioral problems. Other medical consultations, such as dental or neurological, may be required.

Social Worker

Individuals with ID and ASD needing inpatient psychiatric admission on a specialty neuropsychiatry unit require considerable community support and services. The social worker's role is to interface with the patient's support group, be it family, care staff, or individuals from various private and governmental agencies involved with the patient's care. While all members of the treatment team gather collateral information from various parties, the social worker completes a psychosocial evaluation from family and relevant informants about the presenting complaint and other background information about the patient. Often, outside records are required, including copies of physician medication orders and medication administration records from residential settings. As well, the social worker updates the family and caretakers on the progress of treatment, gives support and educates the family and caretakers about the patient's diagnosis and behavioral needs. Supportive therapy with family members not uncommonly occurs, often informally over the phone, including processing the range of difficulties the patient and family must endure. Sometimes it is better for the patient, especially if a young or not-so-young adult, to live outside the family home. These decisions can be difficult for the family and processing decisions and emotions is crucial for a smooth transition. Visits from the family and/or caretakers are an opportunity for evaluation of the patient's condition—how the patient seems to be doing. These visits are processed by the social worker and salient information is reported to other members of the treatment team.

Behavioral Therapist

Because patients with intellectual and developmental disabilities (ID and ASD) are generally admitted for aggressive or self-injurious behaviors and because of the efficacy of behavioral interventions, behavioral therapists play an integral role in the development of applied behavioral analytic interventions on the inpatient neuropsychiatry units (Foxx 2008; Matson et al. 1996). These clinicians are master's- or doctoral-level board-certified behavior analysts who may have assistants working under their license credentialed as registered behavior technicians. A behavioral therapist starts by gaining collateral information from caregivers and the outpatient treatment team regarding target behaviors and begins to observe the patient on the unit while gathering anecdotal data. A functional behavioral assessment is completed after analyzing collected data. A behavioral intervention plan is developed to intervene on the contingencies maintaining a target behavior. Finally, that plan is tested and modeled to direct care staff with follow-up maintenance checks to ensure that fidelity of treatment is followed and that objectives are met. The behavioral therapist will make adjustments to the plan as necessary. Caregivers may come to the inpatient unit to be trained in implementing strategies that have been identified to be successful. Final recommendations are provided to outpatient therapists and caregivers.

Psychologist

Though doctoral-level psychologists are able to determine and develop individual treatment plans targeting problem behaviors, as well as provide direct individual therapy, their major role is in performing a variety of assessments that are of relevance to the neuropsychiatric population. These assessments may provide diagnostic clarity or strengthen the diagnosis of a suspected neurodevelopmental disorder. Intelligence tests may be performed to determine the cognitive ability of an individual. Adaptive behavior assessments determine the strengths or deficits of day-to-day behaviors of an individual as compared to typically developing peers. Informant- and observation-based assessments can be used to determine the impact of psychopharmacological interventions on the individual (Pyles et al. 1997). Psychological assessments of cognitive and functional strengths and weaknesses can guide treatment strategies both inpatient and outpatient and can be followed over time to assess progress in some areas.

Speech and Language Pathologist

SLPs focus on the communication and swallowing aspects of an individual (American Speech-Language-Hearing Association 2016). SLPs can assess and determine a patient's strengths and deficits in speech production and fluency. This assessment can be used to determine whether there is a language delay or if an individual's language deficits are due to a neuropsychological condition. Individuals within the neuropsychiatric population may have more difficulties with utilizing functional communication (Diehl 2003), and as such, an SLP may develop initial interventions that can be generalized and further developed on an outpatient basis. Furthermore, SLPs can assess difficulties associated with feeding and swallowing. Such an assessment may determine if the swallowing difficulty arises from a neurological condition, sensory issues, or behavioral conditioning (Twachtman-Reilly et al. 2008). These findings can help determine the most effective follow-up treatment whether it be further behavioral therapy, occupational therapy, speech and language therapy, or medical treatment.

Occupational Therapist

An OT assesses functional abilities and identifies deficits in adaptive behavior and social skills. As well, the OT seeks to identify activities that are meaningful to the individual. The therapist can help determine what supports are needed and help build on emerging skills. The OT facilitates a wide array of choices based on the patient's needs and promotes a sense of inclusion within a group setting (Umeda et al. 2017). OTs can also ascertain sensory-based disorders and construct strategies to help the individual adapt or grow, while identifying preventive measures on the unit related to the individual's sensory aversions (Schaaf and Miller 2005). This information can be used to address caregivers and the community in taking steps to adapt to the needs of everyone (Umeda et al. 2017).

Educators

Hospitalizations, especially lengthy ones, may be highly disruptive to an individual's education due to missed schoolwork and the risk of falling behind (Eaton 2012). Communication between both settings can be vital to ensure a smooth transition back into school. School personnel have identified a greater need to understand mental health disorders, have access to discharge summaries, and have a greater understanding on how problem behaviors may interfere with academic achievement (Simon and Savina 2010). As such, the educators and school psychologists in a hospital setting play an important role in assessing an individual's general cognitive ability and achievements, facilitating communication between the school and hospital, and making recommendations for additional supports to be put into place for when the individual returns to the school. Furthermore, they serve as an advocate for increased resources and individualized education plans, if warranted, to help reduce the risk of rehospitalization when the main source of difficulties appears in an academic setting.

Inpatient Treatment

Admission

Psychiatric treatment should be provided in the least restrictive environment. This precept determines the admission criteria for neuropsychiatric patients to the acute inpatient unit. Four general levels of care can then be identified, based on clinical stability and safety: 1) outpatient community services, 2) group home settings with therapeutic services, 3) residential treatment facilities, and 4) acute inpatient stabilization unit. The need for an acute inpatient stabilization unit typically occurs when the individual is a danger to self or others or is having a decline in functioning, or when concerted outpatient treatment is failing and acute inpatient treatment is expected to be effective. In the general psychiatric population, *danger to self or others* usually refers to suicidality and aggression. For the ID and ASD population, *danger toward others* usually refers to recurrent physical aggression, and *danger toward self* typically refers to self-injurious behaviors or a significant functional decline from developmental baseline (McGuire and Siegel 2018). The second issue, functional decline, occurs commonly in acute psychiatric exacerbations in general, but it is amplified in individuals with ID and ASD. This phenomenon, termed *cognitive disintegration*, can entail significant regression, from which the individual recovers once the acute psychiatric condition is treated (Sovner 1986; Sovner and Hurley 1986).

With any acute stabilization unit, regardless of specialization, the discharge goal is for transition of the patient to the least restrictive environment once the acute issue is addressed and the patient is psychiatrically stabilized for outpatient treatment. The transition of care is usually to the previous community provider, whether that be the primary guardian or a group home. However, when the patient is unable to transition back to an outpatient community setting because of the chronicity of their behaviors and/or care requirements beyond the capacity of the short-term unit, then a referral to a residential treatment facility may be indicated.

Referral to an acute stabilization unit can occur from a variety of settings, including the patient's primary care physician or psychiatrist, outpatient therapist, social worker, group home, or school, or after an evaluation from a physician in an ED. Although direct admissions to a neuropsychiatric unit can be arranged, the majority of patients are first referred to an ED for an evaluation prior to admission. If the ED determines the patient is a danger to self or others, they may be referred to an inpatient hospital.

Unfortunately, the need for inpatient services for those with ID and ASD is large, and accessibility to a specialized or general unit that is able to address the unique needs of this population is limited (McGuire and Siegel 2018). This increased demand, along with limited resources, often leads to long wait times in an ED. A study of patients with ASD and ID who presented to the ED for a mental health complaint found that these patients were more likely to remain for extended periods in the ED than their neurotypical peers (Wharff et al. 2011).

According to a study by Siegel and colleagues (2014), presentations to a specialized neuropsychiatric unit for youth ranging from 5 to 21 years in age with either an ASD or an ID diagnosis included aggression (at 89%), self-injury (at 2.6%), and functional decline (at 7.9%). The most common presentation has been found to be externalizing problem behaviors, including aggression, self-injurious behavior, property destruction, and severe tantrums (Siegel et al. 2012). Although externalizing behaviors constitute the major reason for admission to a neuropsychiatric unit, an admission to a short-term unit can also assist in diagnostic clarification, benefiting outpatient providers in identifying appropriate treatment goals (Day 1994). Given the high level of aggressive and self-injurious behaviors as a chief complaint, an acute psychiatric unit should be equipped to effectively treat and handle these behaviors. As such, a specialized neuropsychiatric unit should have appropriate support services as well as staff and clinicians who are educated in the unique challenges of patients with neuropsychiatric needs (McGuire and Siegel 2018).

A panel of expert clinicians from six specialized units compiled a list of suggested practices for psychiatric inpatient units treating youth with ASD and ID. These recommendations include the following (McGuire et al. 2015):

1. Obtain information specific to the child with ASD or ID and their support system.
2. Screen for a medical etiology of the presenting problems.
3. Assess for co-occurring psychiatric disorders, and use evidence-informed pharmacotherapy.
4. Assess and support communication and occupational therapy needs.
5. Conduct a behavioral assessment, and collect data on observable target behavior.
6. Adapt the unit environment and programming to create therapeutic spaces and activities appropriate for children with ASD or ID.
7. Provide structured educational services during hospitalization to facilitate the transition back to school.
8. Provide direct care staff with training specific to working with children with ASD or ID.
9. Determine when a longer inpatient length of stay is required for changing patterns of externalizing behavior and facilitating generalization and multidisciplinary work.
10. Interpret standard medical necessity criteria for inpatient psychiatric care in the context of the developmental disorder.

Once a patient is admitted, it is critical for the inpatient team to complete a comprehensive assessment as outlined in steps 1–5 above. This includes interviewing the patient as well as gathering collateral information from the primary guardian, outpatient providers, and school personnel. In addition, coordinating care with any service providers that may be involved with the patient, such as the Department of Social Services (DSS) and/or Developmental Disabilities Administration, should also be done at admission and prior to discharge. Although collateral information should be part of any admission, it is particularly critical to obtain when treating patients with neurodevelopmental disorders such as ID or ASD because this population often has challenges describing their behaviors or internal states regardless of their developmental level and language skills.

An "admission meeting," scheduled at the beginning of the admission, would ideally take place with the patient's primary guardian, outpatient providers, and the inpatient treatment team, including the psychiatrist, social worker, OT, speech pathologist, nursing staff, behavioral therapist, and discharge coordinator. This meeting serves the purpose of gathering historical information, such as prior psychiatric and medical treatment; defining the reason for admission; clarifying expectations from the guardian and outpatient providers; setting treatment goals; and assisting in the coordination of care with the patient's primary treatment providers. Other pertinent information may include the patient's performance of ADLs, primary method of communication (see below), medication administration issues, ability to cooperate with lab draws, sensory sensitivities (e.g., noise, lights, materials/tactile), food preferences and food-related issues (including pica), sleep issues and routines, other routines, tolerance of group situations, general strengths and weaknesses, and likes and dislikes (Pratt et al. 2012). Further, information during this meeting could be gathered to help with developing behavioral intervention plans, help guide psychiatric diagnosis, facilitate the need to contact schools, review past testing, and help target pharmacological interventions. In addition, the meeting can also help foster the development of a therapeutic relationship with the patient's primary guardian, because they are able to meet the entire team in person and have a forum to "be heard."

To facilitate communication with the neuropsychiatric patient at admission, the clinician should consider alternative methods to gather historical information. The first step would be to communicate with the patient's primary guardian and outpatient providers regarding the patient's developmental level during admission or at the admission meeting as recommended above. Also, if the patient had previous neuropsychological testing, this should be reviewed to help determine the patient's baseline developmental level as well as strengths and weakness that could help in communication during their inpatient stay. For example, if a patient has relative strengths in visual processing and weakness in processing speeds, the clinician may try to utilize visual aids. Also, for verbal patients with ID or ASD, it could be beneficial to ask direct questions in a simple, straightforward manner to avoid language that may seem ambiguous and confusing. For nonverbal patients, it may be important to find out if the patient uses Picture Exchange Communication System or sign language, or has another form of communication. If a patient is unable or unwilling to communicate either directly or through alternative methods, the clinician may have to rely completely on collateral information from the admission meeting or guardian report. However, regardless of the patient's ability to communicate either directly or with assistance, it is vital to engage the patient in direct and indirect observation. Critical information can be gathered through a physical examination and observation. Though not exhaustive, examples of information that can be obtained through observation include possible signs or symptoms of neurological issues or catatonia, level of agitation or anxiety, level of alertness and orientation, ability to engage with their environment, social reciprocity, ability to maintain or initiate eye contact, stereotypic behaviors or movements, response to prompts, ability to follow commands, and communication methods and styles, as well as possible triggers for agitation and/or aggression. A complete physical examination should take place on admission to rule out medical issues that may have caused or contributed to the reason for admission.

Diagnostic Evaluation

Diagnosing a psychiatric illness for a patient with ID or ASD on the basis of the current DSM criteria presents several challenges for the inpatient team. Much of the language in DSM is based on patients who are neurotypical and often assumes the patient can reflect their internal state with some degree of certainty (Fletcher et al. 2017; Sovner 1986; Sovner and Hurley 1986). In addition, because patients with ID and ASD often present with externalizing and disruptive behaviors, many clinicians and caregivers tend to attribute these behaviors to the ID or core symptoms of ASD rather than considering that the behavior can also be a manifestation of an underlying psychiatric or medical condition. This tendency, termed *diagnostic overshadowing*, can lead to underdiagnosing of psychiatric illness in this population (Jopp and Keys 2001; Sovner and Hurley 1986). However, higher rates of affective (depression) and anxiety disorders have been reported (McGonigle et al. 2014) compared with the general population. In addition, affective disorders tend to peak in adolescence and young adulthood and can result in deteriorating behaviors (Ghaziuddin et al. 2005; McGonigle et al. 2014).

Since aggression and self-injurious behaviors are some of the most common chief complaints for admission to neuropsychiatric inpatient units (Siegel et al. 2012, 2014), it is important that a full diagnostic evaluation be completed to identify psychiatric causes, medical causes, or environmental causes (e.g., significant social pressures, abuse, bullying, lack of proper management of ID and ASD) or to determine whether the self-injurious behavior is best conceptualized as primarily behavioral with antecedents and maintaining conditions. Self-injurious behavior can also be part of the behavioral phenotype of genetic disorders such as Lesch-Nyhan syndrome, Smith-Magenis syndrome, or Prader-Willi syndrome (Harris 2006; Nyhan 1972, 1976; Shapira et al. 2002; Smith et al. 1998). Issues related to aggression and self-injurious behavior are often a combination of a psychiatric diagnosis with issues primary to ID and ASD and/or communication deficiencies that make it challenging to know how much one aspect is driving the other.

There are several ways to help the clinician organize their thinking related to assessment, diagnosis, and treatment planning related to a chief complaint of externalizing behaviors such as behavioral outbursts with or without aggression and self-injurious behaviors. The following is a starting point and not exhaustive. The first step in evaluating behavioral outbursts is to go through a basic ABC (antecedent-behavior-consequence) analysis with the behavioral therapist. Once this analysis is complete, it would be useful to also define the frequency, duration, and character of the outbursts. One helpful defining approach is to categorize the outbursts in terms of either "temper tantrums" or "meltdowns." We would define a temper tantrum as a reaction to limit setting, wanting to avoid a request or situation or not getting what the patient wants. Temper tantrums are typically goal directed with the purpose of either avoiding a command or engaging in disruptive behaviors until a desired outcome is obtained. A meltdown can also have similar triggers as temper tantrums such as limit setting or wanting to avoid something. However, meltdowns are also more likely to come out of the blue with no obvious trigger, be a reaction to sensory issues, and be a reaction to anxiety or fear. Unlike temper tantrums, meltdowns typically do not resolve when the patient obtains the desired object or outcome and will continue without any clear goal or purpose. Although both temper tantrums and meltdowns can be associated with a co-occurring psychiatric diagnosis such as ADHD, meltdowns are more likely to be a manifestation of an underlying psychiatric diagnosis or medical cause. Differentiating between temper tantrums and meltdowns can be helpful in safety planning, in developing strategies to treat the outbursts, and in determining ways to approach behavioral strategies, and as a guide in diagnosing psychiatric conditions.

The differential diagnosis of behavioral changes regardless of levels of aggression to self or others is broad. Many aspects of irritability and mood changes can be part of the diagnosis of ASD or other neuropsychiatric diagnoses. For instance, patients with ASD can have behavioral issues related to core features such as insistence on sameness, sensitivities in their environment, or tendency to isolate themselves to engage in preferred interests (McGonigle et al. 2014). To identify a co-occurring psychiatric diagnosis, the treatment team must understand the patient's baseline behaviors. The differential diagnosis for increased aggressive behavioral changes includes major depressive disorder, anxiety, disruptive mood dysregulation disorder, impulse-control disorder, ADHD, bipolar I or II disorder, psychosis due to a primary disorder such as schizophrenia, and agitated catatonia. All of these diagnoses can co-occur with the neuropsychiatric diagnosis and either lead to or contribute to increased aggression, self-injurious behaviors, and behavioral outbursts. For example, an adolescent with ID or ASD may develop an irritable depression contributing to decreased frustration tolerance and more difficulty inhibiting impulsive aggression that may already be a challenge at baseline. This phenomenon, termed *baseline exaggeration*, refers to the increase in challenging behaviors, including aggression and self-injurious behavior, during the exacerbation of a psychiatric illness or from some other form of stress (Fletcher et al. 2017; Sovner and Hurley 1986). Or a child with ASD who has baseline struggles with transitions and change in routine may develop an anxiety disorder, leading to even higher levels of behavioral problems or self-injurious behavior when they are upset in reaction to an internal "fight or flight" stimulus. A diagnosis such as bipolar disorder can be more explicit in terms of obvious mood lability leading to behavioral changes and/or aggression. In terms of psychosis, a patient may have increased difficulty with organization of thoughts and may act out behaviorally as a response to auditory or visual hallucinations. Agitated catatonia may be more difficult to identify when a patient has increased impulsive aggression; however, this diagnosis must be part of the differential diagnosis because it can be life-threatening and requires special interventions. A clinician should refer to established guidelines and expert consensus articles when agitated catatonia is suspected. Although it can be challenging to gain narrative descriptions from patients with language delay or those who are nonverbal, the diagnosis can still be made by observation and historical information from their caregivers. Here are some considerations that can differentiate certain diagnoses:

- **Depression:** Does the patient have a decreased lack of interest in preferred activities (anhedonia) or appear irritable or depressed outside of behavioral outbursts? Are there changes in appetite? Energy? Sleep patterns? Are they isolating themselves more than usual, regardless of wanting to engage in preferred interests?

- **Bipolar disorder:** Are there increased goal-directed behaviors different from or increased above baseline? Restricted interest or preferred activities? Are there increased sexualized behaviors such as increased masturbation? Are there changes in sleep patterns, such as being up for days with little to no need for sleep? Does the mood appear different, such as seemingly expansive or grandiose? Are baseline stereotypic behaviors more rapid or engaged at a higher intensity? Are the patient's behaviors more disorganized?
- **Anxiety:** Does the patient appear more anxious than usual when routines are changed? Are they more reactive during difficult social situations? Do they try to avoid certain activities that are different from those at baseline? If verbal, do they ask for reassurance about safety or schedules? Do they have a heightened aversion to sensory triggers?

Medical Evaluation

In addition to screening for psychiatric comorbidities, the clinician should evaluate for medical conditions. Prior to every admission, we recommend that the patient have a full physical examination and screening laboratory tests. The following are recommended at admission:

- Complete blood count with platelets and differential
- Comprehensive metabolic screen
- Thyroid-stimulating hormone test
- Urine toxicology screen
- Urinalysis
- Pregnancy test

The following may be indicated depending on decisions with medications:

- Lipid panel (to include fasting cholesterol, lipids, high-density and low-density lipoprotein)
- Prolactin level
- Vitamin B levels
- Other laboratory testing related to specific syndromes or presentations

In addition, weight and blood pressure readings should be obtained for all patients at admission.

There are two purposes for completing a medical evaluation. The first is to ensure that the patient is medically stable enough to be treated on a psychiatric unit. The second purpose is to screen for causes or contributors to the patient's chief complaint and reason for admission. Neuropsychiatric patients such as individuals with ID or ASD tend to have more difficulty with inhibiting impulses, difficulty expressing themselves, problems with behavioral regulation, and a biological predisposition to physiological arousal (Mazefsky and White 2014). Given the increased propensity to emotional dysregulation, combined with limited communication skills and cognitive impairments, the neuropsychiatric patient is more likely to express physical discomfort or change through externalizing behaviors, which can sometimes manifest as aggression and seemingly "attention-seeking" behaviors. In addition, increased or new self-injurious behaviors could be a sign from nonverbal patients that they are physically distressed. Behavioral outbursts can manifest as medical issues, including constipation, tooth pain, or an ear infection (Woods 2011). For example, in a study looking at ID patients admitted to a specialized unit, it was found that 60% of those with behavioral problems had constipation and 38% had gastroesophageal reflux (Charlot et al. 2011). It is therefore important to assess for possible medical and physical causes that could be driving the behavior. We recommend screening for the following:

- Pain sources, including headaches, poor dentation causing dental pain, eye pain, and ear pain
- Gastrointestinal issues, including constipation and gastroesophageal reflux
- Vision problems
- Seizures
- Sleep apnea leading to increased irritability and poor frustration tolerance
- Hearing loss
- Asthma
- Autoimmune issues
- Thyroid disorders

In addition, for adult patients, a screen for delirium should be considered. This would include conducting a general medical screen as outlined above in addition to reviewing the patient's medications, especially those medications that are highly anticholinergic. As discussed earlier in this chapter, individuals with genetic syndromes, such as Down syndrome, Prader-Willi syndrome, or 22q11DS deletion syndrome, are predisposed to certain medical conditions, which should be emphasized in the medical evaluation.

Treatment Plan

Establishment of Goals as a Team in Coordination With Patient, Family, and Outside Agencies

Treatment plan goals are established early in the admission process. The treatment team gathers an extensive history of the patient and determines current mental health and well-being. Collateral information is collected from caregivers and the patient. Various clinicians of the multidisciplinary team perform a multitude of specialty assessments within the first few days of admission and report their findings in treatment team meetings. This information is used to help develop a comprehensive profile of the patient's current strengths and needs that informs the team on the areas of focus during hospitalization. As a result, highly individualized and measurable goals for hospitalization are determined for each patient. The treatment team can assess the progress made toward fulfilling these goals to help determine when a patient is ready for discharge.

Short-term day-to-day goals can also be established. Patients on neuropsychiatric units should be encouraged to identify their own goals throughout the day. This might include learning how to cope with stressors and maintain better control over target behaviors and attending more group activities. These goals can be measured directly and feedback provided to the patient in the form of reminders and encouragement or positive reinforcement when the patient is successful.

Goals should not be arbitrary or overly general. The purpose of goal setting on an inpatient unit is to determine each individual's measure of success in overcoming a psychiatric crisis and in learning new skills. These goals should be attainable and in coordination with the needs of caregivers and/or outside agencies. Finally, successful goals will be generalizable and maintainable outside the hospital.

Behavioral Plans

Another aspect in determining inpatient success is the implementation of a behavioral intervention plan and analysis of its efficacy in determining objective behavioral outcomes. A behavioral therapist or psychologist can use indirect or direct methods in determining the function of a target behavior through a functional behavioral assessment (Gresham et al. 2001). Observation and collection of data on the occurrence of target behaviors as well as collateral information from caregivers can provide a clue as to what is maintaining these behaviors. Quantitative data collected in the form of frequency or occurrence of a behavior over a period of time give treatment team members baseline information on the frequency of the behavior. Qualitative data collected in the form of ABC (antecedent-behavior-consequence) data give clinicians more descriptive information about each occurrence of a target behavior. For example, quantitatively a clinician may determine that a patient engages in physical aggression eight times per day on average. Qualitatively, that clinician may determine that the antecedent to this physical aggression was being asked to attend a particular activity and the consequence of the physical aggression was to successfully avoid going to that activity. The function of this behavior may be determined to be one of escape or avoidance and can help narrow the focus of what to target in a behavioral intervention plan. To further test functional relationships, a neuropsychiatric inpatient unit can employ a functional analysis of the problem behavior directly by testing various conditions that may elicit a target behavior (Hanley et al. 2003; Iwata et al. 1994). Once these steps have been completed, a behavioral intervention plan can be developed.

A behavioral intervention plan integrates multiple strategies. It operationalizes the exact target behaviors that should be measured and provides a uniform definition that all direct care staff can follow. The behavioral intervention plan includes communication strategies identifying the verbal ability of the patient and how one should respond back verbally. Preventive measures are added that identify specific environmental triggers to be avoided. Skill-building strategies direct staff in teaching and encouraging functional alternatives to target behaviors. Reinforcement strategies help identify preferred items or activities that motivate the patient as well as determine when and how frequently those reinforcers should be used. Finally, management strategies can tie all of these methods together and direct the staff on how to respond to target behaviors while utilizing the aforementioned strategies.

The implementation of a behavioral intervention plan incorporates several steps. It involves training the staff, through discussion and modeling, on how to implement the plan. Clinicians monitor the fidelity of treatment by observing how staff execute the plan and provide them with direct feedback on their implementation. Finally, behavioral therapists elicit feedback from staff and observe the patient's response to the plan in determining whether adjustments need to be made. As adjustments are made, the entire process of training and fidelity checks is repeated.

Finally, a behavioral intervention plan takes into account whether it can be implemented outside the hospital. Caregivers can be brought in and trained to implement a plan that has been shown to effectively intervene on a target behavior. Caregivers can then execute the plan and receive additional support or feedback from the behavioral therapist. Once this process is complete, recommendations can be made for in-home implementation.

Social Work and Family Interventions

Social workers provide a variety of interventions on a neuropsychiatric inpatient unit. They play an important role in collecting information from caregivers and outside agencies and then communicating their findings to the treatment team. Likewise, they will communicate back with caregivers and offer updates on the patient's progress. The support of family members or caregivers is integral to the success of an individual with a neuropsychiatric condition. When possible, the social worker will coordinate several meetings with both caregivers and patient present. This allows for a discussion of the reasons for psychiatric admission and allows all parties to talk with mediation from the social worker. The social worker facilitates the discussion to understand both the caregivers' and patient's concerns and what they hope to achieve from this hospitalization. A future-oriented approach can be taken to help develop realistic expectations from all parties involved. Such an approach can cause a great deal of stress given that reasons for hospitalization can include the victimization of a caregiver or the patient's perceived aversive response to being hospitalized. It is the social worker's goal to have everyone's voice heard and to incorporate everyone's thoughts in finding a solution to prevent future crises and hospitalizations.

Social workers will begin to facilitate sign-outs with objective goals as the patient shows readiness for discharge. Both patient and caregivers will be able to assess if goals discussed during family meetings can generalize out in the community, where stressors may be more unpredictable. Coordination of training with the behavioral therapist and caregivers may be made to strengthen the strategies that can be used to encourage successful transitions. Ensuring that applicable resources and supports are put in place outside the hospital setting can further foster positive outcomes.

Programming

A structured schedule filled with therapeutic groups and activities plays an important role on an inpatient neuropsychiatric unit. OTs provide a variety of structured activities to focus on socialization and daily tasks and to help the patient find enjoyment in recreation. Nurses can provide therapeutic groups on medication management and a variety of hygiene and medical issues. Specialized clinicians can help individuals develop an outlet for expressing themselves or to cope with stressors through art, music, or movement. Psychologists and counselors can provide group sessions on social skills and coping strategies. While each patient receives individualized treatment and goals, making available groups led by members from a multidisciplinary team helps nurture a sense of community among individuals who may face similar issues as well as provides education or sharing of experiences that may help deter future crises.

Pharmacotherapy

Pharmacotherapy is used in the treatment of specific psychiatric conditions such as depression, ADHD, and bipolar disorder. Pharmacotherapy for aggression and self-injurious behavior not clearly linked to diagnoses such as bipolar disorder, depression, psychotic disorders, anxiety disorders, panic attacks, and so forth is a more controversial topic because medications can be misused (Branford et al. 2020). However, if other interventions fail, psychotropic medications may be useful to treat severe aggression and self-injurious behavior in the population of individuals with intellectual and developmental disabilities. Use of these medications should be informed by a biopsychosocial formulation that is based on a functional assessment of behavior. Indications should be clearly identified. Regular monitoring should occur, and the need for continuation or discontinuation of the medication should be regularly evaluated once the individual is stabilized in the community (Devapriam and Alexander 2019; Golombek and King 2010; Sabus et al. 2019). Side effects of medications can also produce behavioral problems with activation or agitation and must be kept in mind as a potential cause of agitation, aggression, self-injurious behavior, or other challenging behaviors (Ruedrich 2016).

Safety

Agitation, aggression, and self-injurious behavior occur on inpatient neuropsychiatric units. These, after all, are the presenting behaviors that could not be managed in a less restrictive setting and required an inpatient level of care. The goal is to provide a safe treatment environment for patients and staff. Proper training of the staff in management and prevention of these behaviors, as-needed medication, and, as a last resort in emergencies, seclusion and restraint all are used to manage dangerous behaviors (Kynoch et al. 2011). As discussed above, understanding the antecedents of the dangerous behaviors and having a de-escalation and management plan are important in preventing aggression or self-injurious behaviors. The assumption is a perturbation is leading to the behavior. This could be physical pain or discomfort, which always must be considered first in language-challenged patients. Other inciting factors include disrupted routines, escape from nonpreferred behaviors, anxiety, emotional upset, and more idiosyncratic reasons. Antecedents are the behaviors or triggers that took place prior to the acts of aggression or perceived agitation. By understanding the antecedents, the treatment team can better understand the causes of agitation and the function of the aggression.

Behavioral data collection on the patients is an important part of the treatment program. These data can be used to identify antecedents to behaviors and guide strategies for reducing or eliminating the behaviors. Regular multidisciplinary treatment team meetings, usually occurring daily, are a forum for reviewing incidents and behavioral data. This process helps to reduce the number of incidents. For more severe incidents, Lean activities, including such process evaluations as a root cause analysis, can be used to identify the factors that likely contributed to the incident, which can then be addressed and, if possible, fixed to minimize the risk of future incidents.

Sensory Issues and Tools

Abnormal sensory-based behaviors are often associated with ASD as well as other developmental disabilities. More than 96% of all patients with ASD report or demonstrate an atypical response to sensorial input. Behavioral responses to hyper- and hypostimulation can result in self-injurious behaviors as well as aggression to others particularly when patients are unable to vocalize their distress (Marco et al. 2011). Champagne (2018) approaches the use of sensory tools as one might approach a diet. She reports that a sensory diet can be developed for an individual who may be craving certain stimulation; this stimulation can be implemented to help facilitate treatment. At times patients might seek calming or organizing stimulation to help them tolerate more familiar tasks. In these moments patients may choose or be directed to steadily rock or listen to soft music or use a comfort wrap. By contrast, when a patient is in sensorial need of high demands, they might choose or be directed to use more alerting sensorial input like a cold washcloth to their face or power walking. Families and treatment teams, especially with the help of occupation therapy, should help patients develop an accessible selection of tools to create a sensory diet. Champagne notes that staff can become better observers and provide strategies for patients when they are in distress with the goal of helping patients self-regulate. Proactive staff on a neuropsychiatric unit can use sensory modulation tools as a means to help de-escalate dysregulated patients, according to Champagne.

Discharge Planning

Discharge planning begins at admission when treatment goals are set. Posthospital residence and support needs are part of this. Coordination with family and multiple providers and agencies, including schools, group homes, and day programs, is necessary for a smooth transition to outpatient care.

Case Example: Youth

CM is a 13-year-old with ASD with intellectual and language impairment as well as moderate ID and is nonverbal. He presented for increased aggression toward others as well as self-injurious behaviors. Though he has a long history of intermittent aggression toward others and self-injurious behaviors, both his aggression and his self-injurious behaviors increased significantly over the 2 months prior to admission. Triggers were unclear, and his parents reported they seem to "come out of nowhere." New behaviors included exhibiting irritability most of the day, impulsively hitting teachers and school aides, and hitting his head aggressively both at school and at home. The self-injurious behaviors and aggression were occurring daily. Self-injurious behaviors to his head were causing bruising to his orofacial region and were very distressing for his parents to observe.

Prior to his admission to the pediatric neuropsychiatric inpatient unit, CM had a medical workup, including a physical examination, basic lab work, and an MRI. Medical etiologies, including otitis media and structural brain causes, were ruled out. On the unit, an admission meeting took place between the parent and inpatient treatment team, information was gathered from the school and patient's outpatient psychiatrist, medical records were obtained, and prior neuropsychological testing was reviewed. CM was observed continuously while on the unit, and the psychiatrist completed an assessment by engaging the patient as well as observing him in the milieu. CM continued to have self-injurious behaviors on the unit and was noted to be consistently irritable and uncomfortable appearing. He had good sleep, no changes in appetite, no increased sexualized behaviors, and nothing that would suggest anxiety. He did not appear to be responding to internal stimuli.

He was started on risperidone because of the high level of aggression and irritability. He had a 1:1 staff member work with him to help block his self-injurious behaviors and redirect him to use preferred sensory objects to help him cope with his distress. The treatment team also put a soft foam helmet on his head and put loose soft mittens on his hands to help decrease injury to self. Although the risperidone decreased his irritability and aggression toward others, he continued to have self-injurious behaviors. The treatment team postulated that CM was having headaches and/or migraines, and he was given doses of acetaminophen when he appeared to be in distress (pain). This intervention led to modest improvement in his self-injurious behaviors. He was put on topiramate to target possible migraines. After topiramate was added, CM's self-injurious behaviors and aggression significantly decreased, and he was discharged home at his baseline.

Case Example: Adult

JP is a 23-year-old with mild ID and a history of bipolar disorder and ADHD. She lived with her biological mother until 8 years ago, when she was removed for neglect and abuse. She had special private schooling as afforded by her adopting parents. In school, she was noted to have hyperactivity, with poor attention, mood lability, and poor judgment. Because of her facial appearance, clinical presentation, and biological mother's putative history of bipolar disorder and alcohol use disorder, the patient was diagnosed with fetal alcohol syndrome. As a teenager and into young adulthood, she had periods of labile mood, irritability, impulsive behaviors, and poor judgment in her interactions with males her own age, seemed highly dependent on male attention, and would become devastated when she felt she was being abandoned by a love interest.

At the time of admission, she was living at a group home funded by the state developmental disabilities agency. She attended a day program but could not advance to any supported employment activities because of the erratic nature of her behavior. Her adoptive parents were closely involved in her care and treatment and acted as her legal guardians. She had been in outpatient psychiatric care since she was in elementary school. She had a previous inpatient psychiatric admission for suicidal ideation. In the several weeks prior to admission, she was increasingly irritable. Her energy was high, and she had a decreased need for sleep. She was hypertalkative. She had become upset about the behaviors of a man her age in her day program. In the weeks prior to admission, she lost her temper and destroyed much of the property in her bedroom, tried to elope from the group home and run into a busy street, and made threats to overdose on a cleaning product. She was being treated with a second-generation antipsychotic and a stimulant.

As her sleep deteriorated, she was put on trazodone, which was subsequently increased. Her condition continued to deteriorate, and she was admitted with suicidal ideation. She was felt by the outpatient provider and others to have borderline personality disorder. The formulation of the treatment team was of bipolar disorder, manic, without psychotic features and with possible mixed features in the setting of ID due to fetal alcohol syndrome. The stimulant was stopped; the trazodone was tapered and then discontinued, since antidepressant doses had been reached when she was an outpatient; and lithium was started. Her mood gradually stabilized, allowing discharge to outpatient care.

On follow-up, her mood was consistently stable, and she was able to benefit from supportive psychotherapy. She advanced in her prevocational activities and was able to work part-time in supported employment, which thrilled her. The diagnosis of borderline personality disorder was no longer made. The treatment team felt JP's difficulties were better explained by her cognitive and emotional deficits related to fetal alcohol syndrome, her life experiences, and diagnosis of bipolar disorder.

Conclusion

Neuropsychiatry is an amalgam of psychiatry and neurology and deals with conditions in this overlapping area, including psychiatric and behavioral conditions in intellectual disability and autism spectrum disorder (or intellectual and developmental disabilities). Modern diagnostic and treatment approaches allow individuals with intellectual and developmental disabilities in psychiatric crisis to be successfully treated and stabilized on acute psychiatric specialty units. Because of multiple adaptive (habilitative), psychiatric, and medical needs in the intellectual and developmental disabilities population, a special approach to evaluation, diagnosis, and treatment involving an expanded inpatient treatment team is required. Behavioral evaluation and intervention are often necessary, and a robust behavioral program is strongly suggested. Special provisions often need to be made in discharge planning that involve agencies tasked with organizing and providing these services.

References

American Psychiatric Association: Diagnostic and Statistical Manual of Mental Disorders, 5th Edition. Arlington, VA, American Psychiatric Association, 2013

American Speech-Language-Hearing Association: Scope of Practice in Speech-Language Pathology [Scope of Practice]. Rockville, MD, American Speech-Language-Hearing Association, 2016. Available at: www.asha.org/policy/sp2016-00343. Accessed September 20, 2021.

Amiet C, Gourfinkel-An I, Bouzamondo A, et al: Epilepsy in autism is associated with intellectual disability and gender: evidence from a meta-analysis. Biol Psychiatry 64(7):577–582, 2008 18565495

Asperger H: "Die autistischen Psychopathen" im Kindesalter. Arch Psychiatr Nervenkr 117(1):76–136, 1944

Asperger H: "Autistic psychopathy" in childhood, in Autism and Asperger Syndrome. Edited by Frith U. New York, Cambridge University Press, 1991, pp 37–92

Baker EK, Godler DE, Bui M, et al: Exploring autism symptoms in an Australian cohort of patients with Prader-Willi and Angelman syndromes. J Neurodev Disord 10(1):24, 2018 30081815

Benvenuto A, Moavero R, Alessandrelli R, et al: Syndromic autism: causes and pathogenetic pathways. World J Pediatr 5(3):169–176, 2009 19693459

Bertrand J, Floyd RL, Weber MK, Fetal Alcohol Syndrome Prevention Team, et al: Guidelines for identifying and referring persons with fetal alcohol syndrome. MMWR Recomm Rep 54(RR-11):1–14, 2005 16251866

Bolton PF, Carcani-Rathwell I, Hutton J, et al: Epilepsy in autism: features and correlates. Br J Psychiatry 198(4):289–294, 2011 21972278

Branford D, Tharian R, Alexander R, Bhaumik S: Pharmacotherapy for mental illness and behaviours that challenge in people with intellectual disabilities, in Oxford Textbook of the Psychiatry of Intellectual Disability. Edited by Bhaumik S, Alexander R. New York, Oxford University Press, 2020, pp 191–202

Caglayan AO: Genetic causes of syndromic and non-syndromic autism. Dev Med Child Neurol 52(2):130–138, 2010 20059518

Centers for Disease Control and Prevention: Fetal Alcohol Spectrum Disorders (FASDs): Data and Statistics. Atlanta, GA, Centers for Disease Control and Prevention, 2016. Available at: www.cdc.gov/ncbddd/fasd/data.html. Accessed November 5, 2021.

Champagne T: Sensory Modulation and Environment: Essential Elements of Occupation, 3rd Edition. London, Pearson, 2018

Charlot L, Abend S, Ravin P, et al: Non-psychiatric health problems among psychiatric inpatients with intellectual disabilities. J Intellect Disabil Res 55(2):199–209, 2011 20546095

Chawner SJRA, Niarchou M, Doherty JL, et al: The emergence of psychotic experiences in the early adolescence of 22q11. 2 deletion syndrome. J Psychiatr Res 109:10–17, 2019 30458299

Chudley AE, Longstaffe SE: Fetal alcohol syndrome and fetal alcohol spectrum disorder, in Management of Genetic Syndromes, 2nd Edition. Edited by Cassidy SB, Allanson JE. Hoboken, NJ, Wiley, 2005, pp 225–238

Clarke DF, Roberts W, Daraksan M, et al: The prevalence of autistic spectrum disorder in children surveyed in a tertiary care epilepsy clinic. Epilepsia 46(12):1970–1977, 2005 16393164

Coleman M: The Neurology of Autism. New York, Oxford University Press, 2009

Cooper S-A, Smiley E, Morrison J, et al: Mental ill-health in adults with intellectual disabilities: prevalence and associated factors. Br J Psychiatry 190(1):27–35, 2007 17197653

Croen LA, Najjar DV, Ray GT, et al: A comparison of health care utilization and costs of children with and without autism spectrum disorders in a large group-model health plan. Pediatrics 118(4):e1203–e1211, 2006 17015508

Dan B: Angelman Syndrome. London, Mac Keith Press, 2008

Dan B: Angelman syndrome: current understanding and research prospects. Epilepsia 50(11):2331–2339, 2009 19874386

Davignon MN, Qian Y, Massolo M, Croen LA: Psychiatric and medical conditions in transition-aged individuals with ASD. Pediatrics 141 (suppl 4):S335–S345, 2018 29610415

Day K: Psychiatric services in mental retardation: generic or specialised provision? in Mental Health in Mental Retardation: Recent Advances and Practices. Edited by Bouras N. Cambridge, UK, Cambridge University Press, 1994, pp 275–292

Day K: Service provision and staff training: an overview, in Treating Mental Illness and Behaviour Disorders in Children and Adults with Mental Retardation. Edited by Dosen A, Leibenluft E, Day K. Washington, DC, American Psychiatric Publishing, 2001, pp 469–492

Devapriam J, Alexander RT: Challenging behaviour and the use of pharmacological interventions, in Seminars in the Psychiatry of Intellectual Disability, 3rd Edition. Edited by Scheepers M, Kerr M. New York, Cambridge University Press, 2019, pp 179–189

Diehl SF: Autism spectrum disorder: the context of speech-language pathologist intervention. Lang Speech Hear Serv Schools 34(3):177–179, 2003 27764319

DiGuiseppi C, Hepburn S, Davis JM, et al: Screening for autism spectrum disorders in children with Down syndrome: population prevalence and screening test characteristics. J Dev Behav Pediatr 31(3):181–191, 2010 20375732

Dykens EM, Roof E, Hunt-Hawkins H, et al: Diagnoses and characteristics of autism spectrum disorders in children with Prader-Willi syndrome. J Neurodev Disord 9(1):18, 2017 28592997

Eaton S: Addressing the effects of missing school for children with medical needs. Pediatr Nurs 38(5):271–277, 2012 23189779 Erratum in: Pediatr Nurs 38(6):330, 2012

Eberhart JK, Parnell SE: The genetics of fetal alcohol spectrum disorders. Alcohol Clin Exp Res 40(6):1154–1165, 2016 27122355

Elsea SH, Girirajan S: Smith-Magenis syndrome. Eur J Hum Genet 16(4):412–421, 2008 18231123

Esbensen AJ, MacLean WE Jr: Down syndrome, in A Comprehensive Guide to Intellectual & Developmental Disabilities, 2nd Edition. Edited by Wehmeyer ML, Brown I, Percy M, et al. Baltimore, MD, Paul H Brookes, 2017

Evans K, Nizette D, O'Brien A: Psychiatric & Mental Health Nursing. Elsevier Health Sciences, 2016

Fletcher R, Barnhill J, Cooper SA (eds): Diagnostic Manual—Intellectual Disability 2 (DM-ID): A Textbook of Diagnosis of Mental Disorders in Persons With Intellectual Disability, 2nd Edition. Kingston, NY, NADD, 2017

Folstein S, Rutter M: Infantile autism: a genetic study of 21 twin pairs. J Child Psychol Psychiatry 18(4):297–321, 1977 562353

Foxx RM: Applied behavior analysis treatment of autism: the state of the art. Child Adolesc Psychiatr Clin N Am 17(4):821–834, ix, 2008 18775372

Gabriels RL, Agnew JA, Beresford C, et al: Improving psychiatric hospital care for pediatric patients with autism spectrum disorders and intellectual disabilities. Autism Res Treat 2012:685053, 2012 22934179

Gaugler T, Klei L, Sanders SJ, et al: Most genetic risk for autism resides with common variation. Nat Genet 46(8):881–885, 2014 25038753

Ghaziuddin M, Quinlan P, Ghaziuddin N: Catatonia in autism: a distinct subtype? J Intellect Disabil Res 49 (Pt 1):102–105, 2005 15634317

Golombek A, King B: Pharmacotherapy, in Developmental Disabilities From Childhood to Adulthood: What Works for Psychiatrists in Community and Institutional Settings. Edited by Dreyden-Edwards R, Combrinck-Graham L. Baltimore, MD, Johns Hopkins University Press, 2010, pp 271–295

Gothelf D, Schneider M, Green T, et al: Risk factors and the evolution of psychosis in 22q11.2 deletion syndrome: a longitudinal 2-site study. J Am Acad Child Adolesc Psychiatry 52(11):1192–1203.e3, 2013 24157393

Gresham FM, Watson TS, Skinner CH: Functional behavioral assessment: principles, procedures, and future directions. School Psych Rev 30(2):156–172, 2001

Haebig E, Sterling A, Barton-Hulsey A, Friedman L: Rates and predictors of co-occurring autism spectrum disorder in boys with fragile X syndrome. Autism Dev Lang Impair 5:1–19, 2020

Haendel M, Vasilevsky N, Unni D, et al: How Many Rare Diseases Are There? Berlin, Nature Publishing Group, 2019

Hagerman RJ: Fragile X syndrome and premutation-associated disorders, in Management of Genetic Syndromes, 3rd Edition. Edited by Cassidy SB, Allanson JE. Hoboken, NJ, Wiley, 2010, pp 397–411

Hagerman RJ, Berry-Kravis E, Hazlett HC, et al: Fragile X syndrome. Nat Rev Dis Primers 3(1):17065, 2017 28960184

Halter MJ: Manual of Psychiatric Nursing Care Planning-E-Book: An Interprofessional Approach. Amsterdam, Elsevier Health Sciences, 2018

Hanley GP, Iwata BA, McCord BE: Functional analysis of problem behavior: a review. J Appl Behav Anal 36(2):147–185, 2003 12858983

Harris JC: Intellectual Disability: Understanding Its Development, Causes, Classification, Evaluation, and Treatment. New York, Oxford University Press, 2006

Iwata BA, Dorsey MF, Slifer KJ, et al: Toward a functional analysis of self-injury. J Appl Behav Anal 27(2):197–209, 1994 8063622

Jones KL, Jones MC, Del Campo M: Smith's Recognizable Patterns of Human Malformation. Amsterdam, Elsevier Health Sciences, 2013

Jopp DA, Keys CB: Diagnostic overshadowing reviewed and reconsidered. Am J Ment Retard 106(5):416–433, 2001 11531461

Kambeitz C, Klug MG, Greenmyer J, et al: Association of adverse childhood experiences and neurodevelopmental disorders in people with fetal alcohol spectrum disorders (FASD) and non-FASD controls. BMC Pediatr 19(1):498, 2019 31842817

Kanner L: Autistic disturbances of affective contact. Nerv Child 2:217–250, 1943

Kanner L: Autistic disturbances of affective contact. Acta Paedopsychiatr 35(4):100–136, 1968 4880460

Kaur S, Christodoulou J: MECP2 disorders, in GeneReviews (internet). Edited by Adam MP, Ardinger HH, Pagon RA. Seattle, University of Washington, 2001

Kidd SA, Berry-Kravis E, Choo TH, et al: Improving the diagnosis of autism spectrum disorder in fragile X syndrome by adapting the Social Communication Questionnaire and the Social Responsiveness Scale-2. J Autism Dev Disord 50(9):3276–3295, 2020 31342442

Kodituwakku P, Kodituwakku E: Cognitive and behavioral profiles of children with fetal alcohol spectrum disorders. Curr Dev Disord Rep 1(3):149–160, 2014

Koren G, Nulman I, Chudley AE, Loocke C: Fetal alcohol spectrum disorder. CMAJ 169(11):1181–1185, 2003 14638655

Kynoch K, Wu CJ, Chang AM: Interventions for preventing and managing aggressive patients admitted to an acute hospital setting: a systematic review. Worldviews Evid Based Nurs 8(2):76–86, 2011 21091980

Lai MC, Lombardo MV, Baron-Cohen S: Autism. Lancet 383(9920):896–910, 2014 24074734

Lai MC, Kassee C, Besney R, et al: Prevalence of co-occurring mental health diagnoses in the autism population: a systematic review and meta-analysis. Lancet Psychiatry 6(10):819–829, 2019 31447415

Lauterbach MD, Schildkrout B, Benjamin S, Gregory MD: The importance of rare diseases for psychiatry. Lancet Psychiatry 3(12):1098–1100, 2016 27889002

Leonard H, Cobb S, Downs J: Clinical and biological progress over 50 years in Rett syndrome. Nat Rev Neurol 13(1):37–51, 2017 27934853

Levy SE, Mandell DS, Schultz RT: Autism. Lancet 374(9701):1627–1638, 2009 19819542

Lishman WA: What is neuropsychiatry? J Neurol Neurosurg Psychiatry 55(11):983–985, 1992 1469416

Lowrey LG: Psychiatry for children: a brief history of developments. Am J Psychiatry 101(3):375–388, 1944

Maenner MJ, Shaw KA, Baio J, et al: Prevalence of autism spectrum disorder among children aged 8 years—Autism and Developmental Disabilities Monitoring Network, 11 sites, United States, 2016. MMWR Surveill Summ 69(4):1–12, 2020 32214087

Manaka D, van der Wath A, Moagi M: People with severe and profound intellectual disability: nurse carer experiences in a South African setting. J Psychol Afr 28(1):69–72, 2018

Mandell DS: Psychiatric hospitalization among children with autism spectrum disorders. J Autism Dev Disord 38(6):1059–1065, 2008 17975720

Mannion A, Leader G: Epilepsy in autism spectrum disorder. Res Autism Spectr Disord 8(4):354–361, 2014

Marco EJ, Hinkley LB, Hill SS, Nagarajan SS: Sensory processing in autism: a review of neurophysiologic findings. Pediatr Res 69(5 Pt 2):48R–54R, 2011 21289533

Matson JL, Benavidez DA, Compton LS, et al: Behavioral treatment of autistic persons: a review of research from 1980 to the present. Res Dev Disabil 17(6):433–465, 1996 8946569

May PA, Chambers CD, Kalberg WO, et al: Prevalence of fetal alcohol spectrum disorders in 4 US communities. JAMA 319(5):474–482, 2018 29411031

Mazefsky CA, White SW: Emotion regulation: concepts and practice in autism spectrum disorder. Child Adolesc Psychiatr Clin N Am 23(1):15–24, 2014 24231164

McDonald-McGinn DM, Emanuel BS, Zackai EH, Hain HS: 22q11.2 deletion syndrome, in GeneReviews. Edited by Adam MP, Ardinger HH, Pagon RA. Seattle, University of Washington, 1999. Available at: www.ncbi.nlm.nih.gov/books/NBK1523. Accessed April 1, 2020.

McDonald-McGinn DM, Kohut T, Zackai EH: Deletion 22q11.2 (velo-cardio-facial syndrome/DiGeorge syndrome), in Management of Genetic Syndromes, 3rd Edition. Edited by Cassidy SB, Allanson JE. Hoboken, NJ, Wiley, 2010, pp 263–284

McDonald-McGinn DM, Sullivan KE, Marino B, et al: 22q11.2 deletion syndrome. Nat Rev Dis Primers 1:15071, 2015 27189754

McGlinchey E, McCallion P, McCarron M: Down syndrome and dementia: advances in the field. Curr Opin Psychiatry 33(3):278–283, 2020 32049764

McGonigle JJ, Venkat A, Beresford C, et al: Management of agitation in individuals with autism spectrum disorders in the emergency department. Child Adolesc Psychiatr Clin N Am 23(1):83–95, 2014 24231169

McGuire K, Siegel M: Psychiatric hospital treatment of youth with autism spectrum disorder in the United States: needs, outcomes, and policy. Int Rev Psychiatry 30(1):110–115, 2018 29537885

McGuire K, Erickson C, Gabriels RL, et al: Psychiatric hospitalization of children with autism or intellectual disability: consensus statements on best practices. J Am Acad Child Adolesc Psychiatry 54(12):969–971, 2015 26598469

McHugh PR, Slavney PR: The Perspectives of Psychiatry. Baltimore, MD, Johns Hopkins University Press, 1998

Mosner MG, Kinard JL, Shah JS, et al: Rates of co-occurring psychiatric disorders in autism spectrum disorder using the Mini International Neuropsychiatric Interview. J Autism Dev Disord 49(9):3819–3832, 2019 31175504

Moss J, Howlin P: Autism spectrum disorders in genetic syndromes: implications for diagnosis, intervention and understanding the wider autism spectrum disorder population. J Intellect Disabil Res 53(10):852–873, 2009 19708861

Moss S, Emerson E, Bouras N, Holland A: Mental disorders and problematic behaviours in people with intellectual disability: future directions for research. J Intellect Disabil Res 41 (Pt 6):440–447, 1997 9430047

Moss J, Howlin P, Hastings RP, et al: Social behavior and characteristics of autism spectrum disorder in Angelman, Cornelia de Lange, and cri du chat syndromes. Am J Intellect Dev Disabil 118(4):262–283, 2013 23937369

Mount RH, Charman T, Hastings RP, et al: The Rett Syndrome Behaviour Questionnaire (RSBQ): refining the behavioural phenotype of Rett syndrome. J Child Psychol Psychiatry 43(8):1099–1110, 2002 12455930

Mount RH, Charman T, Hastings RP, et al: Features of autism in Rett syndrome and severe mental retardation. J Autism Dev Disord 33(4):435–442, 2003a 12959422

Mount RH, Hastings RP, Reilly S, et al: Towards a behavioral phenotype for Rett syndrome. Am J Ment Retard 108(1):1–12, 2003b 12475362

Mukherjee RAS, Hollins S, Turk J: Fetal alcohol spectrum disorder: an overview. J R Soc Med 99(6):298–302, 2006 16738372

Neul JL, Benke TA, Marsh ED, et al: The array of clinical phenotypes of males with mutations in Methyl-CpG binding protein 2. Am J Med Genet B Neuropsychiatr Genet 180(1):55–67, 2019 30536762

Nulman I, Shulman T, Liu F: Fetal alcohol spectrum disorder, in Handbook of Developmental Neurotoxicology. Edited by Slikker W, Paule MG, Wang C. Amsterdam, Elsevier, 2018, pp 427–437

Nyhan WL: Behavioral phenotypes in organic genetic disease: presidential address to the Society for Pediatric Research, May 1, 1971. Pediatr Res 6(1):1–9, 1972 5046967

Nyhan WL: Behavior in the Lesch-Nyhan syndrome. J Autism Child Schizophr 6(3):235–252, 1976 1086851

O'Brien G: Behavioural Phenotypes in Clinical Practice. New York, Cambridge University Press, 2002

Oskarsdóttir S, Belfrage M, Sandstedt E, et al: Disabilities and cognition in children and adolescents with 22q11 deletion syndrome. Dev Med Child Neurol 47(3):177–184, 2005 15739722

Ovsiew F, Jobe TH: Neuropsychiatry in the history of mental health services, in Neuropsychiatry and Mental Health Services. Edited by Ovsiew F. Washington, DC, American Psychiatric Press, 1999, 1–22

Pelc K, Cheron G, Dan B: Behavior and neuropsychiatric manifestations in Angelman syndrome. Neuropsychiatr Dis Treat 4(3):577–584, 2008 18830393

Pontillo M, Menghini D, Vicari S: Neurocognitive profile and onset of psychosis symptoms in children, adolescents and young adults with 22q11 deletion syndrome: a longitudinal study. Schizophr Res 208:76–81, 2019 31056275

Popova S, Lange S, Probst C, et al: Estimation of national, regional, and global prevalence of alcohol use during pregnancy and fetal alcohol syndrome: a systematic review and meta-analysis. Lancet Glob Health 5(3):e290–e299, 2017 28089487

Pratt K, Baird G, Gringras P: Ensuring successful admission to hospital for young people with learning difficulties, autism and challenging behaviour: a continuous quality improvement and change management programme. Child Care Health Dev 38(6):789–797, 2012 22017703

Pyles DAM, Muniz K, Cade A, Silva R: A behavioral diagnostic paradigm for integrating behavior-analytic and psychopharmacological interventions for people with a dual diagnosis. Res Dev Disabil 18(3):185–214, 1997 9220544

Ramirez-Bermudez J, Perez-Esparza R, Aguilar-Venegas LC, Sachdev P: Neuropsychiatry: towards a philosophy of praxis. Rev Colomb Psiquiatr 46 (suppl 1):28–35, 2017 29037336

Ramsay M: Genetic and epigenetic insights into fetal alcohol spectrum disorders. Genome Med 2(4):27, 2010 20423530

Richards C, Jones C, Groves L, et al: Prevalence of autism spectrum disorder phenomenology in genetic disorders: a systematic review and meta-analysis. Lancet Psychiatry 2(10):909–916, 2015 26341300

Rosen TE, Mazefsky CA, Vasa RA, Lerner MD: Co-occurring psychiatric conditions in autism spectrum disorder. Int Rev Psychiatry 30(1):40–61, 2018 29683351

Royal College of Psychiatrists: DC-LD (Diagnostic Criteria for Psychiatric Disorders for Use With Adults With Learning Disabilities/Mental Retardation). OP 48. London, Springer Science and Business, 2001

Ruedrich S: Psychopharmacology, in Psychiatric and Behavioural Disorders in Intellectual and Developmental Disabilities. Edited by Hemmings C, Bouras N. New York, Cambridge University Press, 2016

Sabus A, Feinstein J, Romani P, et al: Management of self-injurious behaviors in children with neurodevelopmental disorders: a pharmacotherapy overview. Pharmacotherapy 39(6):645–664, 2019 30793794

Sachdev PS: An agenda for neuropsychiatry as a 21st century discipline. Acta Neuropsychiatr 19(1):2–5, 2007 26952792

Sandin S, Lichtenstein P, Kuja-Halkola R, et al: The heritability of autism spectrum disorder. JAMA 318(12):1182–1184, 2017 28973605

Sandini C, Eliez S, Schneider M, Armando M: 22q11. 2 deletion syndrome: a neurodevelopmental model of psychosis, in Risk Factors for Psychosis: Paradigms, Mechanisms, and Prevention. Edited by Thompson AD, Broome MR. Amsterdam, Elsevier, 2020, pp 143–164

Sansone SM, Schneider A, Bickel E, et al: Improving IQ measurement in intellectual disabilities using true deviation from population norms. J Neurodev Disord 6(1):16, 2014 26491488

Schaaf RC, Miller LJ: Occupational therapy using a sensory integrative approach for children with developmental disabilities. Ment Retard Dev Disabil Res Rev 11(2):143–148, 2005 15977314

Schalock RL, Borthwick-Duffy SA, Bradley VJ, et al: Intellectual Disability: Definition, Classification, and Systems of Supports, 11th Edition. Edited by Schalock RL, Borthwick-Duffy SA, Buntinx WHE, et al. Silver Spring, MD, American Association on Intellectual and Developmental Disabilities, 2009

Schneider M, Debbané M, Bassett AS, et al: Psychiatric disorders from childhood to adulthood in 22q11.2 deletion syndrome: results from the International Consortium on Brain and Behavior in 22q11.2 Deletion Syndrome. Am J Psychiatry 171(6):627–639, 2014 24577245

Schultz RJ, Glaze DG, Patterson MC, et al: Rett syndrome: genetics, clinical features, and diagnosis (online). Waltham, MA, UpToDate, 2018

Shapira NA, Lessig MC, Murphy TK, et al: Topiramate attenuates self-injurious behaviour in Prader-Willi syndrome. Int J Neuropsychopharmacol 5(2):141–145, 2002 12135538

Shorter E: A History of Psychiatry: From the Era of the Asylum to the Age of Prozac. New York, Wiley, 1997

Siegel M, Gabriels RL: Psychiatric hospital treatment of children with autism and serious behavioral disturbance. Child Adolesc Psychiatr Clin N Am 23(1):125–142, 2014 24231172

Siegel M, Doyle K, Chemelski B, et al: Specialized inpatient psychiatry units for children with autism and developmental disorders: a United States survey. J Autism Dev Disord 42(9):1863–1869, 2012 22189962

Siegel M, Milligan B, Chemelski B, et al: Specialized inpatient psychiatry for serious behavioral disturbance in autism and intellectual disability. J Autism Dev Disord 44(12):3026–3032, 2014 24925543

Simon JB, Savina EA: Transitioning children from psychiatric hospitals to schools: the role of the special educator. Residential Treatment for Children & Youth 27(1):41–54, 2010

Smeets EE, Schrander-Stumpel CTRM: Rett syndrome, in Management of Genetic Syndromes, 2nd Edition. Edited by Cassidy SB, Allanson JE. Hoboken, NJ, Wiley, 2005, pp 457–468

Smith ACM, Dykens E, Greenberg F: Behavioral phenotype of Smith-Magenis syndrome (del 17p11.2). Am J Med Genet 81(2):179–185, 1998

Sovner R: Limiting factors in the use of DSM-III criteria with mentally ill/mentally retarded persons. Psychopharmacol Bull 22(4):1055–1059, 1986 3809370

Sovner R, Hurley AD: Four factors affecting the diagnosis of psychiatric disorders in mentally retarded persons. Psychiatric Aspects of Mental Retardation Reviews 5(9):45–49, 1986

Startin CM, D'Souza H, Ball G, et al: LonDownS Consortium, Strydom A: Health comorbidities and cognitive abilities across the lifespan in Down syndrome. J Neurodev Disord 12(1):4, 2020 31973697

Stevenson DA, Heinemann J, Angulo M, et al: Gastric rupture and necrosis in Prader-Willi syndrome. J Pediatr Gastroenterol Nutr 45(2):272–274, 2007 17667731

Summers JA, Allison DB, Lynch PS, Sandler L: Behaviour problems in Angelman syndrome. J Intellect Disabil Res 39 (Pt 2):97–106, 1995 7787388

Tang SX, Yi JJ, Calkins ME, et al: Psychiatric disorders in 22q11.2 deletion syndrome are prevalent but undertreated. Psychol Med 44(6):1267–1277, 2014 24016317

Taua C, Hepworth J, Neville C: Nurses' role in caring for people with a comorbidity of mental illness and intellectual disability: a literature review. Int J Ment Health Nurs 21(2):163–174, 2012 22034918

Tranfaglia MR: The psychiatric presentation of fragile X: evolution of the diagnosis and treatment of the psychiatric comorbidities of fragile X syndrome. Dev Neurosci 33(5):337–348, 2011 21893938

Trimble M: Neuropsychiatry. CNS Spectr 21(3):221–222, 2016 27322689

Tuchman R, Rapin I: Epilepsy in autism. Lancet Neurol 1(6):352–358, 2002 12849396

Tuchman R, Cuccaro M, Alessandri M: Autism and epilepsy: historical perspective. Brain Dev 32(9):709–718, 2010 20510557

Twachtman-Reilly J, Amaral SC, Zebrowski PP: Addressing feeding disorders in children on the autism spectrum in school-based settings: physiological and behavioral issues. Lang Speech Hear Serv Sch 39(2):261–272, 2008 18420528

Umeda CJ, Fogelberg DJ, Jirikowic T, et al: Expanding the implementation of the Americans with Disabilities Act for populations with intellectual and developmental disabilities: the role of organization-level occupational therapy consultation. Am J Occup Ther 71(4):1–6, 2017 28661376

Veltman MWM, Craig EE, Bolton PF: Autism spectrum disorders in Prader-Willi and Angelman syndromes: a systematic review. Psychiatr Genet 15(4):243–254, 2005 16314754

Verhoeven WMA, Tuinier S, Curfs LMG: Prader-Willi syndrome: the psychopathological phenotype in uniparental disomy. J Med Genet 40(10):e112, 2003 14569135

Vogels A, Matthijs G, Legius E, et al: Chromosome 15 maternal uniparental disomy and psychosis in Prader-Willi syndrome. J Med Genet 40(1):72–73, 2003 12525547

Vorstman JAS, Breetvelt EJ, Duijff SN, et al: Cognitive decline preceding the onset of psychosis in patients with 22q11.2 deletion syndrome. JAMA Psychiatry 72(4):377–385, 2015 25715178

Wehmeyer ML, Brown I, Percy M, et al: A Comprehensive Guide to Intellectual and Developmental Disabilities, 2nd Edition. Baltimore, MD, Brookes, 2017

Weyrauch D, Schwartz M, Hart B, et al: Comorbid mental disorders in fetal alcohol spectrum disorders: a systematic review. J Dev Behav Pediatr 38(4):283–291, 2017 28460370

Wharff EA, Ginnis KB, Ross AM, Blood EA: Predictors of psychiatric boarding in the pediatric emergency department: implications for emergency care. Pediatr Emerg Care 27(6):483–489, 2011 21629148

Whittington J, Holland TH: Prader-Willi Syndrome: Development and Manifestations. New York, Cambridge University Press, 2004

Williams C, Dagli A: Angelman syndrome, in Management of Genetic Syndromes, 3rd Edition. Edited by Cassidy SB, Allanson JE. Hoboken, NJ, Wiley, 2010, pp 53–62

Woods R: Behavioural concerns: assessment and management of people with intellectual disability. Aust Fam Physician 40(4):198–200, 2011 21597528

Yudofsky SC, Hales RE: The reemergence of neuropsychiatry: definition and direction. J Neuropsychiatry Clin Neurosci 1(1):1–6, 1989 2535424

Yuen RKC, Szatmari P, Vorstman JAS: Genetics of autism spectrum disorders, in Autism and Pervasive Developmental Disorders. New York, Cambridge University Press, 2019, pp 112–128

Zhao Y, Guo T, Fiksinski A, et al: Variance of IQ is partially dependent on deletion type among 1,427 22q11.2 deletion syndrome subjects. Am J Med Genet A 176(10):2172–2181, 2018 30289625

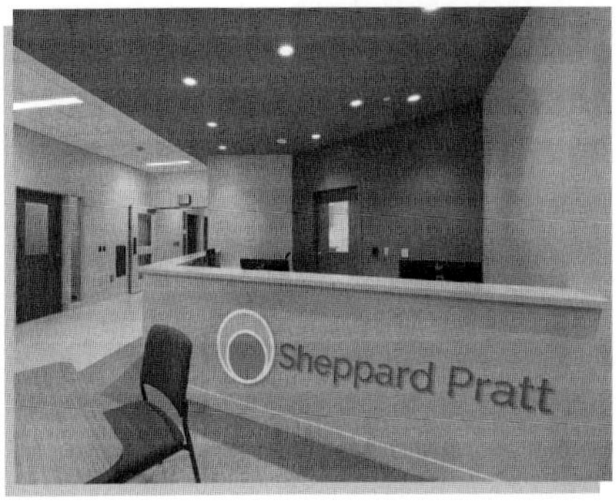

CHAPTER 7

The Eating Disorders Unit

Jennifer L. Goetz, M.D.
Steven F. Crawford, M.D.
Harry A. Brandt, M.D.

While current estimates suggest that at least 30 million individuals suffer from a diagnosable eating disorder (Hudson et al. 2007), substantially more have subthreshold eating disorder–related symptoms. According to a national sample of more than 36,000 U.S. adults from the 2012–2013 National Epidemiologic Survey on Alcohol and Related Conditions, the lifetime prevalence estimates for anorexia nervosa (AN), bulimia nervosa (BN), and binge-eating disorder (BED) were 0.80%, 0.28%, and 0.85%, respectively (Udo and Grilo 2018). According to the 2017 Youth Risk Behavior Survey, 38% of adolescent girls and 25% of adolescent boys believed they were overweight, and 60% of adolescent girls and 34% of adolescent boys were actively attempting to lose weight (Kann et al. 2018). Many of these individuals were within a normal weight range. By age 6 years, girls start to express concerns about their weight or shape, and 40%–60% of elementary school girls (ages 6–12) are concerned about their weight or about becoming too fat, and for some, these concerns endure throughout their life span (Smolak 2011). With the development of an eating disorder come the potentially drastic consequences related to malnutrition, laxative and diuretic abuse, self-induced vomiting, and excessive exercise. The physical and emotional toll that eating disorders take on a person spares no organ system and affects every aspect of that individual's life.

DSM-5 Classification of Eating Disorders

DSM-5 (American Psychiatric Association 2013) recognizes six eating disorders: anorexia nervosa, bulimia nervosa, binge-eating disorder, and avoidant/restrictive food intake disorder (ARFID), as well as two diagnoses previously subsumed under DSM-IV-TR (American Psychiatric Association 2000) "feeding disorders of infancy and early childhood," pica and rumination disorder; along with two categories for clear illness not meeting full criteria of the recognized eating disorders: "other specified feeding or eating disorder" and "unspecified feeding or eating disorder."

Anorexia Nervosa

The DSM-5 criteria for AN include the following:

1. Restriction in energy intake relative to requirements, leading to significantly low body weight in the context of age, sex, developmental trajectory, and physical health. (*Significantly low body weight* is defined as weight less than minimally normal or less than that minimally expected for children/adolescents.)
2. Intense fear of gaining weight or of becoming fat or persistent behavior that interferes with weight gain despite significantly low weight.
3. Disturbance in the way in which one's body weight or shape is experienced; undue influence of body weight or shape on self-evaluation, or persistent lack of recognition of the seriousness of current low body weight.

Two subtypes of AN are recognized: a predominantly restricting type, characterized primarily by extreme restriction of caloric intake as the primary means of weight control; and a binge-eating/purging type, which is marked by regularly engaging in bingeing and/or purging (self-induced vomiting, misuse of laxatives, diuretics, or enemas) episodes to control weight. Often there will be characteristics of both a restricting and a binge-eating/purging type, though the predominating feature will dictate clinical classification. Though BN is also marked by episodes of bingeing and purging, the key difference in patients with binge-eating/purging subtype of AN is that all the criteria for AN listed above are met.

There is no single standard for what constitutes a minimally normal body weight, and determining whether weight is abnormally low depends on individual factors such as frame size, skeletal structure, and ethnicity. The previous version of DSM (DSM-IV-TR) suggested that a minimally normal weight was equal to 85% of "expected" weight for age and height; however, the current criteria do not stipulate any specific weight parameter, and the threshold for expected weight is left to clinical judgment. Individuals lose weight and/or maintain a low body weight in various ways, but reduction of food intake is usually present. They often begin by excluding high-calorie foods, but dietary restraint can progress to a restricted diet that is sometimes limited to only a few foods. Individuals may fast for days and exercise excessively such that these behavioral patterns interfere with important activities, reflecting the obsessive nature of the illness. In addition, about half of individuals with AN may purge by self-inducing vomiting or misusing laxatives, diuretics, or enemas. As the individual continues to lose weight, the fear of gaining weight often paradoxically increases. This fear, coupled with denial of illness, often leads to resistance to seeking treatment.

Disturbed body image manifests in various ways, with some individuals believing they are grossly overweight, and others focusing concern on specific body areas they experience as too large. As a result, individuals may weigh themselves excessively, measure body parts, or examine themselves ritualistically in a mirror. Self-esteem is unreasonably dependent upon body shape, weight, and appearance; weight loss is often viewed as an achievement and sign of self-discipline, whereas weight gain is seen as a failure of self-control. Individuals may occasionally concede that they are emaciated, often while denying the evidence of medical complications of starvation. Thought process may appear nearly delusional in circumscribed areas pertaining to the body, but these cognitive distortions are best viewed as overvalued ideas.

Psychological and behavioral signs and symptoms associated with AN include relentless pursuit of thinness, obsessional preoccupation with food (e.g., collecting recipes, hoarding food), fear of certain foods, restricted repertoire of foods, preference for low-calorie foods, overestimation of number of calories consumed, overuse of condiments and artificial sweeteners, food-related rituals (e.g., cutting food into small pieces, refusing to mix foods or colors on the plate, drinking water after each bite), fear of eating in public, social withdrawal, exercise rituals (e.g., running a set distance each day, swimming a certain number of laps, performing an exact number of abdominal crunches), restlessness/fidgeting/hyperactivity, limited insight/denial of illness, resistance to treatment and weight gain, limited emotional expression, rigidity in thinking and behavior, perfectionism, and an overwhelming need to control one's environment. Some of these features may persist despite weight restoration, reflecting either problems that preceded the onset of the eating disorder or long-term consequences of a persistent starvation state. This raises important questions regarding what symptoms of AN are state related as a direct result of starvation as opposed to reflecting underlying genetically driven traits.

Bulimia Nervosa

The DSM-5 criteria for BN include the following:

1. Recurrent episodes of binge eating.
2. Recurrent inappropriate compensatory measures to prevent weight gain, such as self-induced vomiting; misuse of laxatives, diuretics, or other medications; fasting; or excessive exercise.
3. Binge eating and inappropriate compensatory measures both occur, on average, at least once a week for 3 months.
4. Self-evaluation is unduly influenced by body shape and weight.
5. Disturbance does not occur exclusively during episodes of AN.

Binge eating is a hallmark of BN and is defined in DSM-5 as eating more than most in a discrete period of time; patients will often consume as much as several thousand calories in a 1- to 2-hour time period. Most individuals report that the binge behavior is not pleasurable; rather, it is the purging afterward from which ensues the pleasure or relief and a sense of control. It is not uncommon for bingeing to precede the onset of development of purging by as much as a year. Many report purging serves to alleviate the physical discomfort associated with the binge as well as alleviate fear of weight gain; it is not uncommon for purging to become the goal of the binge itself. Individuals with BN are typically of normal to slightly increased weight, as opposed to those with AN, who are severely underweight.

Binge-Eating Disorder

DSM-5 is the first version of the manual to classify BED as its own diagnosis; it had previously been categorized for research purposes as a "condition for further study" in DSM-IV-TR. BED is characterized in DSM-5 as follows:

1. Recurrent episodes of binge eating.
2. The binge-eating episodes are associated with three or more of the following: eating much more rapidly than normal; eating until feeling uncomfortably full; eating large amounts of food when not feeling physically hungry; eating alone because of feeling embarrassed by how much one is eating; feeling disgusted with oneself, depressed, or very guilty afterward.
3. Marked distress regarding binge eating is present.
4. The binge eating occurs, on average, at least once a week for 3 months.
5. The binge eating is not associated with the recurrent use of inappropriate compensatory behavior as in BN and does not occur exclusively during the course of BN or AN.

Individuals with BED are typically overweight or obese and often eat in private because of the shame they feel in association with bingeing. Triggers for binge eating include negative affect, interpersonal stressors, dietary restraint, and boredom. While binge eating may serve to alleviate certain feelings that precipitated the binge in the short term, dysphoria and negative self-evaluation are often the result of the behavioral pattern. Comorbid medical conditions associated with BED include those associated with being overweight: cardiovascular disease, type 2 diabetes, gallbladder disease, arthritis, and infertility.

Other Specified/Unspecified Feeding or Eating Disorder

DSM-5 reserves use of these diagnoses for when patients have symptoms of a feeding or eating disorder that cause clinically significant distress or impairment in social, occupational, or other important areas of functioning, yet do not meet the full criteria for any of the disorders in the diagnostic categories. The "other specified" category is used in cases in which the clinician chooses to communicate the specific reason that the presentation does not meet criteria for one of the other eating disorders (e.g., bingeing or purging <1 week or for <3 months). The "unspecified" category is used in situations in which the clinician chooses *not* to specify the reason that criteria are not met for a specific disorder and includes presentations in which there is insufficient information to make a more formal diagnosis (e.g., in an emergency room setting).

Avoidant/Restrictive Food Intake Disorder

ARFID was added to DSM-5 to describe the presentation of patients engaged in restrictive eating behaviors without the associated concerns about weight and shape and often without the associated psychological characteristics of those with AN. ARFID is characterized in DSM-5 by the following:

1. An apparent lack of interest in eating or food, avoidance based on the sensory characteristics of food, or concern about aversive consequences of eating, as manifested by persistent failure to meet appropriate nutritional and/or energy needs

associated with one or more of the following: a) significant weight loss or failure to achieve expected weight or faltering growth in children; b) significant nutritional deficiency; c) dependence on enteral feeding or oral nutritional supplements; and d) marked interference with psychosocial functioning.
2. The disturbance is not better explained by lack of available food or by an associated culturally sanctioned practice.
3. The eating disturbance does not occur exclusively during the course of AN or BN, and there is no evidence of a disturbance in the way in which one's body weight or shape is experienced.
4. The eating disorder is not attributable to a concurrent medical condition or not better explained by another mental disorder. When the eating disturbance occurs in the context of another condition or disorder, the severity of the eating disturbance exceeds that routinely associated with the condition or disorder and warrants additional clinical attention.

Individuals in the ARFID category constitute a heterogeneous group, and because ARFID is a more recently defined syndrome, it will likely take some time to better characterize the clinical features and course of individuals with ARFID and to determine whether there are particular subgroups within the broader group.

In a group of adolescents with eating disorders receiving treatment at a specialty clinic, 14% had symptoms that met criteria for ARFID; those with ARFID were more likely to be young and male. Many reported food avoidance, decreased appetite, and abdominal pain (Fisher et al. 2014). Nearly half of children with this diagnosis report fear of vomiting or choking. About one-fifth report that they avoid certain foods because of sensory issues. In one study, one-third of children with ARFID had a comorbid mood disorder, three-quarters had an anxiety disorder, and nearly one-fifth were diagnosed with an autism spectrum disorder (Nicely et al. 2014).

Pica

This eating disorder is diagnosed when the following criteria are met according to DSM-5:

1. Persistent eating of nonnutritive, nonfood substances over the period of at least 1 month.
2. The eating of nonnutritive, nonfood substances is inappropriate to the developmental level of the individual.
3. The eating behavior is not part of a culturally supported or socially normative practice.
4. If the eating behavior occurs in the context of another mental disorder (e.g., intellectual disability, autism spectrum disorder, schizophrenia) or medical condition (including pregnancy), it is sufficiently severe to warrant additional clinical attention.

Rumination Disorder

This eating disorder is characterized by the following:

1. Repeated regurgitation of food over a period of at least 1 month; food may be rechewed, re-allowed, or spit out.

2. The repeated regurgitation is not attributable to an associated gastrointestinal or other medical condition (e.g., gastroesophageal reflux, pyloric stenosis).
3. The eating disturbance does not occur exclusively during the course of AN or BN, BED, or ARFID.
4. If the symptoms occur in the context of another mental disorder (e.g., intellectual disability, autism spectrum disorder), they are sufficiently severe to warrant additional clinical attention.

Comorbid Psychopathology

Psychiatric comorbidities are common in patients with eating disorders, including mood disorders, anxiety disorders, obsessive-compulsive disorder, personality disorders, and substance use disorders (Herzog et al. 1996; Krug et al. 2008). Some of these are a direct result of the eating disorder and often resolve with treatment of the primary eating pathology, whereas others may coexist and persist after treatment. Patients with restricting-type AN often have major depressive disorder, and about 15% will have an obsessive-compulsive disorder unrelated to eating behavior (Braun et al. 1994). Women with eating disorders appear to have had higher rates of obsessive-compulsive personality traits in childhood (Anderluh et al. 2003). Alcohol use disorders are more prevalent among patients with BN than among those with restrictive AN; among AN patients, alcohol use disorders are more common in patients with the binge eating–purging subtype (Halmi et al. 1991). Cluster B personality types (histrionic, borderline, narcissistic) have a higher association with BN and binge-eating/purging–type AN, while Cluster C personality types (obsessive-compulsive, avoidant, dependent) are more prevalent among those with restricting-type AN. AN has among the highest mortality rates of the psychiatric illnesses, with a standardized mortality ratio of 5.35, most commonly due to medical complications of the disorder itself or from the remarkably high rates of suicide seen in the illness (Fichter and Quadflieg 2016). Prompt and early recognition of coexisting conditions is essential to the treatment and recovery of patients, and treatment and recovery should be appropriately addressed within the context of a multidisciplinary team approach.

Epidemiology

Trends in the epidemiology of eating disorders are difficult to assess because the diagnostic criteria have changed over time and detection via self-report measures may not be reliable in an illness marked by secrecy and denial. The lifetime prevalence of AN in women is estimated to be 0.3%–1% (Hoek and van Hoeken 2003), and according to the National Comorbidity Survey Replication, male lifetime prevalence is estimated at 0.3% (Hudson et al. 2007).

AN has a bimodal age of distribution, with the first peak at ages 13–14 and the other at ages 17–18. These two distinct periods of time, marked by biological influences and environmental factors, may be associated with a sense of lack of control. In someone with a biological predisposition, food intake may serve as a way to control some aspect of their life at a time when they feel all other control has been lost.

Lifetime prevalence rates for BN in women are estimated at 1%–3% (Fairburn and Beglin 1990; Hudson et al. 2007). BN is unimodal in its age at onset and tends to affect women in their late teens or early 20s—a time often marked by transitions in living, and pressures regarding life choices in terms of partners, careers, and family planning—all of which may contribute to the development of an eating disorder.

BED has a 1-year and lifetime prevalence of 1.6% and 3.5% among U.S. females and 0.8% and 2.0% among U.S. males, respectively (Hudson et al. 2007). Little is known about the developmental course of BED given its relatively new recognition among the eating disorders in DSM-5. It is not uncommon for dieting to follow the development of binge eating, in contrast to BN, in which dysfunctional dieting typically precedes the onset of binge eating. BED usually develops in young or later adulthood, in contrast to AN and BN, which typically develop in younger individuals; when BED does develop earlier in life, it often does not come to professional attention until later adulthood.

ARFID is more than "picky eating," and children do not simply grow out of it; in fact, they often become malnourished as a result of the limited variety of foods they eat. The prevalence of ARFID remains to be determined but is estimated at 3%–5% of children, with boys potentially having a higher risk than girls for this disorder (Norris et al. 2016).

The previously recognized "eating disorder not otherwise specified," or EDNOS, category of DSM-IV-TR had a relatively high prevalence, occurring in approximately 3%–5% of women between the ages of 15 and 30 in Western countries (Putukian 1994). The EDNOS category constituted the largest proportion of diagnosable eating disorders, reflecting the heterogenic nature in which eating disorders present and manifest. The prevalences of the subsequently delineated categories of "other specified feeding or eating disorder" and "unspecified feeding or eating disorder" are not yet clear and will require more time for study.

Pathogenesis

Eating disorders are complex illnesses, with current models emphasizing a combination of genetic, biological, psychological, family, environmental, and social factors as important contributors to the overall pathogenesis. As an example, an anxious or perfectionist individual may experience decreased self-esteem or self-control because of predisposing factors (biology, family history, traumatic events) and then use dieting behavior or weight loss to provide a sense of stability and control in their life (Garner and Garfinkel 1997). The dynamic interplay of these factors may then be the catalyst for the development of an eating disorder.

Psychological, Family, Environmental, and Social Factors

A variety of factors have been implicated in the development of eating disorders. A history of dieting, childhood preoccupation with a thin body, social pressures encouraging thinness, physical and sexual abuse, sports and artistic endeavors in which a thin physique is emphasized (ballet, running, or wrestling), and sports in which scoring is highly subjective (skating, diving, gymnastics) have all been associated with the development of eating disorders (McKnight Investigators 2003; Nattiv et al. 1994; Patton et al. 1999).

Family distress can be a significant factor in the development of an eating disorder, and certain characteristics, including perceived high parental expectations, poor communication, difficulty managing conflict, and enmeshment or estrangement, often contribute. Families often have a difficult time responding appropriately to the changing physical and emotional needs of their child, and as with other psychiatric disorders, in families that are highly critical of the patient, outcomes tend to be poor (van Furth et al. 1996).

Genetics

A role for genetics in the pathogenesis of eating disorders is supported by studies showing that young women whose first-degree relatives have eating disorders have a 6- to 10-fold increased risk for developing one themselves (Woodside 1995). Monozygotic twins have a higher rate of concordance for eating disorders (up to 50%–80%) compared with dizygotic twins, and there is also a higher prevalence of affective disorders and alcoholism in first-degree relatives of patients with eating disorders (Halmi et al. 1991; Herzog et al. 1996; Kendler et al. 1991; Strober 1991).

A genome-wide association study (GWAS) looking at 16,992 cases of AN and 55,525 control subjects identified eight significant loci associated with AN and found that the genetic architecture of AN mirrors its clinical presentation, showing significant genetic correlations with other psychiatric disorders, physical activity, and metabolic/lipid/anthropometric traits (Watson et al. 2019). Single-nucleotide polymorphism (SNP)–based genetic correlations across the eight loci were found to be highly correlated with known comorbid psychopathology (including obsessive-compulsive disorder, major depressive disorder, anxiety disorders, and schizophrenia). Positive SNP associations were found with physical activity, which is often pathologically elevated in AN, and high-density lipoprotein cholesterol. Negative SNP associations were found with fat mass, BMI, obesity, type 2 diabetes, fasting insulin, insulin resistance, and leptin. Although low BMI has been thought to be a consequence of the psychological features of AN, these data suggest that metabolic dysregulation may contribute to the exceptional difficulty that individuals with AN have in maintaining a healthy BMI despite therapeutic nourishment. These findings are important first steps in elucidating underlying pathological mechanisms of the disease that may thereby direct future therapeutic interventions.

Far less is known about the genetics of BN than is known about the genetics of AN. The heritability of BN is estimated at approximately 60% and is highly correlated with the heritability of AN (46%–79%) (Bulik et al. 1998). BED is also highly heritable, with estimates around 50% (Bulik et al. 1998). There are significant correlations between BED and BN symptoms. Samples are currently being collected from patients with BN for GWAS to test for genetic variants associated specifically with BN.

Because of the relatively recent addition of many of the eating disorders to DSM-5, they have not yet been the subject of twin, family, or genome-wide association studies to elucidate genetics.

Neurobiology

Anorexia Nervosa

While much remains to be learned, much is now known about the neurobiological underpinning of AN and extreme caloric restriction. Enlarged cortical sulci and ventricles have been the most frequently reported structural finding in the literature (Phillipou et al. 2014). Other findings include enlarged cerebrospinal fluid (CSF) spaces and increased total CSF volume. Reduced gray and white matter volumes have frequently been reported, and some recent studies show persistent gray matter abnormalities and greater CSF volumes even with weight restoration. Recent evidence suggests that the core pathological findings of distorted body image and denial/lack of recognition of malnutrition may be related to abnormalities in the insular cortex, which is involved in multiple processes, including taste, visceral sensation, modulation of attention and emotion, self-awareness, and autonomic functions, all prominent abnormalities/features of AN (Schreuder 2011). It is possible that the autonomic dysfunction seen in AN, including bradycardia, orthostasis, sweating, and anxiety, may reflect, at least to some degree, insular lesions. As insular lesions have been shown to reduce cravings for alcohol and drugs, they may similarly reduce cravings for food.

Beyond the structural abnormalities, multiple neurotransmitter systems have been examined in relation to AN, the most frequently studied of which are serotonin and dopamine. Serotonin plays an important role in regulating feeding, satiety, and appetite suppression as well as harm avoidance. Therefore, disturbances in serotonin synthesis and/or function may result in appetite dysregulation, anxious and obsessional behaviors, and difficulty with impulse control. Serotonin is made from tryptophan, an essential amino acid produced from food sources. Dietary restriction lowers the plasma level of tryptophan, and not surprisingly, lower levels are found in patients with AN, potentially resulting in decreased availability to the brain. Downstream effects of this decreased availability include decreased serotonin synthesis, downregulation of serotonin transporters, and compensatory supersensitivity of postsynaptic receptors. Most research has focused on the metabolite of serotonin, 5-hydroxyindoleacetic acid (5-HIAA), and 5-HT_{1A} receptors. Acutely ill patients with AN show significantly lower CSF basal concentrations of 5-HIAA, which have been associated with increased impulsivity and aggression; individuals who have recovered from AN show elevated 5-HIAA levels compared with healthy control subjects (Phillipou et al. 2014). While the role of serotonin in AN is not entirely clear and warrants further study, this neurotransmitter is a likely candidate to influence behavioral inhibition and self-control.

Dopamine, on the other hand, plays important roles in reward, habit formation, affect, decision-making, executive control, motivation/drive, initiation, maintenance of complex movements and behaviors, and stereotyped motor activity. The major metabolite of dopamine, homovanillic acid, has been shown to be decreased in the CSF of individuals with acute AN, and levels return to normal with weight restoration. Weight-recovered individuals with AN have higher binding potential of D_2/D_3 receptors in anteroventral striatum compared with healthy control subjects, and this may be associated with decreased intrasynaptic dopamine concentration and increased D_2/D_3 receptor density, which could contribute to faulty reward processing around food, body image, and weight (Bailer et al. 2007; Frank et al. 2005).

Additionally, it may be useful to focus on abnormalities in the brains of individuals with AN on a systems level, particularly the reward system that encompasses mesolimbic systems, including the midbrain/ventral tegmental area, nucleus accumbens, and orbitofrontal cortex. Patients with AN report less desire for high-calorie foods and slower response times, suggesting lower motivation to seek food, when compared with healthy control subjects (Cowdrey et al. 2013; Scaife et al. 2016). Many functional MRI studies have presented images of food that are presumed to be innately rewarding to patients with AN and have noticed differential activation among individuals with AN in areas of the brain central to reward, although specific regions identified and the status of those regions as hypo- or hyperactive have been inconsistent across studies (Cowdrey et al. 2011; Ellison et al. 1998; Fuglset et al. 2016; Holsen et al. 2012). There have been inconsistent findings on volumetric abnormalities in the orbitofrontal cortex in individuals with AN when compared with healthy control subjects. Among adolescents and adults with AN, functional MRI reveals heightened connectivity between the nucleus accumbens and the orbitofrontal cortex, regions associated with reward and cognitive and behavioral control. There is increased dopamine receptor density in the nucleus accumbens of women with AN after recovery. Given these abnormalities in both the acutely ill and recovered states, the functioning of reward circuitry is likely impacted by food restriction (Steinglass and Walsh 2016).

The dopaminergic system has been the target of the reward-centered model of AN (Steinglass and Walsh 2016). This model posits that habit formation is a process in which goal-directed behaviors are associated with rewards; if practiced enough, these behaviors become automatic and independent of reward (e.g., habitual). The shift from goal-directed to habitual behavior appears to be accompanied by a shift in the supporting neural circuits from the mesolimbic reward system to the dorsal striatum habit system (basal ganglia, caudate, putamen) and dorsolateral prefrontal cortex. Restricted intake is initially reinforced, often in the form of compliments, satisfaction, and sense of self-control. The behavior (restriction) is thus repeated and becomes automatic to the point that it can be elicited by specific stimuli and cues (onset of meals leads to food rituals and minimal intake). There is evidence from PET studies of multiple abnormalities in the dorsal frontostriatal circuits in those with AN: hypermetabolic caudate nucleus, decreased caudate volume, and altered dopamine binding in the caudate. Furthermore, restricted intake in AN has been associated with activity in the dorsal striatum such that a food choice task activated the dorsal striatum in a group of patients with anorexia but not in healthy control subjects and there were no group differences in mesolimbic reward regions. This lends further evidence to the model of shift from a reward-based behavioral paradigm that activates the mesolimbic system to a habitual paradigm that activates the dorsal striatum in those with AN.

Bulimia Nervosa

Studies of individuals with BN indicate an increased reinforcing value of food. This has been exhibited in studies showing that women with BN work harder than healthy control subjects for highly palatable foods, delivered and consumed as they were earned, providing immediate reinforcement (Bodell and Keel 2015). Neural responses to pictures of food or taste are inconsistent across studies in BN; compared with healthy controls, individuals with BN often show greater activation in the medial orbitofrontal cortex, anterior cingulate cortex, visual cortex, and insula in response to pictures of palatable foods, which has been correlated with symptom severity (Brooks et al. 2011; Uher et al. 2004). Some research, however, has suggested a reduced reward response to expected sweet taste and to unexpected taste in individuals with BN compared with healthy controls (Bohon and Stice 2011; Frank et al. 2006, 2011). In the fed versus fasted state, those remitted from BN do not show the decreased basal ganglia and limbic responses to sucrose or water that healthy control subjects show (Ely et al. 2017).

In functional MRI studies related to food, individuals with BN show aberrant neural activation in control-related regions—specifically, decreased activation of left dorsolateral prefrontal cortex in response to food pictures (Bohon and Stice 2011; Uher et al. 2004). Studies of both adolescent and adult BN patients have found decreased activation in frontostriatal control circuits during cognitive conflict tasks, which was also associated with increased bulimic symptoms (Marsh et al. 2009, 2011). Large samples of adolescents and adults with BN show age-associated decreases in volume and cortical thickness of frontal and parietal regions associated with control-related circuits (Berner et al. 2018; Marsh et al. 2015). Individuals with BN show greater preference for immediate reward and difficulty delaying gratification (Bari and Robbins 2013; Kekic et al. 2016).

Psychiatric Levels of Care

Individuals with eating disorders receive care in a variety of settings, from the outpatient to inpatient—both medically and psychiatrically—as well as in partial hospital settings, depending on the medical stability, severity and frequency of symptoms, psychiatric comorbidity, safety of the patient, psychosocial supports, and response to current and prior treatments. A majority of individuals are cared for in the outpatient setting with a multidisciplinary treatment team.

The American Psychiatric Association (APA) *Practice Guideline for the Treatment of Patients With Eating Disorders*, 3rd Edition (Yager et al. 2006), recommends inpatient care on a specialized unit for adults with eating disorders in the following circumstances:

- Weight <85% of individually estimated healthy body weight
- Heart rate (HR) <40 beats per minute (bpm)
- Blood pressure <90/60 mm Hg
- Temperature <97°F
- Dehydration
- Hepatic, renal, or cardiovascular complications
- Electrolyte imbalance
- Potassium <3 mEq/L
- Glucose <60 mg/dL
- Organ compromise requiring acute treatment
- Poorly controlled diabetes
- Hematemesis

The Society for Adolescent Health and Medicine's recommendations for hospitalization for children and adolescents with an eating disorder are as follows (Golden et al. 2015):

- Weight <75% of individually estimated healthy body weight; OR acute weight loss with food refusal; OR ongoing weight loss despite intensive management
- Dehydration

- Electrolyte disturbance (hypokalemia, hypophosphatemia, hyponatremia)
- Electrocardiographic abnormalities (e.g., prolonged QTc or severe bradycardia)
- Physiological instability
- Severe bradycardia (HR <50 bpm daytime; HR <45 bpm night)
- Hypotension (<90/45 mm Hg)
- Hypothermia (temperature <96°F/35.6°C)
- Orthostatic increase in heart rate (>20 bpm) or decrease in blood pressure (>20 mm Hg systolic or >10 mm Hg diastolic)
- Arrested growth and development
- Failure of outpatient treatment
- Acute food refusal
- Uncontrollable bingeing and purging
- Acute medical complications of malnutrition (e.g., syncope, seizures, cardiac failure, pancreatitis)
- Comorbid psychiatric or medical condition that prohibits or limits appropriate outpatient care (severe depression, suicidal ideation, obsessive-compulsive disorder, type 1 diabetes mellitus)

The APA's practice guideline (Yager et al. 2006) further recommends hospitalization in the following circumstances:

- Any existing comorbid psychiatric disorder requiring hospitalization
- Suicide plans and suicidal intent or other concerns suggesting elevated risk of suicide
- Severe co-occurring substance use disorder
- Any existing comorbid medical disorder requiring inpatient management (e.g., diabetes mellitus)
- Poor motivation to recover
- Preoccupation with ego-syntonic or -dystonic thoughts
- Lack of cooperation with treatment
- Need for supervision during and after all meals, in bathrooms and around exercise, that cannot be achieved at home (e.g., failure of treatment in less restrictive environment)
- Acute food refusal
- Uncontrollable binge eating and purging
- Treatment program or provider who is too distant for patient to access
- Presence of additional stressors interfering with ability to eat
- Severe disabling symptoms of bulimia that have not responded to outpatient treatment
- Lack of social support at home to assist patient in abstaining from acting on eating disorder behaviors

Clinical Evaluation

All patients who present with clinical suspicion of an eating disorder should have a thorough evaluation, including a history, physical examination, and laboratory workup with a focus on eliciting components of the diagnostic criteria, associated features, comorbid psychopathology, and medical complications. Medical complications are secondary to caloric restriction and weight loss in AN and to bingeing and purging behaviors in BN.

Patients with AN are often not forthcoming about their illness, and symptoms are typically ego-syntonic. Individuals may present with anxiety, depression, or somatic discomfort due to medical complications such as pain with eating, bloating, or "inability to keep food down." Patients are often ashamed and may attempt to conceal their thinness by wearing bulky clothes, inflate their body weight by hiding objects in their clothes, and drink water excessively to create the illusion that their weight is higher and stable. Denial often delays assessment until family members or friends are compelled to obtain psychiatric and medical care for their loved one. It is often important to engage the family in the initial and ongoing assessment and evaluation of patients.

The clinical evaluation should assess the following:

- Height and weight
- Current body weight and desired weight
- Recent weight changes
- Highest and lowest weights, weight stability, and history of efforts to control weight and shape
- Frequency of self-weighing
- Meal patterns
- Daily caloric intake and pattern of consumption
- Present and past eating disorder symptoms
- Dietary restriction
- Attitudes about food, eating, body weight, and shape
- Binge eating
- Compensatory behaviors
- Food rituals (e.g., cutting food into extremely small pieces or refusing to mix different types or colors of food on the plate)
- Menstrual status (last menstrual period, regularity, weight at which spontaneous menses occur)
- Suicidality
- Comorbid disorders, such as anxiety, mood, impulse-control, substance use, and personality disorders
- Nicotine, caffeine, cocaine, and stimulant use
- Psychosocial functioning
- Family history of eating disorders and other psychopathology

It is critical for the interviewer to ask very specific questions of the patient and gather collateral information from family and others, because many patients can be defensive or evasive regarding their current symptoms. As part of the mental status examination, the clinician should note behavioral restlessness or fidgeting. Impaired attention, concentration, and thought process can indicate cognitive impairment, including delirium related to medical complications of low weight and/or purging. Anxious or depressed affect should be assessed. Insight and judgment can be evaluated by asking about the patient's target weight and treatment-seeking behaviors. Patients with eating disorders are at increased risk for suicide as well as nonsuicidal self-injurious behavior, and determining these risks should be a part of the routine patient assessment.

Physical Examination

Within the context of a complete physical examination, key portions include weight and height, orthostatic vital signs, temperature, skin and oropharyngeal examination, and abdominal and neurological examination (to look for other causes of weight loss or vomiting—abdominal or CNS mass). Other signs that are often present include hair loss, edema, poor dentition, and scarring or calluses on the dorsum of the hand (resulting from use of fingers to induce vomiting).

Laboratory Assessment

Tests should be guided by the symptoms and physical findings and include complete blood count and differential; comprehensive metabolic panel (blood urea nitrogen/creatinine, liver function tests, phosphorus, calcium, magnesium, albumin and prealbumin); amylase and lipase; thyroid function tests (thyroid-stimulating hormone, triiodothyronine [T_3], and thyroxine [T_4]); luteinzing hormone, follicle-stimulating hormone, estrogen, testosterone, prolactin, vitamin D, and urinalysis; stool guaiac; DEXA (dual-energy X-ray absorptiometry) scan; and electrocardiography.

Medical Complications

Many medical complications can occur during starvation or persistent purging, and specific attention should be paid to this portion of the exam, which is critical in acute stabilization and determination of appropriate level of care. AN has the second highest mortality rate of any mental illness, estimated at around 10%, second only to opiate use disorder, and this is due in large part to cardiac dysfunction and the effects of chronic malnutrition (Arcelus et al. 2011; Chesney et al. 2014).

Starvation induces protein and fat catabolism that leads to loss of cellular volume and atrophy of the heart, brain, liver, intestines, kidneys, and muscles. The primary risk factors for developing medical complications in AN are degree of weight loss and chronicity of the illness. Complications of AN include myocardial atrophy, cardiac arrhythmias and conduction abnormalities, mitral valve prolapse, pericardial effusion, bradycardia, hypotension, leukopenia, functional hypothalamic amenorrhea, infertility, osteoporosis, vitamin deficiencies, gastroparesis, constipation, and growth retardation. Complications of BN include dehydration, hypokalemia, metabolic alkalosis secondary to purging, cardiac arrhythmias and conduction abnormalities, menstrual irregularities, Mallory-Weiss syndrome, ipecac-induced myopathy, Boerhaave's syndrome, gastroesophageal reflux disease, hypokalemic ileus, pancreatitis, and erosion of dental enamel. As in AN, these medical complications can be life-threatening, especially those associated with cardiac conduction abnormalities. Treatment for complications includes nutritional rehabilitation and cessation of binge-purge behaviors. Many complications can be expected to resolve with these measures alone.

Model of Inpatient Care

Recovery is often very difficult without a sufficient level of supervision and support when the patient is in a low weight range and/or when uncontrollable bingeing and purging are present. There have been no controlled trials that have evaluated criteria for hospitalization in patients with eating disorders, though several organizations (APA, Society for Adolescent Health and Medicine) have issued guidelines. Weight gain is an essential component of successful outcomes in those who are severely underweight and malnourished, and weight restoration can correct many of the physiological consequences of an eating disorder (Sylvester and Forman 2008). One study examined outcomes after hospitalization and found that those patients who were allowed to remain in the hospital until they regained their necessary weight (90%–92% of ideal body weight) had an improved outcome compared with those who did not regain their weight and were discharged earlier (Baran et al. 1995). Longer initial hospitalization has been shown to be cost-effective and suggests that prolonged initial hospitalization may provide the support necessary to successfully treat patients (Crow and Nyman 2004).

Multidisciplinary Team Approach

The most accepted treatment for eating disorders involves a multidisciplinary team approach, including a psychiatrist, internist/pediatrician, dietitian (with experience in treating eating disorders), and mental health professional (Ph.D., Psy.D., LICSW). The medical provider (either psychiatrist or internist/pediatrician) often serves as the coordinator of care and must rule out other medical causes of weight loss, vomiting, or menstrual irregularity. The psychiatrist or internist/pediatrician monitors immediate medical issues (vital sign stability, electrolyte abnormalities, and hydration status) as well as long-term sequelae, including issues related to bone density, menstruation, and growth issues in younger patients. Daily weigh-in and twice-daily vital sign checks are needed to ensure weight gain (for patients with AN) and medical stability on the inpatient unit. Depending on the specific needs of the individual patient, weights may be blinded or visible but should also be early morning, post-void and in a paper gown. The medical provider provides admission history and physical exams and assists in ruling out and treating concurrent medical conditions in patients. The dietitian plays a major role by providing nutritional education and experiential/exposure therapies. The dietitian engages in directed dialogue with the patient about available dietary options and meal plan requirements. The dietitian, with the medical provider, can help set appropriate weight goals. The mental health professional serves to provide individual and family therapy to patients. On the inpatient unit, this is best accomplished in a cognitive-behavioral therapy (CBT) framework (Fairburn 2008), which complements the overall milieu's therapeutic structure. Therapy addresses underlying issues that may have initiated and perpetuated the eating disorder.

Additional members of the treatment team in many settings include art therapists, movement therapists, music therapists, occupational therapists, and mental health specialists who serve to maintain the therapeutic nature of the milieu. The key features of the team approach include expertise from multiple domains; communication among team members is crucial for optimal treatment.

Core Therapeutic Modalities

Psychological treatment may include psychoeducation, CBT, dialectical behavior therapy (DBT), acceptance and commitment therapy (ACT), and family-based therapy (FBT).

Psychoeducation

No matter at what stage of illness someone presents on the inpatient unit, the backbone of all treatment is psychoeducation about eating disorders. This includes educating patients on the various types of eating disorders, the medical complications of eating disorders, the psychiatric comorbidity, the treatment modalities shown most effective, the nutritional approach on the specific unit, and expectations for the unit especially at mealtimes and regarding pharmacological treatments. Psychoeducation happens across a variety of settings on the inpatient unit, including individual sessions with the psychiatrist, internist, and therapist; nutritional counseling; group settings; and family therapy.

Cognitive-Behavioral Therapy

The most studied form of treatment to date for eating disorders has been CBT, pioneered for eating disorders by Christopher Fairburn (2008). CBT emphasizes the relationship of thoughts and feelings to behaviors and helps patients learn to recognize the thoughts and feelings that lead to disordered eating. CBT has greater evidence to support its use in treating BN than in treating AN and was originally developed as an outpatient therapeutic modality (Bacaltchuk et al. 2001; Whittal et al. 1999).

Nevertheless, the principles of examining cognitions that support and maintain the eating disorder and exposure regarding feared situations involving food form the cornerstone of the therapeutic program of most inpatient eating disorder units. The CBT model for the treatment of eating disorders emphasizes the important role of the cognitive (including attitudes around weight, shape, and their control) and behavioral (including dietary restriction and binge eating and purging) factors that contribute to and maintain the eating disorder and its associated pathology.

The initial emphasis in treatment is on stabilization of symptoms and behavioral change. This is accomplished by placing patients on meal plans that either stabilize weight if current weight is adequate or allow weight to be gained in a controlled and monitored setting. Stabilization and behavioral change also involve blocking access to and participation in behaviors that support the eating disorder, including purging, exercising, and laxative/diuretic abuse. This is accomplished by having locked and supervised bathroom time; preventing access to means to induce vomiting or use laxatives, diuretics, or diet pills; and having supportive time to process emotional and physical discomfort following meals. With progression of treatment, behavioral coping strategies are augmented with cognitive restructuring techniques, including work on interpersonal issues, body image, and affect regulation. The last stage of CBT involves relapse prevention and maintenance planning. Given the highly structured nature of CBT, despite its design as an outpatient model of care, it has been shown to be well suited to the inpatient unit as well, because it emphasizes early behavioral change in a structured and systematic way.

Behavioral strategies are an essential element of the leading empirically supported treatments for eating disorders—including CBT, FBT, and specialist supportive clinical management. Key behavioral elements proven to be effective and important to treatment outcome have been studied. In this regard, establishment of a regular eating pattern (which involves many behavioral techniques, such as operant and classical conditioning and self-monitoring), exposure, behavioral experiments, and behavioral skills training are currently considered core interventions within these evidence-based treatment protocols (Waller and Raykos 2019). The inpatient unit affords individuals repeated opportunities to engage in exposure therapy, including being weighed, eating meals, tolerating fullness without the ability to purge, and being exposed to one's body through mirror work and body tracings. The goal in exposure therapy is for the individual to habituate to feared stimuli and through inhibitory learning incorporate new information that "inhibits" the existing fear. Ultimately, the individual develops a tolerance for negative emotions.

In addition to individual CBT, the milieu and group therapy programs are well suited to CBT-based interventions across a variety of topics, including body image, self-esteem, coping skills training, and motivation to change.

Dialectical Behavior Therapy

In addition to CBT, several other forms of treatment are used in the inpatient setting. DBT, developed by Marsha Linehan, has been shown to be effective in individuals with eating disorders, especially those in whom affective regulation and impulsivity have been especially problematic; it has also shown promising effects in AN for emotional and behavioral overcontrol (Chen et al. 2015). DBT can serve to complement the core CBT-based curriculum on inpatient units with groups and individual therapy sessions that focus on mindfulness, distress tolerance, emotional regulation, and interpersonal effectiveness. This form of therapy was first designed to treat borderline personality disorder and can be especially useful when there is a comorbidity with an eating disorder.

Radically open dialectical behavior therapy (RO-DBT) offers a novel way of understanding how self-starvation in AN is used as a maladaptive regulation strategy to reduce negative affect (negative reinforcement). This form of DBT posits that rather than aiming for emotional regulation, long-term mental health is achieved by increasing social connectedness. This form of therapy teaches skills involved in enhancing flexibility, intimacy and connectedness, and receptivity to openness, and it has shown effectiveness in treating AN (Hempel et al. 2018).

Acceptance and Commitment Therapy

ACT can be a useful adjunctive treatment, especially when patients are struggling to find motivation to change. The core tenets of the therapy involve aligning behaviors with values. Helping patients identify their core values and working to build a life that supports those can be an important part of treatment, especially when there is little apparent motivation to change.

Family-Based Therapy

FBT (Maudsley model) is highly effective for children and adolescents with AN and has been shown to be superior to other forms of therapy in this age group. This type of therapy involves parental control and supervision of meals with gradual return of control to the child or adolescent as weight stabilizes. Although FBT was designed as an outpatient treatment, its principles can be successfully incorporated into the inpatient care of children and adolescents with eating disorders by having family members decide on meals and engaging families in family meals throughout treatment, thereby empowering parents to take over control of their child's nutritional health. Although there are limitations to its use on the inpatient unit, given its superior outcomes in the outpatient setting, its use in a more structured setting may be helpful for easing the transition home—it also allows for families to be more involved and engaged in their child's treatment process.

Nutritional Rehabilitation

The APA *Practice Guideline for the Treatment of Patients With Eating Disorders*, 3rd Edition (Yager et al. 2006) states that a program of nutritional rehabilitation should be established for all patients with AN who are underweight. Expected rates of controlled weight gain have historically been 2–3 pounds (0.9–1.4 kg) per week for most inpatients (compared with 0.5–1 pound [0.2–0.5 kg] per week for most outpatients). Intake levels usually begin at 30–40 kcal/kg (1,000–1,600 kcal/day) and are advanced progressively. Newer research has challenged this slow rate of weight gain and suggests that weight gain closer to 4 pounds (1.8 kg) per week is safe in closely monitored settings; furthermore, risk of hypophosphatemia and refeeding syndrome appears more closely related to admission BMI than to rate of weight gain itself (Redgrave et al. 2015). For patients with BN, the guidelines state that nutritional counseling may be a useful adjunct to other treatment modalities.

While weight gain is the cornerstone of treatment for patients with AN, serious and potentially fatal complications can arise when refeeding is administered too rapidly and/or aggressively, termed the "refeeding syndrome." This constellation of fluid and electrolyte imbalances (hypophosphatemia, hypokalemia, hypomagnesemia) can result in clinical complications, including peripheral and central edema, congestive heart failure, cardiac arrhythmias, and pulmonary edema. For these reasons, careful attention must be paid to the refeeding process, with prompt repletion of electrolytes, ideally under supervised inpatient conditions if patients are severely malnourished.

Other Treatment Components

Various treatment modalities (CBT, DBT, ACT, FBT) have already been discussed above. Here we focus on the various components that make up each individual's treatment program in the inpatient setting.

Nutrition Groups/Meal Planning

Many eating disorder units have unique methods by which they go about meal planning. Some units utilize an exchange system for protein, carbohydrates, and fats; others use a pure caloric system. Both of these systems allow for unlimited flexibility in increasing intake for weight gain purposes. Liquid supplementation may be used in conjunction with meals and snacks to supplement weight gain and/or as supplementation when meals are not completed. No matter the system used, a core feature of the inpatient program is education around nutritional needs for each individual; to that end each patient has individual meetings with the dietitian. Nutrition groups are a cornerstone of the psychoeducation program and allow the opportunity for dietitians to teach patients about intake requirements, intuitive eating, hunger and satiety, and moderation of all types of foods.

Individual Psychotherapy

As outlined above, individual psychotherapy is a key component of the individualized treatment program. Unlike on other inpatient psychiatric units, on the eating disorder unit, intensive targeted individual therapy is a necessary component of the treatment. Treatment is CBT-focused on the individual needs of the patient and usually occurs two to three times per week. Examples of topics addressed include self-esteem, body image, perfectionism, interpersonal difficulties, and emotional regulation, and are in addition to the standard CBT program examining thoughts, feelings, and behaviors related to food, weight, and body image. Again, depending on the individual needs of the patient, the individual therapist may also utilize components of DBT or ACT as augmenting strategies; motivational enhancement therapy may be effective when motivation to change is a barrier to treatment.

Family Psychotherapy

Outside of formal FBT, families are an important component of treatment and should be active participants in their significant other's/child's/parent's care, as developmentally appropriate. In some inpatient settings, the family therapist is also the individual therapist. However, in many settings the family therapist is a separate therapist who is able to focus solely on the needs of the family system, enabling the individual therapist to focus solely on the needs of the patient. Key areas for many families in therapy are psychoeducation around the eating disorder, communication, trust, coping skills, and relapse prevention strategies.

Expressive (Art, Music, and Movement) and Occupational Therapies

Expressive therapies are a useful clinical adjunct to traditional talk therapies in the treatment of eating disorders. These treatment modalities can augment the patient's nutritional goals as they learn appropriate means of tolerating and expressing feelings while reducing anxiety. Specifically, these activities provide an opportunity to practice mindfulness techniques, as well as allow for expression of thoughts/emotions that patients may be unable to verbalize. Each of these modalities provides for holistic treatment in the higher-level care of patients with eating disorders.

Group and Milieu Therapy

The majority of a patient's day-to-day time is spent in the milieu and in groups. Groups are an essential component of the treatment, as information is disseminated widely and then discussed in a more nuanced and personalized way in individual and family therapy sessions. Groups are divided by age and are thus developmentally appropriate. Given the high comorbidity with substance use and trauma, specialty groups for these populations can further augment the treatment.

Pharmacotherapy

Pharmacotherapy for AN has been largely disappointing, with few trials demonstrating efficacy, and those mostly for comorbid depressive and obsessive-compulsive disorders; anxiolytic medications may be helpful before meals for the patient with AN, and there are case reports of successful use of atypical antipsychotics in patients with severe AN, especially with respect to weight gain in controlled settings (most evidence for olanzapine) (Bissada et al. 2008; Dunican and DelDotto 2007). The APA guideline specifies that psychotropic medications should not be used as the sole or primary treatment for AN (and there are currently no FDA-approved medications for AN) but can be considered for the treatment of comorbid conditions such as major depressive disorder or obsessive-compulsive disorder.

Pharmacotherapy for BN has been more successful than pharmacotherapy for AN, with antidepressant drugs having been the most widely studied (Bacaltchuk and Hay 2001). A number of trials have shown reduction in binge eating and vomiting in patients treated with fluoxetine at doses of 20 mg—and even greater reductions at 60 mg—leading to its approval by the FDA for treatment of BN (Fluoxetine Bulimia Nervosa Collaborative Study Group 1992; Goldstein et al. 1995; Walsh et al. 1997).

Pharmacotherapy for BED has been more encouraging than that for the other eating disorders, though psychotherapy is typically viewed as more efficacious. Several medications have been studied, including the selective serotonin reuptake inhibitors, antiepileptics (topiramate and zonisamide), and ADHD medications (lisdexamfetamine). In 2015, lisdexamfetamine became the first FDA-approved medication for the treatment of BED after an expedited review. It has shown efficacy in reducing the number of binge-eating episodes as well as the compulsive behavior associated with binge eating; it has not, however, been studied for treatment of weight loss per se (McElroy et al. 2015).

Physical Structure of the Inpatient Eating Disorder Unit

The design of the eating disorder unit should take into consideration the essential importance of sustained behavioral control and blockade of core eating disorder behaviors, including food restriction/disposal of non-eaten food, compulsive exercise, bingeing, and purging. Extra attention should be given to the dining room space such that patients may be directly monitored during mealtimes, thereby reducing opportunities to hide food and avoid caloric intake. Given the extremely charged and emotional nature of eating for this patient population, careful attention should be given to the decor of the dining room space, and attempts should be made to make it as calming and soothing as possible. There should be a place to process and distract patients once meals are complete. Bathrooms on the unit need to be locked to minimize access for patients to engage in surreptitious purging and/or water loading prior to weigh-ins. One unit has successfully utilized key-flush toilets; this allows for privacy and dignity while simultaneously minimizing destructive eating disorder behaviors. Common areas should be planned to facilitate constant line-of-sight monitoring for all patients by nursing staff. Some programs have utilized closed-circuit television to monitor patients, but this requires explicit informed consent from patients/parents prior to use.

On units where adolescents and adults share the same space, attention should be given to providing space for each population that is private and conducive to healing in an age- and developmentally appropriate fashion.

Staff-to-patient ratios on the inpatient eating disorder unit tend to be higher than on other general psychiatric, medical, or specialty units owing to the secretive and sneaky nature of eating disorder pathology and the need for a highly skilled interdisciplinary team of mental health workers/specialists, nurses, care coordinators, milieu liaisons, individual and family therapists, dietitians, internists/pediatricians, and psychiatrists.

Treatment Consent, Coercion, Capacity, and Commitment

Eating disorders, AN in particular, are often ego-syntonic illnesses, and very frequently patients are unable to distinguish themselves from their illness, often denying the presence of any illness at all. Remarkably, this occurs despite often drastic and medically compromising degrees of malnourishment and medical complexity.

In medicine, adult patients are presumed to have medical decision-making capabilities, even if these decisions are clearly not in their best interest; they are deemed to have *capacity* to make medical decisions, based on the principle of *autonomy*. To demonstrate capacity, patients must communicate a choice regarding their treatment that is unchanged and stable over time. They must demonstrate understanding of the risks, benefits, and alternatives regarding treatment. They must be able to manipulate the information in a manner that is consistent with their values. And finally, they must demonstrate appreciation of the consequences of their decisions. This paradigm for assessing capacity becomes potentially problematic when we look at the way in which patients with AN, in particular, identify with their illness. As such, the decisions they make, as evidenced in their daily decisions around food, weight, exercise, and so forth, may be thought of as reflective of an "anorexic value system" rather than a value system that reflects the individuals' true wishes in absence of the eating disorder.

In a qualitative study looking at semistructured interviews assessing attitudes and values surrounding the illness versus standardized capacity assessments (the MacArthur Competency Assessment Test [MacCAT-T]), several themes emerged from the semistructured interviews: 1) AN appeared to impact attitudes toward death and disability such that thinness was viewed as chiefly important despite the risk of death and that patients viewed medical complications as a sign of success; 2) AN impacted patients' values such that achievement of thinness was more important than all other aspects of life and was seen as part of the person's identity; and 3) patients were ambivalent around treatment and recovery, viewing change as outside their control. When these same patients were administered the MacCAT-T, their performance was indistinguishable from that of healthy control subjects, demonstrating a good understanding of the illness, its consequences, and treatments offered (Tan et al. 2003a). This study suggests that treatment refusal may not occur because patients want to die, but rather because they perceive death and disability as unimportant when compared with AN itself. Thus, if this is a product of the disease itself, it may be a core feature impairing decision-making concerning treatment that would not be present if the patient did not have AN. This has implications for our conceptual understanding of treatment capacity in AN specifically. If one is deemed not to have capacity to make decisions, each state has a system of surrogate decision-maker status, typically starting with either parents or spouses, with frequent reevaluation to determine when capacity has reemerged. Given that patients with AN score no differently on formal capacity assessments, it may be that other, more value-based assessments are required to determine whether a functional deficit exists that could be reasonably expected to return with treatment. When a surrogate decision-maker takes over, the standard by which they are to make decisions is based on what that person would want in the specific situation; in the case of AN, the individual's disorder must be removed from the value-based decisions.

Each state has laws pertaining to involuntary treatment, or civil commitment, for individuals with a mental health condition who are at imminent risk of harm to themselves or others or are unable to care for themselves adequately in the community. These laws, which differ by state, are based on the ethical principle of *beneficence*, or care that is in the best interest of the patient. While individuals with AN often both are at imminent risk of harm via self-starvation and show impaired ability to care for themselves via impaired judgment regarding their nutritional needs, the mental health community has long been hesitant in using these means to hospitalize patients with eating disorders. The reasons for this hesitancy are myriad and include lack of agreement on risk imminence regarding starvation, weight loss, and medical compromise; lack of access to specialty care on most general inpatient units; lack of access to specialty beds on inpatient eating disorder units; and concern regarding the therapeutic relationship (Carney et al. 2008). In the United States use of involuntary commitment is quite rare; this may reflect a willingness of patients to ultimately consent to admission under pressure from clinicians or families, a process known as *coercion*. In informed consent, decisions are to be made without coercion, though in practice, especially in the case of eating disorders, coercion is a frequently employed tactic. Clinicians may actually delay hospitalization in favor of a voluntary admission, which is often viewed as reflective of greater investment by the patient, though this is not always borne out in treatment.

Involuntary admissions may thus be necessary to manage the life-threatening status of a patient with an eating disorder when the individual is unwilling or unable to take steps to work with the treatment team. Core goals should be set for the involuntary portion of the treatment, and when the person is able to consent to treatment in a voluntary status, they should be permitted to do so, assuming they are committing to treatment. Involuntary treatment should be administered only when there is a life-threatening situation (e.g., electrolyte imbalance, cardiac arrhythmia, organ compromise, congestive heart failure) and should not be a part of ongoing care on an eating disorder unit. Involuntary-type treatments include, but are not limited to, seclusion and restraints for severe agitation, especially associated with feeding; use of nasogastric tube feeding when oral feedings are refused and there is acute medical compromise; and use of intramuscular medications to manage coexisting psychiatric illnesses that may be further impairing the medical and psychiatric stability of the individual.

Studies have shown that patients admitted involuntarily have a lower age at illness onset, longer duration to weight restoration, greater psychiatric morbidity, and higher frequency of tube feeding, refeeding syndrome, and use of locked wards. No significant differences have been found in terms of weight at discharge between voluntarily and involuntarily treated patients (Ayton et al. 2009; Clausen and Jones 2014). In one study of adolescents, those admitted voluntarily had a greater rate of premature discharges, higher rates of readmission, and poorer outcomes compared with those admitted involuntarily (Ayton et al. 2009).

Treatment Outcomes

In two qualitative studies of individuals from treatment centers across England, patients and parents viewed involuntary treatment as justified to save a life independent of capacity. When treatment refusal was overridden, patients expressed gratitude in hindsight and viewed involuntary treatment as caring when it was provided in a safe and compassionate environment. They expressed that trusting relationships with parents and professionals helped patients engage and accept treatment and overcome their own ambivalence (Tan et al. 2003b, 2010). Multiple studies have found no differences in weight gain and no negative effects on the treatment relationships between voluntarily and involuntarily treated patients (Ayton et al. 2009; Clausen and Jones 2014). Of course, all of these studies are plagued by small sample sizes, and thus more research is needed in each of these domains.

Discharge Planning

There is limited research on the optimal timing of discharge from an inpatient eating disorder unit. Degree of weight gain has emerged as a clinical indicator of improved eating disorder pathology, specifically earlier weight gain with regard to longer-term outcomes (Accurso et al. 2014).

Depending on the location of the inpatient unit, where the patient lives, local resources, insurance coverage, and the individual needs of the patient, there are multiple step-down options from the inpatient unit.

For those who still require 24/7 care but may no longer require the intensive medical or safety monitoring of an inpatient unit, residential care is an option, though this is not always covered by insurance companies. The partial hospital level of care is useful for patients who need supervision of some meals and a structured day program but are able to live with their families. This level of care is often a very important transition step between being in the hospital and returning to the community/school/work. Many programs offer an intensive outpatient program, which is typically a group-based program for 3–4 hours, 3–4 days per week. These programs allow patients to more fully integrate back into their lives and communities—be it school, work, or home—while remaining in intensive treatment with additional supports. This level of care is most effective for those patients who have a higher motivation to comply with treatment and prevent relapse and those who are not medically or psychiatrically acute. In the outpatient setting, an interdisciplinary team that specializes in eating disorders—preferably one that is colocated and can easily coordinate care—is recommended. The team mirrors that of the inpatient unit and generally consists of a psychiatrist, pediatrician/internist, and individual therapist, with or without a family therapist and a dietitian.

Case managers and discharge coordinators on the inpatient unit serve as liaisons to the medical teams, families, and insurance companies in identifying appropriate next level of treatment programs.

Conclusion

Eating disorders are a complex group of illnesses that require a high level of suspicion and careful evaluation in order to diagnose. Etiologically, they are thought to arise from an interaction of biological, genetic, psychological, environmental, and social factors. The treatment of eating disorders is highly specialized and requires a team approach in order to provide the best chance for a successful outcome. While weight stabilization and/or control of bingeing and purging are necessary, they are not sufficient for a full and long-lasting recovery. Approximately 50% of individuals with eating disorders will fully recover, 20%–30% will have a partial recovery, and the remainder will chronically struggle with their eating disorder. Sadly, about 10% will die within the first

10 years of their illness. Treatment requires psychological counseling, dietary consultation, medical stabilization, and various experiential therapies. Often the greatest barrier to treatment is denial, which is a hallmark of these illnesses. However, with a team approach, there is hope and the great potential for a full and lasting recovery.

References

Accurso EC, Ciao AC, Fitzsimmons-Craft EE, et al: Is weight gain really a catalyst for broader recovery? The impact of weight gain on psychological symptoms in the treatment of adolescent anorexia nervosa. Behav Res Ther 56:1–6, 2014 24632109

American Psychiatric Association: Diagnostic and Statistical Manual of Mental Disorders, 4th Edition, Text Revision. Washington, DC, American Psychiatric Association, 2000

American Psychiatric Association: Diagnostic and Statistical Manual of Mental Disorders, 5th Edition. Arlington, VA, American Psychiatric Association, 2013

Anderluh MB, Tchanturia K, Rabe-Hesketh S, Treasure J: Childhood obsessive-compulsive personality traits in adult women with eating disorders: defining a broader eating disorder phenotype. Am J Psychiatry 160(2):242–247, 2003 12562569

Arcelus J, Mitchell AJ, Wales J, Nielsen S: Mortality rates in patients with anorexia nervosa and other eating disorders: a meta-analysis of 36 studies. Arch Gen Psychiatry 68(7):724–731, 2011 21727255

Ayton A, Keen C, Lask B: Pros and cons of using the Mental Health Act for severe eating disorders in adolescents. Eur Eat Disord Rev 17(1):14–23, 2009 18666096

Bacaltchuk J, Hay P: Antidepressants versus placebo for people with bulimia nervosa. Cochrane Database Syst Rev (4):CD003391, 2001 11687198

Bacaltchuk J, Hay P, Trefiglio R: Antidepressants versus psychological treatments and their combination for bulimia nervosa. Cochrane Database Syst Rev (4):CD003385, 2001 11687197

Bailer UF, Frank GK, Henry SE, et al: Serotonin transporter binding after recovery from eating disorders. Psychopharmacology (Berl) 195(3):315–324, 2007 17690869

Baran SA, Weltzin TE, Kaye WH: Low discharge weight and outcome in anorexia nervosa. Am J Psychiatry 152(7):1070–1072, 1995 7793445

Bari A, Robbins TW: Inhibition and impulsivity: behavioral and neural basis of response control. Prog Neurobiol 108:44–79, 2013 23856628

Berner LA, Stefan M, Lee S, et al: Altered cortical thickness and attentional deficits in adolescent girls and women with bulimia nervosa. J Psychiatry Neurosci 43(3):151–160, 2018 29688871

Bissada H, Tasca GA, Barber AM, Bradwejn J: Olanzapine in the treatment of low body weight and obsessive thinking in women with anorexia nervosa: a randomized, double-blind, placebo-controlled trial. Am J Psychiatry 165(10):1281–1288, 2008 18558642

Bodell LP, Keel PK: Weight suppression in bulimia nervosa: associations with biology and behavior. J Abnorm Psychol 124(4):994–1002, 2015 26191637

Bohon C, Stice E: Reward abnormalities among women with full and subthreshold bulimia nervosa: a functional magnetic resonance imaging study. Int J Eat Disord 44(7):585–595, 2011 21997421

Braun DL, Sunday SR, Halmi KA: Psychiatric comorbidity in patients with eating disorders. Psychol Med 24(4):859–867, 1994 7892354

Brooks SJ, O'Daly OG, Uher R, et al: Differential neural responses to food images in women with bulimia versus anorexia nervosa. PLoS One 6(7):e22259, 2011 21799807

Bulik CM, Sullivan PF, Kendler KS: Heritability of binge-eating and broadly defined bulimia-nervosa. Biol Psychiatry 44(12):1210–1218, 1998 9861464

Carney T, Tait D, Richardson A, Touyz S: Why (and when) clinicians compel treatment of anorexia nervosa patients. Eur Eat Disord Rev 16(3):199–206, 2008 18059050

Chen EY, Segal K, Weissman J, et al: Adapting dialectical behavior therapy for outpatient adult anorexia nervosa: a pilot study. Int J Eat Disord 48(1):123–132, 2015 25346237

Chesney E, Goodwin GM, Fazel S: Risks of all-cause and suicide mortality in mental disorders: a meta-review. World Psychiatry 13(2):153–160, 2014 24890068
Clausen L, Jones A: A systematic review of the frequency, duration, type and effect of involuntary treatment for people with anorexia nervosa, and an analysis of patient characteristics. J Eat Disord 2(1):29, 2014 25414793
Cowdrey FA, Park RJ, Harmer CJ, McCabe C: Increased neural processing of rewarding and aversive food stimuli in recovered anorexia nervosa. Biol Psychiatry 70(8):736–743, 2011 21714958
Cowdrey FA, Finlayson G, Park RJ: Liking compared with wanting for high- and low-calorie foods in anorexia nervosa: aberrant food reward even after weight restoration. Am J Clin Nutr 97(3):463–470, 2013 23364019
Crow SJ, Nyman JA: The cost-effectiveness of anorexia nervosa treatment. Int J Eat Disord 35(2):155–160, 2004 14994352
Dunican KC, DelDotto D: The role of olanzapine in the treatment of anorexia nervosa. Ann Pharmacother 41(1):111–115, 2007 17190846
Ellison Z, Foong J, Howard R, et al: Functional anatomy of calorie fear in anorexia nervosa (letter). Lancet 352(9135):1192, 1998 9777839
Ely AV, Wierenga CE, Bischoff-Grethe A, et al: Response in taste circuitry is not modulated by hunger and satiety in women remitted from bulimia nervosa. J Abnorm Psychol 126(5):519–530, 2017 28691842
Fairburn CG: Cognitive Behavioral Therapy and Eating Disorders. New York, Guilford, 2008
Fairburn CG, Beglin SJ: Studies of the epidemiology of bulimia nervosa. Am J Psychiatry 147(4):401–408, 1990 2180327
Fichter MM, Quadflieg N: Mortality in eating disorders: results of a large prospective clinical longitudinal study. Int J Eat Disord 49(4):391–401, 2016 26767344
Fisher MM, Rosen DS, Ornstein RM, et al: Characteristics of avoidant/restrictive food intake disorder in children and adolescents: a "new disorder" in DSM-5. J Adolesc Health 55(1):49–52, 2014 24506978
Fluoxetine Bulimia Nervosa Collaborative Study Group: Fluoxetine in the treatment of bulimia nervosa: a multicenter, placebo-controlled, double-blind trial. Arch Gen Psychiatry 49(2):139–147, 1992 1550466
Frank GK, Bailer UF, Henry SE, et al: Increased dopamine D2/D3 receptor binding after recovery from anorexia nervosa measured by positron emission tomography and [11c]raclopride. Biol Psychiatry 58(11):908–912, 2005 15992780
Frank GK, Wagner A, Achenbach S, et al: Altered brain activity in women recovered from bulimic-type eating disorders after a glucose challenge: a pilot study. Int J Eat Disord 39(1):76–79, 2006 16254868
Frank GKW, Reynolds JR, Shott ME, O'Reilly RC: Altered temporal difference learning in bulimia nervosa. Biol Psychiatry 70(8):728–735, 2011 21718969
Fuglset TS, Landrø NI, Reas DL, Rø Ø: Functional brain alterations in anorexia nervosa: a scoping review. J Eat Disord 4:32, 2016 27933159
Garner DM, Garfinkel PE: Handbook of Treatment for Eating Disorders, 2nd Edition. New York, Guilford, 1997
Golden NH, Katzman DK, Sawyer SM, et al: Position Paper of the Society for Adolescent Health and Medicine: medical management of restrictive eating disorders in adolescents and young adults. J Adolesc Health 56(1):121–125, 2015 25530605
Goldstein DJ, Wilson MG, Thompson VL, et al: Long-term fluoxetine treatment of bulimia nervosa. Br J Psychiatry 166(5):660–666, 1995 7620754
Halmi KA, Eckert E, Marchi P, et al: Comorbidity of psychiatric diagnoses in anorexia nervosa. Arch Gen Psychiatry 48(8):712–718, 1991 1883254
Hempel R, Vanderbleek E, Lynch TR: Radically open DBT: targeting emotional loneliness in anorexia nervosa. Eat Disord 26(1):92–104, 2018 29384459
Herzog DB, Nussbaum KM, Marmor AK: Comorbidity and outcome in eating disorders. Psychiatr Clin North Am 19(4):843–859, 1996 9045226
Hoek HW, van Hoeken D: Review of the prevalence and incidence of eating disorders. Int J Eat Disord 34(4):383–396, 2003 14566926

Holsen LM, Lawson EA, Blum J, et al: Food motivation circuitry hypoactivation related to hedonic and nonhedonic aspects of hunger and satiety in women with active anorexia nervosa and weight-restored women with anorexia nervosa. J Psychiatry Neurosci 37(5):322–332, 2012 22498079

Hudson JI, Hiripi E, Pope HG Jr, Kessler RC: The prevalence and correlates of eating disorders in the National Comorbidity Survey Replication. Biol Psychiatry 61(3):348–358, 2007 16815322

Kann L, McManus T, Harris WA, et al: Youth Risk Behavior Surveillance—United States, 2017. MMWR Surveill Summ 67(8):1–114, 2018 29902162

Kekic M, Bartholdy S, Cheng J, et al: Increased temporal discounting in bulimia nervosa. Int J Eat Disord 49(12):1077–1081, 2016 27301653

Kendler KS, MacLean C, Neale M, et al: The genetic epidemiology of bulimia nervosa. Am J Psychiatry 148(12):1627–1637, 1991 1842216

Krug I, Treasure J, Anderluh M, et al: Present and lifetime comorbidity of tobacco, alcohol and drug use in eating disorders: a European multicenter study. Drug Alcohol Depend 97(1–2):169–179, 2008 18571341

Marsh R, Steinglass JE, Gerber AJ, et al: Deficient activity in the neural systems that mediate self-regulatory control in bulimia nervosa. Arch Gen Psychiatry 66(1):51–63, 2009 19124688

Marsh R, Horga G, Wang Z, et al: An FMRI study of self-regulatory control and conflict resolution in adolescents with bulimia nervosa. Am J Psychiatry 168(11):1210–1220, 2011 21676991

Marsh R, Stefan M, Bansal R, et al: Anatomical characteristics of the cerebral surface in bulimia nervosa. Biol Psychiatry 77(7):616–623, 2015 23978404

McElroy SL, Hudson JI, Mitchell JE, et al: Efficacy and safety of lisdexamfetamine for treatment of adults with moderate to severe binge-eating disorder: a randomized clinical trial. JAMA Psychiatry 72(3):235–246, 2015 25587645

McKnight Investigators: Risk factors for the onset of eating disorders in adolescent girls: results of the McKnight longitudinal risk factor study. Am J Psychiatry 160(2):248–254, 2003 12562570

Nattiv A, Agostini R, Drinkwater B, Yeager KK: The female athlete triad: the inter-relatedness of disordered eating, amenorrhea, and osteoporosis. Clin Sports Med 13(2):405–418, 1994 8013041

Nicely TA, Lane-Loney S, Masciulli E, et al: Prevalence and characteristics of avoidant/restrictive food intake disorder in a cohort of young patients in day treatment for eating disorders. J Eat Disord 2(1):21, 2014 25165558

Norris ML, Spettigue WJ, Katzman DK: Update on eating disorders: current perspectives on avoidant/restrictive food intake disorder in children and youth. Neuropsychiatr Dis Treat 12:213–218, 2016 26855577

Patton GC, Selzer R, Coffey C, et al: Onset of adolescent eating disorders: population based cohort study over 3 years. BMJ 318(7186):765–768, 1999 10082698

Phillipou A, Rossell SL, Castle DJ: The neurobiology of anorexia nervosa: a systematic review. Aust N Z J Psychiatry 48(2):128–152, 2014 24194589

Putukian M: The female triad: eating disorders, amenorrhea, and osteoporosis. Med Clin North Am 78(2):345–356, 1994 8121215

Redgrave GW, Coughlin JW, Schreyer CC, et al: Refeeding and weight restoration outcomes in anorexia nervosa: challenging current guidelines. Int J Eat Disord 48(7):866–873, 2015 25625572

Scaife JC, Godier LR, Reinecke A, et al: Differential activation of the frontal pole to high vs low calorie foods: the neural basis of food preference in anorexia nervosa? Psychiatry Res Neuroimaging 258:44–53, 2016 27866012

Schreuder M: Insula function in anorexia nervosa. Unpublished bachelor's thesis, Utrecht University, Utrecht, the Netherlands, 2011

Smolak L: Body image development in childhood, in Body Image: A Handbook of Science, Practice, and Prevention, 2nd Edition. Edited by Cash T, Smolak L. New York, Guilford, 2011, pp 67–75

Steinglass JE, Walsh BT: Neurobiological model of the persistence of anorexia nervosa. J Eat Disord 4(4):19, 2016 27195123

Strober M: Family genetic studies of eating disorders. J Clin Psychiatry 52(suppl):9–12, 1991 1938990
Sylvester CJ, Forman SF: Clinical practice guidelines for treating restrictive eating disorder patients during medical hospitalization. Curr Opin Pediatr 20(4):390–397, 2008 18622192
Tan J, Hope T, Stewart A: Competence to refuse treatment in anorexia nervosa. Int J Law Psychiatry 26(6):697–707, 2003a 14637209
Tan JO, Hope T, Stewart A, Fitzpatrick R: Control and compulsory treatment in anorexia nervosa: the views of patients and parents. Int J Law Psychiatry 26(6):627–645, 2003b 14637206
Tan JO, Stewart A, Fitzpatrick R, Hope T: Attitudes of patients with anorexia nervosa to compulsory treatment and coercion. Int J Law Psychiatry 33(1):13–19, 2010 19926134
Udo T, Grilo CM: Prevalence and correlates of DSM-5-defined eating disorders in a nationally representative sample of U.S. adults. Biol Psychiatry 84(5):345–354, 2018 29859631
Uher R, Murphy T, Brammer MJ, et al: Medial prefrontal cortex activity associated with symptom provocation in eating disorders. Am J Psychiatry 161(7):1238–1246, 2004 15229057
van Furth EF, van Strien DC, Martina LM, et al: Expressed emotion and the prediction of outcome in adolescent eating disorders. Int J Eat Disord 20(1):19–31, 1996 8807349
Waller G, Raykos B: Behavioral interventions in the treatment of eating disorders. Psychiatr Clin North Am 42(2):181–191, 2019 31046921
Walsh BT, Wilson GT, Loeb KL, et al: Medication and psychotherapy in the treatment of bulimia nervosa. Am J Psychiatry 154(4):523–531, 1997 9090340
Watson HJ, Yilmaz Z, Thornton LM, et al: Genome-wide association study identifies eight risk loci and implicates metabo-psychiatric origins for anorexia nervosa. Nat Genet 51(8):1207–1214, 2019 31308545
Whittal ML, Agras WS, Gould RA: Bulimia nervosa: a meta-analysis of psychosocial and pharmacological treatments. Behav Ther 30:117–135, 1999
Woodside DB: A review of anorexia nervosa and bulimia nervosa. Curr Probl Pediatr 25(2):67–89, 1995 7768115
Yager J, Devlin MJ, Halmi KA, et al: Practice Guideline for the Treatment of Patients With Eating Disorders, 3rd Edition. Arlington, VA, American Psychiatric Association, 2006

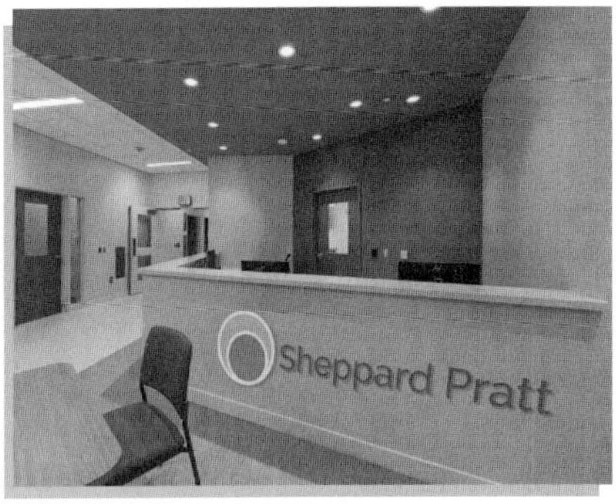

CHAPTER 8

The Forensic Unit

Tobias D. Wasser, M.D.
Charles C. Dike, M.D., M.P.H., FRCPsych
Michael A. Norko, M.D., M.A.R.

The forensic unit serves most of the same clinical functions as acute or long-term-care units in general psychiatric hospitals. In addition to those functions, the forensic unit must be able to manage the mostly mandated nature of the care provided and the dual nature of forensic treatment—namely, serving both the treatment needs of the individual patient and the security and safety needs of the facility and the society in which it operates (Evans and Bader 2020). As a consequence of the dual mandate of this work, the forensic unit is positioned in the middle of the many competing and often adversarial postures of various social agents.

Forensic units regularly admit acutely ill patients who are often psychotic, agitated, and aggressive. Some patients, like those found not guilty by reason of insanity, may also stay many years on forensic units because of concerns about their risk to the community.

The dual nature of forensic treatment means that all staff members on a forensic unit (including security staff) need to attend to both treatment and safety/security concerns, because effective treatment can never be delivered in an environment in which people feel unsafe or security is compromised. A collaborative model usually works best in balancing treatment and safety/security concerns (Seppänen et al. 2018).

Even when such balance is achieved, however, forensic clinicians find themselves responding to contrasting and adversarial pressures as sociolegal agents pursue varied objectives in their scrutiny of care provided and decisions reached by the hospital treatment team. These opposing forces challenge clinicians to simultaneously enhance and restrict patient freedoms; decrease length of stay and keep patients sequestered longer; support patient recovery and autonomy and control their behavior more fully; provide patient-centered care and respond to victims' concerns; and integrate patients into the community and respect community opposition. And clinicians must negotiate all of these demands while attempting to maintain hope and the momentum of personal development for their patients, with little acknowledgment of the stresses of the conflicting demands.

Admission Criteria

Patients who are admitted to forensic units generally fall into one of four categories: individuals admitted for restoration of competency to stand trial; insanity acquittees (those found not guilty, or not criminally responsible, by reason of mental disease or defect) who are undergoing evaluation and receiving treatment; inmates transferred from correctional facilities for evaluation, acute care, or placement at end of sentence; and civil patients admitted (either voluntarily or involuntarily) because of agitation and risk of assault that cannot be managed in other environments.

Although many jurisdictions permit outpatient or jail-based competency restoration, most often this work is accomplished in secure inpatient settings because of concerns about custody as well as treatment compliance. These defendant-patients are sent to the forensic unit by order of a criminal court because they have been found not competent to stand trial. The goal of treatment for these patients is to restore the individual's abilities to understand the legal proceedings and to assist in the defense process. This means that this treatment is not directed at holistic or "client centered" goals, because as soon as the relevant capacities are restored, the individual is returned to court. This does not mean, however, that forensic units do not have to do adequate discharge planning, because many defendants (e.g., those with low-level charges) may be released from custody or even have their charges disposed of at the time that they are found restored to competence by the court; they are thus returned to the community, where they will need ongoing services to help them maintain their health and functioning. It also does not mean that the forensic unit is relieved of the responsibility for providing services to meet immediate needs that are not directly related to competency to stand trial; for example, the unit may have to provide for long-neglected psychiatric, medical, or even surgical interventions.

Despite the fact that a successful insanity defense requires that the individual both admit the criminal act and prove a serious mental illness, the successful acquittee will often arrive at the hospital denying both propositions emphatically (Zonana and Norko 1993). This complicates therapeutic engagement and treatment planning. Periods of potential commitment may be quite long (e.g., decades), creating challenges for instilling hope for recovery and release.

Patients are referred from correctional settings to forensic units to be provided acute hospital-level psychiatric care that cannot be adequately provided in the prison or jail (American Psychiatric Association 2016). It can be very difficult to provide important features of hospital units (where the primary goal is treatment) within a correctional setting (where the primary goal is custody). These include a therapeutic milieu, trauma-sensitive care, and a full range of consultative and intensive clinical services to meet diverse needs (Dike 2017; Kapoor et al. 2018; Norko et al. 2015). The concept of "fitness for imprisonment" has been proposed as an algorithm to help determine when transfer to a hospital is necessary (Vogel et al. 2013).

Incarcerated patients are also sometimes referred to hospitals for various statutorily created evaluations as part of the criminal justice process. Often inmates with continuing serious psychiatric disabilities may be referred for admission to forensic units upon completion of their prison sentence. These admissions are best accomplished through a collaborative approach between mental health colleagues in the hospital forensic unit and the correctional settings.

Finally, the forensic unit is used in many jurisdictions as a tertiary referral site for civil patients whose aggressive behavior is difficult to manage in other inpatient settings. This happens because forensic units are generally more secure, have increased security staffing, and have experience in dealing with aggressive behaviors among individuals admitted through various stages of the criminal justice system. Their admission most often also prompts additional scrutiny by legal advocates because admission to forensic units may entail additional curtailment of liberties, invite increased stigma, subject the civil patient to an environment of criminally committed patients, and delay or deter later successful discharge to the community.

Diagnostic Workup

The diagnostic process in a forensic psychiatric inpatient unit is necessarily comprehensive. It involves not only an assessment of the psychiatric condition but also an ongoing assessment of needs and risks. Therefore, a multidisciplinary team approach to diagnosis is emphasized and advocated.

Immediately after admission assessments by psychiatry and nursing (and sometimes social work, psychology, and rehabilitation therapy if the admission occurs during regular hours), a presumptive diagnosis is made. Thereafter, the various disciplines begin an intense period of discipline-specific assessment of needs that will culminate in the development of a more comprehensive treatment plan within a few days of the admission.

Every team member is involved in the assessment of risks, which includes assessing risk-relevant needs and deficits of the individual, so that interventions can be delivered to target those needs and enhance protective factors (Dvoskin and Heilbrun 2001). The patient's behavior is closely monitored on and off the unit and in group settings for risks of suicide, violence, or elopement. Later in the assessment process, a decision is made about the necessity for psychological or neuropsychological testing to assess malingering, personality characteristics, intelligence, cognitive disorders, mood disorders, or psychosis.

Obtaining collateral information is especially important in a forensic psychiatric hospital. Patients often arrive directly from court, sometimes with minimal documentation of psychiatric history or current mental state. If the admission is directly from corrections, it is helpful to note if the patient was involuntarily medicated, attempted suicide, or received any "tickets" for disciplinary problems. This information is helpful in the immediate assessment of severity of psychiatric disorder and current risk of suicide or violence.

A problem often encountered during off-hours admissions from the courts is the unavailability of records. Most of these patients were in jail or prison before going to court and often arrive at the forensic hospital late at night because of the logistics of transport. As a result, it is often difficult to contact health care workers from other agencies, and there can be delays in receiving needed information.

Treatment

Treatment of individuals on a forensic unit serves two purposes: to treat severe mental illness and to treat challenging, often dangerous behavior to decrease the risk of violence (Davoren et al. 2015; McInerny and Minne 2004). Psychiatric disorders in this population are often severe and refractory to treatment, hence the need for broad and comprehensive treatment approaches that address biological, psychological, social, spiritual, and cultural factors that influence the development of psychiatric disorders or recovery from them.

In recent years, there has been an increasing recommendation to employ patient-centered and recovery-oriented care into forensic units (Dorkins and Adshead 2011; Livingston et al. 2012). This principle empowers patients to take an active role in their treatment as they work collaboratively with clinical staff; it emphasizes patients' autonomy, as they are essentially in charge of their treatment. In reality, most patients on forensic units have limited authority because their detention in the hospital (and sometimes treatment) is court mandated. Further, a third party, usually a judicial body, makes decisions regarding access to the community. Despite these challenges, however, there is evidence that patient-centered care can be applied successfully on forensic units (Dike 2017; Kapoor et al. 2018). In one study, while forensic patients had a positive attitude to recovery-oriented care, staff were more likely to perceive it as creating a potentially unsafe environment (Livingston et al. 2012). The authors concluded that enhancing recovery-oriented care may improve patient engagement in services. This growing opportunity for access to recovery-oriented care is another advantage of the forensic hospital unit compared with correctional mental health units (Norko et al. 2015).

Biological Treatment

Biological treatment includes pharmacological and nonpharmacological interventions. Psychotropic medications are used for treating psychotic and mood disorders, but some are also used off-label for insomnia, impulsivity, agitation, and aggression, as well as for sexual disorders.

Antipsychotics are commonly used, not only for psychosis but also for agitation (Zimbroff 2003), mood stabilization, aggression, and impulsivity (Glancy and Knott 2003). Mood stabilizers are prescribed for agitation, aggression, and impulsivity (Glancy and Knott 2002), and as augmentation of antipsychotic and antidepressant medications, in addition to being prescribed for mood stabilization. Antidepressants are used for depression, anxiety disorders, sexual disorders, and compulsivity/impulsivity (Coccaro and Kavoussi 1997). Hormonal therapy is indicated for sex offenders

(Saleh and Guidry 2003) and includes antiandrogens (e.g., medroxyprogesterone acetate), synthetic gonadotropin-releasing hormone analogues, and oral estrogens. Ketamine, a medication that has recently gained FDA approval for treating severe depression and suicidal thoughts, is not yet widely prescribed on forensic units.

The high prevalence of refractory psychiatric disorders and aggression fosters the use of high dosages of psychotropic medications as well as antipsychotic polypharmacy, despite limited evidence of the usefulness of this approach (Stahl 2002). There is recent evidence, however, that antipsychotic polypharmacy could be beneficial in certain situations; it is associated with slightly lower risk of psychiatric rehospitalization than monotherapy, with clozapine plus aripiprazole having the best outcome (Tiihonen et al. 2019). Use of high doses of psychotropic medications coupled with polypharmacy increases the risk of serious side effects and drug-drug interactions. A relatively sedentary lifestyle due to the patients' illnesses and the structure and nature of forensic units, and the tendency to indulge in excessive eating, complicates the problem of obesity, a common side effect of psychotropic medications.

In some instances, potentially dangerous side effects or drug-drug interactions may limit medication choices available for vigorously treating psychosis or aggression. The risk of physical aggression to other patients and staff due to inadequate treatment must then be balanced against the dangers of treatment to the patient. On some occasions, patients admitted for restoration to competency have been recommended to the courts as not competent to stand trial and not restorable because concerns about side effects or adverse drug interactions have limited the treatment. Medical comorbidity could also limit options for psychotropic medication treatment and lead to inability to restore competency.

A unique characteristic of forensic units that affects medication use is the wide age range of the unit population, from the late teens to the geriatric. Some acquittees spend decades in the hospital, and as they get older, dosages of their psychotropic medications should be adjusted to avoid gradual toxicity that may sometimes appear to be sudden and inexplicable. Although there is no restriction regarding prescription of controlled substances such as benzodiazepines, opioids, and stimulant medications, clinicians should be vigilant because high drug-seeking behavior in prison can transfer to the forensic unit.

In terms of nonpharmacological treatment interventions, electroconvulsive therapy is effective for treating severe and refractory depression, mania and psychosis, catatonia, agitation, and aggression in dementia (Tang and Ungvari 2003; van den Berg et al. 2018) and aggression and self-injurious behavior in autism with catatonia (Haq and Ghaziuddin 2014).

Psychotherapies

Psychotherapeutic techniques are useful adjuncts to medications and in some cases are the primary treatment intervention. Commonly used psychotherapeutic treatments include cognitive-behavioral therapy (CBT), dialectical behavior therapy (DBT), behavior therapy, trauma-specific therapies, supportive therapy, psychoanalysis, and various other forms of dynamic psychotherapy. Psychotherapy may be accomplished in individual, group, family, or couples settings. The effectiveness of psychotherapeutic techniques in treating forensic patients has long been recognized (Doctor 2008; Pfafflin and Adshead 2004).

Forensic units manage a high proportion of individuals with treatment-refractory psychiatric disorders, cognitive deficits, or developmental or acquired brain disorders that increase their likelihood of exhibiting behavioral excesses and violence. In addition, a high proportion of forensic patients have been exposed to severe and prolonged trauma (Mueser and Rosenberg 2001), more so if they were admitted from corrections (Kristine 2011). As a result, psychological evaluation on admission can both generate a psychological profile of the patient and offer indications of appropriate psychotherapy modalities to employ in the patient's treatment.

For insanity acquittees who have committed heinous crimes against others, psychotherapeutic techniques will help the patient and hospital understand the rationale behind the crimes and subsequently guide decisions about treatment and risk (Papapietro 2019). Group therapy has been shown to instill hope in a unique group of acquittees, those who have killed a parent, and subsequently encourage their active participation in their recovery (Hillbrand and Young 2008).

DBT groups to target patients with emotional/behavioral dysregulation related to personality disorder, and START NOW, an evidence-based skills therapy adapted from DBT for corrections, are also useful interventions on forensic units (Trestman 2016). In addition, patients participate in groups that are specifically directed to forensic topics, such as competency to stand trial, not guilty by reason of insanity, family homicide, legal education, and problem sexual behavior.

Behavior therapy can be helpful in managing difficult personality disorders, refractory psychosis, developmental disabilities, and aggression. Interventions range from basic behavioral guidelines for responding to aggressive or self-injurious patients to a comprehensive positive behavior support plan shown to be effective in forensic settings (Tolisano et al. 2017). Effective behavioral interventions require consistent application of behavioral plans through all shifts, which may be difficult when regular, trained staff are absent or when staff are reluctant to fully engage in the program. Behavioral plans are often more involved than routine care and require vigilance and active participation of staff to be effective. The relative scarcity of behaviorally trained psychologists further compounds the problem. Some hospitals have established a behavioral intervention service staffed by experienced behavioral psychologists to provide consultation to unit staff across the facility, as well as supervision and monitoring of the plans.

Patient and Family Education

Education services on a forensic unit provide information and support for family members, who are often confused about the differences between a forensic unit and a prison. Family members may also be frustrated by limits on the food or other items they may bring to their loved one, and have difficulty appreciating the potential danger the items pose. Therefore, family education is necessarily broad in scope and includes an understanding of specific major mental illnesses as well as the special processes of a forensic unit. Family members of patients on forensic units may experience being neither included in decisions about their relative's future nor provided with information (Hörberg et al. 2015). Involving families in patients' treatment has positive effects, not only for the patient but also for their family members and relationships within the family (Richards et al. 2019).

Family support and education meetings can be run by any designated member of the treatment team, at a regular interval of time. The meetings sometimes have a social flavor, and in that context, information is shared informally among attendees. Opportunities are provided for family members to mutually support one another, share experiences, and offer advice. It is believed that the more equipped and the more confident family members feel, the more helpful they will be to both the treatment team and their loved ones.

Rehabilitation and Recreational Therapies

Psychosocial rehabilitation is a broad term that includes socialization, recreation, vocational rehabilitation, and financial management (Ladds 1996). Recreational therapies are used to treat and maintain the physical, mental, and emotional well-being of patients through a variety of techniques, including music, relaxation, arts, sports, games, dance, drama, and community outings. These therapies help individuals reduce depression, stress, and anxiety; develop better social skills; and become more confident. The goal is for patients to express their feelings in a therapeutic setting and to experience meaningful and pleasurable activities despite the limitations imposed on them by the hospital environment.

In addition, therapists help long-stay patients reintegrate into the community by teaching them how to use community resources and recreational activities. Community trips are planned for patients who have progressed through the maximum-security units to less secure units and who have low risks of aggression or elopement. Patients are taught how to utilize relaxation techniques to relieve anxiety. They are also encouraged to develop adaptive leisure activities and hobbies. Leisure activities, especially structured group programs, are particularly helpful not only to maintain patients' general health and well-being but also to decrease opportunities for aggressive behavior.

There is a risk that patients in forensic units will spend time mainly sleeping and in passive unstructured leisure occupations (Farnworth et al. 2004). Too much time spent in their rooms can hinder patients' rehabilitation (Dvoskin et al. 2002). When patients are involved in structured activities, they may be less likely to provoke each other out of the frustration of inactivity. Exercise and sports programs help in dissipating energy and in generating an overall feeling of well-being. Through team sports patients learn to work collaboratively with others to achieve a common goal. These activities also provide opportunities for therapists to teach patients anger management and appropriate methods of coping with frustration. For certain patients, especially those with communication difficulties, art therapy may provide an avenue for self-expression, and pet therapy may help the patient establish a connection not only with the pet but also with the staff handler.

In some facilities, forensic patients with an appropriate safety level (and under close monitoring by staff) may have access to a library, computers, and vocational rehabilitation activities such as woodcraft, leather shop, sewing and mending, and cooking. A teacher may be available for those patients who want to pursue further education to obtain a general equivalency diploma. The issue of free access to the internet remains an area of concern for forensic unit administrators, and therefore, such access is not widely offered at present.

Other rehabilitation therapies, such as physical therapy, occupational therapy, and speech therapy, are available as necessary to help patients achieve their highest level of function. Sensory modulation tools (e.g., weighted blankets) and comfort rooms (with limited stimuli and soothing atmosphere) are useful adjuncts for managing agitation.

Milieu Management

In addition to the usual requirements of maintaining an effective therapeutic milieu on an inpatient unit, the staff and managers of forensic units must attend to safety and control of aggression. Forensic patients have often committed serious and frightening acts of violence as the basis of their referral, and many exhibit ongoing aggressive behavior that may have been unresponsive to management in other settings. (This includes male patients who have histories of sexual aggression or physical assault on females, which must also be considered in placement decisions.) In addition, forensic patients may have significant pro-criminal attitudes; individuals transferred from correctional settings may also exhibit behaviors such as making a weapon or affiliating with gang members.

In such an environment, it is easy for staff and patients alike to experience fear, which leads to anger and potentiates the eruption of violence (Evans and Bader 2020). It is thus important to acknowledge and manage staff fear in order to mitigate countertransference and patient aggression. Direct care staff may wish to manage safety by creating structure through rules and schedules, although patients may experience this as an excess of staff control (Caplan 1993). The notion of relational security addresses staff-patient relationships, staff knowledge of individual patients' histories, and general experience and knowledge about forensic populations (Seppänen et al. 2018). Research demonstrates that it is possible for mandated treatment providers to develop affiliative relationships with patients that are fair, caring, firm, and authoritative without becoming authoritarian (Manchak et al. 2014).

All staff must understand the importance of being mindful of safety and security as well as the need to achieve the therapeutic goals of the unit (Long et al. 2012). Ongoing discussions and training among treatment and security staff may help keep both these tasks operationalized in practice. (Staff training on milieu therapy can produce desirable outcomes in ward atmosphere and patient satisfaction; see Nesset et al. 2009.)

One of the ways in which security concerns are operationalized by all staff is by attention to the environmental risks. This begins with careful selection of furniture, building materials, hardware, windows, bathroom fixtures, and other physical elements (Shaw 2014). It also includes regular searches for contraband, weapons, broken items, missing hardware, and so forth in all areas accessible to patients. Items that can be used for cutting, for creating fire, or as a weapon should be identified as nonpermitted items, and this information should be made available to patients and visitors in writing (Kaltiala-Heino and Kahila 2006). The mitigation of ligature risk is as important on forensic units as on any other psychiatric unit (Hunt et al. 2012). Other important environmental considerations are noise level, census, use of single versus double rooms, and creation of comfortable spaces.

Staffing is a significant component of effective milieu management on the forensic unit. It is often perceived that higher staffing ratios should generally be available on forensic units (Kaltiala-Heino and Kahila 2006; Seppänen et al. 2018). Direct care staff members feel more comfortable when higher staff-to-patient ratios are maintained; patients perceive a higher level of staff control of the environment under such conditions (Phillips and Caplan 2003). Patients' perception that the environment is safe and well controlled has a calming effect on the unit by decreasing fears and negative stimulation. Too great a perception of rigid control, however, increases the sense of hostility among patients and decreases safety. Effective communication among staff and patients in community meetings is important to maintaining this delicate balance of a controlled environment while permitting individuals to experience some needed levels of privacy and freedom (Tomlin et al. 2018). Models of milieu management are available to help reduce conflict, aggression, and perceived coercion, and improve hope and unit atmosphere (Bader and Evans 2015; Bowers 2014; Maguire et al. 2018).

Programmatic interventions can also play a major role in the development and maintenance of a therapeutic milieu in forensic environments. Behavioral programming can be very effective when it rewards nonaggressive behavior, improvement in social skills and cooperation, and participation in treatment and educational activities. Social learning programs have been instituted effectively in several forensic settings, reducing aggression and use of restraint and seclusion and leading to improvements in milieu management and discharge success (Goodness and Renfro 2002; Newbill et al. 2011). Although these programs require a significant investment in staff training and maintenance of program integrity, they provide a model of staff intervention that is interactive, continuous, and positive, which contributes to recovery.

An important recent development for forensic units has been the architectural design and construction of new facilities. Contemporary designs maximize visibility on the unit, patient dignity and privacy, smaller social groupings, daylight and views of and access to natural spaces, and a "normalized" routine of living at "home" and going out to work, education, health care appointments, and recreation (Dvoskin et al. 2002; Seppänen et al. 2018; Shaw 2014).

Finally, it is worth recognizing that even when the physical environment is well designed, safely maintained, and appropriately staffed with effective milieu models and therapeutic programs, staff members must still cope with a group of individuals with seriously disturbed behavior and histories of extraordinary violence. Providing settings in which staff can process stressful events (e.g., in debriefings or supervision) and safely unload the effects of chronic stress and exposure to negative thoughts and feelings can be very helpful (Dickinson and Wright 2008; Kuhlman 1988).

Management of Suicidal and Aggressive Behaviors

The management of violence in correctional facilities is generally conceptualized as a security matter, whereas in forensic hospitals, milieu management and positive behavioral support plans become viable options (Dike 2017; Kapoor et al. 2018). Some patients are transferred directly from correctional settings, some from maximum-security or "super-max" prisons, with a history of being in segregation for violent behaviors or with multiple "tickets" for aggression. These patients are suddenly placed onto units with patients who may be in the early phase of their justice involvement or still trying to make sense of their legal situation and who are vulnerable by virtue of serious mental illness or developmental disability. In addition, patients who present unmanageable risks of suicide in general hospitals are sometimes sent to forensic hospitals for management because forensic hospitals are more secure. Thus, the mix of patients on a forensic unit makes it inherently a high-risk environment. Staff in forensic units must therefore be more vigilant to cues that indicate high potential for suicide or physical aggression in their patients.

Specific interventions to decrease risk of self-harm include a combination of pharmacological treatment, environmental manipulation, and close monitoring. The presence of psychiatric (or dangerous personality) disorders should be noted, carefully evaluated, and vigorously treated. History of suicide attempts and other self-injurious behaviors should be thoroughly explored to understand potential triggers.

As on any inpatient psychiatric unit, careful attention should be paid to environmental ligature risks throughout the unit. There should be no access to windows that open.

Depending on the degree of risk of suicide, patients may be placed under a level of increased observation such as continuous observation or 1:1 monitoring at all times. There should be open and clear communication between unit leadership and line staff across all shifts about specific risks and plans to manage the risk.

Management of aggression also includes pharmacotherapy, psychotherapy, and environmental manipulation. Pharmacotherapeutic techniques used for treating aggression include mood stabilizers, antipsychotics, and antidepressants (Felthous and Stanford 2015; Glancy and Knott 2002, 2003). These often need to be combined with behavioral interventions to be successful.

For acutely agitated patients, taking a time-out—in either their bedroom, a comfort room, or other de-escalation area—may help to diffuse their distress and symptoms (Seppänen et al. 2018). Such use of a time-out must be voluntary and may be one of the actions listed by the patient on their preferred methods for de-escalation ascertained at the time of admission. When such measures are ineffective or the patient is unable to avail themselves of this option, involuntary seclusion may be necessary to maintain safety.

The use of seclusion and restraints to manage aggression (both self- and other-directed) on a forensic unit must be managed thoughtfully and judiciously, as in any other setting. The Joint Commission and the Centers for Medicare & Medicaid Services standards restrict the use of restraints and seclusion to emergency situations in which there is imminent risk that the individual may physically harm self or others. Restraints are to be used only as a last resort and discontinued as soon as the imminent risk is resolved. Not only are there restrictions on the initial application of restraint, there are also policies regarding duration in restraints, monitoring of restrained or secluded patients by a licensed independent practitioner, and monitoring of the physical health of the patient during and after restraints/seclusion (Recupero et al. 2011). In fact, several regulatory agencies and professional organizations, including the National Association of State Mental Health Program Directors, have advocated for and identified strategies to reduce the use of such measures in inpatient psychiatric settings, including forensic units (National Association of State Mental Health Program Directors 2006).

Advocates for some continued use of restraints and seclusion maintain that there are certain situations when a patient loses control and becomes imminently dangerous to self and others, during which the use of restraints and seclusion is appropriate to maintain safety (Liberman 2006). Opponents argue that there are no indications for the use of restraints and seclusion to manage aggression. They suggest that the best practice is to train line staff in verbal de-escalation methods, mediation techniques, and conflict resolution and to detect aggressive behavior in its early phases and ideally mitigate it before it becomes uncontrollable (Curie 2005). A balanced approach may seek to reduce the use of seclusion and restraint maximally via programmatic developments and staff training, yet still recognize that, particularly in environments faced with the challenge of violent patients who have been refractory to interventions in other settings, some use of these procedures may still be necessary.

For forensic patients with a high risk of aggressive behavior, the unit staff should generate a list of behavioral cues that indicate increasing agitation or psychosis that have historically been associated with violence for the individual. Early detection of these behavioral cues could lead to immediate removal of the patient from the aggravating situation or allow the utilization of the patient's preferred method of decreasing their agitation. Training of line staff on verbal de-escalation techniques is useful. For some patients, the early use of medications for agitation, in addition to interventions discussed earlier, is successful at decreasing aggression.

In emergency situations when a patient's level of aggression does not sufficiently diminish in response to the measures described above, seclusion and/or restraint may be necessary to safely manage the patient's behavior. Such restrictive methods should be implemented using a least restrictive methodology and only for the shortest duration necessary to manage the psychiatric emergency (Recupero et al. 2011). The continuum of such interventions typically spans from locked seclusion to physical (manual) restraint to mechanical restraint. When employing mechanical restraints, most forensic units utilize restraint beds, though recent evidence suggests beneficial safety outcomes with the use of restraint chairs (Visaggio et al. 2018). In the most extreme circumstances, preventive aggression devices, also known as "ambulatory restraints," can be considered (Maier et al. 1994), but it is very challenging to justify their ongoing need after the acute emergency has passed and, once started, difficult to assess when it is safe to discontinue their use.

Discharge Planning

As with all inpatient units, discharge planning on the forensic unit ideally begins at the time of admission, when strengths and supports available to the patient in the community are assessed and the trajectory of care is being plotted. There are many special variations of discharge planning within a forensic setting; however, discharging patients with a history of serious violence requires additional carefulness (Davoren et al. 2015).

Patients transferred from correctional settings often return to those settings (Norko et al. 2015), so housing, employment, insurance, and availability of health care are not immediate concerns. For these patients, correctional treatment staff will be provided necessary follow-up information to ensure successful continuity of care. Long-term patient care for individuals with serious mental illness involved in the criminal justice system is shared among forensic hospitals, correctional facilities, and community providers in complex interactions, requiring communication and collaboration among colleagues in the various settings (Kapoor et al. 2018).

Patients restored to competency to stand trial will be returned to court; for serious charges, they will likely be returned to correctional settings. However, the forensic unit staff can never know what might transpire in court, as patients could be discharged precipitously. Therefore, staff must prepare contingency discharge plans for all patients restored to competency as they return to court. This includes a place of residence, psychiatric and medical appointments in the community, with a supply of medications; and other supports as needed.

For insanity acquittees, decisions about discharge are made by a third party, usually a judicial body. As a result, individuals might remain hospitalized long after the treatment team determines they can be safely discharged with supports. Successful discharge requires collaboration with community providers to craft a detailed plan for appropriate monitoring and delivery of treatment services. Often this starts with graded exposures to the community through therapeutic passes before conditional release, not just to provide an opportunity to assuage the anxieties of the patient and the community providers, but also to offer the patient a chance to practice basic skills needed to survive in the community (e.g., shopping, learning bus routes). Family, friends, and community providers are involved in the coordination of these carefully constructed plans. For most patients in maximum security settings, it would be prudent to start the discharge process by stepping down to a less secure treatment setting before accessing the community (Dike 2017).

An element of this planning that is unique to this population is the need to overcome the fears and special concerns of community providers, or even the public, that may accompany the release of a well-known insanity acquittee who caused great anguish for the community. These fears will often limit the range of placement opportunities normally available to patients with chronic psychiatric disabilities and often require skillful negotiations on the part of treatment team staff and community providers to assuage fear and promote willingness to engage with a notorious acquittee. In some cases, this will require placement in homes with 24-hour staffing, line-of-sight staffing while in public areas outside of the residence, peer support staffing as they access community areas away from their home, and other resources that increase the financial cost of discharging these patients. Not infrequently, it requires the intervention of senior management of a state's department of mental health to facilitate acceptance of the patients into a community program.

Civil patients on a forensic unit, especially those who have been treated in maximum security facilities, are not free from the stigma associated with being labeled "forensic." Once these patients are identified as being on a forensic unit, discharge planning becomes an uphill task because the forensic label implicates dangerousness. Hence, every effort should be made to discourage admission of these patients into an identified forensic unit, and once admitted, to discharge them as soon as possible. Successful transitioning requires the elaboration of a relapse prevention plan, detailing measures to avoid circumstances leading to potential harm, contingencies for containing risk when those circumstances are encountered, and strategies for reducing harm should containment plans fail (Dvoskin 2002).

In all of this planning, it is necessary to be mindful of an ethics of risk assessment and management practices. Clinicians must be vigilant to focus their concerns on the clinical care of their patients, avoiding the all-too-easy lapse into becoming agents of social control (Mullen 2000).

Special Challenges of the Forensic Unit

The dual mandate of the forensic unit to provide clinical care of the individual and to ensure protection of the public can often be successfully negotiated by providing good treatment that is focused on the patients' clinical needs. This is most likely to occur when the patients are appropriately admitted for treatable psychiatric conditions that are the source of the risk to the community.

At times, however, a patient's level of violence may become so intense and/or predatory that it cannot be safely managed in this setting. In such rare circumstances, having a mechanism to transfer such patients to correctional settings is beneficial as this may be the only environment that can safely manage the patient's behavior. For example, housing in a standard prison cell may be an effective intervention to prevent interpersonal violence, representing a less restrictive intervention than frequent use of seclusion or restraint that might be required for the same individual in a hospital setting (Norko et al. 2015). Such transfers should not be undertaken lightly though, given the disparate missions of hospitals and correctional institutions and potential risks to patients (Piel and Goldenberg 2012). A particularly difficult challenge for forensic units is how to manage individuals who are too aggressive for the unit staff to handle but cannot be transferred to any other setting. In such instances, it can be helpful to explore creative strategies for utilizing security personnel to provide additional support to clinical staff.

The challenge of this dual mandate can become quite tangible when transporting patients from forensic units to the community for court appointments and/or medical appointments. Forensic units are tasked with ensuring the safe transport of the patient but also balancing this against their liberty interests in not having undue physical restraint. Transportation options range from transport solely with clinical staff to transport with handcuffs, leg irons, and multiple police officers. Ideally, risk assessment processes permit the balancing of these competing interests (Dike et al. 2015).

The treatment of sex offenders is another challenge unique to the forensic unit. Most of these individuals have a primary diagnosis of paraphilia, or paraphilia with comorbid psychotic disorder or substance use disorders. These patients are often admitted to forensic units after being found not guilty by reason of insanity or at the conclusion of a period of incarceration, particularly in states with sexually violent predator laws allowing the commitment of individuals with such offense histories to hospitals after completion of their term of incarceration. Available evidence suggests that sex offender treatment is evidence based and effective at reducing recidivism (Bradford et al. 2013). Biological treatments (surgical castration, antiandrogens, gonadotropin-releasing hormone analogues, and selective serotonin reuptake inhibitors) have demonstrated a larger effect size than psychological treatments (generally cognitive-behavioral approaches), but both are effective, and the combination of the two demonstrates the most promising results (Thibaut et al. 2010). Hormonal treatment may be associated with serious side effects, so such agents should be used cautiously (Gooren 2011). A 2002 meta-analysis suggests that sexual offence recidivism rates are lower for sex offenders treated with CBT or multisystemic therapy (Hanson et al. 2002). Unfortunately, in most locales there is a dearth of psychologists trained to provide psychotherapy specifically for sex offenders.

Clinical administrators of forensic units must guard against the admission of individuals who pose risk by virtue of criminality and antisocial personality, because there is no credible end point for hospitalization of such individuals. The admission of some such individuals is often politically and legally unavoidable, but their presence is debilitating to the therapeutic milieu and staff morale. The misuse of forensic units for preventive detention of dangerous individuals who would otherwise not require hospital-level care contributes to the stigma of mental illness and wastes the finite resources available to treat people with serious mental illness who require conditions of enhanced security. The barriers to discharge (and demands on staff time) of inappropriately placed individuals are extraordinary and contribute to poor bed utilization and patient flow to aftercare placements.

Recruitment and Retention of Staff

Forensic units are often faced with high rates of staff turnover across disciplines. These increased rates of turnover are often attributed to the increased risk for patient assault, need for physical intervention (e.g., restraint and seclusion), and subsequent staff injury. Further, the physical environment and restrictive nature of such units can become demoralizing over time. Recruiting and retaining psychiatrists to work on such units can be extremely difficult. Given the existing national shortage of psychiatrists (National Council Medical Director Institute 2017), recruiting psychiatrists to work in any setting can be hard, but particularly so in such highly specialized settings where the risk for violence, legal entanglements, testimony requirements, and clinical complexity are all increased and rates of compensation may not be significantly different than in other settings. This challenge can be compounded by the misperception that only those with forensic training can work in such settings.

In addition to the milieu management strategies described above to reduce the risks of such settings, particular interventions have been found to be useful to enhance retention and recruitment. For example, Thorpe et al. (2009) described a clinical coaching program for forensic nurses in a Canadian forensic hospital that paired veteran nurses with recent graduates, leading to significant increases in new forensic nurse retention. For psychiatrist recruitment and retention, there are also several strategies that can be employed (Reynolds 2017). These may include cultivating relationships with local academic institutions to provide opportunities for teaching and scholarship, increasing engagement with local and national professional organizations to build camaraderie and a larger recruitment network, highlighting advantages of state employment (e.g., absence of managed care pressures), and, if possible, providing financial bonuses for forensic board certification.

Conclusion

Several characteristics distinguish the forensic unit from other inpatient psychiatric units, including the need to address psycholegal questions in evaluation and treatment; the explicit specialization in the management of aggression; a patient population with histories of often extraordinary levels of violence; and the need to balance treatment and recovery concerns for patients with security and safety concerns for patients, staff, and visitors to the facility and the outside community. Forensic units can be challenging places to work, especially when staff members find themselves at the center of various competing advocacies and adversarial processes. When balanced approaches are taken to the special tasks of the forensic unit, and when productive teamwork can be fostered, the work can nonetheless be very rewarding.

References

American Psychiatric Association: Psychiatric Services in Correctional Facilities, 3rd Edition. Washington, DC, American Psychiatric Publishing, 2016

Bader SM, Evans SE: Implementing an ecological approach to violence reduction at a forensic psychiatric hospital: approaches and lessons learned. CNS Spectr 20(3):177–181, 2015 25882371

Bowers L: Safewards: a new model of conflict and containment on psychiatric wards. J Psychiatr Ment Health Nurs 21(6):499–508, 2014 24548312

Bradford JM, Fedoroff P, Gulati S: Can sexual offenders be treated? Int J Law Psychiatry 36(3–4):235–240, 2013 23702350

Caplan CA: Nursing staff and patient perceptions of the ward atmosphere in a maximum security forensic hospital. Arch Psychiatr Nurs 7(1):23–29, 1993 8476314

Coccaro EF, Kavoussi RJ: Fluoxetine and impulsive aggressive behavior in personality-disordered subjects. Arch Gen Psychiatry 54(12):1081–1088, 1997 9400343

Curie CG: SAMHSA's commitment to eliminating the use of seclusion and restraint. Psychiatr Serv 56(9):1139–1140, 2005 16148330

Davoren M, Byrne O, O'Connell P, et al: Factors affecting length of stay in forensic hospital setting: need for therapeutic security and course of admission. BMC Psychiatry 15:301, 2015 26597630

Dickinson T, Wright KM: Stress and burnout in forensic mental health nursing: a literature review. Br J Nurs 17(2):82–87, 2008 18414278

Dike CC: Management of forensic hospitals: bearing witness to change in forensic psychiatry and psychology practice. Edited by Griffith EEH, Norko MA, Buchanan A, et al. Boca Raton, FL, CRC Press, 2017, pp 219–233

Dike CC, Nicholson E, Young JL: Transporting forensic psychiatric patients. J Am Acad Psychiatry Law 43(4):468–475, 2015 26668224

Doctor R: Murder: A Psychotherapeutic Investigation. Forensic Psychotherapy Monograph Series. Brett Kahr, Series Editor. London, Routledge, 2008

Dorkins E, Adshead G: Working with offenders: challenges to the recovery agenda. Adv Psychiatr Treat 17:178–187, 2011

Dvoskin JA: Knowledge is not power—knowledge is obligation. J Am Acad Psychiatry Law 30(4):533–540, 2002 12539909

Dvoskin JA, Heilbrun K: Risk assessment and release decision-making: toward resolving the great debate. J Am Acad Psychiatry Law 29(1):6–10, 2001 11302389

Dvoskin JA, Radomski SJ, Bennett C, et al: Architectural design of a secure forensic state psychiatric hospital. Behav Sci Law 20(5):481–493, 2002 12239707

Evans SE, Bader SM: The indistinguishables: determining appropriate environments for justice involved individuals. CNS Spectr 25(2):122–127, 2020 31599217

Farnworth L, Nikitin L, Fossey E: Being in a secure forensic psychiatric unit: every day is the same, killing time or making the most of it. Br J Occup Ther 67:430–438, 2004

Felthous AR, Stanford MS: A proposed algorithm for the pharmacotherapy of impulsive aggression. J Am Acad Psychiatry Law 43(4):456–467, 2015 26668223

Glancy GD, Knott TF: Psychopharmacology of violence, Part II: mood stabilizers. AAPL Newsl 27:14, 2002

Glancy GD, Knott TF: Psychopharmacology of violence, Part III. AAPL Newsl 28:14, 2003

Goodness KR, Renfro NS: Changing a culture: a brief program analysis of a social learning program on a maximum-security forensic unit. Behav Sci Law 20(5):495–506, 2002 12239708

Gooren LJ: Clinical review: ethical and medical considerations of androgen deprivation treatment of sex offenders. J Clin Endocrinol Metab 96(12):3628–3637, 2011 21956411

Hanson RK, Gordon A, Harris AJ, et al: First report of the collaborative outcome data project on the effectiveness of psychological treatment for sex offenders. Sex Abuse 14(2):169–194, discussion 195–197, 2002 11961890

Haq AU, Ghaziuddin N: Maintenance electroconvulsive therapy for aggression and self-injurious behavior in two adolescents with autism and catatonia. J Neuropsychiatry Clin Neurosci 26(1):64–72, 2014 24515677

Hillbrand M, Young JL: Instilling hope into forensic treatment: the antidote to despair and desperation. J Am Acad Psychiatry Law 36(1):90–94, 2008 18354129

Hörberg U, Benzein E, Erlingsson C, Syrén S: Engaging with families is a challenge: beliefs among healthcare professionals in forensic psychiatric care. Nurs Res Pract 2015:843717, 2015 26448874

Hunt IM, Windfuhr K, Shaw J, et al: Ligature points and ligature types used by psychiatric inpatients who die by hanging: a national study. Crisis 33(2):87–94, 2012 22343063

Kaltiala-Heino R, Kahila K: Forensic psychiatric inpatient treatment: creating a therapeutic milieu. Child Adolesc Psychiatr Clin N Am 15(2):459–475, x, 2006 16527666

Kapoor R, Dike CD, Norko MA: Psychiatric treatment in forensic hospital and correctional settings. Psychiatr Ann 48:102–108, 2018

Kristine LM: Gangs and violence in prisons, in Corrections. Edited by Chambliss WJ. Thousand Oaks, CA, Sage, 2011. Available at: https://edge.sagepub.com/system/files/Ch12RennisonGangsandViolenceinPrisons.pdf. Accessed October 30, 2021.

Kuhlman TL: Gallows humor for a scaffold setting: managing aggressive patients on a maximum-security forensic unit. Hosp Community Psychiatry 39(10):1085–1090, 1988 3229742

Ladds B: Forensic treatment and rehabilitation: the growing need for more services and more research. Int J Ment Health 25(4):3–10, 1996

Liberman RP: Elimination of seclusion and restraint: a reasonable goal? Psychiatr Serv 57(4):576, author reply 576–578, 2006 16603760

Livingston JD, Nijdam-Jones A, Brink J: A tale of two cultures: examining patient-centered care in a forensic mental health hospital. J Forens Psychiatry Psychol 23(3):345–360, 2012 22815648

Long CG, Knight C, Bradley L, Thomas M: Effective therapeutic milieus in secure services for women: the service user perspective. J Ment Health 21(6):567–578, 2012 23216224

Maguire T, Ryan J, Fullam R, McKenna B: Evaluating the introduction of the Safewards Model to a medium- to long-term forensic mental health ward. J Forensic Nurs 14(4):214–222, 2018 30433910

Maier GJ, Van Rybroek GJ, Mays DV: A report on staff injuries and ambulatory restraints: dealing with patient aggression. J Psychosoc Nurs Ment Health Serv 32(11):23–29, 1994 7884688

Manchak SM, Skeem JL, Rook KS: Care, control, or both? Characterizing major dimensions of the mandated treatment relationship. Law Hum Behav 38(1):47–57, 2014 23834388

McInerny T, Minne C: Principles of treatment for mentally disordered offenders. Crim Behav Ment Health 14 (suppl 1):S43–S47, 2004 16575787

Mueser KT, Rosenberg SD: Treatment of PTSD in persons with severe mental illness, in Treating Psychological Trauma and PTSD. Edited by Wilson JP, Friedman MJ, Lindy LD. New York, Guilford, 2001, pp 354–382

Mullen PE: Forensic mental health. Br J Psychiatry 176:307–311, 2000 10827876

National Association of State Mental Health Program Directors: Six Core Strategies for Reducing Seclusion and Restraint Use. Alexandria, VA, National Association of State Mental Health Program Directors, 2006. Available at: www.nasmhpd.org/sites/default/files/Consolidated%20Six%20Core%20Strategies%20Document.pdf. Accessed October 18, 2019.

National Council Medical Director Institute: The Psychiatric Shortage: Causes and Solutions. Washington, DC, National Council for Behavioral Health, 2017. Available at: www.thenationalcouncil.org/wp-content/uploads/2017/03/Psychiatric-Shortage_National-Council-.pdf. Accessed January 10, 2020.

Nesset MB, Rossberg JI, Almvik R, Friis S: Can a focused staff training programme improve the ward atmosphere and patient satisfaction in a forensic psychiatric hospital? A pilot study. Scand J Caring Sci 23(1):117–124, 2009 19170956

Newbill WA, Paul GL, Menditto AA, et al: Social-learning programs facilitate an increase in adaptive behavior in a forensic mental hospital. Behav Interv 26(3):214–230, 2011

Norko MA, Burns CG, Dike C: Hospitalization, in Oxford Textbook of Correctional Psychiatry. Edited by Trestman RL, Appelbaum KL, Metzner JL. New York, Oxford University Press, 2015, pp 141–145

Papapietro DJ: Involving forensic patients in treatment planning increases cooperation and may reduce violence. J Am Acad Psychiatry Law 47:35–41, 2019

Pfafflin F, Adshead G: A Matter of Security: That Application of Attachment Theory to Forensic Psychiatry. London, Jessica Kingsley, 2004

Phillips RTM, Caplan C: Administrative and staffing problems for psychiatric services in correctional and forensic settings, in Principles and Practice of Forensic Psychiatry, 2nd Edition. Edited by Rosner R. London, Arnold, 2003

Piel J, Goldenberg E: Washington's Senate Bill 6610 on transferring provisions for persons found not guilty by reason of insanity. J Am Acad Psychiatry Law 40:253–260, 2012 22635299

Recupero PR, Price M, Garvey KA, et al: Restraint and seclusion in psychiatric treatment settings: regulation, case law, and risk management. J Am Acad Psychiatry Law 39(4):465–476, 2011 22159974

Reynolds J: Staffing forensic hospital units: a burden on the medical director. AAPL Newsl 42(3):2, 31, 2017

Richards M, Doyle M, Cook P: A literature review of family interventions for dual diagnosis: implications for forensic mental health services. Journal of Forensic Practice 11:39–49, 2019

Saleh FM, Guidry LL: Psychosocial and biological treatment considerations for the paraphilic and nonparaphilic sex offender. J Am Acad Psychiatry Law 31(4):486–493, 2003 14974804

Seppänen A, Törmänen I, Shaw C, Kennedy H: Modern forensic psychiatric hospital design: clinical, legal and structural aspects. Int J Ment Health Syst 12:58, 2018 30377440

Shaw MA: The secure residential psychiatric facility: process, design, and results for behavioral healthcare, in Forensic and Ethical Issues in Military Behavioral Health. Edited by Ritchie EC. Fort Sam Houston, TX, Office of the Surgeon General, Borden Institute, 2014, pp 217–243

Stahl SM: Antipsychotic polypharmacy: squandering precious resources? J Clin Psychiatry 63(2):93–94, 2002 11874226

Tang W-K, Ungvari GS: Efficacy of electroconvulsive therapy in treatment-resistant schizophrenia: a prospective open trial. Prog Neuropsychopharmacol Biol Psychiatry 27(3):373–379, 2003 12691772

Thibaut F, De La Barra F, Gordon H, et al; WFSBP Task Force on Sexual Disorders: The World Federation of Societies of Biological Psychiatry (WFSBP) guidelines for the biological treatment of paraphilias. World J Biol Psychiatry 11(4):604–655, 2010 20459370

Thorpe G, Moorhouse P, Antonello C: Clinical coaching in forensic psychiatry: an innovative program to recruit and retain nurses. J Psychosoc Nurs Ment Health Serv 47(5):43–47, 2009 19489514

Tiihonen J, Taipale H, Mehtälä J, et al: Association of antipsychotic polypharmacy vs monotherapy with psychiatric rehospitalization among adults with schizophrenia. JAMA Psychiatry 76(5):499–507, 2019 30785608

Tolisano P, Sondik TM, Dike CC: A positive behavioral approach for aggression in forensic psychiatric settings. J Am Acad Psychiatry Law 45(1):31–39, 2017 28270460

Tomlin J, Bartlett P, Völlm B: Experiences of restrictiveness in forensic psychiatric care: systematic review and concept analysis. Int J Law Psychiatry 57:31–41, 2018 29548502

Trestman R: Development of a skills-based psychotherapy for forensic psychiatric hospital settings. Presented at the Joint Conference of the Southern States Psychiatric Hospital Association and the NASMHPD Forensic Division, Nashville, TN, October 2016. Available at: www.nasmhpd.org/sites/default/files/START%20NOW%20NASMHPD%20Forensic%20Division%20Presentation_Trestman.pdf. Accessed November 11, 2019.

van den Berg JF, Kruithof HC, Kok RM, et al: Electroconvulsive therapy for agitation and aggression in dementia: a systematic review. Am J Geriatr Psychiatry 26(4):419–434, 2018 29107460

Visaggio N, Phillips KE, Kichefski K, et al: Is it safe? The restraint chair compared to traditional methods of restraint: a three hospital study. Arch Psychiatr Nurs 32(5):723–728, 2018 30201200

Vogel T, Lanquillon S, Graf M: When and why should mentally ill prisoners be transferred to secure hospitals: a proposed algorithm. Int J Law Psychiatry 36(3–4):281–286, 2013 23706656

Zimbroff DL: Clinical management of agitation. Medscape Psychiatry Clinical Update, April 2003. Available at: www.medscape.com/viewprogram/2311_pnt. Accessed July 11, 2007.

Zonana HV, Norko MA: Mandated treatment, in Clinical Challenges in Psychiatry. Edited by Sledge WR, Tasman A. Washington, DC, American Psychiatric Press, 1993, pp 249–291

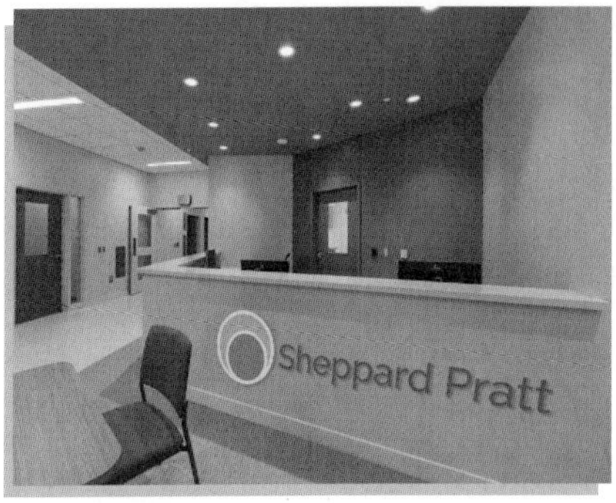

CHAPTER 9

The Psychotic Disorders Unit

Edward Zuzarte, M.D.
John J. Boronow, M.D.
Harsh K. Trivedi, M.D., M.B.A.

Most hospitals have psychiatric units that are nonspecialized, also referred to as *general adult units*. Patients of different age groups and with a variety of diagnoses are treated on one unit. This is the crisis intervention model of care. It is akin to treating a patient with a myocardial infarction next to a patient who is in labor next to a patient who is in septic shock—it is easy to see why it becomes very difficult to render individualized care for each patient.

Unlike medical and surgical environments, where care is provided in the patient's room, psychiatric environments are, by their very nature, milieu based, and this can lead to suboptimal care based on the mix of patients and their level of destabilization at any given moment. Likewise, there are certain conditions in psychiatry that truly require dedicated teams and specialized skill sets, as can be seen in the chapters in Part I of this textbook on inpatient care units designated by diagnostic cohorts. Milieu-based settings can be a particular disadvantage for patients with severe psychotic illnesses, who are more likely to be aggressive, cognitively limited, and/or lower functioning; to have poor insight; and/or to take longer to improve and stabilize.

The result is that seriously mentally ill patients with psychosis, when treated on a general unit, are rarely stabilized enough to achieve successful remission of psychotic symptoms or resumption of baseline functioning to prevent rehospitalization. Many of these patients have treatment-refractory conditions and are functionally impaired. They have had numerous trials of antipsychotic medication with less than an adequate response. Some of these patients may need a trial of clozapine or electroconvulsive therapy (ECT) and much closer monitoring for compliance and therapeutic response.

Acute inpatient psychiatric units are rarely able to keep these patients long enough to give them an adequate trial of these lifesaving medications and treatment. The loss of state hospital beds across the nation has compounded this issue, as more of these patients with complex needs present for admission onto acute-stay general psychiatric units. For appropriate care of such individuals, a dedicated psychotic disorders unit with specialized treatment requires a milieu that can provide a proper environment designed to meet their care needs and with specialized staff to provide evidence-based and effective treatment.

Sheppard Pratt established an inpatient psychotic disorders unit in 1984 to provide state-of-the-art diagnosis and treatment for this special patient population. At the time, it was seen as very controversial because of the focus on a particular clinical population of adults, the deemphasis of psychodynamic approaches, and the focus on evidence-based care. The key to improved clinical outcomes would be a focus on observable, constructive behaviors and positive consequences while incorporating evidence-based medication and treatment plan regimens.

Why then should we consider a specialty program targeting psychosis today? The mission of a specialized psychotic disorders unit is to serve the needs of patients with severe and persistent mental illness whose psychosis is likely to be chronic and whose resulting disability is both widespread and profound.

The history of American inpatient psychiatry is very much bound up in the story of caring for these patients (see Chapter 1). Ever since Pennsylvania Hospital volunteered to care for "the sick-poor and the insane who were wandering the streets of Philadelphia" in 1751 (University of Pennsylvania Health System 2007), there has been a recognition in American society that there is a population of severely disturbed people whose illness is both chronic and refractory to treatment. The asylum movement was begun in the nineteenth century to provide humane care, if not cure, for these unfortunate people. By the end of the twentieth century, this national enterprise, implemented on a state-by-state basis as the state hospital system, had been largely dismantled under the rubric of deinstitutionalization. This historic change was fueled by advances in treatment, especially the promulgation of antipsychotic medication; by social concerns about the rights of patients to live unsegregated in society in the least restrictive manner; by documented abuses of patients within the confines of total institutions; and by powerful economic pressures to reduce the cost of care.

Deinstitutionalization coalesced with managed care in recent decades, yet the challenge of how to best provide services for the chronically psychotic patient at all levels of care has not been resolved. Many, if not most, such patients receive so-called crisis stabilization for their acute psychotic relapses on general inpatient units within local community hospitals. The restrictions on length of stay placed by commercial managed care organizations, using severely curtailed and often arbitrary criteria for hospital care, can result in patients being discharged prematurely, with consequent readmissions and the evolution of the all-too-familiar "revolving door" scenario. In addition, the mixing of severely psychotic chronic patients with younger, higher-functioning patients and/or with older, more fragile geriatric patients leads to a predictable additional pressure within the milieu to extrude patients with illnesses characterized by disruptive behavior by discharging them early.

The mission, then, of a specialized psychotic disorders inpatient unit is to implement state-of-the-art diagnostic and therapeutic techniques, coupled with a sophisticated appreciation of the patient's illness in its community context, for the treatment of some of the most ill patients with the most treatment-resistant disorders. That community context includes social (family, friends, care providers, and all manner of outpatient treatment team members), historical (onset of illness, precipitators of relapse or noncompliance, motivators of positive change, response to past treatments), economic (available therapeutics of all sorts, from medications to assertive community treatment teams and cognitive-behavioral therapy–competent therapists), and even legal (restraining orders, criminal charges, mandated treatment orders) considerations. The vision of such a unit is to accurately diagnose the acutely ill or relapsed patient, implement the optimal therapeutics that can be realistically expected to be followed up within the patient's community setting, control inpatient behavioral problems with the greatest efficiency for the patient and the least adverse impact on other patient groups, and coordinate the handoff of treatment to the next level smoothly on the continuum of care with minimal disruption to the flow of treatment and the greatest chance for immediate, intermediate, and long-term therapeutic success.

Unit Structure

The psychotic disorders unit is a treatment unit. Individuals come into our care when experiencing a psychotic and/or delusional episode and cannot be safely managed outside the hospital. The median length of stay is about 2 weeks, with a range between 3 days and 2–3 months. The state of Maryland has zero adult nonforensic state hospital beds; hence, in states where such beds do still exist, there may be a point in treatment when these patients are transferred to the state hospital to complete their admission. Even in states where nonforensic capacity exists, transfers are often difficult, and thus the full course of treatment will occur as described in this chapter.

This program does not treat forensic patients (i.e., patients who are involved in the legal system on the basis of committing a crime in the context of being psychiatrically ill) or patients who are primarily connected with the Veterans Health Administration system. It is no small achievement that this program treats very ill and chronically impaired patients. The staff here are dedicated and have special skills and interest to work with patients who have such a disabling illness and very little support system.

The unit is a 22-bed unit, with a central nursing station and three corridors projecting from it. There are individual patient rooms with their own attached private bathrooms. There is a central kitchen where meals are served, as well as a multifunctional group room. There is also a terrace, which is open but is secure so that patients can be "outside" without the need to leave the unit. The unit also includes a laundry room, where patients can do their own laundry with assistance from staff and gain functional mastery over instrumental activities of daily living (IADLs). Examples of IADLs that patients master to varying degrees based on illness severity include using the telephone, doing laundry, managing medications, and handling finances. The availability of occupational therapists and a robust multidisciplinary team is key to patients attaining these skills.

The unit staff includes all disciplines working collaboratively and in sync to treat this population. These include the nursing staff (three to four RNs per shift), nurse aides (also referred to in our setting as mental health workers), occupational therapists, social workers, a discharge coordinator, behavior specialists, psychiatrists, nurse practitioners, and nurse managers. Medical consultants and smoke cessation counselors are also actively involved. This collaboration is very critical to provide proper treatment and education when treating this very difficult and vulnerable population.

The entire unit is composed of wide-open corridors with spacious individual patient rooms and bathrooms. This gives the impression of a comfortable and welcoming hotel rather than an acute inpatient psychiatric unit and leads to a comfortable and relaxing environment for the patients. The unit has large windows, allowing plenty of light to come through. There are two entrances, both of which have two sets of doors. There are also several offices throughout the unit where our four distinct treatment teams meet for patient interviews, family meetings, and treatment planning.

Academic Structure

This unit is the flagship unit for our Sheppard Pratt/University of Maryland Psychiatry Residency Program. We have first- and second-year psychiatry residents who rotate through this unit every month. There are also medical students, nursing students, and occupational therapy students from several universities who work and train on the unit as part of clinical rotations. The ability to engage in regular teaching rounds strengthens the milieu, while lectures on the current state-of-the-art ensure a high level of expertise across all disciplines.

Beyond the Unit Walls

For such a program to be successful, it requires active referral to step-down programs and proactive linkages to support structures for postdischarge success.

Substantial risk of decompensation and readmission can occur during transitions of care with this population. We have created extensions of our program at non-inpatient levels of care to facilitate the ongoing treatment of psychotic patients after they have been stabilized on the inpatient unit. These programs include the Sullivan Day Hospital, which is a day program specializing in treating patients with psychotic illnesses, and the Weinberg Residential Crisis Program, where patients are able to step down and live temporarily until a more permanent arrangement for their housing has been identified. Both of these programs are based on the Sheppard Pratt campus in Baltimore, Maryland, adjacent to the inpatient hospital so as to provide maximum patient support and ease ability to transition between programs as clinically necessary.

Admission Criteria

The admission criteria for such a program can be formulated both diagnostically and functionally. Diagnostically, the core target population would include patients with schizophrenia and its spectrum disorders; bipolar and related disorders; substance-induced psychotic disorders (with the drug being in most cases amphetamines or LSD, or occasionally cannabis); developmental disorders; neuropsychiatric disorders, including psychoses due to epilepsy, head injury, or Wilson's disease; and personality change due to medical etiologies, especially paranoid, aggressive, and disinhibited types. Some geriatric patients with dementia and behavioral dyscontrol may at times be more successfully treated in a psychotic disorders milieu as well. The common presentation across these diagnoses is the presence of psychosis and displaying of more aggressive and violent behaviors.

Functionally, diagnosis notwithstanding, the hallmark of a patient treated in an inpatient psychosis program is the patient's cognitive dysfunction, including other negative symptoms, and its attendant disability. Nursing staff view such patients as requiring "hands on" nursing, compared with higher-functioning patients on general units where verbal interaction is a much more important medium of therapeutics. By *hands-on*, we mean the need to guide such patients through many, if not all, of their activities of daily living; prompt them continually to attend to the milieu schedule; set limits, including physically, around boundaries and socially inappropriate behavior; and restore order and good hygiene on the unit if there is destruction of property or soiling of linen, clothing, or the unit environment. On the basis of functional inability to care for themselves, imminent risk of harm to self or others, and general poor insight into their illness, the majority of patients on this unit are admitted involuntarily or "on certificate."

Special Populations

One specific population that bears mentioning comprises patients with intellectual disabilities. The management of psychotic disorders in this population can often be considerably problematic. The clinical presentation may be due to an underlying medical condition, or these patients may also have personality disorders, like anyone else. The impact on treatment, and on the rest of the milieu, of such patients can be great, particularly if they present with labile, disinhibited, aggressive, apathetic, or paranoid behaviors. They not only may present with hallucinations, delusions, a formal thought disorder, negative symptoms, and/or a mood syndrome but also may be impulsive, perseverative, attention-seeking, histrionic, childish, and/or grossly primitive, superimposed on the cognitive limitations, which makes communication, learning, and participation in higher-functioning groups difficult. Additional complexity may also come from not-uncommon physical disabilities, ranging from frequent expressive language and speech disorders to more disabling problems such as ataxia or spasticity, and the need to assist the patient with most activities of daily living, from toileting to feeding. Such patients often are unable to take advantage of the programming designed for the rest of the psychotically ill peers in the milieu; and while the services of a behavioral psychologist are often very helpful, they are rarely available on most inpatient units across the nation. Access to the outpatient behavioral treatment plan, often forgotten by psychiatrists unfamiliar with this population, can be enlightening, especially in framing the patient's baseline behaviors before the psychotic disorder episode developed, but it can be practically very difficult to implement such a plan in an inpatient milieu, where the staffing and training may be incongruent with the context of the outpatient behavioral plan.

Aggressive patients constitute another challenging population. The increase in patient-to-worker violence in hospitals, particularly in emergency departments and psychiatric units, is an issue across all hospital settings (Arnetz et al. 2017). Although aggression is common in the untreated psychotic population (Krakowski et al. 1999; Steinert et al. 1999), the psychosis program must not allow itself to become the de facto intensive care unit for the whole hospital, where every violent patient is sent to keep the other units safe. There tends to be a dynamic of the "state hospital ward" even within a single hospital. This is deleterious to preventing violent behavior and deteriorates the therapeutic milieu such that treatment progress becomes difficult. It is important that clinical staff throughout the hospital have the skills to successfully manage non-psychotic aggressive patients without triaging them to a psychosis program. Similarly, a psychosis unit is not (necessarily) a forensic unit. Unless there are additional specialized resources available for the safe management of potentially violent forensic patients, it is necessary to screen out such patients at the point of admission. Screening criteria that we have found useful include what the most serious violence up to that point has been; whether there is a criminal history; whether a weapon was used; whether the violence was self-limited or sustained; whether it was in the context of a clear and avoidable precipitant, such as substance intoxication or the presence of specific conflict with another person; whether the referral is coming from an unreliable source; and what the patient's behavior in the emergency department was subsequently. The balance of this determination is that any remote history of legal involvement or recent misdemeanor for a petty offense is not judged as an exclusion for admission to the psychosis unit. While some best practices have emerged from work done at Sheppard Pratt (Roca et al. 2016), additional research into managing patient-to-worker violence is necessary.

Dual Diagnosis

The patient with co-occurring, and, particularly, active, substance abuse presents a clinical challenge. Although comprehensive programming for chemical dependency may exist on other specialty units, the psychotic patient may not be able to take full advantage of it, at least during the first part of the hospitalization. There is also a concern that psychotic patients may be victimized by certain street-savvy patients on a chemical dependency unit. Even when they are stabilized, there is well-documented evidence that patients with co-occurring severe and persistent mental illness and substance use disorders can have trouble accessing medication-assisted treatment for chemical dependency because of such obstacles as residual paranoia and thought disorder, which make the mandatory participation in verbal 12-step groups in some programs highly problematic (Green et al. 2007). As with the first-episode psychotic patient, the decision of where to admit the dually diagnosed psychotic patient is often a difficult one, and the flexibility to transfer the patient (in either direction) should be anticipated based on patient presentation, patient functional status, milieu patient mix, and likelihood of treatment success based on staffing and culture within your programs.

Dissociative Identity Disorder and PTSD

The psychotic patient with dissociative symptoms and a history of physical abuse is another unique challenge. There are both differential diagnostic considerations (Is the patient truly dissociative? Is what appears to be PTSD essentially a complicating factor in an otherwise clear-cut case of schizophrenia?) and practical considerations (If the patient has dissociative identity disorder, is the thought disorder so severe that a trauma disorder specialty unit would not be appropriate, because the patient would not be able to make use of the higher-order cognitive/behavioral therapies employed on such a unit?). The triaging of such patients is further complicated by the fact that the dissociative or psychotic elements are in many cases only uncovered subsequent to the admission, so a certain amount of collegial reassessment and cross-consultation between programs is required.

Other Considerations

Finally, certain nonmedical considerations such as insurance and placement resources cannot be dismissed from a complete understanding of why some patients are not admitted. A specialty psychosis unit has a very specific set of skills and objectives to bring to the care of patients with some of the most disabling illnesses in psychiatry. Depending on the setting, it may have an intermediate or long-term average length of stay. State hospitals, U.S. Department of Veterans Affairs hospitals, and forensic settings may all have programs explicitly designed for a length of stay measured in months. Likewise, specialty units will understandably at times receive referrals of the most ill patients in the state, if not the country, and yet the patients will not have the portfolio of resources needed to support any kind of adequate treatment planning. With the advent of value-based contracting and gain sharing among commercial insurance plans, informed and progressive health plans have begun understanding the substantial financial savings and improvement in clinical outcomes that can come through the combination of a specialty admission on a psychosis unit and a robust continuum of services, as provided at Sheppard Pratt. In fact, we have operated a successful capitation program, named Chesapeake Connections, for nearly two decades that provides a per-member-per-month allocation for us to manage all aspects of care for seriously mentally ill adults.

Diagnostic Workup

The first 24 hours of admission are a critical period with regard to the patient's diagnosis and treatment. Patients arrive on the psychosis unit from a multitude of potential referral sources. In our experience, many of these psychotic patients have been homeless, living on the streets, or living in shelters for some period of time before coming to the hospital and arrive extremely disheveled, with extremely poor hygiene, and with poor nutritional status. Establishing rapport, restoring dignity, and providing a welcoming and safe orientation to the unit are important first steps. *Safe* refers to the patient's subjective experience as well as the staff's objective experience that a safety search has been conducted, that no weapons or forbidden items have entered the milieu, and that the right resources are available for them to maintain a therapeutic milieu. An important aspect of the orientation is a tour of the unit, explanation of the unit schedule, and communication of key behavioral expectations to help establish boundaries for accepted behavior from the patient and to reassure the patient about how they will be kept safe from any potential behavior of peers on the unit.

The patient is then encouraged to shower, change clothes, and acclimate to their new surroundings. The nursing admission assessment is an invaluable tool for paving the foundation for a successful admission. The ability to establish rapport, to help the patient "let their guard down," and elicit key information about current symptomatology, recent functioning, and potential risks is key. A full body exam helps to identify any injuries, bruises, and any other physical problems that were missed in the emergency department. Discussion about recent substance use to avoid withdrawal and understand triggers, and effective de-escalation techniques for aggressive behavior, are key.

The patient is then seen by a physician for a full physical exam and orders are written for any physical problems. These orders may consist of ordering labs, finger sticks, and special diets; reviewing nursing assessment and vital signs; requesting follow-up medical consults; and ordering medications after medication reconciliation. Likewise, a thorough social work psychosocial evaluation can assess patient strengths, determine key supports, identify key treatment providers, inform discharge planning, and help the team better understand the immediate context of the patient's admission. The patient then undergoes a detailed diagnostic psychiatric assessment. The chart is reviewed and collateral information is obtained from the family and the patient's outpatient providers. All of this information is then compiled and a psychiatric diagnosis is made, followed by the development of a detailed biopsychosocial formulation and a treatment plan.

The differential diagnostic evaluation of the psychotic patient can be extensive (Sheitman et al. 1997; Skikic and Arriola 2020), particularly when all the rare but possible neuropsychiatric manifestations of a host of medical and neurological disorders are considered. One cannot stress enough the importance and value of the two most basic evaluation tools: a good history and a neurological examination. These alone, when combined with basic laboratory tests (comprehensive metabolic profile, complete blood count, urinalysis, toxicology screen, syphilis serology), will identify the vast majority of "organic" psychoses that warrant medical-surgical, rather than psychiatric, triage. The addition of computed tomography scanning or MRI, often now routinely done in urban emergency departments for any mental status changes, further improves such screening, although these tests can sometimes be ordered by the busy emergency physician in lieu of a good history and neurological examination. A lumbar puncture is warranted for the catatonic or deliriously psychotic patient, again usually done in the emergency department prior to admission. The only other routine test not usually available in the emergency setting is the electroencephalogram, and here history is usually able to at least identify epilepsy as a diagnosis needing further assessment. In addition, electroencephalograms are usually readily available on the psychiatric inpatient service. Copper and other heavy metal assays, urine porphobilinogens, chromosome testing for Huntington's disease or specific intellectual disability diagnoses, antinuclear antibody test, and other more obscure testing can be performed on the inpatient psychiatric unit as needed, once the clinical presentation and history are clarified after admission. Brain metabolic studies such as PET, single-photon emission computed tomography, and functional MRI, as well as brain electrical activity mapping, remain primarily research investigations.

Psychological testing, when done properly by skilled doctoral-level psychologists in sufficient depth, can shed important light on matters of diagnosis, prognosis, and rehabilitation. Projective testing can document the severity of otherwise "sealed over" paranoia, the extent of formal thought disorder and its impact on functioning, and the otherwise hidden delusional themes that motivate the patient. The Rorschach Inkblot Test, a projective psychological test consisting of 10 inkblots printed on cards, is helpful in revealing any underlying paranoid thinking, delusions, and thought disorder that may not be obvious otherwise. The Continuous Performance Test (Beck et al. 1956) and the Wisconsin Card Sorting Test (Berg 1948) can document the degree of attentional and frontal deficit in the medicated patient as a guide to appropriate discharge and rehabilitation planning. IQ testing and even simple proxies for IQ, such as the Wide Range Achievement Test—Reading subtest (Jastak et al. 1993), give a snapshot of both overall cognitive functioning and the degree to which that functioning has declined over the course of the illness. More specific neuropsychological testing, such as tests of memory and praxis, can further clarify the specific domains of cognitive deficit, which in turn have immediate bearing on disposition planning and rehabilitation.

Taking a good history is important on the inpatient unit. The focus here is not to rule out the occasional outlier with a neuropsychiatric illness but rather to deepen the understanding of the course of illness, once confirmed as primarily psychiatric in nature. The timeline, first championed by Emil Kraepelin (Kraepelin and Quen 1990) and later expanded upon by Adolf Meyer (Meyer and Winters 1950), is a very helpful tool in this regard. One draws a line from birth to the present and identifies key historical dates, such as developmental milestones (e.g., preschool problems, school problems, highest level of education, marriage/divorce/loss of a parent), as well as psychiatric history (e.g., first contact with any mental health provider, first treatment with medications, first hospitalization, any legal problems). Below the line one documents treatments, including names and dosages of medications as available, episodes of psychotherapy, residential placements, and so on. Inspection of the timeline makes it clear what necessary data are still lacking (e.g., Why was the patient at the state hospital for 5 years? What did the state hospital do to be able to discharge the patient eventually?). It also reveals trends, such as the increase in treatment failures (six hospitalizations in the past 8 months compared with two in the previous 5 years). The timeline also can reveal episodes of wellness, an especially important datum in the clinical history (e.g., Why was the patient stable between 1999 and 2004? Was there a certain medication, or certain psychosocial support, that enabled stability during that time?).

The timeline usually results in the need to request old records from previous treatments in order to answer some of these questions, because it is virtually impossible to do so directly with this patient population, owing to the fundamental brain deficits that afflict them in the first place. Our treatment algorithms are all predicated on knowledge of historical facts regarding prior response to treatment, and the lack of such knowledge severely constricts the likely accuracy of any cross-sectional treatment decisions. Patients being transferred to a specialty unit from another inpatient setting should always have their medication record sent along. One can immediately understand what exactly was being tried, and what exactly the patient actually received, without having to wait for a discharge summary to be dictated. The central premise here is that the inpatient hospitalization is not a self-contained island but rather a point along a temporal continuum of care for a chronic condition. It must address itself to what happened before, and what will happen after, the hospitalization, if it is to be successful.

The genogram is another underutilized tool that is useful for understanding the chronically mentally ill patient as well as most other psychiatric populations. The genogram quickly enables the clinician to understand the social reality of the patient in terms of family and other intimate relationships as well as living arrangements, which are often paramount in undertaking discharge planning and understanding relapses. Knowing who the players are in the patient's family nexus, including the sad possibility that there are none, as well as what their attitudes toward the patient and treatment are, is an indispensable part of evaluating the patient in the broader psychosocial context, and this knowledge is usually necessary in order to develop a realistic aftercare plan.

Hence, the crucial part of this exercise is connecting with current outpatient treatment providers and the patient's current support structure. Outpatient providers can contribute substantial knowledge about the patient and about past treatments, and can help the patient with adopting changes in the treatment plan to achieve better stability. Members of the patient's support system, such as family members, are integral to care planning and provide a scaffolding to help their loved one succeed postdischarge. Keeping all privacy issues in mind, being able to include outpatient treatment providers and psychosocial supports involved during the inpatient stay in treatment planning and in family meetings can be a significant strength in the postdischarge transition.

Treatments

Medication

Most patients admitted to this unit suffer from psychosis. Some are floridly psychotic, whereas others are quietly psychotic and guarded. Many of these patients also suffer from other comorbid conditions, the most common being mood disorders, and others being trauma-related conditions, substance abuse, and impulse-control disorders.

A comprehensive discussion of antipsychotic therapeutics is well beyond the scope of this chapter; the focus here is on certain core principles of treatment. The most important single point to make about psychopharmacology with this population is not about the pharmacology itself. It is, simply stated, that no amount of pharmacology will be helpful if the patient does not take the medication reliably. The problem of nonadherence is the single biggest obstacle to outpatient success in this population (Lacro et al. 2002; Wade et al. 2017). Noncompliance is related to patient knowledge, attitudes toward their illness, past treatment experiences, perceived risks and benefits of treatment, lack of support systems, financial and insurance issues, and a host of other factors (Kane et al. 2013). The challenge on the inpatient unit is to assess the reasons for nonadherence and develop a treatment plan that can optimally address them.

Concerns about side effects certainly rise to the top of patients' expressed reasons for nonadherence and should be actively elicited and responded to by the inpatient psychiatrist. Complaints about weight gain, sedation, and extrapyramidal symptoms can all be responded to in a rational way with alternative medications, although helping the patient appreciate nuances may be difficult if paranoia causes the patient to disparage all medications with a broad brush. First and foremost, however, the psychiatrist should present patients with the clearest possible message that they can exercise choice over the medications and that their opinion about side effects is sincerely respected and responded to. Equally difficult may be sorting out whether prior failures with certain medications were true medication failures (described as common in the Clinical Antipsychotic Trials of Intervention Effectiveness studies [Lieberman et al. 2005]) or were due to noncompliance, partial compliance, or heavy cigarette smoking leading to lower medication levels (Iglesias Garcia et al. 2017). Many times, patients respond to and do well with the same medication that was considered a treatment failure while in the outpatient setting, the only difference being that we were able to monitor their compliance. In such cases, it may be helpful to think about nonmedication portions of the treatment plan, such as the support system or structure around the patient postdischarge. Successful treatment with clozapine, for example, can be sustained by discharging the patient to a supervised residential setting that better supports adherence. Likewise, we firmly believe that trying the newest medication or a different medication trial is not necessarily the best option. Many times, patients who have done well on a certain regimen of medication in the past and who are agreeable to staying on this medication should be continued on the same medication, and there is no clinical reason to subject them to other trials.

Identification of nonadherence early in the admission process should alert the psychiatrist to considering depot antipsychotics as a pharmacological strategy. This technology, although more than 50 years old (Kurland and Richardson 1966), is still much underutilized in the United States compared with Western Europe (Glazer and Kane 1992). The inpatient setting is often a good place to initiate such treatment. The hospitalization often brings with it a certain impetus for change from the patient, the family, or the outpatient treatment team. The patient's resistance to recommendations for depot treatment in a 15-minute clinic "medication check" visit may change over a period of several days, with daily psychoeducation from doctors, nurses, and activity therapists with access to videos and pamphlets and with input from family and outpatient treatment team members. (Bringing to bear such a "full-court press" to motivate the patient about an important treatment decision is another unique advantage of the specialized psychotic disorders unit.) If the patient does indeed cooperate with initiating depot antipsychotics, careful consideration needs to be given to the details of treatment in terms of initial dosing; choice of drug, including payment limitations; and the handoff to the next level of care. Choosing a drug that cannot be delivered after discharge is a serious but avoidable error.

Long-acting depot antipsychotic medication is the medication of choice for patients who have a history of noncompliance (Pacchiarotti et al. 2019). These medications include older long-acting typical antipsychotic medications like haloperidol decanoate and fluphenazine decanoate. Newer long-acting depot medications include Invega Sustenna, Abilify Maintena, and Aristada. The older depot antipsychotics are more readily available but have more side effects, including akathisia, extrapyramidal side effects, and increased risk of tardive dyskinesia. We prefer the new atypical long-acting injectables, which are as effective and can get the patient to a therapeutic dose.

If depot antipsychotics are not indicated or agreed to, the inpatient team must still ensure that oral medications are being swallowed during the hospitalization. Some nonadherent patients will appear to take their medications but will not, in fact, do so, and this may necessitate administration of the medications in liquid form for a period of time. Medications utilized in liquid form include haloperidol, fluphenazine, risperidone, and lorazepam. The next best choice of medication is medication in the rapid dissolving form. Risperdal M-Tab and Zyprexa Zydis are some examples of this. These medications rapidly dissolve in the mouth in a few seconds and are difficult to cheek.

Mouth checks may be needed for some patients at the time of medication administration, or patients may need to be kept in view of staff for an hour or so. Administering the medication just once a day may be helpful, as well as writing an order to reoffer all refused doses of medications for the next three medication times within the next 24-hour medication cycle before documenting that day's medications as refused. This latter tactic has proved extremely helpful over the years. Many acutely relapsed patients are so disorganized that medication refusal is not really a rational decision. Offering the same medication that was refused at 9 A.M. again at 1 P.M., at 6 P.M., and at bedtime often results in successful administration as the patient's mood or suspiciousness fluctuates during the course of the day and with ongoing interaction with the other therapeutic aspects of the milieu, including one-to-one talks, peer conversations, illness educational classes, and family visits.

The second most important psychopharmacological principle is to find out what has or has not worked previously. Patients who are known to have done well on a certain regimen and who are agreeable to continuing that regimen should not be subjected to trials of newer medications unless there is a persuasive (preferably evidence-based) rationale for making a change.

In our experience, the patient population admitted to a psychotic disorders unit responds better to the older atypical antipsychotic medications, which are time tested and proven to be effective over and over again. These include olanzapine, risperidone, and quetiapine.

Dosing is occasionally an issue with successful antipsychotic treatment. There is good evidence that first-episode patients may respond to lower-than-average dosages of antipsychotics (Lieberman et al. 2003; McEvoy et al. 1991). However, a common problem in patients with persistent mental illness is that they receive dosages of medication that are too low and therefore insufficiently effective. Tobacco dependence may exacerbate this problem in some patients whose liver enzymes are induced by the effects of tar in the smoke, resulting in increased metabolism and clearance of antipsychotics. There is also a less well documented but nevertheless strongly held clinical observation that many patients with persistent mental illness have developed a tolerance to antipsychotics, resulting in a remarkable persistence of symptoms and lack of side effects in the face of objectively monitored robust dosing.

One strategy worth considering with such a scenario is to obtain antipsychotic serum levels. Such levels are not routinely available for the atypical antipsychotics and many of the typical agents, and even if available, they are not easily interpretable unless the result is zero or very high, given the lack of studies of clinical correlation. The one drug for which levels are reliably interpretable is haloperidol, which is fortunately a widely used product. The therapeutic plasma level is between 5 and 20 ng/mL. For example, obtaining a steady-state haloperidol level of 2 ng/mL in a patient taking 40 mg/day of elixir in a well-supervised inpatient setting suggests that rapid metabolism may indeed play a role in nonresponse. Such a finding might well lead to a decision to pursue an ultra-high-dosage strategy or switch to a product or a route (e.g., depot) that is more likely to achieve a therapeutic level. This problem can be further compounded by the artificially imposed vicissitudes of cigarette availability. In the contemporary environment, cigarette smoking is being eliminated altogether from many hospital campuses. The lack of access to cigarettes, coupled with the relatively longer length of stay with this population, may result in de-induction of liver enzyme metabolism during the course of inpatient treatment, with subsequent lowering of antipsychotic dosages. However, the patient may then have a relapse within a week of discharge because they return to smoking two packs a day or more and, as a result, the liver enzymes are re-induced.

Duration of treatment with antipsychotics cannot be emphasized enough in the assessment of response to treatment. Managed care has artificially distorted what has otherwise been extremely well documented since the 1960s (Casey et al. 1960)—namely, that antipsychotics take time to work. Even if rapid response to initial treatment results in quick behavioral improvement in some critical target behaviors, such as violence, the overall response to antipsychotic treatment can take up to 3 months to optimize and even as long as 6 months for clozapine (Conley et al. 1997). No amount of dosage increase will speed up this process once the dosage has reached the therapeutic threshold for a particular patient. Finding each patient's threshold has become a bit more difficult with the atypical antipsychotics, because there are often no side effects for documenting bioavailability of the dosing. Nevertheless, once an optimal dosage has been settled on, there is much value in waiting for the antipsychotic to show benefit before making changes, although the waiting may often be done at a lower level of care.

Because the illness of patients in the chronic population is by definition so characteristically treatment refractory, a structured, rational, and evidence-based approach to psychopharmacology is necessary. Between the complexity of the clinical presentation and the host of medications available, there is a very real danger of these patients winding up on all sorts of irrational polypharmacy regimens prescribed by well-intentioned but time-stressed psychiatrists or other physicians. It is quite common for patients to be admitted to the psychosis unit while taking two antipsychotics, and those taking three or even four can even be seen. Partly owing to the increased tolerability of the atypical antipsychotics, to the fact that antipsychotic medications are still frequently carved out from otherwise managed formularies, and also perhaps to the aggressive marketing of products, psychiatrists are often adding multiple antipsychotics for patients who continue to display refractory symptoms. It has been our experience that regimens of three and four antipsychotics are almost never necessary and that even combinations of typical and atypical antipsychotics beg the question, If the patient improved only after adding a full dose of a typical antipsychotic to an atypical one, what is the added value of continuing the atypical agent? The Texas Implementation of Medication Algorithms (TIMA) has provided a readily accessible web-based resource for guiding clinicians in the evidence-based sequential treatment of patients with refractory psychosis (Texas Department of State Health Services 2007). One may quibble with a detail here or there, but overall the TIMA is vastly superior to the ad hoc and idiosyncratic treatment combinations that arrive at our doorstep on admission. It also has built into it the same fundamental assumptions about adequate length of treatment trials described earlier.

Because the severely and persistently mentally ill population has illnesses that are so often treatment refractory, there is always a risk of unwarranted complacency with suboptimal outcomes. This is only further bolstered by the medical necessity standards of some commercial managed care companies, which appear to be structured to contain long-term risk with their psychotic patients, because such patients often transfer from the commercial policy risk pool to the public-sector risk pool (either Medicare, Medicaid, or local state hospital). We have often seen commercial managed care companies deny continued inpatient care for the sickest of young psychotic patients, not because these patients are not sick enough but because they are not making progress and thus are categorized as "custodial" and not meeting the contractual definition of "acute care."

Nevertheless, one should not succumb to economic pressures or despair. Rather, when faced with a failure in treatment, one must continue to take care of the patient, and the first medical consideration should always be a reevaluation of the diagnosis. The major differential diagnosis to consider when otherwise appropriate treatment for psychosis fails is a mood disorder. Kraepelin (1921) himself continued to reevaluate the validity of his famous dichotomy between dementia praecox and manic depression even at the end of his career, and mood disorders remain today the most common confounding syndromes in assessing persistently psychotic patients. Many of the patients admitted carry a diagnosis of schizoaffective disorder or severe bipolar disorder with psychotic symptoms. These patients are also treated with a mood stabilizer; the most common mood stabilizers are lithium and valproic acid. These medications are much easier to initiate on the unit. Valproic acid can be started as a loading dose regimen of 30 mg/kg body weight and then reduced to 20 mg/kg body weight (Martinez et al. 1998). This achieves mood stabilization much more rapidly than other medication, but it is not very effective in treating the depressive phase of patients with mood disorders. Lithium is more complicated to initiate and titrate, and takes longer to achieve a therapeutic response (Keck et al. 2000), but is much more effective in treating mania and depression.

Aggressive treatment for atypical mania, atypical depression, and coexisting anxiety disorders (including obsessional states and panic disorders) should always be considered in refractory cases. Other potential but harder-to-treat complications that may thwart forward progress in inpatient treatment include co-occurring personality disorders, personality changes due to other neurological disorders, dissociative disorders, and even malingering.

An additional item to manage and not to lightly dismiss is the somewhat vague but all-too-real problem of demoralization (Clarke and Kissane 2002). The ravages of chronic psychosis, which extend across the biopsychosocial continuum from cognitive decline at the biological level to the crushing of self-esteem and hope at the psychological level and to loss of friends, family, vocation/role, and income at the social level, can so converge and impact patients that they are left with virtually no reason or motivation to get out of bed every day and face the bleakness of current life circumstances. Such patients are extremely difficult to engage in any setting and represent the greatest collective fear we all experience when we hear that someone we love has schizophrenia.

Clozapine

Many of the patients admitted to this unit have been suffering from chronic psychotic illnesses for years, sometimes even decades. Some of them have not taken medication in months to years. The longer their duration of untreated psychosis, the poorer the prognosis and the longer it takes for them to respond to treatment (some may not respond at all). Our unit is a specialized unit that treats these very challenging patients in a relatively short period of time. Many of these patients present to the inpatient unit on a wide variety of medications. They are sometimes on "polypharmacy regimens," taking two to four antipsychotic medications at one time. These patients clearly have treatment-refractory illness and have been put on many medications in an effort to treat their symptoms, much to the frustration of their outpatient providers. These patients clearly meet the criteria to be started on clozapine, the one drug that is proven to be effective in treatment-refractory schizophrenia.

Clozapine is a complicated medication that is specifically indicated for treatment-refractory schizophrenia (Siskind et al. 2016). It has given patients with the most difficult to treat symptoms a chance to recover and improve their quality of life. Although this medication is difficult to initiate and titrate, the key message to understand is this: if your unit admits and treats patients with refractory schizophrenia, clozapine must be an available option in your pharmacological armamentarium. Not utilizing clozapine is a disservice to your patients. We routinely place patients on clozapine.

Although not the "magic bullet" it was originally touted to be (Wallis and Willwerth 1992), clozapine remains the gold standard for the treatment of refractory psychosis. The difficulty of using the drug is not to be minimized, however, because the problems with agranulocytosis are only the tip of the iceberg. Sedation, hypotension, tachycardia, constipation, drooling, enuresis, hyperthermia, myoclonic jerking, and generalized seizures are also common side effects, as are the more recently documented complications of weight gain, diabetes, acute myocarditis, and chronic cardiomyopathy. However difficult this drug can be to tolerate, many patients do so, and some patients have indeed been saved by it, remaining out of the hospital and living independently. Clozapine therefore remains an important therapeutic tool to offer the patient with a treatment-refractory illness. We believe that initiating patients on clozapine and managing the initial side effects of this drug on the psychotic disorders unit is one of the greatest services that we can do for these very seriously ill patients. The baton is then passed to the outpatient treatment team to continue with medication and monitor long-term side effects.

Chronic Psychoses and Nicotine

Another important point to add is the powerful role that cigarette smoking has had in the treatment of patients with chronic psychoses. The powerful attraction to nicotine observed in many patients with chronic illnesses has led to some fascinating research on the possible role of nicotinic receptors in the pathogenesis of psychotic symptoms (Simosky et al. 2002). The nursing management challenges associated with smoking are daunting and include problems such as theft, contraband, patient conflicts and assaults, and a never-ending barrage of smoking-related demands. We have made available to patients all forms of nicotine replacement (e.g., patch, lozenge, gum, inhaler). There are regular groups addressing cigarette smoking. There is a staff member who specializes in treating nicotine dependence and is available to speak to the patients if requested by the patient or staff member. Asking patients to make it a goal to quit cigarettes is an important part of the discussion during team meetings. Together, such interventions can significantly reduce the hostility and demandingness of the occasional patients for whom the smoke-free hospital is truly an additional stress compounding their already exacerbated illness.

Management of Side Effects

Managing medication side effects is an important consideration because it impacts patient safety, optimizes the patient's care experience, allows even the most thought-disordered patient to have a voice in their treatment, and can prevent future medication noncompliance.

Patients who are treated with typical antipsychotic medication are routinely started on anticholinergic medication as prophylaxis. The most common medication is benztropine; other options are diphenhydramine and trihexyphenidyl. There are some patients who may develop extrapyramidal symptoms, even if they are treated with a standing dose of prophylactic anticholinergic medication. The extrapyramidal symptoms are managed by adjusting the dose of the anticholinergic or antipsychotic medication. Other side effects of typical antipsychotics include akathisia, which is treated with β-blockers, anticholinergics, and benzodiazepines. Dystonic reactions, now relatively uncommon, are treated with injectable diphenhydramine or benztropine.

Patients treated with atypical antipsychotic medications experience fewer and less severe side effects than those treated with typical antipsychotic medication. Common side effects of these medications are sedation, orthostatic hypotension resulting in dizziness, unsteadiness, and increased risk of fall. These side effects are best managed by a slower titration of the medication and dosing medication mostly at night. Another common side effect is constipation, which is managed with prophylactic stool softeners and osmotic agents.

Other common side effects of medication are tremors from lithium and sodium valproate, sedation and increased risk of falls from benzodiazepines, and dry mouth, blurred vision, and constipation from anticholinergic medication.

Electroconvulsive Therapy

In addition to the utilization of clozapine, ECT is another option that must be considered in the treatment of difficult schizophrenia spectrum cases. Catatonic symptoms (Taylor and Fink 2003) and mood symptoms in schizophrenia will respond to ECT, as in any other mood disorder, and the same criteria should apply in both instances: severe symptoms, urgency of lifesaving treatment, and failure of pharmacological treatment. It should be remembered, however, that unlike bipolar I disorder, schizophrenia spectrum disorders will have enduring psychotic symptoms that persist even as the acute mood disorder remits with ECT. It is particularly important not to unduly continue ECT after the mood disorder symptoms have improved or to inappropriately target the residual schizophrenic positive and negative symptoms, which are unlikely to respond in any fundamental way to ECT. On the other hand, catatonic symptoms, especially frank stupor, whether seen in a pure mood disorder or in schizoaffective disorder or catatonic schizophrenia, usually respond well to ECT (Taylor and Fink 2003). Catatonic excitement is also a legitimate target for ECT. Some patients with schizophrenia or schizoaffective disorder who are unresponsive to psychopharmacology may also benefit from ECT (Fink and Sackeim 1996), including maintenance ambulatory ECT (Chanpattana and Andrade 2006).

Psychotherapies

The inpatient unit is designed to bring specialized care to the treatment of very sick patients, but it must not be forgotten that the setting is quite intentionally designed within a larger continuum of care. The criteria for inpatient treatment nowadays are extremely narrow and focused on the most acute and disturbed behaviors that threaten life and safety of the patient and/or others. Patients in such a state are, for the most part, deeply psychotic, and their capacity to engage in psychotherapy is consequently gravely diminished. By the time they are stabilized adequately to be able to engage in psychotherapy, they are usually considered ready for treatment at a lower level of care, such as partial hospitalization coupled with supervised residential care. In addition, the demands of contemporary inpatient medical practice, which place tremendous time and productivity pressures on psychiatrists in the context of high volumes of service, extensive documentation requirements, managed care reviews, and collateral meetings with team members and families, leave little time in the day for psychotherapy.

Evidence-based cognitive-behavioral psychotherapies have been utilized as components of treatment for patients with schizophrenia in Great Britain and Europe (Dickerson 2000); however, such modalities are difficult for the short-term crisis-oriented inpatient setting as it presently exists in the United States.

Learned behaviors may persist even after the patient has received stellar psychiatric treatment and superior psychopharmacological medication management. Identifying, strategizing, and analyzing critical elements of action is the focus of the behavior specialist. Through the use of a systematic scientific approach of applied behavior analysis, often referred to as ABA, the facilitator researches and thereby pinpoints crucial elements in behavior. Depending on the function of behavior, responses may need to be either increased or decreased to develop a suitable manner by which action is socially congruent with societal norms and allows the person to be rewarded with consequences that reinforce future positive responses.

Newly acquired skills are then relayed to community support members (e.g., relatives, friends, associates) so that they might gain a better understanding of how best to relate to their loved one and, in turn, not practice old and unrewarding behavior with the patient. It is essential to not only educate the community support structure but also provide practices before patients return to the community. This further strengthens the patient's ability to positively function well in society as they have in the inpatient environment. The goal of every plan is to use and generalize newly acquired skills in their home environment.

One of the most helpful things the inpatient team can do is to educate the patient and family about the existence of these therapies and to ensure a positive frame of their importance as the patient transitions to outpatient resources as part of comprehensive discharge planning.

Patient and Family Education

If intensive individual psychotherapy is not practicable for the acute inpatient setting, one can nevertheless attempt to educate patients and families about the core issues surrounding a diagnosis of schizophrenia or other severe and persistent mental illnesses. Particularly in the case of families experiencing a first episode of psychosis in their loved one, family members are often confused and scared and having difficulty understanding the enormity of what is happening. Beyond psychoeducation and treatment planning, they also need support and space to process. Will their loved one go back to who they were prior to the first break? Will they be able to resume college or maintain their job? What happens to all the hopes and dreams that the person had? And how does the family best support their loved one in staying healthy? These are important questions because the family's ability to better understand both the nature of the illness and how they can support their loved one is key to preventing nonadherence to treatment, preventing familial strain, and fortifying the support system for your patient postdischarge.

There has been significant progress in the availability of educational materials and existence of family support groups over the past generation. A variety of tools are available for illness education, including pamphlets, books, videos, and internet sites. It is important to help family members understand about good places to turn to for trusted information. The Sheppard Pratt website includes a "Knowledge Center" that provides information that has been reviewed by our experts and is updated regularly. Referral of patients and their families to their local chapter of NAMI (National Alliance on Mental Illness) and its excellent website is an equally important intervention in this regard. Personal support from other families managing the difficulties of schizophrenia should be recommended and has proven very helpful to many families.

Occupational and Recreational Therapies

Sheppard Pratt is considered the birthplace of occupational therapy. The practice of occupational therapy was formally developed in 1921 by Sheppard Pratt psychiatrist Dr. William Rush Dunton. Dr. Dunton was inspired by the use of purposeful activities and events to restore individuals' levels of functioning; he was also a proponent of the idea that "occupation is a basic human need, and that occupation is therapeutic." At Sheppard Pratt, these meaningful, therapeutic activities took place within the halls, on the grounds, and in dedicated spaces for such activities. Patients engaged in activities that were meaningful to them, such as gardening, farming, art, dancing, music, sports, and picnics.

The primary content focus of our rehabilitation groups is on illness and medication education. Patients leaving inpatient status should at least have a rudimentary grasp of what their illness is all about and the integral role of medication in their lifelong self-management of the illness. Because of these patients' cognitive deficits and psychotic symptoms, achieving such "psychoeducation" effectively is no small task and requires a good deal of flexibility and creativity on the part of the group leader. In addition to traditional group and didactic modalities, group leaders may rely on the same kind of multimodal sensory learning used in the education of children with ADHD, including rapid rotation from one modality to another and use of video, interactive educational games, and writing exercises to communicate a few essential teaching objectives. More ambitious goals, such as vocational assessment, social skills training, and life skills associated with successful independent living, must wait for lower levels of outpatient care in the continuum. The rehabilitation group leader is in an excellent position to provide the treatment team with valuable data about the patient's cognitive level, degree of disorganization, motivation, and negative symptoms, all of which can guide disposition planning to the extent that a continuum of different outpatient programming is actually available in the patient's geographical location.

Purely recreational groups, on the other hand, can be tremendously important. Contemporary psychiatric hospital design can provide secure, enclosed, but very attractive outdoor courtyard space that can offer patients fresh air and an opportunity to walk and experience the outdoor weather as well as offer quiet private space on a bench in the sun. Within the confines of the indoor unit, gross motor therapeutic activities associated with music and group participation, such as exercise and dance groups, can decrease tension and lead to a sense of community. The long hallways in hospitals lend themselves to a variety of bowling and pitching games with soft, quiet equipment. Arts and crafts activities are often nonthreatening and appealing to psychotic patients when they can experience mastery and pleasure and pride at creating something attractive that they can even proudly wear and call their own. In our setting, the television is usually not a primary focus of patient attention or interest. Likewise, reading is seldom the preferred activity of choice for most patients, usually because of significant impairment of attention and concentration. Music can be particularly soothing, and judicious use of relaxation music with natural sounds of waterfalls or rain or beach sounds can be very effective in quieting a milieu that has become overstimulated.

Other Modalities

The psychotic disorders unit is often the venue for treating patients with highly treatment-refractory conditions, often of considerable complexity. The ability to work with such patients in a safe, coherent, and controlled inpatient setting with an experienced multidisciplinary team is much needed for effective care for the chronically mentally ill. The inpatient stay in such a setting can be viewed as a unique opportunity, like the eye of a storm, to pause and reflect thoughtfully and, if possible, breathe new life into the treatment. For this to happen, of course, a certain vision must be established and maintained under the leadership of the psychiatrist as team leader. This vision is based on a deep commitment to empiricism and evidence-based diagnosis as well as evidence-based treatment. Time is spent in team meetings revisiting preliminary assessments of the patient during the course of the current treatment. The goal of such a comprehensive and synthesizing approach is to provide the patient, the family, and the outpatient team with a new perspective on the nature of the problem(s), the treatment, and the prognosis. At its best, such an inpatient stay serves as an extended consultation for the ongoing treatment of the patient, which, if well documented in an in-depth discharge summary that is proactively distributed to all the relevant members of the patient's treatment team, can provide an ongoing guidepost to future clinicians as they wrestle with an illness that is notoriously chronic and confusing.

Milieu Management

Managing a unit composed of psychotic people, particularly when the milieu has multiple agitated, disorganized, and aggressive patients, can be challenging. Despite progress in psychopharmacology in the past 50 years, effective inpatient management cannot be reduced to just aggressive medication practices (Coffman et al. 1987); in fact, overutilization of medication as the only strategy leads to unintended consequences for patients, greater risk of adverse reactions to medications, and increased risk of medication noncompliance based on the patient's experiences with receiving intramuscular injections or high dosages of sedating medications and their side effects.

Principles of a more generic "milieu therapy" may apply fruitfully in any inpatient setting, but a specifically behavioral focus for a psychotic disorders program remains helpful. General principles include 1) defining the patient and the target psychopathology using a robust behavioral perspective, with specific behavioral descriptors of the precipitants, reinforcers, and contingencies surrounding the target behaviors; 2) paying close attention to the degree of expressed emotion (Wearden et al. 2000) used by staff and making continuous efforts to minimize and re-express that emotion in more neutral ways; 3) minimizing reliance on complex higher-order verbal interpersonal interactions (such as might occur in confrontational or interactive community meetings) in favor of a simpler, more concrete problem-oriented review of the day's events and requirements; 4) avoiding any purposeful, although artificial, therapeutic "neutrality" in favor of a more globally affirming and continuously positive stance toward the patient; and 5) focusing on core activities of daily living that are typically disrupted in the course of an acute psychotic episode and that can often be taken for granted in higher-functioning nonpsychotic patient populations.

One tool that we have found to be useful is the incorporation of structured behavioral observations into the daily charting of the staff. Certain frequent and clinically urgent target behaviors are routinely queried and documented on every shift and include nighttime sleep, use of as-needed medication (and for which specific behaviors and contexts), incontinence, vomiting, and the use of any limit-setting interventions such as time-out in the bedroom or quiet room or use of seclusion or restraint. In addition, a dictionary of patient-specific target behaviors is used for any staff to spontaneously add to ongoing tracking of specific patients, including such things as yelling, cursing, threats, sexual self-stimulation, inappropriate touching of others, intrusive attention seeking, failure to get out of bed, or medication refusal. Such documentation can be readily reviewed, provide insight into whether treatment interventions (be they medical or behavioral) are helpful, and guide ongoing treatment planning.

The management of such a milieu, while challenging, can be done in a manner that provides better patient care, reduces risk of patient adverse events, minimizes risk of staff injury, and leads to a milieu that is conducive to the therapeutic process.

As in any other specialized setting, staff education is a necessary foundation. A common understanding of the illness, its symptoms, the cognitive deficits it manifests, and how a brain dysfunction impacts decision-making, impulsivity, aggression, and insight can lead to staff with greater understanding of the patient, greater empathy, and better ability to manage the milieu and work as a team.

This common understanding of psychosis informs how your unit is structured, the daily schedule, how to manage new admissions, and every other detail of unit functioning. We have found the following items to specifically aid in milieu functioning:

1. Having a core and committed staff that takes ownership for the well-functioning of the unit across all shifts

2. Training staff on behavior management (de la Fuente et al. 2019)
3. Practicing mock codes for high-risk events, such as aggression, to ensure that all staff are proficient and working in unison
4. Eliminating the situation in which patients are waiting in a line for medications or for meals
5. Identifying precautions for specific patients at greater risk for aggression and discussing management plans at each shift
6. Having an organized code process and identifying specific roles, similar to what occurs for CPR
7. Utilizing a root cause analysis structure to better understand through a fish-bone diagram the multiple areas for potential improvement
8. Enabling every member of the team to be involved in performance improvement activities, including utilization of Lean projects, that belong at the front line of care.

Management of Suicidal and Aggressive Behaviors

The psychotic patient presents certain unique challenges in terms of suicidal and aggressive behaviors. The suicidal impulses of an acutely psychotic person with schizophrenia can be particularly powerful, in part because of the compelling force of auditory and other hallucinations, which bring a whole new level of "reality" to the already depressed and/or frightened patient. Patients with schizophrenia may hurt themselves in a panic of violence in order to appease the command of "God" or the "Devil," or to escape the (mis)perceived threat from the paranoid "other," in which case death itself is viewed as a better outcome than the horror of being trapped by the other. The power of such delusions, coupled with tremendously real affective and often religious energy, can result in such acts as throwing oneself through a window, cutting (not scratching) clear through tendons and arteries, shooting oneself in the head with a shotgun, putting a knife into one's heart, setting oneself on fire, jumping in front of a subway train, or castrating oneself or removing one's eyes ("cast off the offending organ"). Simple overdosing is often not the schizophrenic way of suicide (Hunt et al. 2006).

Similarly, aggression directed toward others can be extreme and quite dangerous. In general, it is fair to say that violence comes with the territory when running a psychotic disorders inpatient program. Persecutory delusions, ideas of reference, and thought broadcasting can all create a state of panic or hostility in patients that makes them a potential risk to themselves, peers, visitors, and staff. Although scrupulously careful and appropriate psychopharmacology can certainly mitigate such violence, it is not a panacea, especially for the acutely admitted patient. First-episode patients, substance-intoxicated patients, patients who have suffered abuse, manic patients, head-injured patients, patients with intellectual disability, antisocial patients, and patients with treatment-refractory illnesses all can present an increased risk of violence.

The psychopharmacological approach to violence is straightforward and evidence based and has been well described repeatedly in the literature (Petit 2005). Besides such psychopharmacological interventions, it is imperative for the staff to have training and confidence in behavioral approaches to the agitated patient. Principles of effective management of the potentially violent patient include 1) transparency and clarity in explaining the rules of the milieu and the patient's legal rights; 2) a neutral but respectful attitude toward the patient at all times, even when the patient is menacing or grossly out of control; 3) avoidance of any threats, coupled with clear limits on what is and is not tolerated in the milieu; 4) recognition and management of staff countertransference that can impact the therapeutic relationship and poison any treatment alliance; and 5) availability of expertly trained staff to ensure safety in as humane and safe a way as possible.

Perhaps the single most important rule to follow, but not always the easiest, is the prompt and effective confrontation of threatening behavior when it first occurs. The failure to intervene immediately, with a clear expression to the patient of the nature and reason for the limit, the possible consequences, and the need to accept additional therapeutics from the staff, almost invariably leads to "escalation" of the aggressive behavior until it reaches a crisis that may, by that point, unavoidably result in someone being injured. The choices of additional therapeutics that should be presented to the out-of-control patient are diverse and include providing as-needed medication, adding a new medication, changing to a different medication, taking a time-out, making restitution to a peer, and removing oneself from the milieu in general or from a specific peer or staff member. Teaching staff to be facile with any and all of these options, either singly or in combination, can greatly enhance the therapeutic leverage of the team and is certainly more helpful than merely relying on as-needed medications.

Seclusion and restraint in particular are often considered when dealing with the acutely psychotic patient. This can begin before the hospitalization, if the police need to subdue a violent patient emergently or if the emergency department staff need to seclude or restrain the patient. To be sure, seclusion and restraint are, and should always be, the last resort in responding to the potential for violence in psychotic patients. Restraints can at times exacerbate fear because of the total helplessness and consequent vulnerability the patient experiences, coupled with the psychotic distortions that convince the patient that the people in control are lying and wish to kill him or her. Every effort should be made to avoid using seclusion and restraint or, if not possible, to minimize their duration and address any iatrogenic morbidity that they may introduce. Nevertheless, it must be said that in our experience, complete renunciation of seclusion and restraint with the psychotic population has never been possible, and seclusion and restraint remain a necessary option in the safe management of psychotically aggressive patients.

Discharge Planning

Involvement of Community Providers, Resources, and Significant Others

The effective treatment of the persistently psychotic patient must always be considered within the broader context of the patient's ongoing outpatient treatment and rehabilitation/housing situation. It is incumbent upon the inpatient program to reach out to the outpatient treatment team, including family and significant others, to do more than merely check a box; rather, the purpose is to support and strengthen a complicated biopsychosocial system in crisis. Remarkably, despite the ravages of managed care, the inpatient team usually still has more resources at its disposal than the beleaguered outpatient team and can create a kind of therapeutic shelter or interlude during which the relevant parties can afford to (briefly) pause and reassess the entire treatment system, determining what may need to be changed. We routinely arrange team conferences with family, outpatient case managers, housing care providers, and service coordinators from other agencies such as developmental disabilities services, social services, protective services, vocational services, educational services, and mobile treatment (or assertive community treatment) teams. We also find that utilizing technology such as videoconferencing is an invaluable way to engage concerned outpatient parties who cannot physically attend such conferences and to keep the discussion totally transparent to the patient. We have found that direct contact with the outpatient treatment providers, including the outpatient psychiatrist, is paramount to effective and collaborative treatment which then leads a warm handoff that is for the patient's benefit.

Families are always relevant in helping the chronically mentally ill. We always begin with the view of the family as an ally. We try to join with them, form a shared therapeutic alliance, and learn from them as much as we can: What motivates the patient? To whom is the patient closest? To whom will he or she listen? Why does the patient feel this way or that?

Working with the patient's family is one of the most important aspects of patient care and discharge planning. Patients come from all over the country and from different situations. Some are homeless, some have families that are "burnt out" because of the patient's illness, some have families that want to be involved but have very few resources, and some patients live in residential programs and group homes and have no involved family members and the group home provider or the residential staff may be closest thing to a family for them. Establishing a shared therapeutic alliance with the family is one of the best steps that we can take to help the patient, especially with regards to discharge planning.

If supporting the patient in the home of 80-year-old parents has become too much, we try to facilitate disengagement and transition to a new developmental level. If the patient's risk of violence has become too great, we provide specific warning and legal advice. Although one must of course obtain the patient's consent to collaborate with the family in this way, such collaboration is critical to long-term success.

When families are actively caring for their relative with persistent mental illness, the old-fashioned "individual therapy" patient-centric model may be completely inappropriate and even hurtful; it should be utilized only on a case-by-case basis when there are specific clinical reasons for following such a model (Glynn et al. 2006).

Transition to Next Level of Care

Despite the economic pressures to discharge patients as soon as they cease being aggressive or self-destructive, the clinical fact remains that psychotic patients remain fragile for some time even after the more florid symptoms remit. Finding appropriate transitional levels of care is imperative; however, in most communities across the nation, this can be quite challenging. In our uniquely American health insurance paradigm, so-called acute treatment (i.e., short-term hospital care) is paid for by most commercial insurances, but "chronic" or "rehabilitation" or "custodial" services are viewed as uncovered and hence the responsibility of the public sector, the family if they have resources, or no one at all in many instances.

The classic Kraepelinian failure to ever fully recover (*restitutio ad integrum*) from what Adolf Meyer later called "the life break" (Meyer and Winters 1950) is a concept that in contemporary America translates functionally into chronic disability and poverty. Disabled patients may become eligible for Social Security Disability Insurance (which comes with Medicare) or Supplemental Security Income (which comes with Medicaid), but getting these entitlements is no small task, and the difficulty in obtaining these benefits varies depending on who happens to fill the seat of the president for federal entitlements, or which governor is deciding state policy such as criteria for who qualifies for Medicaid or whether the state will expand Medicaid access. Without these entitlements, paying for long-term ancillary services in the community can be impossible.

It is not uncommon, for example, for the newly psychotic child of middle-class parents with good commercial insurance to be unable to access the local psychiatric rehabilitation program because it is not possible to get Medicaid and neither the commercial insurer nor Medicare will pay for it. Commercial insurers, to this day, astoundingly refuse to approve long-acting injectable medications that have now become the hallmark for treatment of patients with medication noncompliance. Likewise, paying for housing can be a tremendous obstacle to successful community adjustment for the person with persistent mental illness. Although some states may have dedicated funding lines to provide supervised residential care for the mentally ill, access often requires years of being on waiting lists. In urban areas of many states, a literal cottage industry has evolved in the past 30 years in which local homeowners will rent out rooms and provide meals and sometimes medication supervision ("board and care"). In our setting, Sheppard Pratt has understood the value of investment in a continuum of services, including residential services. Across our system of care, we now have more than 1,200 temporary and long-term supportive housing slots throughout our geography.

Crisis Bed Stabilization

Our hospital is fortunate to have established a crisis bed stabilization program at strategic locations across the state. Each program has 16–20 crisis beds that can be utilized for patients who are being discharged from the hospital and need some level of supervision and structure. Patients are able to reside at this program for 1–3 weeks. This is a temporary but much needed option. Our unit works closely with crisis bed staff and has an open line of communication, which helps a great deal in facilitating the patients' discharge to this level of care. Medication is supervised by staff, although the patients are expected to take their medication on their own. Case management is provided by staff in order to help patients transition back into the community.

Specialty Day Hospital

Because the transitional period can be a vulnerable one for patients recovering from an acute psychosis, there is a role for a day hospital model, also known as *partial hospital,* that delivers programming specifically tailored to the persistently ill patient. General partial hospital programs, which are run out of a psychiatric unit embedded in a general hospital, are typically geared for higher-functioning patients, with programming that emphasizes recovery and return to work and family. The persistently ill patient struggles in this environment, precisely because the high-functioning patients are no longer so symptomatic and wish to focus on higher-level problem solving.

We have a specialized partial hospital program that is specifically designed for and focuses on the treatment of patients who suffer from psychosis and other chronic mental illnesses, are intellectually limited, and in general are "lower functioning." This is one of the few partial programs in the country that specialize in treating the chronic psychotic population. The staff are trained and specialize in working with this cohort of patients. Whereas patients on the inpatient unit are not there long enough when they are stable to benefit from social skills groups, such as a cooking group, they can definitely take advantage of such occupational therapy programming in a partial setting. Coordinating such a day hospital with the inpatient unit allows for continuity of physician coverage as the patient is stepped down to a lower level of care and exposed to a higher level of psychosocial stress and performance demands. This can be invaluable when medications need to then subsequently be adjusted. A registered nurse can coordinate closely with the care provider, and a social worker can do family work now that the patient is back at home.

Conclusion

Treating patients with psychotic disorders is difficult and challenging. Treating these patients in a private, non–state hospital setting on a specialized unit for a shorter period of time and using an evidence-based approach—which is more than just crisis intervention—presents our definition of specialty care that you would want if it was your loved one.

Over the past 35 years, this unit has developed a specialized set of skills and programming to treat this difficult population, who in the past were only treated adequately for long periods of time, in state hospital settings. Utilizing a combination of evidence-based psychopharmacology, behavior modification, various psychosocial interventions, specialized nursing care, and our step-down programs as an extension for this very impaired and vulnerable population helps us to provide state-of-the-art, evidence-based treatment.

In summary, the treatment of psychotic patients requires specialty care. Specialty care is provided in chronic disease programs across medicine, such as a cystic fibrosis program in a children's hospital, a high-risk pregnancy program in maternal-fetal medicine, and an oncology unit in a general hospital. Although length of stay in the hospital has been greatly shortened, the severity of illness and psychosocial needs of this very vulnerable population have not decreased. Creative programming that targets these patients with specialized services can result in better outcomes, occasionally dramatically so. Such programming speaks well of the progress that the mental health professions together have made over the years in bringing rational, caring, and effective therapeutics to the sickest patients we treat. There are still too many seriously mentally ill individuals in communities across our nation who are unnecessarily homeless or incarcerated because of an absence of access to such care. This is work we can all be proud of, and work that we must all engage in across our nation, for these patients and their families need us to create access to meaningful, high-quality care.

References

Arnetz JE, Hamblin L, Russell J, et al: Preventing patient-to-worker violence in hospitals: outcome of a randomized controlled intervention. J Occup Environ Med 59(1):18–27, 2017 28045793

Beck LH, Bransome ED Jr, Mirsky AF, et al: A continuous performance test of brain damage. J Consult Psychol 20(5):343–350, 1956 13367264

Berg EA: A simple objective technique for measuring flexibility in thinking. J Gen Psychol 39:15–22, 1948 18889466

Casey JF, Bennett IF, Lindley CJ, et al: Drug therapy in schizophrenia: a controlled study of the relative effectiveness of chlorpromazine, promazine, phenobarbital, and placebo. AMA Arch Gen Psychiatry 2:210–220, 1960 13808145

Chanpattana W, Andrade C: ECT for treatment-resistant schizophrenia: a response from the Far East to the UK. NICE report. J ECT 22(1):4–12, 2006 16633199

Clarke DM, Kissane DW: Demoralization: its phenomenology and importance. Aust N Z J Psychiatry 36(6):733–742, 2002 12406115

Coffman JA, Nasrallah HA, Lyskowski J, et al: Clinical effectiveness of oral and parenteral rapid neuroleptization. J Clin Psychiatry 48(1):20–24, 1987 3542982

Conley RR, Carpenter WT Jr, Tamminga CA: Time to clozapine response in a standardized trial. Am J Psychiatry 154(9):1243–1247, 1997 9286183

de la Fuente M, Schoenfisch A, Wadsworth B, et al: Impact of behavior management training on nurses' confidence in managing patient aggression. J Nurs Adm 49(2):73–78, 2019 30633062

Dickerson FB: Cognitive behavioral psychotherapy for schizophrenia: a review of recent empirical studies. Schizophr Res 43(2–3):71–90, 2000 10858626

Fink M, Sackeim HA: Convulsive therapy in schizophrenia? Schizophr Bull 22(1):27–39, 1996 8685661

Glazer WM, Kane JM: Depot neuroleptic therapy: an underutilized treatment option. J Clin Psychiatry 53(12):426–433, 1992 1362569

Glynn SM, Cohen AN, Dixon LB, Niv N: The potential impact of the recovery movement on family interventions for schizophrenia: opportunities and obstacles. Schizophr Bull 32(3):451–463, 2006 16525087

Green AI, Drake RE, Brunette MF, Noordsy DL: Schizophrenia and co-occurring substance use disorder. Am J Psychiatry 164(3):402–408, 2007 17329463

Hunt IM, Kapur N, Windfuhr K, et al: Suicide in schizophrenia: findings from a national clinical survey. J Psychiatr Pract 12(3):139–147, 2006 16732132

Iglesias Garcia LE, Iglesias Alonso A, Bobes J: Concentrations in plasma clozapine levels in schizophrenic and schizoaffective patients. Rev Psiquiatr Salud Ment 10(4):192–196, 2017 28844295

Jastak JF, Jastak SR, Wilkinson GS: The Wide Range Achievement Test, Revised 2. Wilmington, Guidance Associates of Delaware, 1993

Kane JM, Kishimoto T, Correll CU: Non-adherence to medication in patients with psychotic disorders: epidemiology, contributing factors and management strategies. World Psychiatry 12(3):216–226, 2013 24096780

Keck PE Jr, McElroy SL, Bennett JA: Pharmacologic loading in the treatment of acute mania. Bipolar Disord 2(1):42–46, 2000 11254019

Kraepelin E: Manic-Depressive Insanity and Paranoia. Edinburgh, Scotland, Churchill Livingstone, 1921

Kraepelin E, Quen JM: Psychiatry: A Textbook for Students and Physicians. Canton, MA, Science History Publications, 1990

Krakowski M, Czobor P, Chou JC: Course of violence in patients with schizophrenia: relationship to clinical symptoms. Schizophr Bull 25(3):505–517, 1999 10478785

Kurland AA, Richardson JH: A comparative study of two long acting phenothiazine preparations, fluphenazine-enanthate and fluphenazine-decanoate. Psychopharmacology (Berl) 9(4):320–327, 1966 4871473

Lacro JP, Dunn LB, Dolder CR, et al: Prevalence of and risk factors for medication nonadherence in patients with schizophrenia: a comprehensive review of recent literature. J Clin Psychiatry 63(10):892–909, 2002 12416599

Lieberman JA, Tollefson G, Tohen M, et al: Comparative efficacy and safety of atypical and conventional antipsychotic drugs in first-episode psychosis: a randomized, double-blind trial of olanzapine versus haloperidol. Am J Psychiatry 160(8):1396–1404, 2003 12900300

Lieberman JA, Stroup TS, McEvoy JP, et al: Effectiveness of antipsychotic drugs in patients with chronic schizophrenia. N Engl J Med 353(12):1209–1223, 2005 16172203

Martinez JM, Russell JM, Hirschfeld RM: Tolerability of oral loading of divalproex sodium in the treatment of acute mania. Depress Anxiety 7(2):83–86, 1998 9614597

McEvoy JP, Hogarty GE, Steingard S: Optimal dose of neuroleptic in acute schizophrenia: a controlled study of the neuroleptic threshold and higher haloperidol dose. Arch Gen Psychiatry 48(8):739–745, 1991 1883257

Meyer A, Winters EE: The Collected Papers of Adolf Meyer. Baltimore, MD, Johns Hopkins University Press, 1950

Pacchiarotti I, Tiihonen J, Kotzalidis GD, et al: Long-acting injectable antipsychotics (LAIs) for maintenance treatment of bipolar and schizoaffective disorders: a systematic review. Eur Neuropsychopharmacol 29(4):457–470, 2019 30770235

Petit JR: Management of the acutely violent patient. Psychiatr Clin North Am 28(3):701–711, 710, 2005 16122575

Roca RP, Charen B, Boronow J: Ensuring staff safety when treating potentially violent patients. JAMA 316(24):2669–2670, 2016 28027370

Sheitman BB, Lee H, Strous R, Lieberman JA: The evaluation and treatment of first-episode psychosis. Schizophr Bull 23(4):653–661, 1997 9366001

Simosky JK, Stevens KE, Freedman R: Nicotinic agonists and psychosis. Curr Drug Targets CNS Neurol Disord 1(2):149–162, 2002 12769624

Siskind D, McCartney L, Goldschlager R, Kisely S: Clozapine v. first- and second-generation antipsychotics in treatment-refractory schizophrenia: systematic review and meta-analysis. Br J Psychiatry 209(5):385–392, 2016 27388573

Skikic M, Arriola JA: First episode psychosis medical workup: evidence-informed recommendations and introduction to a clinically guided approach. Child Adolesc Psychiatr Clin N Am 29(1):15–28, 2020 31708044

Steinert T, Wiebe C, Gebhardt RP: Aggressive behavior against self and others among first-admission patients with schizophrenia. Psychiatr Serv 50(1):85–90, 1999 9890585

Taylor MA, Fink M: Catatonia in psychiatric classification: a home of its own. Am J Psychiatry 160(7):1233–1241, 2003 12832234

Texas Department of State Health Services: Texas Implementation of Medication Algorithms. Austin, Texas Department of State Health Services, 2007. Available at: www.dshs.state.tx.us/mhprograms/TIMA.shtm. Accessed April 21, 2007.

University of Pennsylvania Health System: In the Beginning: The Story of the Creation of the Nation's First Hospital. Philadelphia, University of Pennsylvania Health System, 2007. Available at: www.uphs.upenn.edu/paharc/features/creation.html. Accessed April 15, 2007.

Wade M, Tai S, Awenat Y, Haddock G: A systematic review of service-user reasons for adherence and nonadherence to neuroleptic medication in psychosis. Clin Psychol Rev 51:75–95, 2017 27838461

Wallis C, Willwerth J: Awakenings: schizophrenia: a new drug brings patients back to life. Time, July 6, 1992, p 57

Wearden AJ, Tarrier N, Barrowclough C, et al: A review of expressed emotion research in health care. Clin Psychol Rev 20(5):633–666, 2000 10860170

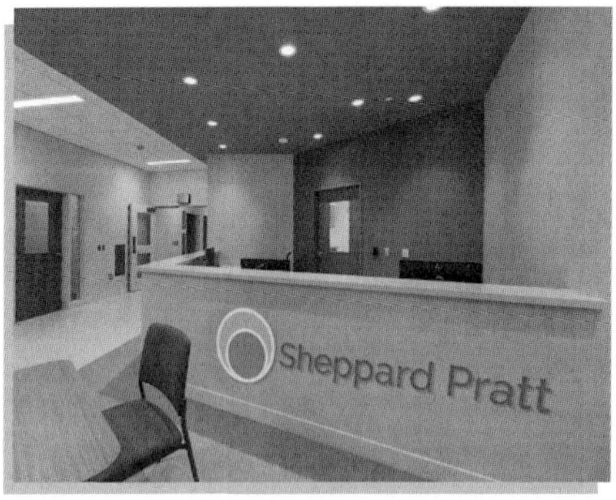

CHAPTER 10

The Substance Use Disorders Co-occurring Unit

Sunil Khushalani, M.D., DFAPA, FASAM
George Kolodner, M.D., DLFAPA, FASAM

The co-occurring disorders inpatient unit focuses on the treatment (stabilization) of patients with co-occurring disorders of a severity that has caused them to become too unsafe or unstable to be treated at an outpatient level of care. We describe one such unit in a freestanding psychiatric hospital. Units that deal with co-occurring disorders exclusively are not very common.

What *co-occurring* refers to here is the co-occurrence of psychiatric and substance use disorders. Unlike general adult units, where some patients might have co-occurring disorders, all patients on a co-occurring disorders unit have co-occurring disorders but may exhibit different degrees of comorbid conditions. A co-occurring disorders unit also focuses on dealing with and stabilizing the psychiatric conditions of its patients. This differs from an addiction-only unit, which might focus solely on withdrawal management and getting patients ready for recovery. It would be difficult for any patient to focus on their recovery unless their psychiatric condition was stabilized.

This may seem straightforward on the surface because all patients with co-occurring disorders would have similar issues, but it is actually challenging because the variety of combinations of psychiatric and addictive disorders is tremendous. This endless variety can make group programming on the unit challenging. In addition, the needs of this population can be incredibly diverse, and the overall care ultimately depends on what resources are available on the unit and what is available to the patients when they are discharged back into their communities.

The presence of an active substance use disorder (SUD) in a patient with another psychiatric disorder can be challenging and even daunting to behavioral health clinicians. While recovery from SUDs is common, many clinicians have not encountered such a positive outcome. The therapeutic pessimism that can accompany the negative previous experiences can provide an additional obstacle to treatment.

While the behavior of such patients demands attention and requires skillful limit setting, maintaining an empathic focus on the patient's experience can facilitate the establishment of the trusting, therapeutic relationship that is so critical to successful treatment and full recovery in the long haul.

Case Vignette

Shirley had been struggling with recurrent depression, social anxiety, and PTSD for years. She had a history of sexual trauma as a child and physical trauma as an adult. She reported multiple adverse childhood experiences. Whenever her depression got worse, she also would become more anxious. At such times, she would drink alcohol to obtain temporary relief from these symptoms. She would often have suicidal thoughts and gestures when intoxicated, leading her to be referred to the co-occurring unit by her outpatient team. Whenever she would try to stop drinking and receive treatment for withdrawal on the inpatient unit, her flashbacks and nightmares would get worse. If she drank regularly, her depression would get worse. She was never completely comfortable in group settings. She had always been shy as a person and felt more anxious in the company of strangers. Speaking up had always been hard in school. She could not easily engage in 12-step meetings or in intensive outpatient programs because of her discomfort with groups. Shirley and her physician on the inpatient unit were both in a quandary as to finding appropriate outpatient structured programs for her in the early stages of her recovery that would provide her with the support that was necessary for her at this early stage.

Conceptual Framework

SUDs are best understood as a complex interplay of biological, psychological, and social factors. Excluding any of these elements reduces the likelihood of a positive treatment outcome.

The biological vulnerability to SUDs has generated skepticism in the past despite corroborating evidence from well-executed twin and adoption studies. More recently, neuroimaging studies have provided an opportunity to correlate patients' response to substances with visualization of brain activity. The result has been a substantial increase in our understanding of the neurobiological correlates of clinical experiences (Volkow et al. 2016).

The concept of a preexisting "addictive personality" persists despite the absence of evidence to support it. The best prospective studies of alcohol use disorder found that the personality traits often cited (dependency, depression, and sociopathy) are the *result of* rather than the precursors of the disorder (Vaillant 2012).

SUDs are best regarded as chronic conditions with acute features, akin to diabetes. The goal of treatment is *recovery*, not "cure," in that a return to normal substance use (effortless non–problem use) is unlikely. Discussions of what qualifies as "recovery" and "abstinence" can spark debate, particularly since the use of opioid agonist medications has become more widespread. Most definitions attempt to incorporate, but do not limit themselves to, the issue of substance use. Here is one definition of recovery as articulated by the American Society of Addiction Medicine (ASAM):

> A process of sustained action that addresses the biological, psychological, social and spiritual disturbances inherent in addiction. Recovery aims to improve the quality of life by seeking balance and healing in all aspects of health and wellness, while addressing an individual's consistent pursuit of abstinence, impairment in behavioral control, dealing with cravings, recognizing problems in one's behaviors and interpersonal relationships, and dealing more effectively with emotional responses. An individual's recovery actions lead to reversal of negative, self-defeating internal processes and behaviors, allowing healing of relationships with self and others. The concepts of acceptance and surrender are also useful in this process. (American Society of Addiction Medicine 2013)

Because recovery is seen as a never-ending, lifelong process, referring to someone as "recovering" or "being in recovery" is preferred to "recovered." For the same reason, the use of the prefix "ex-," as in "ex-alcoholic," is to be avoided.

One exception to the use of the prefix "ex-" is in the context of tobacco, where the term *ex-smoker* is commonly used. Tobacco use disorder is included in DSM-5 (American Psychiatric Association 2013), although the term "nicotine use disorder" would be more accurate given the recent increase in the use of nontobacco inhalers such as vaping. Both the recovery community and the professional addiction treatment community have downplayed any danger that continued tobacco use poses to abstinence from other addictive substances. Evidence to the contrary, however, is beginning to emerge (Weinberger et al. 2017).

Abstinence from all addictive substances is the strategy that is associated with the most favorable treatment outcomes. Even if a substance has been used nonaddictively, continued use increases the likelihood that patients will return to using their "drug of choice." Furthermore, many of these substances can be deleterious to another psychiatric disorder that the co-occurring patient is struggling to manage.

Harm reduction is an approach that focuses on reducing the damage caused by the substance rather than on abstinence. The evidence for the benefits of needle exchange, for example, is clear—reducing the transmission of infectious diseases without increasing the incidence of addiction. Nevertheless, political controversy persists and can create obstacles for public funding and broader acceptance.

Description of the Co-occurring Unit

A co-occurring inpatient unit is not a rehabilitation facility ("rehab"), but it could be a starting point in the process of recovery. It is generally a short-term unit. The average length of stay on the unit we describe is 7–8 days. Since this is such a short period, and there could be an interplay of variables such as intoxication or withdrawal syndromes, unstable psychiatric conditions, and biomedical conditions, treatment on such a unit requires highly skilled assessments, effective management, and careful planning.

There is no fixed length of stay on this unit. The length of stay varies depending on several factors, some of which are patient related and others of which are dependent on the resources available to each patient for their aftercare. Available resources can vary by patients' geography and insurance, and this can affect a patient's length of stay.

Unlike an inpatient or outpatient program that deals just with patients who come in voluntarily, a co-occurring inpatient unit could receive patients admitted either voluntarily or involuntarily. Management of the milieu and conducting groups on such a unit are complex because the unit usually ends up having a mixture of both voluntary and involuntary patients.

Some psychiatric patients who are undergoing treatment for alcohol or opioid withdrawal are also in need of monitoring for suicidal or aggressive behavior. Some other patients who misuse stimulants or synthetic cannabis, for instance, can present in very disorganized, agitated, or psychotic states that might require management on a co-occurring disorders unit. Each of these patients could be in a different stage of alertness, stability, or motivation.

Staff on such units need to be familiar with the psychopathology of addiction, substances that cause addiction, associated problems that accompany addictions, and presentations during intoxication and withdrawal management phases. Staff also need to understand the nature of psychiatric disorders, from mood disorders to psychotic disorders, trauma disorders, and personality disorders, as well as their treatments. There is a bidirectional relationship between addiction and psychiatric disorders, such that an understanding of just one set of issues is not enough in the adequate management of these complex cases.

Case Vignette

Paul was admitted as a psychiatric inpatient for the first time for his first manic episode. He had also been using crack cocaine on a daily basis for the last 2 weeks, and he had not slept for more than an hour or two since the misuse started. He presented to the unit as an involuntary patient with rapid speech and labile and irritable mood. He had a very hard time getting along with everyone on the unit and could become loud and disruptive. At night, he would pace the hallways on the unit, screaming loudly and demanding beverages and snacks because he felt very hungry. "I would not mind a cold beer, it's so hot in here," he once said. When he attended groups, he tended to dominate or interrupt others as they tried to speak. He also would confront others and insisted on telling them "the truth," which he insisted others should hear. The other patients were very upset at him and thought of him as very arrogant and rude. Two other male patients wanted to beat him up because they felt that he had insulted them. They also felt that he should not be on the unit because he was not interested in his recovery.

Social issues such as legal charges or homelessness may lead to the admission of such patients to inpatient units. These issues can make discharging back into the community challenging. Psychiatric, addictive, and medical conditions can also make disposition difficult because not all aftercare facilities are equipped, staffed, or willing to deal with such challenges. Sometimes, social issues are underlying the patient's psychological distress, such as when a patient continues to verbalize suicidal ideation until a residential program becomes available. These conditional suicidal thoughts may stop once a disposition becomes clearly available. Cases like these can often increase the average length of stay on the inpatient unit.

A *multidisciplinary team* that includes physicians, nurses, social workers, addiction counselors, pharmacists, rehabilitation therapists, and mental health technicians provides *integrated* care for patients on this unit.

Clinicians often lack the combined expertise for treating both psychiatric and addictive disorders (Wüsthoff et al. 2014). In the past, this led to either *sequential* or *parallel* treatment.

In *sequential* treatment the thinking was that the treatment of both psychiatric and addictive disorders should be separate. The expectation was that the individual would stabilize one kind of disorder prior to enrolling in treatment for the other. Usually, the patient was expected to have their addictions stabilized first, before their psychiatric conditions could be addressed. Such a treatment model was usually a way to exclude such patients rather than welcome them into treatment (Mueser 2003). While it defended its own programmatic boundaries, this approach did not serve the needs of the individual or the needs of the larger system. It also disregarded the interactive nature of co-occurring disorders, which led to poor outcomes.

In *parallel* treatment, the patient was expected to address both of these disorders concurrently, either in different settings or with different teams. The approach did not amount to a cohesive treatment approach. The coordination of care was left up to the patient because the two sets of providers or teams rarely communicated. Sometimes the two kinds of programs had conflicting treatment philosophies. For instance, providers in the addiction program could be confrontational with the patient, hoping that such a strategy would overcome the denial or the rationalizations of a patient suffering from addictions. On the other hand, providers in the mental health program would believe that confrontation could have harmful effects on the patient and lead to their worsening. Parallel treatment, like sequential treatment, led to poor outcomes.

Since the 1980s, integrated treatment has been recommended for the treatment of co-occurring disorders; in this approach, the same team provides care for both kinds of disorders at the same place concurrently (Minkoff 1989).

The ASAM Criteria (Lindner et al. 2013), formerly known as the ASAM Patient Placement Criteria, constitute a nationally recognized set of comprehensive guidelines. These criteria can guide placement, continued stay, and transfer or discharge of patients with co-occurring disorders. The ASAM Criteria facilitate the development of treatment plans through a multidimensional assessment of patients. From this assessment, various levels of treatment can be recommended depending on the extent of direct medical management provided as well as the structure, safety, and intensity of treatment services.

An ASAM level 4, which typically describes care that patients receive in co-occurring inpatient units, is labeled as a "medically managed intensive inpatient service." This level offers 24-hour nursing care and daily physician care for severe, unstable problems in what ASAM considers the first three of the six dimensions of multidimensional assessment. Dimension 1 refers to assessment of a patient's past and current use and need for withdrawal management. Dimension 2 refers to a patient's biomedical history and complications of their biomedical condition. Dimension 3 refers to emotional, behavioral, and cognitive conditions that require stabilization. As one can see from these first three dimensions, many patients on a co-occurring inpatient unit may require help in one or more of these dimensions. Dimension 4 deals with a patient's readiness to change or interest in changing. Dimension 5 addresses the potential for relapse, continued use, or continued problem potential. Finally, Dimension 6 assesses an individual's recovery or living situation, and the surrounding people, places, and things. The last three dimensions can help the treatment team in creating an individualized plan of care for a patient.

Inpatient psychiatric units can be *co-occurring capable* (COC) or *co-occurring enhanced* (COE) (Gotham et al. 2010). The unit we describe belongs to the latter category. COC treatment programs accommodate individuals with SUDs that are relatively stable. COE treatment programs accommodate individuals with acute and unstable substance use disorders.

Goals of Treatment

Typically, patients are admitted to a co-occurring inpatient unit because of *safety* concerns or because *acute stabilization* is needed. Safety concerns are articulated either by the patient or by others. There could be concerns of suicide, homicide, aggression, poor ability to care for self, or issues of safety due to withdrawal from alcohol or other substances. Withdrawal from opioids can be very uncomfortable, and withdrawal from alcohol, benzodiazepines, and barbiturates (which are rarely a reason for admission today) can be life-threatening and require immediate intervention. Many admissions today are prompted by opioid overdoses (due to heroin that with increasing frequency is being admixed with or replaced by fentanyl analogues). Sometimes addictive or psychiatric disorders can destabilize medical conditions like diabetes or a seizure disorder that, as a result, may need to be monitored or managed on an inpatient unit. A determination is made prior to admission regarding whether the medical needs of the unstable patient can be managed on the inpatient psychiatric unit.

Patients can present with a variety of problems, including mood or anxiety disorders, psychotic disorders, and cognitive disorders, that can be antecedents to their presenting symptoms. They could be in withdrawal from alcohol and/or other substances, which can complicate their presentations. Patients can also be suffering from chronic pain, severe insomnia, or flashbacks that can be very distressing to them. *Symptom reduction* usually then becomes an initial goal for treatment for the patient or their family.

One of the initial tasks for the treatment team is to aim for *diagnostic clarification*. Sometimes, patients have underlying primary psychiatric disorders that began prior to the onset of addictions. At other times, the misuse of alcohol or other substances leads to psychiatric presentations. Sometimes, when patients present in a crisis emergently, it is hard to distinguish what is primary or what is secondary because patients cannot remember what started first or they are poor historians and are not able to provide comprehensive details. One of the guiding principles of integrated treatment is to not get into the primary versus secondary debate and to treat both kinds of conditions as if they are primary (Mueser 2003). Nevertheless, as patients come to the inpatient unit acutely, decisions have to be made regarding choice and timing of medications in order to guide treatment and discharge planning. If the provider is not sure that the patient has a primary psychiatric condition, then the patient, the family, and the outpatient provider need to be alerted to the fact that the medications prescribed may not be needed soon after the stabilization is completed. In such cases, medication doses could be reduced to see if the psychiatric symptoms reemerge. If they do not, then the initial presentation could have been mainly substance induced.

Families and caretakers, too, who have been bearing the burden of these conditions also could be seeking explanations or diagnostic clarification that might help them obtain benefits as well as gain a better understanding of the conditions so that they can care better for their loved ones.

Sorting out co-occurring disorders can occur over time with ongoing monitoring of treatment. Most patients fall into one of four clinical scenarios.

Two primary disorders

- People with psychiatric disorders will at times use potentially addictive substances to temporarily relieve their psychiatric symptoms. For a subset of vulnerable individuals, this use will progress to the extent that a separate SUD will develop and complicate their original psychiatric disorder.
- People who have already developed a SUD will subsequently develop another psychiatric disorder.

One primary and one secondary disorder

- When the original psychiatric disorder is effectively treated, the patient's problematic use of the addictive substance will resolve without specific treatment.
- When the SUD is effectively treated, the patient's other psychiatric symptoms will resolve without specific treatment.

Sorting out which of these scenarios is accurate is very difficult as long as the patient continues to use addictive substances. One of the goals of admission to a co-occurring treatment unit is to stop the use of the substance in a medically safe manner so that this diagnostic process can be initiated.

The treating physician in consultation with the team usually makes the provisional diagnosis, articulates the formulation, and creates the initial treatment plan. The formulation includes more than just the diagnosis. It includes the presenting problem, pattern of problems, predisposing factors, precipitating events, perpetuating factors, protective or positive factors, prognosis, and plan (Sperry et al. 1992). The multidisciplinary treatment plan evolves as the formulation evolves. It is important to keep sharing this formulation with the patient and give them an opportunity to interact with the treatment team about the formulation presented to them. Sometimes, the patient might suggest modifications or additions that might make the formulation richer. A good formulation is essential and is a very useful tool to guide the care of patients in such complex cases.

It is very important to ascertain directly from the patients and families their expectations of treatment. This usually clarifies the patients' self-understanding, their level of insight into their own predicament, and their level of motivation to deal with the specific problem.

Interestingly, a patient could be in an earlier stage of motivation of change for working on their mental illness but in a later stage of change for working on their addiction, or they could be in an earlier stage of motivation to change for giving up one drug (e.g., cannabis) but in a later stage of change for giving up another drug (e.g., cocaine) (see "Addressing Abstinence From Addictive Substances" later in this chapter). This is a useful framework to help provide a *stage-based treatment* plan for the patient and the staff on the unit (Velasquez et al. 2015). Often treatment providers tend to suggest interventions appropriate to later stages of change to patients who are in an early stage of change, only to see the interventions not succeed or the patients resist their recommendations.

For some patients, an admission to the inpatient unit could be their first attempt at recovery, and for others it could be one of many admissions to such a unit for a remitting and relapsing course of the condition. The needs of each of these kinds of patients are different. The former need diagnostic clarity, an adequate formulation that they can align with, and an introduction to the world of recovery. They may need education, not only about their psychiatric condition and their addiction but also about the interaction between these two conditions. The latter may need help in exploring the reasons for relapses and need work on relapse prevention skills. *Psychoeducation* plays a large role for each of these two kinds of patients.

Once again, it is challenging to design programming that addresses every patient's individual needs. Ideally, a comprehensive set of groups is available on the unit, and the treatment team can help individualize the offerings to match the needs of each patient and their stage of change.

In addition to the patient, the family also needs education and support. These can be offered contiguously to the visiting hour, or in a family meeting with the social worker, over the phone, or in a group designed to address the needs and frequently asked questions of family members.

Since many programs in the community do not provide integrated treatment, it is common to see either the psychiatric disorder or the addiction disorder ignored. The interaction between the two can be a mystery to the patient when the patient first arrives. Others, who have had a few or many relapses, need to gain an understanding of the kinds of factors that make it hard for them to stay stable. An inadequate focus on either of the two kinds of conditions can keep their co-occurring disorder unstable. Unfortunately, many co-occurring patients may have lost connections to families, homes, and jobs and may not have insurance or a source of income. They may have incurred legal or medical problems. All these become significant roadblocks to recovery that necessitate the help of trained professionals.

Discharge and aftercare planning is an important focus right from the time a patient arrives. A big overlay of social problems calls for the expertise of a social worker or a discharge coordinator who can connect the patient to the known resources in the community, such as recovery housing, benefits, and help with employers or legal entities, while the patient's co-occurring disorder is being stabilized. In addition, since these conditions can be chronic, and there is the potential for relapsing and remitting, patients need aftercare teams and programs to help them maintain their stability. There is a vast range of programs, from partial hospitalization programs and intensive outpatient programs to residential programs, that are available as aftercare options, in addition to a traditional outpatient team. Programs vary considerably by geography, definition, admissions, exclusion criteria, and coverage. Hence, a large part of knowing how to care for patients is knowing the resources available in the patient's surrounding context. It also takes knowledge, experience, patience, and skill to be able to guide patients and their families through this confusing and bewildering maze. Each patient at the time of discharge needs aftercare providers, programs, and prescriptions. They may also need help with housing, transportation, and linkages to community resources. Transitions can be more successful if representatives from community programs are willing to come and meet the patient on the inpatient unit, so that there can be a warm handoff, or at least have a phone conversation with a patient. A patient can have many questions about the aftercare program, questions that are best addressed by the staff of the aftercare program.

Even though relapses may be episodic, the impact of the addictive disorders and the vulnerabilities are chronic and ongoing support is required. Unlike the mental health system, the system that takes care of addictions is not generally set up to provide ongoing care with all the wraparound needs of patients with co-occurring disorders. Therefore, aftercare planning often involves combining features of more than one aftercare program to meet all the needs of a patient. Currently, the overall health care system is very fragmented. A single location at the outpatient level of care is usually unable to provide for all of a patient's needs in a comprehensive manner.

Patients can also be introduced to recovery resources such as *mutual help meetings* (e.g., Alcoholics Anonymous [AA], Narcotics Anonymous [NA], SMART Recovery) on the inpatient unit so that they can have these resources in their recovery armamentarium. Patients with co-occurring disorders need to be given advice on how to navigate these mutual help meetings. Specifically, they may need guidance on what to disclose, or not disclose, with respect to their psychiatric conditions and their medications. Some individuals in these mutual help groups have a limited understanding of psychiatric conditions. They may advise patients about how to take care of their psychiatric conditions and specifically discourage them from taking medications. This can obviously affect patients' ability to avoid destabilization of their psychiatric conditions.

Co-occurring disorder patients have a high percentage of *medical conditions that need monitoring and management*. These conditions are sometimes very closely linked to either the psychiatric condition or its treatment or are a sequela of their addiction. It is useful for patients to have access to medical consultants who can address their somatic needs. A significant number of medical conditions, ranging from minor infections or allergic reactions to chronic conditions like hypertension, diabetes, and hypothyroidism, can be managed on the co-occurring unit while the patients are being stabilized. Inpatient units have access to ancillary services such as phlebotomy, portable imaging, nutrition counseling, and physical therapy, all of which could play a vital role in stabilizing a patient (such services can vary considerably depending on the location of the inpatient unit). The treating psychiatrist or the medical consultant can also decide on what problems need to be referred out, in case there are medical problems of a higher complexity or urgency. This decision will depend on what services or resources are available within the hospital. Inpatient units also have access to rapid response teams whose members can assess emergencies such as injuries, seizures, respiratory depression, or chest pain.

Case Vignette

Jorge had been drinking for years. In addition to depression, alcohol use disorder, and tobacco use disorder, he also had hypertension, gastroesophageal reflux disease, and peripheral neuropathy. His neuropathy was particularly distressing. He could not sleep at night because of his burning pain and was frustrated because it affected his ability to function. His friend introduced him to Percocet, which eventually led to an opioid addiction. When his liver enzymes were quite high upon admission, the admitting nurse practitioner ordered a hepatitis panel. The patient was diagnosed as having been infected with hepatitis C. The treatment team helped him find a primary care provider close to his residence and educated him about how to take care of hepatitis C.

In addition to symptomatic improvement, patients are looking for functional improvement. They would benefit from *skills training* that will help them with various challenges like dealing with stress, managing sleep or anxiety, and preventing relapses. Distress tolerance and refusal skills, as well as education on the importance of sleep hygiene, could help patients in their recovery.

More than anything else, since many patients come to the unit very demoralized, one of the essential goals of treatment is to provide patients and families with a sense of *hope and optimism*.

Admissions to the Co-occurring Unit

As patients are referred for admission to the co-occurring unit, it is important to screen patients carefully to ensure that one can safely meet the multiple needs of the patient on the unit. Units in freestanding psychiatric hospitals do not have easy access to medical and surgical services. Emergency departments (EDs) generally conduct a history and physical examination, which includes basic labs, vital signs, and baseline functional evaluations. The commonly ordered laboratory tests in EDs include a complete blood count (CBC), a basic or comprehensive metabolic panel, a pregnancy test, a urinalysis and urine toxicology, and a blood alcohol level. Medical conditions can be identified in anywhere from one-half to three-fourths of patients. Therefore, one important consideration is the "medical clearance" of patients referred to the unit. Four scenarios are common (Anderson et al. 2017):

1. A medical condition(s) is masquerading as a psychiatric condition. Sometimes this condition can be exclusively cared for in a medical setting, whereas at other times this medical condition could be treated on the psychiatric unit. A common obstacle is that freestanding psychiatric units do not usually handle conditions needing intravenous medications.
2. The medical condition(s) is complicating the psychiatric condition significantly, such that the medical condition has to be stabilized first. Examples of such a condition are uncontrolled seizures and delirium in the context of alcohol withdrawal.
3. The medical problem(s) is coincidental but has to be managed while the patient is psychiatrically hospitalized. Unstable hypertension is an example of such a condition.
4. The medical condition(s) can be deferred to outpatient care but cannot be ignored while the patient is under one's care. Examples of such a condition are eczema and anemia.

It is important to try to only accept patients who can be safely cared for on the psychiatric unit, based on the capabilities and resources available on the unit or in the particular hospital. A good team of medical consultants can be very useful in helping differentiate between what can be and what cannot be treated on the unit.

Case Vignette

A patient with uncontrollable mania had been tough to manage on the unit and was not responding to standard medication regimens. The attending asked for a second opinion consultation. The consultant noticed that the patient had refused admission labs. He asked that the treatment team try once again to obtain labs, including tests for thyroid-stimulating hormone and rapid plasma reagin. When the results came back, everyone was surprised that the patient tested positive for syphilis and had a very high titer. It was recommended that the patient get treatment for syphilis, which could improve the patient's treatment response and prognosis.

There is a group of patients for whom medical assessment in the emergency room is warranted prior to their arriving to the unit—patients older than 65, those who have abnormal vitals and disorientation, those with no previous history of psychiatric disease, and those who have a history and physical exam that suggest a medical illness (Wilson et al. 2017). For most other patients, vitals, a thorough history and physical exam, some basic labs, and assessment of mentation will be enough to catch most medical conditions.

If a pregnant patient is being referred to an inpatient unit, one needs to know the gestational age. If a patient is in the first trimester, it is important to inquire about a history of bleeding. An ultrasound could be done for gestational age and viability. If a patient is in the second or third trimester, one could request a fetal ultrasound using a fetal Doppler. Normal fetal heart rate for previable fetuses is between 120–160 beats per minute. In the third trimester, fetal monitoring could also be requested via a nonstress test. There should be a thorough assessment for evaluation of high-risk obstetrical parameters such as preeclampsia or vaginal bleeding. If patients are presenting to the ED with symptoms of preterm labor or are found to have high-risk findings or abnormal fetal monitoring, one should request an obstetrical consultation. If the ED medically clears the patient, it would be helpful to get specific recommendations for the management of the pregnancy on the inpatient psychiatric unit (Lee et al. 2016).

Safety on the Co-occurring Inpatient Unit

Safety is a very important focus on the inpatient unit—safety not just of the patient but also of the staff who care for the patient. Safety concerns are what get patients hospitalized and are very important to demonstrate at the outset to gain approval for an admission or for meeting continued medical necessity criteria.

It is important to pay attention to safety right from the outset of an inpatient stay. On the Co-occurring Unit at Sheppard Pratt, upon admission, each patient goes through a manual safety search, which is done in a sensitive and caring way so as not to make the patient too uncomfortable or retraumatize them if the patient has a history of trauma. All the belongings they bring are thoroughly checked as well. Some units also use metal detectors to detect weapons or sharp objects that are brought in and could be dangerous to the patient themselves or others.

Another focus of these two searches is to detect any contraband in the form of substances of abuse or paraphernalia that could become a safety concern for the patient or others. We have seen instances in which patients bring in contraband from outside, receive contraband from visitors, or have shared or sold their administered medications.

For a while when our unit was seeing a high degree of influx of contraband, we instituted some safe practices that reduced the instances of discovered contraband on the unit. As countermeasures, we restricted food and beverages that were being brought in by visitors. Staff also began checking everything that was being brought in before it was handed to the patients. If visitors requested to come outside of visiting hours, staff monitored these visits. Finally, we provided lockers to visitors in which to keep their bags and other belongings. Implementing a few of these measures significantly reduced the instances of contraband on our unit.

There are other safety concerns on such a unit. Sometimes patients present in a verbally or physically aggressive manner. We have seen instances of destruction of property by unstable patients, as well as physical aggression toward staff or other patients. The key is getting a good history from the referring source such as the ED; observing patients at frequent intervals; and medicating them proactively. The aim is to manage both their psychiatric condition and withdrawal symptoms to calm and stabilize patients quickly. The clinician also needs to narrow down the patient and system determinants of each aggressive event to determine factors that are actionable. Analyzing each event over time makes patterns visible, and this could lead to specific countermeasures.

Other safety concerns center on the possibility that patients will be experiencing delirium, seizures, or oversedation that leads to respiratory depression during the withdrawal management phase of their treatment. All of these conditions can be potentially dangerous. Sometimes patients are admitted and in need of simultaneous treatment with opioids (in the form of buprenorphine or methadone) or benzodiazepines (as part of withdrawal management). When these need to be co-prescribed, the risk of overdose and respiratory depression rises. As a result, on our unit, we began monitoring the patient's respirations round the clock in a diminishing frequency over a 3-day period. If no respiratory concerns were elicited, we would stop this monitoring. One can also monitor the patients using the Pasero Opioid-Induced Sedation Scale (Nisbet and Mooney-Cotter 2009) to pick up cases of oversedation in patients early and intervene accordingly by either dose reduction or, if necessary, naloxone administration. Oversedation and respiratory depression can also be a risk for other reasons. Many patients may be nonadherent with their psychiatric medications as outpatients. When patients are admitted to the unit, their outpatient medications are often restarted at their original dose. There could be a synergistic interaction between all the administered medications and residual substances that the patient might have been using prior to admission. It is important to remember, also, that psychiatric patients may be at greater risk, especially if they are receiving other medications that can be sedating, such as certain antipsychotics, antidepressants, sedative-hypnotics, and α_2 agonists. Other factors can contribute to oversedation and heightened risk of respiratory depression, such as when patients being prescribed both benzodiazepines and opioids have chronic obstructive pulmonary disease or obstructive sleep apnea. It is important to be careful in the initial phases of each patient's treatment. The physician can start a patient's medications conservatively after obtaining collateral information and checking the prescription drug-monitoring program, and titrate the dose up slowly, especially when the patient is also getting medications for withdrawal management.

Another situation that requires vigilance and care is the continuation of methadone for the first time on the inpatient unit. The clinician should confirm the dose with the patient's outpatient methadone program directly and not just rely on records sent with the patient. Sometimes when an outpatient methadone program is called, the program's version of the doses that the patient received does not match what the patient actually took. Methadone can be initiated on inpatient units for patients already enrolled in a methadone program for the treatment of an opioid use disorder. In the case of patients on methadone maintenance, it is given to the patients as a liquid. It can also be initiated in hospitals for pregnant patients who have opioid use disorder (although buprenorphine is replacing methadone as the treatment of choice for pregnant patients with opioid use disorder).

Case Vignette

Carlos, a patient in an outpatient methadone program, was admitted to the inpatient unit after he voiced suicidal ideation. According to the outpatient methadone program, the patient was taking 150 mg of methadone. The patient was given his dose as confirmed. Three days into this treatment regimen the patient was found to be in respiratory depression and had to be given naloxone nasal spray to reverse his condition. When the patient recovered, he admitted to lying. He admitted that as an outpatient he had been using only half of the prescribed dose. He had been selling the rest of his dose to supplement his income.

We have also instituted a safety checklist to monitor safety events on the unit. This checklist is currently being completed by the nurse in charge during each shift. If any safety situations occur, they are acted upon, communicated to the next shift, and discussed at a brief meeting daily. Keeping track of each of these safety events, including near misses, allows the unit leadership and staff to notice emerging safety concerns. We noticed an increase in ED send-outs due to severe constipation. Seeing this trend led to a discussion about monitoring patients for this concern and using prophylactic agents for patients taking opioids and medications like clozapine reliably in order to prevent constipation. Earlier, we discovered contraband as a major safety concern in the same way.

Assessments

As patients are admitted to the unit round the clock, one of the first assessments they receive is the nursing assessment. The nursing staff can set the tone for the unit. They can orient the patient to the unit and attend to all their immediate needs. The nurse conducts an assessment that evaluates the various needs and risks associated with the patient, including vital signs, safety, allergies, dietary needs, nutritional status, fall risk, and withdrawal status, and does a physical and psychiatric review of systems. The nurse communicates and hands off the summary of their assessment to the physician (who may or may not be on the unit) and gives their input on the observation level of the patient. The patient may need to resume their medications right away and may need medications for withdrawal management. Some of the commonly used scales for withdrawal management on the inpatient unit are the Clinical Institute Withdrawal Assessment for Alcohol—Revised (CIWA-Ar; Sullivan et al. 1989) and the Clinical Opiate Withdrawal Scale (COWS; Wesson and Ling 2003).

Another assessment is the review of systems and physical examination, which can be conducted by a physician assistant or resident. This review is important in order to establish a baseline of the patient's somatic status and needs, and it acts as a guide for a part of the care plan that focuses on somatic needs. Patients with co-occurring disorders can have various significant somatic sequelae of their substance use, ranging from those related to withdrawal and its management to conditions that worsen or are caused by substance use such as hypertension or infectious diseases.

Next, at the time of the psychiatric assessment, one of the first steps prior to assigning a working diagnosis and initiating a treatment plan is to gain a good understanding of the patient by gathering a thorough history. It is important to start with the chief complaint, which usually gives an idea of what has precipitated the present episode of treatment and the patient's expectations from the treatment team.

It is important to understand the exact circumstances that brought the patient to the hospital. Gathering this history gives the treatment team a sense of the presenting crisis, the antecedent factors, some key players in the patient's life, whether the patient or someone else initiated this referral, the patient's level of understanding and motivation, and their level of organization as they provide their narrative. It is then easy to quickly understand whether this is the first time the patient has attempted treatment or whether this is one of many admissions that follows a particular pattern. In addition to what precipitated the admission, it is also important to understand what maintains a patient's problems.

Through this process, it is possible to witness a mix of multiple psychiatric conditions in addition to multiple addictions affecting the patient's presentation. It is like trying to untangle a mass of intertwined multicolored threads. A useful technique is to take a piece of paper and draw multiple swim lanes. Each lane can be used to trace the progression of a particular category of symptoms, such as mood, anxiety, or psychotic symptoms. As the psychiatric assessment progressively elucidates the progression and timelines for various conditions, one below the other, the psychiatrist can also understand the occurrence of each condition chronologically with respect to one another. For example, if one discerns that the social anxiety started very early in life and worsened in middle school, and was then followed by episodes of recurrent depression in the teenage years, followed by a progressively severe course of alcohol use, one gets a good sense of the evolution of the patient's co-occurring conditions. We can then predict that there is a better chance of addressing the depression after the phase of managing withdrawal and attaining early sobriety. It is then necessary to deal with the underlying social anxiety, which was present at the outset and which might be interfering with any group treatment or referral to mutual help groups.

As these conditions evolve, often over years, patients can accumulate layers of problems that all interact with one another. It is useful to get information from multiple sources—the patient, the referring entity, the patient's family, relevant outpatient providers if the patient has some, programs that the patient might be attending, and their other medical providers. Information can also come from past records, the prescription drug monitoring program, judiciary case search, and outpatient pharmacies, among other resources. Such information gathering can take time; however, given that psychiatry lacks diagnostic laboratory tests or imaging studies, a richer and nuanced understanding of the patient does require paying attention to multiple perspectives. In addition, there are complex biopsychosocial disorders that defy simplistic solutions. As information keeps pouring in, the treatment team has to reconcile that new information with the unit-based observations in order to keep revising the formulation of the patient and the treatment plan.

One of the main tasks of the psychiatrist's assessment is also to attempt to arrive at a provisional working diagnosis. A psychiatrist is trying to assess the presence or absence of one or many psychiatric conditions, which could be leading to the patient's current distress or affect the patient's overall functioning. Sometimes even this seemingly clearly defined task is not easy to accomplish. For example, the patient may come in saying that they have been diagnosed with multiple psychiatric conditions at once while they are also dependent on multiple substances. They could also be withdrawing from each of these substances. As a diagnostician, one might also notice borderline personality traits or become aware of the psychosocial pressures of homelessness, poverty, legal problems, and a lack of insurance, making the job of arriving at a working diagnosis very challenging. There is also an additional time pressure, because the physician has to make decisions about medications to initiate that the patient is claiming to be on.

Case Vignette

A patient presented to the unit saying he was depressed and suicidal. He gave a history of bipolar disorder, PTSD, anxiety disorder, ADHD, and chronic pain. He said he was on buprenorphine maintenance. He also said that he was being prescribed lithium, quetiapine, prazosin, zolpidem, mixed amphetamine salts, and gabapentin. The patient gave a history of drinking a pint of alcohol daily; he was using cocaine intravenously a few times a week and was smoking cannabis regularly, having obtained a medical cannabis card. The admitting resident was baffled by the sheer number of prescriptions and felt tremendous pressure from the patient as the patient angrily demanded that all his outpatient medications be resumed right away.

The use of alcohol and substances just prior to admission can definitely color the initial presentation. Different substances behave differently during phases of intoxication and withdrawal, and it is important for treatment providers to be familiar with such presentation profiles of commonly used substances of abuse. Some of these presenting problems begin clearing up in hours or days after the admission. This might be indicative of a substance-induced condition. Some substances, such as stimulants or synthetic cannabis used chronically, may take time to clear, and often a 7- to 8-day stay is insufficient to clearly demarcate what is substance induced and what is attributable to the underlying condition. Family history is often not very helpful because families, too, can be genetically loaded with both mental illness and addiction. Incarceration or pregnancies can provide a respite from heavy alcohol and substance use, which may offer some clues, but sometimes patients claim using substances even during those periods and in controlled environments.

It is also important to ascertain a history of adverse childhood experiences and history of trauma, which are often found in patients with co-occurring disorders. A very significant history of trauma can have a big impact on treatment outcomes and can make everything from alliance building, to diagnosis of a number of associated conditions, to response to treatments much more challenging. Trauma-informed units and systems have to offer safety, trustworthiness, choice, collaboration, and empowerment of the patient. Often patients use substances as a way to cope with histories of very significant and often repeated trauma. The design and programming of the unit, and its approach to such patients, have to ensure that all staff understand the impact and implications of trauma on the patient. Staff should not conduct themselves in ways that make the patient feel powerless or vulnerable. A very rigid adherence to and a heavy-handed application of rules without any flexibility often iatrogenically creates frequent crises on the unit and can retraumatize the patient. Trauma-informed units can lead to fewer seclusions and restraints and can enhance the safety of both patients and staff. All staff may need to be trained about trauma. They need to know de-escalation techniques, understand how to help patients identify triggers, and demonstrate facility in instituting calming strategies that do not exclusively focus on the use of medication to deal with various crises.

As part of the initial assessment, a psychiatrist may have to order some laboratory tests. If patients are medically cleared and referred from an ED, they often come with results of a CBC with a differential and a basic or comprehensive metabolic panel (if they come in with a basic metabolic panel, a hepatic function panel should also be ordered), a urinalysis, a pregnancy test, and a blood alcohol level. If patients come from non-ED settings, then the admitting physician can order these laboratory tests.

The number of tests ordered by each ED and how the results are reported can vary across EDs and their respective laboratories. Occasionally, the patient also comes with an electrocardiogram and some imaging tests if there is a history of injuries or altered mental status changes. It is useful for the admitting psychiatrist to order thyroid function tests and tests for syphilis and other sexually transmitted diseases, such as gonorrhea and chlamydia (recently there has been an increase in some of these diseases). It is also important to test for HIV and hepatitis because they often occur as a result of unsafe sexual behaviors or risky substance use behaviors. If a patient is a chronic alcohol user, it is also helpful to test for vitamin B_{12} and folate levels. On our unit, we have also found a very high incidence of vitamin D deficiency in the patients with co-occurring disorders. The admitting psychiatrist can also order a lipid panel and hemoglobin A_{1c}, because many patients with serious mental illnesses have poor physical health, which can be worsened by the use of antipsychotics and can lead to metabolic syndrome.

Other useful testing in the treatment of patients with addictions is urine drug screening, which is typically done in the ED. In some treatment settings, such as outpatient clinics, these tests are underutilized. These drug screens are based on different types of immunoassays. They can be fast, sensitive, and inexpensive. Their limitations are that they can yield false-positive and false-negative results. They generally indicate the presence or absence of a class of substances (such as benzodiazepines). It is also important to know for a particular screening tool what substances it is capable of testing for and what substances it is unable to detect. For instance, not all screens test for buprenorphine, fentanyl, methadone, or synthetic cannabis.

The drug screening results can be confirmed with either gas chromatography/mass spectrometry or liquid chromatography/mass spectrometry. These confirmatory tests are highly sensitive and specific and can offer quantitative measurement. They can be used for serial measurements to see if patients have truly discontinued the substance or if there is continued use. The downside of these confirmatory tests is that they can be expensive and can have a turnaround time of up to a week. This time delay to get confirmatory results can be limiting for use in inpatient settings because stays can be brief and results may come back after the patients are discharged. These tests can identify a particular analyte as opposed to a class of substances. For example, they can pick up alprazolam in a patient who has just been prescribed chlordiazepoxide, indicating illicit use. For these results to be interpreted correctly, it is important to know the kinds of substances used by patients, their half-lives, and their metabolic pathways. Results can be expected or unexpected. Unexpected results could indicate the presence of substances that were not expected or the absence of medications such as buprenorphine or lorazepam that might be on the patient's active medication list, raising the possibility of diversion or binge use. Immunoassays are considered presumptive, and confirmatory tests based on mass spectrometry are considered definitive. This is a rapidly advancing field, and it might be helpful to discuss hard-to-interpret findings with laboratory professionals (Li et al. 2019).

The aim of all these assessments is to gather a comprehensive history of the types, extent, and pattern of substance use. The progression of the patient's addiction history and the impact of these addictions on various aspects of the patient's life are important to understand. It is also important to understand the patient's level of motivation to change their own condition, their strengths and weaknesses, and the recovery environment. One must assess what the patient knows and what they have tried to do about their own condition. In addition to their lived experience of interventions tried, it is also important to learn about the barriers they have experienced. Embodying the spirit of motivational interviewing, all treatment providers need to convey a sense of acceptance and hope, evoke from the patient what they may already know about changing their lifestyle, collaborate to elicit motivation to change, and coach them on what they want to learn. Ultimately, this approach to assessment of the patient respects the patient's autonomy and what they decide for themselves.

These assessments allow treatment providers to assess all six ASAM dimensions for each patient, a process that can allow the treatment team to come up with a comprehensive care plan.

Two additional points here. Confidentiality laws that affect addiction treatment (42 C.F.R. Part 2) are more stringent than HIPAA laws and can hinder communication between all treating providers and at times shield patients' problematic behaviors to their own detriment if the patients do not provide consent for such communication.

In addition, mental health laws allow involuntary treatment based on dangerousness due to mental illness in emergent situations but do not afford the same leeway to providers to treat patients involuntarily if it is deemed that the patients' dangerousness is a result of their addictions. Both these factors at times limit what treatment providers can do, and this can cause terrible consternation for families, who may not know how to stop the patient's self-defeating and high-risk behaviors. Often, only the judicial system can set these limits and mandate treatment.

Assessment is a continuous process. It does not just end with the admission assessments. One can broadly conceptualize three broad tasks or phases of treatment: First, the treatment team arrives at an initial assessment and formulation. Then, they strive to stabilize both the psychiatric and the addictive disorders. Finally, they prepare a road map and comprehensive care plan for the patient based on the resources available to the patient, their family, and their community. Each of these tasks and phases needs its own ongoing assessment. The early withdrawal management process can be challenging for both patients and staff because the patients can be both unstable and uncomfortable. The treatment team has to watch for complications like delirium, seizures, infections, and autonomic instability, in addition to safety concerns about whether patients might hurt themselves or others. Ongoing assessments by social workers and discharge coordinators during and after discharge planning can be helpful to ensure that patients have access to programs, providers, medications, a safe place to live, recovery resources, and transportation.

Psychotic, suicidal, aggressive, oversedated, or delirious patients can all pose unique challenges to the staff. Staff have to stay focused and hypervigilant to changes that each patient is going through in addition to gauging the day-to-day atmosphere on the unit. Sometimes two or three unstable patients can make it challenging for the entire unit to focus on everyone's recovery because these patients can take up the bulk of staff time and attention. A brief daily meeting can focus on safety issues, the flow of patients through the system, and the quality of care on the unit. Safety, delivery, and quality issues are best solved when they are small and addressed on a daily basis. Paying attention to how the unit system behaves on a daily basis can be instrumental in staying prepared for upcoming challenges and make the unit staff more cohesive and competent to handle these challenges. The unit leadership has to work on the psychological safety of the staff and create a just culture so that safety concerns can regularly come to the surface and promptly be addressed. The nursing staff needs to feel comfortable escalating matters, and the unit leadership needs to support such a practice of uncovering problems and to treat these problems as opportunities for continuous improvement.

Treatment Planning

Most patients with co-occurring disorders receive at least some care from the mental health service system, with a minority receiving services from substance abuse treatment providers. According to Minkoff (1989), there are philosophical differences between traditional systems of care for persons with addictions compared with persons with mental health disorders. In the traditional mental health system, medical professionals provide treatment. There is a bigger emphasis on diagnosis, laboratory tests, medications, case management, and a continuous treatment framework. Addiction is viewed as secondary to psychopathology in this model. In the traditional system of care for addictions, treatment is offered via a peer counselor model. There is more emphasis on spiritual recovery, self-help, detachment and empowerment, and an episodic treatment framework. Often, psychopathology is viewed as secondary to addiction (Mueser 2003). These philosophical differences can pose challenges for patients depending on which professional or paraprofessional provider they encounter along their journey to recovery. As a multidisciplinary team, it is important to be attentive to such paradigmatic differences and try to pragmatically blend the perspectives offered by both systems.

Closely related to the stages of change based on the transtheoretical model are the stages of treatment for co-occurring disorders first described by Osher and Kofoed (1989). They observed that co-occurring patients progress through four stages: *engagement*, *persuasion*, *active treatment*, and *relapse prevention* (relapses to prior stages of treatment are common). On the basis of the patient's stage of treatment, appropriate goals and treatment plans can be offered. The engagement stage of treatment overlaps with the precontemplation stage of change (see the discussion of Prochaska and DiClemente's stages of change model in subsection "Addressing Abstinence From

Addictive Substances"). The persuasion phase of treatment overlaps with the contemplation and preparation stages of change. The active treatment stage corresponds to the action stage of change, and the relapse prevention stage of treatment matches the maintenance stage of change.

The engagement stage is defined by a lack of regular contact with a clinician or absence of a working alliance between the patient and clinician. In the engagement stage, the clinician can provide monitoring and crisis stabilization and practical assistance with necessities like food, clothing, and shelter; emotional support to patients and their families can also be provided.

Patients who come under the care of a provider, such as those involuntarily admitted to an inpatient unit or coerced by a family member, often are behaviorally unmotivated to receive care. Such patients are in the persuasion stage of treatment. In this stage, providers can provide education through individual and group work, motivational interviewing, structured activities, and medications to stabilize psychiatric conditions.

On inpatient units, most commonly, patients are in one of these two stages of treatment—engagement or persuasion. The treatment team has to prepare them for active treatment and relapse prevention stages of treatment. The patients are believed to be in the active treatment stage when they have been free of addiction for at least a month. For them to be in the relapse prevention stage, they have to be free of addiction for 6 months. Most of the time if the patients are in one of these two latter stages, they are not admitted to the co-occurring inpatient unit.

Treatment

The limited time frame of the patient stay on the co-occurring unit necessitates a primary focus on having a provisional diagnosis and stabilization. The use of medication assumes a more prominent role in the treatment plan than will be the case in post-discharge care.

Withdrawal Management

Basic Issues

The onset of withdrawal symptoms can provide a unique opportunity to engage patients in addressing problematic substance use. While wishful thinking can prevent patients from acknowledging the existence of the problem, the distress associated with the onset of withdrawal can be a therapeutic wake-up call.

Effectively relieving a patient's withdrawal discomfort, in addition to reducing morbidity and mortality, can also be an opportunity to build a trusting therapeutic relationship. What is conveyed to the patient is that the clinician both cares about their distress and is competent at relieving it. This experience can be helpful later in the treatment process when the clinician asks the patient to bear psychological pain as part of the recovery process.

Withdrawal protocols are frequently being updated, rendering any specific protocols placed in this chapter quickly out of date. One reliable source for the most recent guidelines is the American Society of Addiction Medicine. Certain basic principles, however, are worth reviewing.

1. Several effective withdrawal protocols exist for each substance. Choose one with which you are comfortable and have a backup for when the patient has had a negative reaction in the past or has a strong aversion to using a particular medication. The ideal medication is long-acting, less toxic, and less reinforcing than the substance on which the patient has become dependent.
2. Be prepared for high tolerance. One of the hallmarks of the addictive use of substances is the insensitivity of the patient to some of their effects. This translates into a need to use large doses of withdrawal management agents.
3. Medicate aggressively and minimize discomfort. There is no evidence that subjecting a patient to a painful withdrawal reduces the likelihood of a later relapse. Current medications and protocols allow symptoms to be reduced rapidly and often eliminated entirely. Stay ahead of the evolving withdrawal syndrome. Proactively administer medication before symptoms become severe.

Accurate tracking of the progress of the withdrawal symptoms and the response of the patient to medication interventions is essential. Many scales exist and will be referenced below for each substance. Another simple approach for all substances is to ask the patient, "On a scale from zero, being completely comfortable, to 10, being the worst withdrawal symptoms you have ever had, what number would you put on your withdrawal discomfort right now?" After a baseline value is established, the question is then repeated regularly to determine if the medication is working. The goal is for the patient to reach a level of zero to 1. While every person's frame of reference is different, having a number placed on this global subjective parameter gives the clinician more guidance than does the simple verbal indication of feeling better or worse.

Management of Withdrawal From Specific Substances

Alcohol. Although many patients with alcohol use disorder experience no or minimal withdrawal symptoms, the potential seriousness of the alcohol withdrawal syndrome mandates that the possibility be addressed early and aggressively. Grand mal seizures and delirium tremens are much easier to prevent than to treat after they develop.

The tendency of patients with alcohol use disorder to minimize their withdrawal symptoms can add to the difficulty of making an accurate assessment. For example, withdrawal anxiety is commonly rationalized as being due to being in an unfamiliar environment. Patients will sometimes respond negatively to questions about "shakiness" but then be found on physical exam to have a hand tremor with arms outstretched and fingers spread. Sometimes the tremor is so fine that it can only be detected by touching the patient's fingertips.

Multiple questionnaires have been developed to predict the likelihood of severe withdrawal, but at this time no consensus exists about the best one. An excellent single predictor of severe withdrawal is a previous history of severe withdrawal, seizures, or delirium tremens. Such a history justifies a more aggressive medication approach, with whatever medication protocol is used.

The choice of medications has been the source of some disagreement. Benzodiazepines have been the gold standard of treatment since the 1960s. Addiction specialists prefer nonreinforcing, long-acting agents such as chlordiazepoxide. Diazepam is another option but is more reinforcing than chlordiazepoxide. Its slightly faster onset of action is not usually of clinical significance. When liver failure is present, oxazepam is a preferred alternative. Nonspecialists tend to use lorazepam for all patients despite the fact that its shorter half-life creates a greater likelihood of rebound symptoms after it is discontinued, which can trigger a relapse. The use of lorazepam should be restricted to when oral medications are not an option. Lorazepam and diazepam also have a greater street value as opposed to chlordiazepoxide or oxazepam.

Medication protocols are divided into two types. In a front-loaded, symptom-driven protocol, most of the medication is given in the first 24–48 hours. This allows for a more rapid control of the alcohol withdrawal syndrome and ultimately the administration of less medication. This approach, however, is more complex to manage well and requires an experienced withdrawal management nurse to examine the patient every 1–2 hours during the first 4–8 hours. On an inpatient unit that admits patients round the clock, this can translate into needing an experienced nurse at all times. This can be challenging to accomplish in hospitals that inevitably involve multiple shifts and changes in nursing staff of various degrees of expertise. In those settings, a practical alternative is a fixed-dose or symptom-triggered benzodiazepine regimen.

Once a medication protocol has been instituted, the next task is to adjust the medication to the most effective level, trying to avoid both under- and overmedicating. Vital signs, although being commonly relied upon, are often not relevant except in the most extreme circumstances. Elevated blood pressure, for example, can be a result of long-term heavy drinking and may require weeks or months to return to normal. The most important symptoms to monitor are agitation, anxiety, restlessness, and insomnia.

While multiple scales exist, the one most broadly referenced is the Clinical Institute Withdrawal Assessment for Alcohol—Revised (CIWA-Ar). Clinical discontent with this scale has, however, been widespread, leading to alternatives that are simpler to administer, such as the Brief Alcohol Withdrawal Scale (Lindner et al. 2019).

Because benzodiazepines can be addictive and sedating and cause delirium, anticonvulsant medications such as carbamazepine, gabapentin, and valproate have emerged as alternative agents. These medications remediate the glutamatergic hyperactivity that contributes to alcohol withdrawal syndrome. Their effectiveness and safety for mild to moderate levels of withdrawal syndromes have been well studied. The lower incidence of sedation when these medications are properly dosed renders patients available more quickly for psychosocial interventions such as group sessions.

A more recent development has been the addition of alpha-adrenergic agonists, such as clonidine and guanfacine. These medications address the adrenergic hyperactivity that plays a role in the development of delirium. Some treatment centers have been able to eliminate entirely the use of benzodiazepines through the use of this combination of medications. This has been particularly welcome because of the relative ineffectiveness of benzodiazepines once full delirium tremens has developed.

A hybrid option can also be considered given that the severity of withdrawal can be so difficult to predict, and many nonspecialist clinicians are not comfortable with the complexity of adding α_2-adrenergic agonists. In this approach, a long-acting benzodiazepine is used the first day and then discontinued in favor of an anticonvulsant medication beginning on the second day of treatment.

Anticonvulsants can be continued, usually at lower doses for a period of weeks or months, to reduce protracted withdrawal symptoms related to craving, sleep, and anxiety.

Vitamin and nutritional supplements are standard parts of alcohol withdrawal syndrome treatment protocols on either a routine or an individualized basis. Medications such as baclofen have been less studied but are commonly used to address discomfort and reduce the likelihood of relapse.

Although alcohol itself was used historically in tapering doses to treat alcohol withdrawal syndrome before the development of less toxic alternatives, it should no longer be used. Some physicians, especially surgeons in the surgical intensive care unit, persist in using it despite the presence of preferable medications (Blondell et al. 2003).

Opioids. While several scales exist to track the progress of opioid withdrawal, the most widely used one is the Clinical Opiate Withdrawal Scale (COWS).

For many years, an α-adrenergic agonist such as clonidine, supported by other "comfort medications," was the only legal option for treating opioid withdrawal. This changed with the passage of the Drug Addiction Treatment Act of 2000 and the actual availability of sublingual buprenorphine on the market in 2003. The use of buprenorphine grew gradually, and buprenorphine has now become the gold standard for managing opioid withdrawal syndromes. Its effectiveness allows patients to quickly become more comfortable, often feeling "normal" within a few hours. As in the case with alcohol, this renders the patient available for psychosocial interventions sooner. In contrast to patients with alcohol withdrawal, patients withdrawing from opioids are less likely to minimize their symptoms and can be irritable and problematic to manage until they become more comfortable. Another difference is that unlike benzodiazepines, buprenorphine has a stabilizing effect on patients with opioid use disorder and can be continued for months to years for relapse prevention.

The molecular shape of buprenorphine affords it unique clinical advantages over other opioids. Respiratory depression does not progress after a dose level of 24 mg is reached. Because of this "ceiling effect," accidental overdose from sublingual administration is rarely a problem, in contrast to methadone. The one caution is that the simultaneous use of benzodiazepines slowly lifts this ceiling effect. This has led some clinicians to maintain that the simultaneous use, when the patient is also withdrawing from alcohol, is contraindicated. Enhanced monitoring for possible respiratory depression, however, is an adequate adjustment to allow both to be used safely.

Delaying administering buprenorphine until withdrawal symptoms appear avoids the danger of precipitating instead of relieving intense withdrawal symptoms. This issue arises from buprenorphine having a high receptor affinity but being a partial rather than a full opioid receptor agonist. If given prematurely, the buprenorphine will displace the prior opioid from the receptor site but not replace the full agonist activity. Creating this degree of displeasure in a patient is a predictable way to damage a developing therapeutic relationship. Many patients who have already experienced such precipitated withdrawal by using illicitly obtained buprenorphine on their own are understandably apprehensive and may respond to clinical education and encouragement in order to be willing to try the medication again.

In past years, a delay of several hours from last opioid use has been sufficient. An exception has been for methadone, which, because of the long half-life of its active metabolites, can require 48 hours or more after the daily dose has been tapered to 30 mg. Management of this issue, however, has been complicated in recent years by the widespread prevalence of illicit fentanyl. Having adulterated and even replaced street heroin as well as counterfeit opioid pills, these compounds will lead to precipitated withdrawal even after the passage of 24 hours and the appearance of substantial withdrawal symptoms. Preliminary efforts are underway to reduce this problem by using micro or macro doses of buprenorphine, although published studies so far are limited (Herring et al. 2021).

Pregnant addicts can benefit from buprenorphine, but as of this writing methadone is still the standard of care. Studies have in fact shown that the neonatal abstinence syndrome is less severe and of shorter duration with buprenorphine than when the mother has been taking methadone.

Clinicians differ, as is the case with alcohol withdrawal management, on the dose that they are willing to provide to patients. The experience of the authors is that there is wide variability in patient dose requirements, depending on tolerance and absorption patterns. Establishing a therapeutic relationship is facilitated by attending sensitively to patient discomfort. Fine-tuning the dose until cravings are minimal or eliminated entirely can reduce physical distractions from psychosocial interventions. Studies documenting optimal doses are still lacking at this time.

Nausea is a problem with some patients. This may be due to the accidental intestinal absorption of the naloxone that is compounded with the buprenorphine. The compounding has been done to discourage intravenous use, in which case the naloxone would become active and blunt the action of the buprenorphine. One option is to have the patient, after the sublingual medication has dissolved, spit out their saliva rather than swallow it. If this is ineffective, the "mono" formulation of buprenorphine, which lacks the naloxone component, is another option. This formulation is primarily intended for use in pregnancy, and its use is otherwise discouraged because of its greater susceptibility for abuse. Ondansetron is another option to manage nausea.

Despite the clear advantages of buprenorphine for withdrawal management, there are three circumstances when an alternative is necessary. First, some patients are not able to tolerate buprenorphine or report feeling "high" on it. Second, some patients desire to take naltrexone for ongoing relapse prevention. Using buprenorphine would delay the time when naltrexone could be started because of the 7-day interval needed between them to avoid precipitated withdrawal. Third, philosophical opposition to buprenorphine continues to exist, leading some patients to request an alternative to an opioid agonist. The best choice in that circumstance is an α_2-adrenergic agonist along with other symptomatic medications. Because the time immediately after discharge is particularly high risk in terms of overdose deaths, these patients are advised to take naltrexone and receive a depot injection prior to discharge if time allows.

Once withdrawal symptoms have been reduced or eliminated, the next decision is how long the patient should continue taking the buprenorphine. Many patients are eager to taper off the medication immediately, often equating this with progress. Outcomes using this approach have been so consistently poor that a clinical consensus has evolved that a duration of at least several months and ideally greater than 1 year is preferable. Patients and their families are often resistant to this approach. Supportive education and reassurance by the clinician can be effective. Parameters to monitor for deciding when to taper include the reestablishment of a stable life, the implementation of a strong recovery program, and the presence of an alternative strategy for managing the stress and distress caused by the co-occurring psychiatric disorder.

Benzodiazepines. When benzodiazepines have been used addictively, the preferred strategy is to establish abstinence from their use. If they have been used in the treatment of a co-occurring anxiety disorder, alternative medications should be explored. If the use has not been addictive, clinical disagreement exists about the advisability of continuing to prescribe low doses.

If the decision is made to stop them, a choice needs to be made between withdrawing the patient using the same benzodiazepine or transitioning to an alternative medication. Tapering with the same medicine is sometimes the simplest approach when the dose is low.

For patients who have been taking high doses, especially for a lengthy period of time, keys to a smooth process are switching to another medication, establishing a taper schedule, and limiting patient access to the medication. The choice of an alternative medication is between phenobarbital and a longer-acting benzodiazepine.

The optimal time frame of the taper is several weeks rather than the limited number of days in which the patient will be in the hospital. This strategy requires the existence of a relationship with a prescriber who is willing to assume responsibility for the taper postdischarge. In this scenario, one of the advantages of using phenobarbital is that a return to benzodiazepine use is more easily detected by urine screening. When benzodiazepines are being used, confirmatory drug testing is important to determine if the patient is taking medication other than the one being prescribed.

Tobacco. Numerous safe and effective nicotine replacement medications are available to relieve the stress of tobacco withdrawal. Because of overconcern about nicotine toxicity, the doses used are sometimes too low to provide adequate relief. For patients who only desire temporary relief until they resume smoking after discharge, short-term options include nonprescription gum and lozenges. Instructing patients about the proper technique for chewing the gum is important for it to be effective. Another option is called an "inhaler" but actually involves sucking through a plastic mouthpiece that contains a cartridge of nicotine liquid, which is absorbed through the buccal mucosa rather than through the lungs.

A medium-term option is a nicotine patch. The guideline for dosing is to equate 1 mg of the patch with one cigarette per day. For example, someone smoking two packs per day would start with two 21-mg patches. The blood nicotine levels reached by the use of these medications is so much lower than the levels reached by the use of tobacco that patches can be supplemented safely with gum and lozenges to address breakthrough symptoms.

Another complicating factor is the use of e-cigarettes. This can also affect the nicotine concentration that the patient is used to and must be considered when calculating the dose of nicotine replacement therapy. Some patients know the concentration of the e-juice they are using and providers can collaborate with them to find the most comforting dose of nicotine replacement therapy.

If the patients can learn to make themselves comfortable in an inpatient environment where smoking is not possible for their entire course of inpatient treatment, they can paradoxically get motivated to quit smoking as they begin to feel a little more confident in their ability to give up smoking.

Hospitals can also invest in a smoking cessation coordinator who can use individual and group work to help patients deal with their tobacco use disorder. The coordinator are able to use psychoeducational and motivational approaches to help patients with this very hard-to-treat addiction.

If patients can find a dose of nicotine replacement therapy or another combination of medications that works for them, these can be continued at the time of discharge. They are also referred to quitlines (1-800-QUIT-NOW) to give them ongoing support and access to nicotine replacement therapy after discharge. (For example, access to free nicotine replacement therapy and a few counseling sessions is available to patients in Maryland through the quitline.)

Cannabis. Despite popular belief to the contrary, the existence of a cannabis withdrawal syndrome has been well documented and the syndrome was therefore included in DSM-5. The symptoms have become more clinically significant as the available tetrahydrocannabinol (THC) concentrations have increased considerably. Anxiety and insomnia are common. Persistent cravings can lead to relapse. Limited studies have found that the use of synthetic THC (dronabinol and nabilone) can relieve the symptoms but has not led to any improvement in long-term recovery outcomes.

Stimulants. No medication has been found to consistently reduce the symptoms that occur following the cessation of stimulants. Although depression can on occasion reach suicidal intensity, symptoms are usually transient and self-limiting.

Multiple substances. The primary decision is whether to withdraw the patient from all substances simultaneously or to break the process into stages. One common clinical scenario is physical dependence on both opioids and alcohol. Some clinicians are concerned about the simultaneous use of buprenorphine and benzodiazepines because the latter can gradually lift the ceiling effect, causing respiratory depression. This issue can be managed by less aggressive dosing of benzodiazepine and monitoring of respiratory status. When patients undergo withdrawal management from alcohol or benzodiazepines and opioids simultaneously, they may be medicated with both chlordiazepoxide and buprenorphine.

Psychosocial Interventions

Addressing Abstinence From Addictive Substances

The use of addictive substances complicates the treatment of other psychiatric disorders whether or not that use meets the criteria for a SUD. For patients who cannot be diagnosed with a SUD, abstaining from these substances would be optimal. For patients reluctant to agree to do this, clarifying the reasons for this recommendation and motivating them to follow this recommendation (see discussion of motivational interviewing below) require skillful clinical interventions.

If the assessment has determined that a patient has a SUD, the next clinical task is to identify the patient's willingness to address this issue. Most clinicians have experienced frustration at encountering patients whose problem with a substance was clear but who were not willing to address the issue effectively. Many clinicians have found that their work with these patients becomes more tolerable and effective through adopting the Stages of Change (transtheoretical) model of James Prochaska and Carlo DiClemente (DiClemente 2018). Their research into how people stopped smoking tobacco led them to some insights about the process of intentional behavior change with practical significance. They concluded that change is best considered to be an extended process rather than an event. They artificially divided the process into five stages.

In the first stage (*precontemplation*), the patient is not seriously considering a particular behavior change in the foreseeable future. In the second stage (*contemplation*), the person is considering change and needs to resolve ambivalence and make a decision to change. In the third stage (*preparation*), patients make a commitment and have an effective and acceptable plan for change. The fourth stage (*action*) is marked by behavior directed toward implementing the change and revising the plan when needed. The fifth and final stage (*maintenance*) is one in which the person takes follow-up steps to sustain the change.

An important aspect of this cycle is that patients typically traverse the stages multiple times before a stable state of recovery is established. Being aware of this phenomenon can be useful in helping both patients and clinicians persevere and not surrender to the discouragement and even hopelessness that can interfere with the long-term recovery process.

The stages of change model provides a road map so that the most effective interventions can be tailored to the patient's current stage. For hospitalized SUD patients, the most clinically challenging and most commonly encountered stages are precontemplation and contemplation. These patients frequently elicit feelings of frustration and even animosity in clinicians. Their lack of acknowledgment of needing assistance with a substance use problem that seemed obvious to others led in the past to characterizing them as being "in denial" about their addiction. Clinical interventions intended to "break through the denial" would often result in an adversarial relationship.

The advent of *motivational interviewing*, developed by William Miller and Stephen Rollnick (Miller and Rollnick 2013), provided an alternative clinical approach that is more collaborative. The foundation of this approach is the establishment of an empathetic relationship with the patient. Described as "a person-centered counseling style for addressing the common problem of *ambivalence* about change," motivational interviewing replaces "denial" with "ambivalence" as the central psychological issue. Ambivalence is considered to be not pathological but rather a normal part of the process of change. The patient wants to keep using the substance because of its positive effects and at the same time stop using it because of the problems it creates.

The task of the clinician is to support the side of the ambivalence that moves the patient in the direction of recovery. One specific way to accomplish this is to be alert to and positively reinforce "change talk," which is anything that patients say that moves them in the direction of recovery. This would include positive statements about the benefits of stopping substance use and negative statements about the problems associated with continued use. By contrast, "sustain talk," which moves patients away from recovery, is to be ignored. Examples would be statements about the relative impossibility of stopping use and the pleasures of continuing to use. Efforts by the clinician to counter sustain talk typically trigger the patient to engage in more sustain talk, thus reinforcing the undesirable side of the ambivalence. Miller and Rollnick point out that trying to argue the patient into recovery is a strategy with little likelihood of success.

Addressing Cravings for Substance Use (Relapse Prevention)

When a patient is admitted to the co-occurring unit, abstinence from addictive substances is established. A return to substance use following discharge is highly likely unless a relapse prevention strategy is designed and implemented. The relapse path consists of a series of relatively predictable steps. Educating patients about this process can be a useful way of reducing the likelihood of a relapse following discharge.

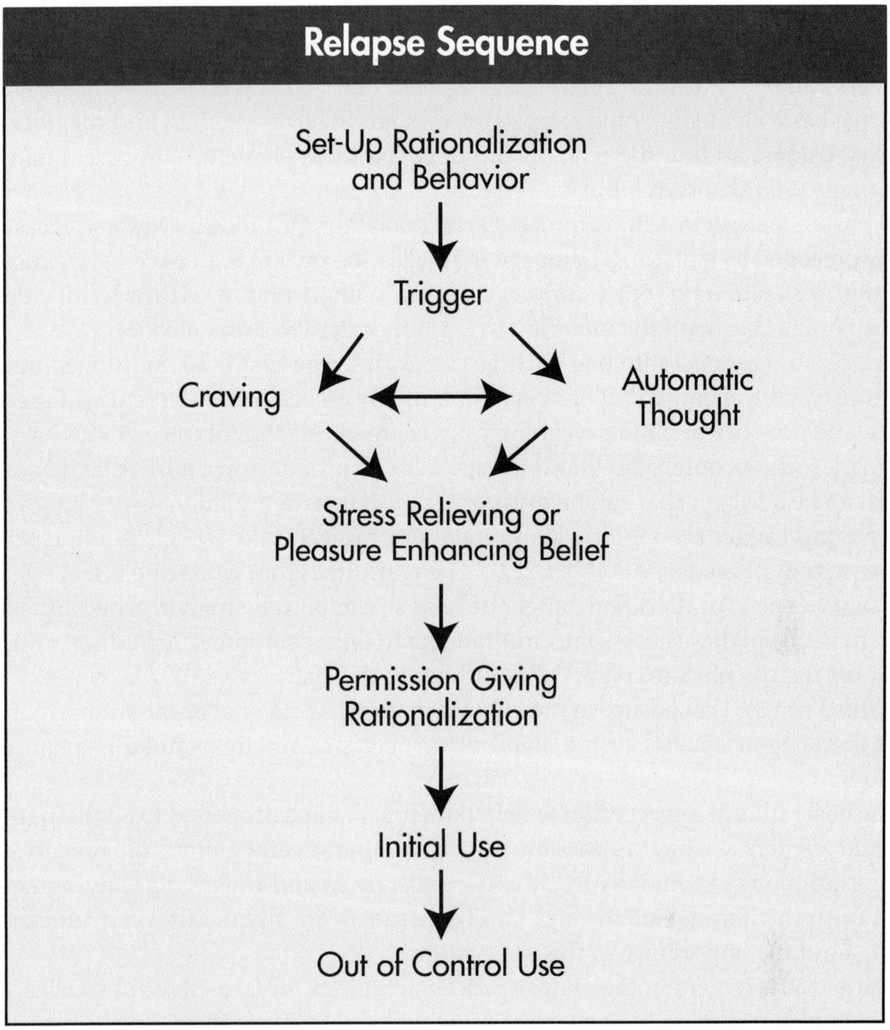

FIGURE 10–1. Relapse sequence.

The transient cognitive impairment frequently seen in newly admitted SUD patients will render many psychotherapeutic interventions ineffective in the short term. On the other hand, a psychoeducational introduction to the relapse process can be at least partially comprehended by these patients and is well worth the effort, with the understanding that repetition will be necessary as the patient improves.

One way of describing the relapse sequence is through the use of the language of cognitive-behavioral therapy (CBT). The concepts of CBT have provided clinicians with a useful tool to use to promote abstinence: language with which to communicate with each other as well as with patients (Beck et al. 1993; Marlatt and Donovan 2005). Figure 10–1, adapted from the work of Marlatt and Beck, is one example of how to diagram the progression of this process.

One of the fundamental points to convey to patients is to consider relapse as a process rather than an event. They often experience a relapse as something that happens to them without warning. Demonstrating to them, by reviewing their own past experiences, that early warning signs exist provides them with multiple opportunities for early intervention. Thus, the confusion and feelings of helplessness that interfere with recovery can be reduced.

Three basic elements of the relapse process are *triggers*, *cravings*, and *cognitive distortions*. Understanding the relationship between these elements empowers patients to manage their disorder more successfully.

Exposure to triggers is the common starting point for the process. On some occasions, this is preceded by a distorted thought that leads the person to unnecessary exposure to a high-risk situation. For example, a person with alcohol use disorder decides to visit a familiar bar with the intention to eat rather than to drink alcohol.

Relapse triggers fall into one of three categories. The first is a conditioned cue—a previously neutral entity that has been repetitively associated with the use of the substance and now has become psychologically charged. Alcoholics Anonymous (AA) refers to these as "people, places, and things." The time of day on a particular day of the week can be a trigger that can be mystifying until it is identified.

A second trigger is an internal emotional or physical state, especially if it is stressful. An acronym used by AA is "HALT." The warning is that when one is feeling hungry, angry, lonely, or tired, the danger of relapse can become higher, especially when more than one of these is present simultaneously. Other emotions, including guilt and shame as well as physical pain, can be added to this list.

A third trigger is exposure to the substance itself. Accidental or intentional contact with the taste of alcohol or the smell of tobacco or cannabis smoke is a common example.

The basic clinical intervention to help patients manage triggers is to advise patients to avoid triggers as much as possible during the first several months of recovery. One basic example is to remove all addictive substances and the accompanying equipment from the home. Patients and family members are frequently very reluctant to understand the importance of this suggestion.

The second element in the relapse process, cravings for addictive substances, is of sufficient importance to have been included in the ICD-10 diagnosis and to have been added as a criterion in DSM-5. The definition used in DSM-5 is "an intense desire or urge for the drug." A suggested query is to ask "if there has ever been a time when they had such strong urges to take the drug that they could not think of anything else" (American Psychiatric Association 2013, p. 483).

Clinical understanding of the psychological and physiological bases of craving is unfortunately limited. Despite the development of several scales to measure craving intensity, none have been scientifically validated. Furthermore, great variability exists between patients in the frequency and intensity of the symptoms. Although patients are usually uncomfortable about their struggle with craving, they do not always spontaneously complain about this. Specifically asking about the presence and intensity of craving is therefore advisable. Patients are sometimes misled by the disappearance of cravings in the contained setting of a hospital and will wishfully assume that cravings will not be a problem after discharge.

Fortunately, practical clinical interventions have evolved and can be useful to discuss with SUD patients during their usually brief stays. Because these interventions are concrete and specific, patients can begin to understand and apply them quickly.

A basic psychotherapeutic intervention to manage cravings is to educate patients about them. The first step is to sensitively inform the patient of the likelihood of the recurrence of cravings following discharge and enlist the patient in trying to make a plan to deal with them. The next step is to review the process by which relapses occur and in which cravings play a central role.

The third element in the relapse process, a variety of types of distorted thinking, typically accompanies the triggers and cravings. This phenomenon has long been known in the 12-step community, where it is referred to as "stinking thinking." (For a detailed discussion of the varieties of thoughts and beliefs, see Beck et al. 1993.) Briefly, the thoughts, known generally as "cognitive distortions" or more specifically as "addiction thinking," contain a kernel of accuracy. They are, however, flawed in critical ways that can lead to a return to substance use. Patients are taught to recognize these thoughts and counter them.

Participation in the Recovery Support Community

The isolation and hopelessness often experienced by people with active SUDs can be moderated by meaningful engagement in the recovery support community. Patients sometimes act as though they need to make a choice between these support groups and professional follow-up treatment. An optimal treatment plan, however, involves both, because of the different contributions each brings to the recovery process.

While involvement in the recovery community comes easily for some people, for others this requires skillful facilitation by clinicians. Resistance can come from actual negative experiences or just expectations based on secondhand information. Encouraging or expecting a willingness to "give meetings a try" is preferable to mandates, which can trigger increased resentment in patients whose stage of change is precontemplation or early contemplation.

Making an early introduction is usually preferable to waiting until later in treatment. This can sometimes be done by means of an "institutional meeting," which some 12-step fellowship mutual support programs, such as AA and Narcotics Anonymous (NA), are willing to bring into hospital wards. Higher-quality experiences may result if the local 12-step organization establishes a regular "open" meeting in a room off the treatment unit but still within the building.

For many years, 12-step fellowship mutual support groups were the only abstinence-oriented community recovery support options. While these groups are still the most widespread options, the evolution of alternative groups has been an important addition. These groups have heterogeneous orientations ranging from the secular (e.g., SMART Recovery, Women for Sobriety) to explicitly religious or Buddhist based (e.g., Celebrate Recovery, Refuge Recovery). As these other options began to emerge, competition and even animosity made it potentially more complicated for a patient to negotiate this landscape. This tension has fortunately been diminishing in recent years, and participation in multiple types of recovery organizations is becoming more common.

At a leadership level of community recovery support organizations, the importance of working collaboratively with professional treatment organizations is recognized. Approved literature is distributed to ensure consistency. Individual members, however, will sometimes violate the written positions of the organization and give patients unsolicited negative advice about treatment, particularly in regard to the use of medication. The most unfortunate example of this has been the opposition to buprenorphine and methadone by members of NA, as well as the organization itself. Ideally, the clinician will be knowledgeable about which meetings are more supportive and direct patients to them. Another option is to suggest that patients taking opioid agonist medication attend AA instead of NA, even if alcohol has not been a problem, because AA is more tolerant of the use of those medications. As long as the NA problem persists, it is advisable to warn patients to be prepared for this response. While not ideal, patients can be counseled to not disclose their medication use, or to work with a sponsor who is supportive of the proper use of medication.

Another unfortunate problem to be avoided is the exploitation of young women in early recovery by predatory male group members. This is particularly relevant for women who are sexual abuse survivors and, as a result, may be insufficiently self-protective. Some 12-step groups are restricted to women, and suggesting that attendance be initially limited to these groups can be useful.

Involvement of Significant Others

Treatment outcomes are improved when clinicians are able to engage those individuals who are important in the patient's life. Because patients with SUD are often incomplete historians, admission assessments will be more accurate if additional information is obtained from collateral sources. Relationships are frequently under stress and in need of clinical intervention. At times, significant others have become enablers by attempting to be helpful in ways that in fact perpetuate the addiction. On occasion, others may have their own active addiction problem. A postdischarge treatment plan is more likely to be effective if these issues are identified and incorporated into the plan.

The Importance of Long-Term Follow-Up

Treatment outcomes for patients with SUD are significantly enhanced when the chronic nature of the disorders is addressed. Planning for appropriate treatment following the resolution of the acute presenting symptoms is essential yet problematic given the short-term limitations of the inpatient unit. Moreover, SUD patients, now relieved of their acute discomfort and chagrined about the substance use that contributed to their admission, often do not appreciate the magnitude of the task of establishing a stable long-term recovery. When follow-up treatment is not adequate, the likelihood of relapse and readmission is high.

A traditional way to address this issue is through the work of internal discharge coordinators who are employed by the hospital. Representatives from insurance companies are sometimes involved as well, in which case coordination on a staff level can become an issue. When feasible, an additional option is for representatives of addiction treatment programs to meet with patients prior to discharge. These meetings can occur in person or by phone.

Deciding on the level of care to refer the patient to for continued care is a challenging task. Based on the ASAM dimensional assessment, placement in an appropriate inpatient or outpatient treatment setting is recommended. The complexity of this process has led to the development of a more user-friendly computerized version called Continuum.

Important practical considerations enter into the final decision, such as the preference of patients and family members, financing, and availability of treatment slots.

Future Directions

The magnitude of the opioid problem will continue to diminish. As the move toward decriminalizing cannabis continues and potency increases, problems with cannabis use will become more prominent. Research findings in neuroscience will lead to a better understanding of and more effective treatment interventions for SUDs. Increased evidence of the neurobiological roots of behavioral addictions will lead to increased attention by the treatment community. Substances that are misused or that individuals get addicted to will offer us an opportunity to understand neurobiology better and also provide a window to future therapeutics. Technological advances like apps, telemedicine, and social media will become more important and better integrated in the treatment of co-occurring disorders.

References

American Psychiatric Association: Diagnostic and Statistical Manual of Mental Disorders, 5th Edition. Arlington, VA, American Psychiatric Association, 2013

American Society of Addiction Medicine: Terminology related to addiction, treatment, and recovery. July 2013. Available at: www.williamwhitepapers.com/pr/dlm_uploads/ASAM-Recovery-Terminology-2013.pdf. Accessed October 31, 2021.

Anderson EL, Nordstrom K, Wilson MP, et al: American Association for Emergency Psychiatry Task Force on Medical Clearance of Adults, part I: introduction, review and evidence-based guidelines. West J Emerg Med 18(2):235–242, 2017 28210358

Beck AT, Wright FD, Newman CF, Liese BS: Cognitive Therapy of Substance Abuse. New York, Guilford, 1993

Blondell RD, Dodds HN, Blondell MN, et al: Ethanol in formularies of US teaching hospitals (letter). JAMA 289(5):552, 2003 12578486

DiClemente CC: Addiction and Change: How Addictions Develop and Addicted People Recover, 2nd Edition. New York, Guilford, 2018

Gotham HJ, Claus RE, Selig K, Homer AL: Increasing program capability to provide treatment for co-occurring substance use and mental disorders: organizational characteristics. J Subst Abuse Treat 38(2):160–169, 2010 19717273

Herring AA, Vosooghi AA, Luftig J, et al: High-dose buprenorphine induction in the emergency department for treatment of opioid use disorder. JAMA Netw Open 4(7):e2117128, 2021 34264326

Lee S, Tucci V, Moukaddam N, et al: Pregnant and virtually abandoned: the multiple hurdles of medically clearing and admitting a pregnant patient to an inpatient psychiatric unit. Journal of Psychiatry and Mental Health 1(1), 2016

Li X, Moore S, Olsen C: Urine drug tests: how to make the most of them: Effective use of UDTs requires carefully interpreting the results, and modifying treatment accordingly. Curr Psychiatr 18(8): 2019

Lindner BK, Gilmore VT, Kruer RM, et al: The ASAM Criteria. Chevy Chase, MD, American Society of Addiction Medicine, 2013

Lindner BK, Gilmore VT, Kruer RM, et al: Evaluation of the Brief Alcohol Withdrawal Scale protocol at an academic medical center. J Addict Med 13(5):379–384, 2019 30741834

Marlatt GA, Donovan DM (eds): Relapse Prevention: Maintenance Strategies in the Treatment of Addictive Behaviors, 2nd Edition. New York, Guilford, 2005

Miller WR, Rollnick S: Motivational Interviewing: Helping People Change, 3rd Edition. New York, Guilford, 2013

Minkoff K: An integrated treatment model for dual diagnosis of psychosis and addiction. Hosp Community Psychiatry 40(10):1031–1036, 1989 2807203

Mueser KT (ed): Integrated Treatment for Dual Disorders: A Guide to Effective Practice. New York, Guilford, 2003

Nisbet AT, Mooney-Cotter F: Comparison of selected sedation scales for reporting opioid-induced sedation assessment. Pain Manag Nurs 10(3):154–164, 2009 19706353

Osher FC, Kofoed LL: Treatment of patients with psychiatric and psychoactive substance abuse disorders. Hosp Community Psychiatry 40(10):1025–1030, 1989 2807202

Sperry L, Gudeman JE, Blackwell B, et al: Psychiatric Case Formulations. Washington, DC, American Psychiatric Press, 1992

Sullivan JT, Sykora K, Schneiderman J, et al: Assessment of alcohol withdrawal: the revised Clinical Institute Withdrawal Assessment for Alcohol scale (CIWA-Ar). Br J Addict 84(11):1353–1357, 1989 2597811

Vaillant GE: Triumphs of Experience. Cambridge, MA, Harvard University Press, 2012

Velasquez MM, Crouch C, Stephens NS, DiClemente CC: Group Treatment for Substance Abuse: A Stages-of-Change Therapy Manual. New York, Guilford, 2015

Volkow ND, Koob GF, McLellan AT: Neurobiologic advances from the brain disease model of addiction. N Engl J Med 374(4):363–371, 2016 26816013

Weinberger AH, Platt J, Esan H, et al: Cigarette smoking is associated with increased risk of substance use disorder relapse: a nationally representative, prospective longitudinal investigation. J Clin Psychiatry 78(2):e152–e160, 2017 28234432

Wesson DR, Ling W: The Clinical Opiate Withdrawal Scale (COWS). J Psychoactive Drugs 35(2):253–259, 2003 12924748

Wilson MP, Nordstrom K, Anderson EL, et al: American Association for Emergency Psychiatry Task Force on Medical Clearance of Adult Psychiatric Patients, Part II: controversies over medical assessment, and consensus recommendations. West J Emerg Med 18(4):640–646, 2017 28611885

Wüsthoff LE, Waal H, Gråwe RW: The effectiveness of integrated treatment in patients with substance use disorders co-occurring with anxiety and/or depression: a group randomized trial. BMC Psychiatry 14(1):67, 2014 24597469

Specialty Settings

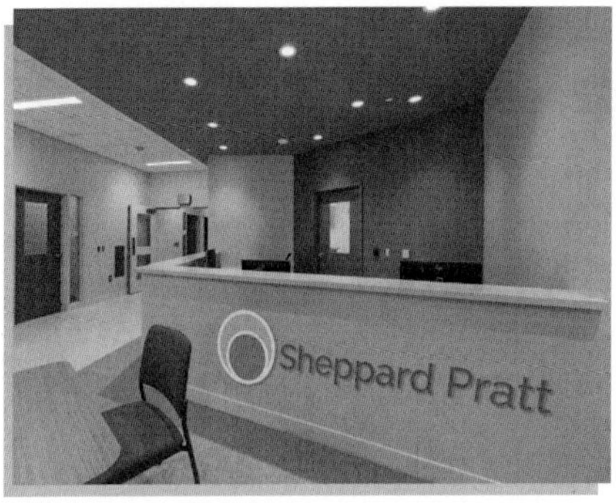

CHAPTER 11

The State Hospital

Debra A. Pinals, M.D.
Brian M. Hepburn, M.D.
Ted Lutterman, B.A.

History of Inpatient Psychiatric Service in the United States

State hospital psychiatry has changed dramatically over the past 75 years. With these changes, differences have evolved in hospitals from state to state. Populations served in the height of the state hospital movement by the mid- to late nineteenth century struggled with a variety of conditions, ranging from epilepsy, Huntington's disease, inebriation, and tertiary syphilis to intellectual disability (intellectual developmental disorder) and neurocognitive conditions, to name a few (Lutterman et al. 2017). For well over a century, however, the state hospitals in the United States were developed primarily to provide the great predominance of inpatient services for individuals with severe mental illness (Geller 2000; Goldman et al. 1983; Talbott 2004). However, since the introduction of community mental health and of Medicare and Medicaid in the 1960s, there has been a dramatic increase in inpatient services at acute general and private psychiatric hospitals. In fact, these settings now provide the bulk of hospital psychiatric care. Although many people still speak about the need for "more [state hospital] beds," there is increased recognition that with development of a full continuum of psychiatric services, ranging from crisis services to inpatient level of care, there could be less reliance on institutional settings (Pinals and Fuller 2020). The state hospitals have thus come to be seen as only one end of the continuum and primarily serve the severely and persistently ill population who cannot be managed in or gain access to the private sector, or more commonly, these facilities serve forensic populations sent by criminal courts.

Populations in the twenty-first century within state hospitals are often divided categorically by their legal status into "civil" and "forensic" populations (Parks and Radke 2014). The forensic categorizations typically include those persons found incompetent to stand trial and those found not guilty by reason of insanity (NGRI). There are other related populations that might be served, such as those undergoing forensic evaluation sent by the courts, though most evaluations are now done on an outpatient basis in communities, including in jails (Wik et al. 2017). Some state hospitals evaluate and treat individuals who are sent from jails and prisons when a hospital level of care may be needed. After several landmark legal decisions (see, e.g., *Kansas v. Hendricks* 1997), many states began to utilize and build hospitals to treat individuals who were civilly committed after being found sexually dangerous because of some type of "mental abnormality" after serving sentences for sex-offending behavior, but who are still often referred to or managed as forensic populations. There are also individuals served by state hospitals who do not have a forensic status but whose behavior is dysregulated or predatory, violent, or chronically self-injurious, and for whom it might be difficult to find a setting in the community that is equipped to support them.

State hospitals generally also represent the safety net for individuals who are uninsured and whose illness does not respond to briefer forms of intervention. With more individuals insured across the country, private and acute hospitals tend to be the mainstay of acute psychiatric care. Still, most states maintain some level of state hospital supports for adults age 21 and older as well as youth younger than 18 or 21, depending on the age cutoff the state sets. Children's units in state hospitals are complex environments. Many youth will have child welfare and even juvenile justice involvement.

With state hospitals left to manage a complicated and deep-end population, the range of behavioral, legal, and social issues faced by patients admitted to state hospitals raises numerous challenges in the landscape of state hospital management. Much of this chapter focuses on the adult populations within state hospitals, although some further aspects of child and adolescent services are highlighted below.

It is well known that the number of persons served in state hospitals dramatically declined in the twentieth century for a variety of social policy and financial reasons. In 1970 there were 369,969 state and county psychiatric hospital beds, and in 2018 there were 39,276 (Substance Abuse and Mental Health Services Administration 2019b). In 1970, 78% of all psychiatric beds were in state psychiatric hospitals. With the elimination of state psychiatric hospital beds and an increase in private psychiatric hospitals and general hospital psychiatric units, by 2018, state psychiatric hospitals represented only 23% of all psychiatric beds. Overall number of state hospitals shifted from 310 in 1970 (Lutterman et al. 2017) to 206 in 2018 (Substance Abuse and Mental Health Services Administration 2019b). Private psychiatric hospitals increased from 150 to 482. (The number of private psychiatric hospitals grew from 1970 to 1990, before declining until the early 2000s, and then increasing 91% from 2002 to 2018.) The influence of managed care on length of stay likely contributed greatly to the decrease in private psychiatric hospitals in the 1990s and early 2000s. Nonfederal general hospitals with separate psychiatric units increased from 664 to 1,053, peaking at 1,593 hospitals with psychiatric beds in 1998 (but decreasing 34% from 1998 to 2018) (Substance Abuse and Mental Health Services Administration 2019b; see Figure 11–1).

Between 1970 and 2004, state hospital admissions were reduced from 487,000 to 266,000, whereas private psychiatric hospital admissions increased from 92,000 to 599,000, and general hospital psychiatric admissions increased from 478,000 to 1,533,000 (Figure 11–2). There were approximately 1.2 million psychiatric admissions in 1969 and 2.7 million admissions in 2004 (Substance Abuse and Mental Health Services Administration 2010). With more people insured and, therefore, able to get their care in the community, there has also been an evolving expectation that individuals will get services in hospitals placed in the community regardless of their ability to pay. Also, laws like the Emergency Medical Treatment and Active Labor Act require sending and receiving hospitals to accept patients regardless of ability to pay.

These various changes in financing have contributed to major shifts in inpatient psychiatric care delivery, which have impacted state hospital admissions. For example, from 2005 to 2018, the number of admissions to state psychiatric hospitals declined by 62%. In 2018, state psychiatric hospitals had 40,473 residents on the first day of the year (Substance Abuse and Mental Health Services Administration 2019a). The utilization rate dropped from 16.5 per 100,000 in 2005 to 12.6 in 2018, with rates steady through 2021. Every state operated psychiatric inpatient beds in 2018, although one state operates their psychiatric inpatient beds as part of a state-operated general hospital (Lutterman et al. 2017).

In 2018, 83% of individuals in state hospitals were adults ages 21–64. Thirty years ago, persons older than 64 years made up more than 25% of the state hospital population. Today, they make up 5.5%. Women compose 33% of the state hospital population, and men make up 67% of the population (Substance Abuse and Mental Health Services Administration 2019a).

The majority of the adults in state hospitals have serious mental illnesses, such as schizophrenia and affective disorders (Substance Abuse and Mental Health Services Administration, Center for Behavioral Health Statistics and Quality 2020). In 2018, in state and county psychiatric hospitals serving adults, approximately 40% of inpatients had co-occurring mental health and substance use disorders (Substance Abuse and Mental Health Services Administration 2019b).

Types of State Hospital Units

Although there is variation between states depending on the number of state psychiatric hospitals and the number of beds, state hospital units may be identified as follows (Santoni and Sundeen 2007):

- *Acute units* are admission units where intensive intervention and treatment and discharge planning occur. Because state hospitals are often not in the business of acute care as the private hospital system is, these units are sometimes designated simply "admission units" because they receive patients being transferred for longer care, often from acute psychiatric hospitals.
- *Continuing care units* are units in which nursing and rehabilitation services are provided in addition to treatment for individuals who require inpatient care beyond

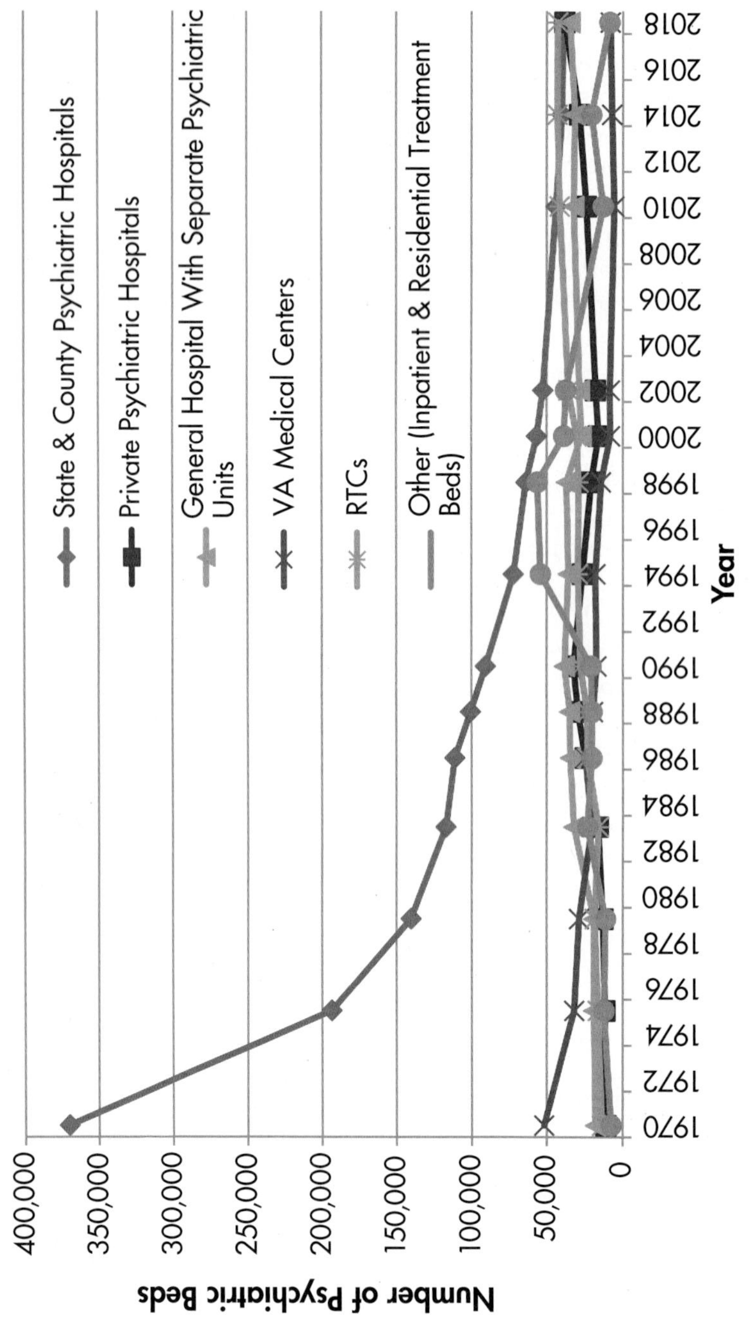

FIGURE 11–1. Distribution of psychiatric beds by type of hospital, 1970–2018.
Source. Adapted by NRI with original data from Substance Abuse and Mental Health Services Administration 2019b.

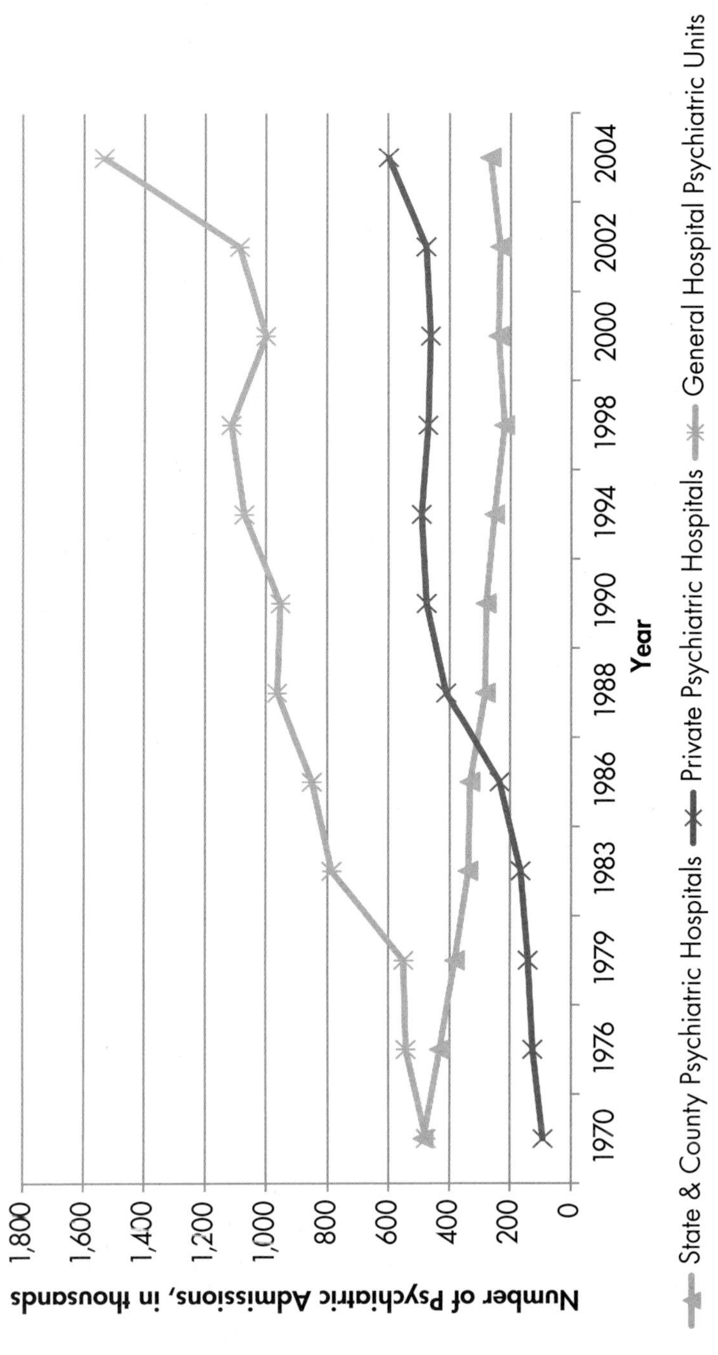

FIGURE 11–2. Admissions to psychiatric beds by type of hospital, 1970–2004.
Source. Adapted by NRI with original data from the National Institute of Mental Health and the Substance Abuse and Mental Health Services Administration.

the acute phase of their mental illness or the initial phase of adjustment to the state hospital.

- *Forensic admission units* are often more secure acute units to which individuals are admitted for pretrial evaluations, such as for competence to stand trial, and posttrial evaluations and for treatment after a court adjudication of an individual as not criminally responsible or NGRI.
- *Forensic continuing care units* are typically more secure units that treat and house those members of the population identified in forensic admission units as having service needs similar to those of individuals treated in continuing-care nonforensic units.

In some states, the civil status and forensic populations are evaluated and treated separately, and in other states they are combined on the same unit. Some states will have units designated for more medically frail, often older adult, populations. Of note, persons with intellectual and/or developmental disability with and without concomitant serious mental illness—often admitted because of some forensic involvement or serious behavioral dysfunction—have once again increasingly been noted as a unique population on psychiatric state hospital units (Pinals et al. 2017). This is likely due to a variety of system shifts and other factors.

Civil Status Population in State Hospitals

The civil status population in state hospitals is made up of individuals identified as typically having met civil commitment criteria as a risk of harm to self or others or unable to care for themselves as a result of mental illness. They may be voluntary or certified (i.e., committed by a court). The limitation of commitment to populations deemed "dangerous" as a result of mental illness has become a source of newly emerging discussion; some proponents have advocated for broadening of commitment criteria, and some states have modified their commitment criteria to account for more need for treatment and risk of deterioration-type issues and have expanded use of outpatient commitment, commonly referred to as *assisted outpatient treatment* (AOT; American Psychiatric Association 2015). At the same time, states are also expanding laws pertaining to *psychiatric advance directives*, which would potentially allow individuals to assert their preferences about hospitalization prior to becoming symptomatic.

With the state-by-state variability in the legal regulation of psychiatric admissions, individuals may be certified as meeting criteria for admission in one state but not another. Nevertheless, the trend for civil patients in state hospitals has been to only admit certified individuals, especially as the individuals typically have already been certified in their acute hospital stay, and the state hospital becomes a site for transfer and continuing care. With more attention to self-directed care, however, there may be some shifts in this trend.

Lengths of stay vary considerably for civil patients but tend to be longer than what is seen in the private system. Those individuals who have stable community supports and resources will generally be able to leave the hospital sooner. Linkage to community services can be challenging, because with fewer state hospitals, geographical distances from natural community environments can create barriers to discharge planning.

Treatment within state hospitals focuses on stabilization, medication treatment, individual and group therapies, and discharge planning (including finding stable housing and securing entitlements). One of the important features of state inpatient care has been the inclusion of rehabilitation services in addition to traditional treatment services. Rehabilitation services aim to improve communication, work capability, and daily living skills (Dhillon and Dollieslager 2000). These have been a focus of the state hospital work, especially given the generally longer lengths of stay in these facilities.

Child and Adolescent Population in State Hospitals

Some states do not provide state hospital services to individuals younger than 21 years. With the expansion of Medicaid and the Children's Health Insurance Program (CHIP), almost every child or adolescent has insurance and can receive their services in the community. The exception is increasingly those youth who are under the order of courts. That said, state hospitals for children and adolescents continue to exist across the country, with individuals younger than 21 years making up 7.1% of the individuals in state hospitals (Substance Abuse and Mental Health Services Administration 2019a). Many have a mix of mental disorders such as ADHD, neurodevelopmental disorders, conduct disorder, oppositional defiant disorder, and affective and psychotic disorders, as well as trauma histories.

Diagnostic assessment, symptom management, and community reintegration are often the primary focus of child and adolescent treatment within state hospitals. Work with youth requires collaboration between parents and/or the legally authorized representative for the youth, the educational setting, and other agencies. In addition, crisis management can sometimes lead to state psychiatric hospitalization, as more youth are boarded in emergency departments awaiting admission, which often is elusive in the private system, especially for youth with more complex conditions or more complex dispositional needs (Nordstrom et al. 2019). State-operated child units provide the opportunity for more extensive diagnostic evaluations, complex medical management, and coordination of care with other state agencies (dosReis et al. 2003).

Similar to those for the adult population, the public inpatient mental health facilities for children and adolescents have moved in the direction of providing court-ordered evaluation and/or treatment. A recent change in the use of public psychiatric child and adolescent units is their role in determining competence to stand trial. Youth found to be not competent are referred to competency restoration services, which may be inpatient. After an inpatient stay and restoration of competency, these individuals are then referred back to the court (Wall et al. 2018).

Forensic Population in State Hospitals

As noted in the overview above, many state hospitals have responsibility for court-ordered evaluations of criminal defendants' competence to stand trial or criminal responsibility (legal "insanity"). Evaluations have for the most part shifted to community settings, but commitment for treatment of forensically involved individuals has become increasingly common (Parks and Radke 2014). Many of these individuals will initially be placed on an admissions unit for evaluation for the courts as well as an assessment of their clinical and behavioral health needs. In many states, individuals charged with higher-level crimes, such as murder, rape, arson, armed robbery, kidnapping, or carjacking, may be evaluated or treated only on a secure forensic unit or within a dedicated secure forensic hospital.

Individuals admitted for forensic evaluation or treatment are offered treatment during their stay, and patients will often take medications and participate in programs voluntarily. With regard to administering medications to patients who prefer not to take them, all states allow for emergency involuntary medication when indicated. All states also have provisions with different laws and legal cases that drive process for medication over objection in the nonemergency situation. For individuals admitted for forensic evaluation, the evaluation is typically done on a designated forensic unit, and the evaluators' reports are then submitted to the court. Following the forensic evaluation period, the court determines whether the individual is competent to stand trial (Wall et al. 2018) or not criminally responsible or NGRI (Janofsky et al. 2014). State hospital beds are increasingly used to admit individuals who are ordered for competence to stand trial restoration after they have been found incompetent to stand trial (Wik et al. 2017), though states are also exploring mechanisms to divert individuals out of the competency system (Pinals and Callahan 2020) or at least into community-based restoration services (Wik 2018). If an individual is found not criminally responsible, state hospitals are often also used for initial assessments to determine if they should be committed to the state hospital for further treatment, and then state hospital beds are used for that treatment, often for years. Patients retained in the state hospitals as not criminally responsible are held generally if determined a risk of harm to themselves or others based on mental disorder.

Discharge for forensic patients can be as complicated as admission processes, as courts are often involved and can even be the ultimate decision maker in some jurisdictions. For individuals found incompetent to stand trial, once competence is restored, they will typically return to court and possibly jail, though a hearing regarding their competence to stand trial may be required before discharge. If competence is deemed unrestorable, the patients may be switched to a civil commitment and held in the hospital, or their criminal case may be disposed of and they may end up released from court. There are a host of systemic issues related to the current system for individuals in the competency system (Callahan and Pinals 2020).

Individuals found not criminally responsible after a period of time can be committed (if found to be a risk of harm because of a mental disorder), released (if not deemed at substantial risk), or, in many jurisdictions, placed on "conditional" release (if safe to be in the community with services in place and other conditions imposed). These individuals will often have periodic reviews with a court or an administrative authority and/or with clinical risk assessments informing discharge decisions. In many states, only the court may release the individual. In some states, an agency or facility-based forensic review board will review the treatment team's findings and advise the state hospital regarding its opinion for the court on the individual's readiness for release or conditional release. Although the legal and security issues are prominent, it is important to note that the focus of the treatment team and the forensic review board is on the patient's psychiatric illness and rehabilitation needs. Conditional release can be confused with the recent iterations of AOT. The former involves the criminal courts, and the latter is a civil court process.

For individuals found incompetent to stand trial, release decisions generally depend on whether their capacities as pretrial defendants have been improved enough for them to be found competent. In those instances, they will be returned to jail in most instances to await trial. For some individuals who are not able to be restored to competence, some other process might ensue, like a civil commitment to the state hospital (Pinals and Callahan 2020).

Nearly all state mental health agencies (SMHAs) provide forensic mental health services Ninety-four percent of states use their psychiatric hospitals to provide services to forensic patients. Fifteen percent of individuals admitted to state hospitals in 2015 had forensic status, and 34% of residents in state hospitals at the end of 2015 had a forensic status (Substance Abuse and Mental Health Services Administration 2017).

One of the more knotty areas of involvement for public mental health has been working with the forensic population referred by the courts after conviction for a sexual offense (Fitch and Hammen 2003). As of 2016, 20 states have laws providing for the special civil commitment of sex offenders, typically called *sexually violent predators*, according to National Association of State Mental Health Program Directors state profiles (Lutterman et al. 2017). Generally, these laws provide for civil commitment after an individual has completed their criminal sentence and is about to be released (Pinals et al. 2011). Although the SMHA is typically responsible for evaluation and treatment, at times it may also provide or administer the facility or purchase security services. The treatment of sexually violent individuals is similar to that of other state hospital patients when an underlying severe psychiatric illness exists. However, only a small percentage of these individuals have severe mental illness, whereas the majority are diagnosed with paraphilias and personality disorders (Becker et al. 2014; Galbreath et al. 2002). The main reason for their commitment is related to community safety. These individuals receive postsentence commitment that may result in indefinite confinement with little opportunity to return to the community (*Karsjens et al. v. Minnesota Department of Human Services et al.* 2018). Their confinement may take resources away from the mental health system and further stigmatize the individuals with mental illness. This is an evolving area of development.

Impact of the State Hospital in the Overall Continuum of Care for Civil Status and Forensic Patients

State hospitals are generally an important part of the continuum of psychiatric care and affect the overall health care system, but as noted above they are only one part of it (Pinals and Fuller 2020). The reduction of state hospital beds in addition to the recent declines in the number of general hospital and private psychiatric hospital beds has resulted in 76% of states reporting a shortage of psychiatric beds (Lutterman et al. 2017), though there is also a growing effort to expand services beyond beds and across the continuum of care (Pinals and Fuller 2020)

Certain populations, including those with intellectual and developmental disability, violence histories, and other challenges, have a more difficult time accessing psychiatric hospital beds. The opioid crisis and the complexities of co-occurring substance use disorder are another factor impacting the continuum of care. The state hospitals have nevertheless continued to be a safety net for additional populations at a time when the supply of beds is decreasing.

In addition to the increased emergency department pressure, courts, jails, and prisons often cite the reduction in state hospital beds as a reason for having higher numbers of persons with mental illness in those justice settings. The phenomenon of individuals with mental illness in the justice system is complex (Lutterman et al. 2017; Pinals and Fuller 2017). There is much discussion taking place about the need to expand the crisis services continuum to fully build out the front end, as opposed to solely focusing on state hospitals as the back-end solution to some of the societal challenges that have contributed to current circumstances (Pinals 2020; Substance Abuse and Mental Health Services Administration 2020). The Sequential Intercept Model (Abreu et al. 2017; Munetz and Griffin 2006) was developed to try to address and reshift individuals with mental illness, intellectual disability, and substance use disorder from justice settings to treatment. For example, states and communities have responded by setting up diversion strategies, crisis intervention teams, mental health courts, reentry services, and the like (Abreu et al. 2017; Pinals 2014).

The relationship between state hospital and community services varies among the states. Across the country, 75% of expenditures of SMHAs are for community services, and approximately 22% are for state hospitals (Lutterman et al. 2017). Despite greater funding for community services, there continues to be a shortage of them. As indicated previously, because of persistent psychiatric symptoms, the need for intensive levels of community services (e.g., assertive community treatment), housing, and/or other services to address complicating social issues remains. Other programs designed to address mental illness earlier, such as first-episode psychosis programs, are also emerging (Kazandjian and Lutterman 2018) but are not as widely available as might be needed.

Importantly, for many years the hue and cry to solve problems was that there needed to be more state hospital psychiatric beds. As noted, more recently the discourse has shifted toward examining on a community, state, and federal level the adequacy of crisis services and other supports along the full continuum of care to support individuals of all ages who require different levels of clinical services at different phases of their illness (Pinals and Fuller 2017.

Accreditation, Patient Rights, and Legal Issues

Joint Commission Accreditation and Performance Measurement

Since 1971, the Joint Commission has been evaluating organizations that provide mental health services, including state hospitals. In 2016, over 80% of state psychiatric hospitals were accredited by the Joint Commission (Lutterman et al. 2017). Two of the primary areas of the Joint Commission's focus are performance and safety.

In February 1997, the Joint Commission began its ORYX initiative to integrate outcomes and other performance measurement data into the accreditation process. However, reporting of data for behavioral health organizations, including state hospitals, was deferred until core measures were identified. The Joint Commission and various mental health organizations worked together to identify and implement a test set of core performance measures (Joint Commission 2008). To date, agreement has been reached on testing the following measures: assessment of violence risk, substance use disorder, trauma, and patient strengths; hours of restraint use; hours of seclusion use; number of patients discharged on multiple antipsychotic medications; and discharge assessment and aftercare recommendations sent to providers at the next level of care upon discharge. The Hospital-Based Inpatient Psychiatric Services core measure set now includes a number of standardized measures for freestanding psychiatric hospitals to help them meet Centers for Medicare & Medicaid Services requirements (see Jointcommission.org; Joint Commission 2021). Measures include screening for risk of violence to self and others, substance use, and psychological trauma history, and assessment of patient strengths. Also, duration of restraint, duration of seclusion, and the number of patients discharged on multiple antipsychotic medications with appropriate justification are included in the core measures.

The Joint Commission's National Patient Safety Goals aim to promote specific improvements in patient safety, including in state hospitals (Joint Commission 2007). The Joint Commission emphasizes goals that focus on system-wide solutions. One recent example includes the recent increased attention to reducing inpatient suicides through reducing lethal means for suicide, addressing ligature risks, and emphasizing protocols to assess patient risks (Joint Commission 2018). Many state hospitals are in older buildings, making this requirement regarding ligature risk reduction challenging and costly. For this and a variety of environment-of-care concerns, several states are investing in newer facilities.

State Regulatory Accreditation and Quality Monitoring

Each state has a government office that licenses and regulates hospitals and health-related institutions. State hospitals might be licensed or fall outside the licensure provisions of private hospitals, and quality usually flows from the SMHA or a bureau of state hospitals. For those state hospitals that do not have Joint Commission accreditation, a state office would generally perform regular inspections. This office also is responsible for inspection and certification of state hospitals participating under the deemed compliance authority from the Centers for Medicare & Medicaid Services. The office may initiate administrative action against state hospitals that violate state rules and regulations, and then it coordinates its actions with the Joint Commission and the Centers for Medicare & Medicaid Services. When hospital quality of care is in question, and after a sentinel event, hospitals perform a root cause analysis (RCA), as required by the Joint Commission. The RCA focuses primarily on systems and processes, not individual performance. The state hospital identifies risks and contributing factors for problem recurrence and determines what improvements are needed.

Protection and Advocacy for Individuals With Mental Illness

In 1975, the U.S. Department of Health and Human Services established a program to protect and to advocate for the rights of persons with disabilities (Protection and Advocacy for Individuals with Mental Illness [PAIMI] program; see SAMHSA.gov) (Substance Abuse and Mental Health Services Administration 2011). In 1986, Congress passed the Protection and Advocacy for Individuals with Mental Illness (PAIMI) Act. Protection and advocacy systems are authorized to access consumers and records for the purpose of conducting independent investigations of abuse, neglect, and rights violations in various types of public and private facilities, including state hospitals. PAIMI-eligible individuals include those diagnosed with a significant mental illness who were abused, were neglected, or had their rights violated or were in danger of abuse, neglect, or rights violations while receiving care or treatment. The Civil Rights of Institutionalized Persons Act was enacted into law in 1980 to help protect the rights of individuals within various settings, including mental health facilities. State hospitals can fall under U.S. Department of Justice review through the Special Litigation Section of the Civil Rights Division, which has the authority to investigate and prosecute complaints related to this legislation.

Court Oversight, Receivership, and Decrees

Court decisions have had a major impact on state hospitals. The *Wyatt v. Stickney* decision (Byrne 1981) gave patients the right to receive treatment that would result in a cure or would improve their mental condition. This landmark decision resulted in increased funding for state hospitals and also contributed to the movement to have treatment in the community. For many years after that case, court decisions and mental health law often reflected the tension between the interests of persons with mental illness and the community's fear of them (Appelbaum 2006).

Probably the most significant court case that has catalyzed the movement of care into community-based settings is *Olmstead v. L.C.* (1999) (which involved class action litigation stemming from Georgia), in which the U.S. Supreme Court indicated it was a violation of the Americans with Disabilities Act to keep people in institutions who were otherwise clinically ready and willing to live in the community. The *Olmstead* claims against states have been numerous and have touched on both civil and forensic populations (Bloom 2012). Major legal areas continuing to impact state hospital psychiatry include the right to refuse treatment, the insanity defense, and confining sex offenders postsentence.

In summary, the accreditation, regulatory, and legal environment has gained prominence in state hospitals over the past decades. State hospitals are under substantial scrutiny in all of these areas and need to effectively staff offices to attend to these oversight requirements. Although there may be concern on the part of state hospital clinicians and administrators that there is too much oversight and that the additional monitoring takes needed resources from clinical care, there is no indication that this will change in the near future, and history would suggest that oversight provides checks and balances to some of the challenges that can result in substandard care in large institutions.

Consumers, Advocates, Providers, and the State Hospital

There continues to be debate within the mental health community regarding state hospitals. Consumer groups, family organizations, employees, unions, community providers, mental health associations, and disability law advocacy organizations have differing opinions on state hospitals. There is not a consensus on the future role of state hospitals among these organizations, but it is clear these facilities continue to serve a vital role at one end of the overall psychiatric continuum (Parks and Radke 2014). The size and bed numbers needed, however, are not clear, and no formula has been fully accepted for this figure (Pinals and Fuller 2017).

In the 1950s, nearly 35% of private-sector employees were union members, and public employees in unions were almost nonexistent (Barone 2005). However, by 2005 about 8% of private-sector employees were union members, and 30%–40% of public employees were union members, making public sector unions a powerful voice in the future of state hospitals. State hospital employees and unions have expressed concern at the trend toward state hospitals providing care for an increasingly forensic population at the same time that there is pressure to stop the use of restraint and seclusion. There are concerns about violence in the state hospitals (Treatment Advocacy Center 2018). There is also concern about the shortage of staff (Parks and Radke 2014) and the lack of training for staff in dealing with forensic patients. At the same time, state hospital staff typically are part of unions, and there can be back and forth between management and staff about balancing needs.

The NAMI (National Alliance on Mental Illness; nami.org) position has been in support of adequate hospital beds and community-based services and expanded funding mechanisms, especially for shorter-term stays currently prohibited from federal reimbursement through the exclusion of Medicaid funding for care within "institutions for mental diseases." It supports involuntary care when safety is at stake and for those who will not agree to treatment because their illness impairs their judgment. NAMI also holds a similar position regarding involuntary medication: people should have a choice about medications, although there are times when individuals with severe symptoms of mental illness are not able to act in their own best interest. NAMI also expresses concern that incarceration or victimization may result if an individual does not get needed hospital treatment, including either private acute or state hospital care.

Mental Health America (mhanational.org) is a strong advocacy group dedicated to improving the quality of life for individuals with severe mental illness. It also advocates for an end to seclusion and restraint, except in rare circumstances. It supports state hospitals being included as part of the continuum of care but also supports vigorous adherence to the U.S. Supreme Court decision in *Olmstead v. L.C.* (1999) that allows individuals with mental illness to live in the community with adequate supports.

The Disability Law Center advocacy organizations are private, nonprofit organizations staffed by attorneys and paralegals to ensure that people with disabilities are accorded the full rights and entitlements afforded to them by state and federal law. They may assert that individuals' rights are not being protected in state hospitals. For example, they may argue that restraint and seclusion are used punitively and for the convenience of the staff. They argue that individuals with mental illness can be successfully treated in the community if appropriate resources are in place. Their advocacy agendas generally include removing barriers to independence; preventing seclusion and/or restraint of children, adolescents, or adults in state psychiatric hospitals; protecting the rights of persons diagnosed with a mental illness to receive care in the least restrictive manner and location; and advocating the enforcement of the right of persons diagnosed with a mental illness to live in the community with adequate supports, as set forth by the *Olmstead* decision (see, e.g., Bazelon Center for Mental Health Law at www.bazelon.org). The tension between individual rights, family rights, and community safety is often played out in discussions between legal advocacy and other stakeholders.

The stakeholders in the mental health community hold varied views regarding the role of state hospitals. Some argue for the current status, some for state hospitals to be downsized but continue to be part of the continuum of mental health care, and others for the closure of state hospitals. However, state hospitals appear to be an essential part of the continuum of care in most states. Therefore, it will be important for stakeholders and SMHAs to reach consensus about the transformation of state hospitals and work toward a best practices model (Parks and Radke 2014).

Budget and Legislative Issues

The majority of state hospital costs are covered by state budgets, through the SMHA, through a separate state hospital division, or through some other governance arrangement. Expenses include staffing for psychiatric and medical services, pharmacy, grounds, and maintenance, to name a few. Several strategies have been used historically to maximize Medicaid reimbursement through the Disproportionate Share Hospital (DSH) program—payments to age groups outside of the institution for mental diseases (IMD) exclusion (18–21, or older than 65)—and through managed care waivers to the IMD exclusion. In 1981, Congress established the Medicaid DSH program (Mechanic 2004) for hospitals that serve a significant number of low-income patients with special needs. At one time, DSH programs became a major source of funding for the nation's state hospitals. In 2010, 10% of the DSH payments (~$2.6 billion) went to state hospitals (Glover and Miller 2013). The "Medicaid IMD exclusion" has been part of federal Medicaid law since its 1965 enactment (42 CFR § 431.620 1979). As summarized above, the IMD exclusion refers to the rule that Medicaid will not pay for the inpatient treatment of individuals ages 22–64 in "institutions for mental diseases," defined as any hospital, nursing facility, or other institution with more than 16 beds that is primarily engaged in providing diagnosis, treatment, or care of persons with mental diseases, including substance use disorders and mental illness, and including care provided regarding their medical needs, nursing care, and related services. Individuals younger than 21 years make up 11.1% of the state hospital population, and individuals older than 64 years make up 5.5% of the state hospital population (Substance Abuse and Mental Health Services Administration 2017). State facilities can collect from Medicaid for these two age groups. In addition, many states have used federal Medicaid managed care waivers to bill for patients ages 22–64 years. This has allowed those states to receive Medicaid payments for hospital care in an IMD. Approximately 22% of the funding for state psychiatric hospitals is estimated to come from Medicaid (Substance Abuse and Mental Health Services Administration 2017). These important payment methods have seen marked shifts and reductions over the last decade. That said, there is increasing attention to removing the IMD exclusion, even if for short-term hospital bed coverage. With the IMD exclusion still in place, however, financing state hospitals largely out of state general fund dollars has created tremendous strain for states (Buck 2003; Draper et al. 2003).

Since World War II, state hospitals have been seen as very costly, and there has been a trend to close hospitals and use the savings to reduce government spending and support community-based care. In non-inflation-adjusted spending, state hospitals went from $3.8 billion in 1981 to $9.7 billion in 2015 (a 151% increase), while community mental health went from $2 billion to $32.7 billion (a 1,528% increase) during the same time period. However, when adjustment was made for inflation and population growth, expenditures for state psychiatric hospitals decreased by 66.7% from 1981 to 2015, while expenditures for community mental health increased by 116% (National Association of State Mental Health Program Directors Research Institute 2017). It is worth noting that a major cost to many state hospital systems has been the growing population of individuals who are postsentence and civilly committed as sexually violent predators. The U.S. Supreme Court in 2019 denied hearing a case that involved an appeal examining the difficulty in discharging these individuals (*Karsjens et al. v. Minnesota Department of Human Services et al.* 2018). Given that only a small number of individuals actually are discharged from these programs, the costs of caring for them will likely continue to increase.

Also, populations with complex needs, such as those with intellectual disability, who often start in the forensic system but then are not easily supported with the model of care delivery of a state hospital and become difficult to discharge, can drive up the cost of care. The stigma of all these populations and the mix of different treatment support needs can strain the care and treatment for individuals with mental illness. Populations within state hospitals also already are known to have high trauma histories (Parks and Radke 2014), and environments where individuals with behavioral challenges or predatory tendencies are encountered can heighten risks of further trauma. With budgets shrinking for state hospitals and costs escalating, the balance for caring for individuals with serious mental illness in these settings can be threatened.

Another issue separate from special populations includes the fact that many state hospital structures are older and even crumbling, making it harder for the environment of care to support the needs of the patients and staff. Some states have invested or are investing in new construction of state hospitals to obviate these problems, which may further enforce that these facilities will continue to be utilized for years to come. Overall, the costs of funding state hospitals continue to be an important issue that needs to stay on the radar of policy-makers.

The Future of State Hospitals

The future of state hospitals has been debated for decades. The hospitals are often demonized and looked upon as archaic relics of an embarrassing past, despite the fact that they are most often Joint Commission accredited, more states are building modern state hospital structures, and these institutions often provide the safety net function for individuals with serious mental illness in addition to providing inpatient care to populations in the forensic system that balances individual needs and public safety. With the outbreak of COVID-19 impacting state hospitals just like other settings, the importance of their work to ensure infection control and safe practices and remain as a safety net has been highlighted (Pinals et al. 2020). There is no indication that state hospitals are going to disappear in the near future, because they have their role in the vital continuum of psychiatric care. Perhaps in thinking more about how to enhance their care and coordination with state hospitals and community-based services, the focus should be on how state hospital leaders should work with stakeholders to provide services consistent with today's science and consistent with a recovery-based model following the goals set out by the President's New Freedom Commission on Mental Health years ago, including that mental health is essential to health, family, and consumer-driven care is critical, and excellent care should be provided (Hogan 2003). Even though those recommendations were crafted more than 15 years ago, their themes continue to forge a path forward and resurface in ongoing work looking at the public mental health system. These efforts go beyond beds alone as a single solution but include state psychiatric beds as part of the overall public mental health service delivery system.

Conclusion

Currently, state hospitals are an important part of the continuum of mental health care in each state. They vary in the amount of civil and forensic populations under their care and in the amount of acute and long-term care that is provided. In some discussions, transformation assumes an end to state hospitals, with a view that everyone will be maintained in the community and close to their natural supports. However, the limits of science today, coupled with the gravity of disorders in a small but enduring proportion of people with serious mental illness and related challenges, still require secure and longer-stay environments for some individuals. In addition, because state hospitals are being used increasingly for forensic care, they serve as an essential element in a full spectrum of state-supported services. Effort and resources therefore continue to be needed to ensure ongoing high-quality care within state hospitals. At the same time, efforts at various levels of government and in the private sector will continue to be needed to enrich services across the broader psychiatric care continuum to support individuals with serious mental illness and other challenges within community settings.

References

42 CFR § 431.620, Agreement with State mental health authority or mental institutions (1979)

Abreu D, Parker TW, Noether CD, et al: Revising the paradigm for jail diversion for people with mental and substance use disorders: Intercept 0. Behav Sci Law 35(5–6):380–395, 2017 29034504

American Psychiatric Association: Resource Document on Involuntary Outpatient Commitment and Related Programs of Assisted Outpatient Treatment. Arlington, VA, American Psychiatric Association, 2015. Available at: www.psychiatry.org/psychiatrists/search-directories-databases/library-and-archive/resource-documents. Accessed December 15, 2020.

Appelbaum PS: Law and psychiatry: twenty-five years of law and psychiatry. Psychiatr Serv 57:18–20, 2006 16403725

Barone M: Public employee unions rule—or do they? US News and World Report, August 12, 2005. Available at: www.usnews.com/blogs/barone/2005/8/12/ public-employee-unions-rule151or-do-they.html. Accessed April 22, 2007.

Becker JV, Johnson BR, Perkins A: Paraphilic disorders, in The American Psychiatric Publishing Textbook of Psychiatry, 6th Edition. Edited by Hales RE, Yudofsky SC, Roberts LW. Washington, DC, American Psychiatric Publishing, 2014, pp 895–925

Bloom JD: CRIPA, Olmstead, and the transformation of the Oregon Psychiatric Security Review Board. J Am Acad Psychiatry Law 40(3):383–389, 2012 22960921

Buck JA: Medicaid, health care financing trends, and the future of state-based public mental health services. Psychiatr Serv 54(7):969–975, 2003 12851432

Byrne G: Wyatt v Stickney: retrospect and prospect. Hosp Community Psychiatry 32:123–126, 1981

Callahan L, Pinals DA: Challenges to reforming the competence to stand trial and competence restoration system. Psychiatr Serv 71(7):691–697, 2020 32237984

Dhillon AS, Dollieslager LP: Rehab rounds: overcoming barriers to individualized psychosocial rehabilitation in an acute treatment unit of a state hospital. Psychiatr Serv 51(3):313–317, 2000 10686236

dosReis S, Barnett S, Love RC, Riddle MA: A guide for managing acute aggressive behavior of youths in residential and inpatient treatment facilities. Psychiatr Serv 54(10):1357–1363, 2003 14557521

Draper D, McHugh M, Achman L, et al: Medicaid Financing of State and County Psychiatric Hospitals (DHHS Publ No SMA 03-3830). Rockville, MD, U.S. Department of Health and Human Services, 2003. Available at: http://download.ncadi.samhsa.gov/ken/pdf/SMA03–3830/CMHS11A.pdf. Accessed April 22, 2007.

Fitch LF, Hammen D: The new generation of sex offender commitment laws: which states have them and how do they work? in Protecting Society From Sexually Dangerous Offenders: Law, Justice, and Therapy. Edited by Winick BJ, La Fond JQ. Washington, DC, American Psychological Association, 2003, pp 27–39

Galbreath NW, Berlin FS, Sawyer D: Paraphilias and the internet, in Sex and the Internet: A Guidebook for Clinicians. Edited by Cooper A. Oxfordshire, UK, Brunner-Routledge, 2002, pp 187–205

Geller JL: The last half-century of psychiatric services as reflected in psychiatric services. Psychiatr Serv 51(1):41–67, 2000 10647135

Glover RW, Miller JE: The Interplay Between Medicaid DSH Payment Cuts, the IMD Exclusion and the ACA Medicaid Expansion Program: Impacts on State Public Mental Health Services. Alexandria, VA, National Association of State Mental Health Program Directors, 2013. Available at: www.nasmhpd.org/sites/default/files/TheDSHInterplay04_26_13WebsiteFINAL.pdf. Accessed October 24, 2021.

Goldman HH, Adams N, Taube CA: Deinstitutionalization: the data demythologized. Hosp Community Psychiatry 34:129–134, 1983 6860396

Hogan MF: The President's New Freedom Commission: recommendations to transform mental health care in America. Psychiatr Serv 54(11):1467–1474, 2003 14600303

Janofsky JS, Hanson A, Candilis PJ, et al: AAPL Practice Guideline for forensic psychiatric evaluation of defendants raising the insanity defense. J Am Acad Psychiatry Law 42(4 suppl):S3–S76, 2014 25492121

Joint Commission: 2007 National Patient Safety Goals. Oakbrook Terrace, IL, The Joint Commission, 2007. Available at: www.jointcommission.org/PatientSafety/NationalPatientSafetyGoals/07_npsgs.htm. Accessed April 22, 2007.

Joint Commission: Performance Measurement Initiatives: Hospital-Based, Inpatient Psychiatric Services (HBIPS) Candidate Core Measure Set, last updated February 15, 2008. Oakbrook Terrace, IL, The Joint Commission, 2008. Available at: www.jointcommission.org/PerformanceMeasurement/PerformanceMeasurement/Hospital+Based+Inpatient+Psychiatric+Services.htm. Accessed April 22, 2008.

Joint Commission: FAQs: suicide risk recommendations. The Joint Commission Perspectives 38(7), July 2018. Available at: www.jointcommission.org/-/media/tjc/documents/resources/patient-safety-topics/suicide-prevention/suicide_risk_recommendations_faqs_july_perspectives.pdf?db=web&hash=7A89FF8D01CC6D8D4A84A389C30F4F03&hash=7A89FF8D01CC6D8D4A84A389C30F4F03. Accessed October 24, 2021.

Joint Commission: Hospital-based inpatient psychiatric services (HBIPS), in Specifications Manual for Joint Commission National Quality Measures (v2015B). Oakbrook Terrace, IL, The Joint Commission, 2021. Available at: https://manual.jointcommission.org/releases/TJC2015B/HospitalBasedInpatientPsychiatricServices.html. Accessed October 24, 2021.

Kansas v. Hendricks 521 US 346 (1997).

Karsjens et al. v Minnesota Department of Human Services et al., No. 0:2011cv03659—Document 1108 (D. Minn. 2018). Available at: https://law.justia.com/cases/federal/district-courts/minnesota/mndce/0:2011cv03659/123875/1108. Accessed October 24, 2021.

Kazandjian M, Lutterman T: Fiscal Year 2018: Snapshot of State Plans for Using the Community Mental Health Block Grant Ten Percent Set-Aside to Address First Episode Psychosis. Alexandria, VA, National Association of State Mental Health Program Directors for the Substance Abuse and Mental Health Services Administration, 2018

Lutterman T, Shaw R, Fisher W, Manderscheid R: Trend in Psychiatric Inpatient Capacity, United States and Each State, 1970 to 2014. Alexandria, VA, National Association of State Mental Health Program Directors, 2017. Available at: www.nri-inc.org/media/1319/tac-paper-10-psychiatric-inpatient-capacity-final-09-05-2017.pdf. Accessed October 24, 2021.

Mechanic RE: Medicaid's Disproportionate Share Hospital Program: Complex Structure, Critical Payments (National Health Policy Forum Background Paper). Washington, DC, National Health Policy Forum, 2004. Available at: www.nhpf.org/pdfs_bp/BP_MedicaidDSH_0914–04.pdf. Accessed April 22, 2007.

Munetz MR, Griffin PA: Use of the Sequential Intercept Model as an approach to decriminalization of people with serious mental illness. Psychiatr Serv 57(4):544–549, 2006 16603751

National Association of State Mental Health Program Directors Research Institute: State Mental Health Agency Revenues and Expenditures Study, Fiscal Years 1981 to 2015. Alexandria, VA, National Association of State Mental Health Program Directors Research Institute, 2017

Nordstrom K, Berlin JS, Nash SS, et al: Boarding of mentally ill patients in emergency departments: American Psychiatric Association resource document. West J Emerg Med 20(5):690–695, 2019 31539324

Olmstead v L.C., 527 U.S. 581 (1999)

Parks J, Radke AQ: The Vital Role of State Psychiatric Hospitals. Alexandria, VA, National Association of State Mental Health Program Directors Medical Directors Council, July 2014.

Pinals DA: Forensic services, public mental health policy, and financing: charting the course ahead. J Am Acad Psychiatry Law 42(1):7–19, 2014 24618515

Pinals DA: Crisis Services: Meeting Needs, Saving Lives. Alexandria, VA, National Association of State Mental Health Program Directors, 2020

Pinals DA, Callahan L: Evaluation and restoration of competence to stand trial: intercepting the forensic system using the Sequential Intercept Model. Psychiatr Serv 71(7):698–705, 2020 32237983

Pinals DA, Fuller DA: Beyond Beds: The Vital Role of the Full Continuum of Psychiatric Care. Alexandria, VA, National Association of State Mental Health Program Directors, 2017. Available at: https://nasmhpd.org/content/tac-assessment-paper-beyond-beds-vital-role-full-continuum-psychiatric-care. Accessed September 1, 2017.

Pinals DA, Fuller DA: The vital role of a full continuum of psychiatric care beyond beds. Psychiatr Serv 71(7):713–721, 2020 32321386

Pinals DA, Glancy G, Lee L: Civil and sex-offender commitment, in The Psychiatric Report: Principles and Practice of Forensic Writing. Edited by Buchanan A, Norko M. Cambridge, UK, Cambridge University Press, 2011, pp 128–144

Pinals DA, Hovermale M, Mauch D, et al: The Vital Role of Specialized Approaches: Persons With Intellectual and Developmental Disabilities in the Mental Health System. Alexandria, VA, National Association of State Mental Health Program Directors, 2017. Available at: www.nasmhpd.org/sites/default/files/TAC.Paper_.7.IDD_.Final_.pdf. Accessed October 24, 2021.

Pinals DA, Hepburn B, Parks J, Stephenson AH: The behavioral health system and its response to COVID-19: a snapshot perspective. Psychiatr Serv 71(10):1070–1074, 2020 32781926

Santoni T, Sundeen S: Staffing Study. Baltimore, Maryland Department of Health and Mental Hygiene, 2007

Substance Abuse and Mental Health Services Administration: Mental Health, United States, 2008 (HHS Publ No SMA 10-4590). Washington, DC, U.S. Department of Health and Human Services, 2010, Table 11.9

Substance Abuse and Mental Health Services Administration: Evaluation of the Protection and Advocacy for Individuals with Mental Illness (PAIMI) Program: Phase III: Evaluation Report. Washington, DC, U.S. Department of Health and Human Services, 2011. Available at: https://store.samhsa.gov/sites/default/files/d7/priv/pep12-evalpaimi.pdf. Accessed October 24, 2021.

Substance Abuse and Mental Health Services Administration: Funding and Characteristics of Single State Agencies for Substance Abuse Services and State Mental Health Agencies, 2015 (HHS Publ No SMA 17-5029). Rockville, MD, Substance Abuse and Mental Health Services Administration, 2017

Substance Abuse and Mental Health Services Administration: 2018 Uniform Reporting System (URS) Output Tables. CBHSQ Data. Rockville, MD, Substance Abuse and Mental Health Services Administration, 2019a. Available at: www.samhsa.gov/data/report/2018-uniform-reporting-system-urs-output-tables. Accessed July 20, 2020.

Substance Abuse and Mental Health Services Administration: National Mental Health Services Survey (N-MHSS): 2018, Data on Mental Health Treatment Facilities. Rockville, MD, Substance Abuse and Mental Health Services Administration, 2019b

Substance Abuse and Mental Health Services Administration: National Guidelines for Behavioral Health Crisis Care. Implementing Behavioral Health Crisis Care. Rockville, MD, Substance Abuse and Mental Health Services Administration, 2020. Available at: www.samhsa.gov/find-help/implementing-behavioral-health-crisis-care. Accessed October 24, 2021.

Substance Abuse and Mental Health Services Administration, Center for Behavioral Health Statistics and Quality: Mental Health Annual Report: 2013–2018. Use of Mental Health Services: National Client-Level Data. Rockville, MD, Substance Abuse and Mental Health Services Administration, 2020

Talbott JA: Deinstitutionalization: avoiding the disasters of the past. 1979. Psychiatr Serv 55(10):1112–1115, 2004 15492071

Treatment Advocacy Center: Eliminating barriers to the treatment of mental illness. Research Weekly, July 17, 2018. Available at: www.treatmentadvocacycenter.org/fixing-the-system/features-and-news/4020-research-weekly violence-in-hospitals-by-people-with-serious-mental-illness. Accessed October 24, 2021.

Wall BW, Ash P, Keram E, et al: AAPL practice resource for the forensic psychiatric evaluation of competence to stand trial. J Am Acad Psychiatry Law 46(3):373, 2018 30368470

Wik A: Alternatives to inpatient competency restoration programs: jail-based competency restoration programs. Falls Church, VA, NRI, October 2018. Available at: www.nri-inc.org/media/1500/jbcr_website-format_oct2018.pdf. Accessed October 24, 2021.

Wik A, Hollen V, Fisher WH: Forensic patients in state psychiatric hospitals: 1999–2016. Alexandria, VA, National Association of State Mental Health Program Directors, August 2017. Available at: www.nri-inc.org/media/1318/tac-paper-9-forensic-patients-in-state-hospitals-final-09-05-2017.pdf. Accessed October 24, 2021.

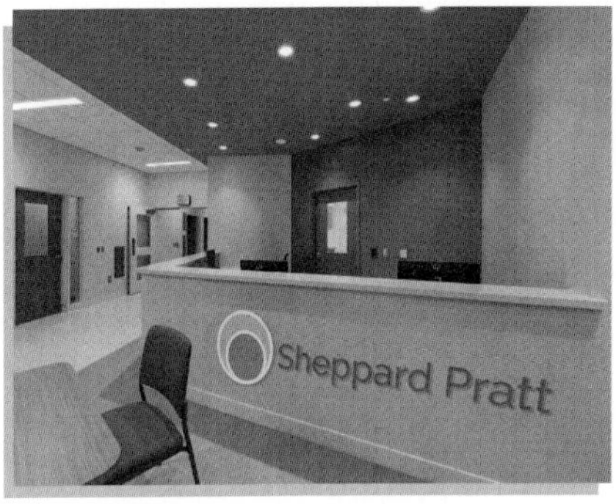

CHAPTER 12

The Veterans Hospital

Anne Marie Stoline, M.D.
Marsden McGuire, M.D., M.B.A.

More than half of all U.S. physicians train and/or practice in the U.S. Department of Veterans Affairs (VA) health care system. Even physicians who never work for VA are likely to encounter veteran patients in the civilian sector; thus, some understanding of the VA system can be helpful to any practitioner and beneficial to the veterans they care for. Given that many veterans struggle with mental health issues, familiarity with VA, the psyche of veterans, and postmilitary psychiatry is particularly relevant to psychiatrists. This chapter explores VA inpatient psychiatric care, noting similarities and highlighting differences in care between VA and other U.S. health care sectors.

U.S. Department of Veterans Affairs: A Brief History

With earlier roots in medical care for disabled soldiers dating back to the 1600s, the first federal hospital for veterans was authorized in 1811. However, President Lincoln is credited with laying out the mission for what would become VA in the 1860s: "To care

---

A.M.S. has worked at the U.S. Veterans Administration (VA) for 18 years. The views represented are her own and do not represent those of the VA. M.M. has worked with the VA for 12 years. The views represented are his alone and do not represent those of the VA.

for him who shall have borne the battle, and for his widow, and his orphan" (Lincoln 1865/1989).[1] VA was formally established in 1930 to provide health care to veterans.[2] VA's scope has broadened since then, with addition of VA federal benefits in the 1950s and the VA National Cemetery Administration (NCA) in the 1970s. Together they operate nationwide programs for health care, financial benefits, and burial assistance. In 1989, VA was elevated to Cabinet status, and it currently has the second largest budget of the 15 Cabinets, after the Department of Defense (DoD).

The Veterans Health Administration (VHA) is currently the largest integrated health care system in the United States. It currently has locations in every state, Washington, D.C., and the U.S. territories of Puerto Rico, U.S. Virgin Islands, Guam, and American Samoa. The only VA facility in a foreign country is in the Philippines, where it is located on U.S. Embassy property. As of 2020, the VHA operates 1,255 health care facilities, including 170 VA medical centers (VAMCs) (over 110 of which have inpatient psychiatric units) and 1,074 outpatient clinics. The Veterans Benefits Administration manages a variety of financial programs, the most significant of which is disability compensation known as service-connected (SC) benefits (U.S. Department of Veterans Affairs 2019a). SC benefits include monthly payments to veterans in recognition of the financial impact of disability due to injuries, diseases, or other conditions incurred or aggravated during active military service. SC disability ratings range from 0% (no disability) to 100% (total disability). Non-service-connected benefits include veteran pensions (a needs-based benefit providing supplemental income to qualifying veterans) and survivor pensions (for qualifying spouses and children of deceased veterans with wartime service). NCA operates 148 national cemeteries and 33 soldiers' lots and monument sites in 42 states and Puerto Rico. NCA also manages burial benefits for eligible veterans and their families.

Since the attacks of 9/11, support for veterans has increased and become less of a partisan issue than in previous years. This support has translated into major legislation and generous federal spending for veterans' care that has helped transform VA into a modern, popular choice for veterans' care. "The [spending] increases over time have reflected the impact of increases in the number of veterans as the result of wars and other conflicts, the aging of the veteran population, and changes in benefits and services provided for veterans" (Scott 2012, p. 2). VA continues to be favored in the congressional budgeting process, with its regular budget increases also reflecting an area of rare political alignment between the major congressional parties and effective political advocacy by veterans, families, and their support groups.

Among the broad responsibilities of VA health care is the care of veterans with conditions related to military service, veterans with catastrophic disabilities, and impoverished veterans. The specific qualifying criteria for enrollment in VA services (and therefore eligibility for care) change regularly. Enrollment generally is available only to those with "other than dishonorable" military discharges, including honorable discharge, general discharge under honorable conditions, medical discharge, and others.

---

[1]The term *soldier* in this chapter is used in three contexts: 1) generically, referring to all members of the army, navy, air force, marines, and coast guard; 2) referring to deployed or ground forces; and 3) referring to combatants.

[2]Unless otherwise noted, data are taken from official VA and other federal government websites, including www.va.gov.

An exception was made through legislation passed in 2018, offering mental health care services to veterans with "other than honorable" (OTH) discharges (this group remains disqualified from receiving other VA services). Under this program, veterans with OTH discharges are encouraged to seek mental health evaluation at VA if they believe their mental health issues are related to military service. Those veterans whose claims are supported by evaluation qualify to receive service-related ongoing VA mental health treatment. As of this writing, it is too early to gauge the effect of this initiative on veterans who were previously excluded from VA mental health care.

Although women have served in the U.S. military since the Revolutionary War, fundamental gender differences in preceding centuries shaped postmilitary care and the VA system. It was not until 1901 that Congress established the Army Nurse Corps, officially assigning women to active-duty roles. Subsequent growth in female participation in U.S. military ranks has been slow; in 1973 only 2.5% of active-duty military were women, with the proportion increasing by 2004 to 15%. A Government Accountability Office report released in May 2020 indicates that the proportion of U.S. active-duty women is now 16.5%—a growth of only 1.5% in the last 16 years (U.S. General Accounting Office 2020).

In the early 1980s, Congress passed legislation granting veteran status to women who had served in the Women's Army Auxiliary Corps during World War II (U.S. Department of Veterans Affairs Advisory Committee on Women Veterans 2012). VA programs specifically for female veterans followed (U.S. Department of Veterans Affairs National Center for Veterans Analysis and Statistics). The goal of the VA Women Veterans Health Care program, established in 1988 when women made up 4.4% of the veteran population, is to improve nationwide medical and psychosocial care for women through careful attention to and support of women veterans' specific needs and preferences (this includes single-sex clinics for women veterans at some medical centers as well as single-sex wings with added security measures in many inpatient and residential programs). Although women are still in the minority in the military, more women in military service translates into more female veterans; as of September 2019, 9.7% of all veterans were women. As one would expect, the preponderance of women veterans is in the younger cohorts. For example, in 2020, 18.70% of living U.S. veterans who had served since September 11, 2001 were female (see www.va.gov/vetdata/Veteran_Population.asp).

In 1995, the national health care cost crisis catalyzed a major change in the VA system when Congress passed legislation requiring VA psychiatric deinstitutionalization, one goal of which was cost savings through transitioning veterans to lower-intensity (and less costly) levels of care when clinically appropriate. The national VA health care system then was divided into 22 Veterans Integrated Service Networks (VISNs) intended to consolidate resources, avoid duplication of services, and optimize access to services at appropriate levels of care. Added benefits of this change included simplified administration and oversight through establishment of administrative offices within each VISN that provide regional leadership and oversight while streamlining reporting from individual facilities to the national administration. As of this writing, the VA system is divided into 18 VISNs, illustrated in Figure 12–1.

Continuing an already established trend of decreasing inpatient psychiatric admissions, deinstitutionalization and decentralization to VISNs occurred hand in hand with an expansion of the continuum of care from inpatient to residential care and spe-

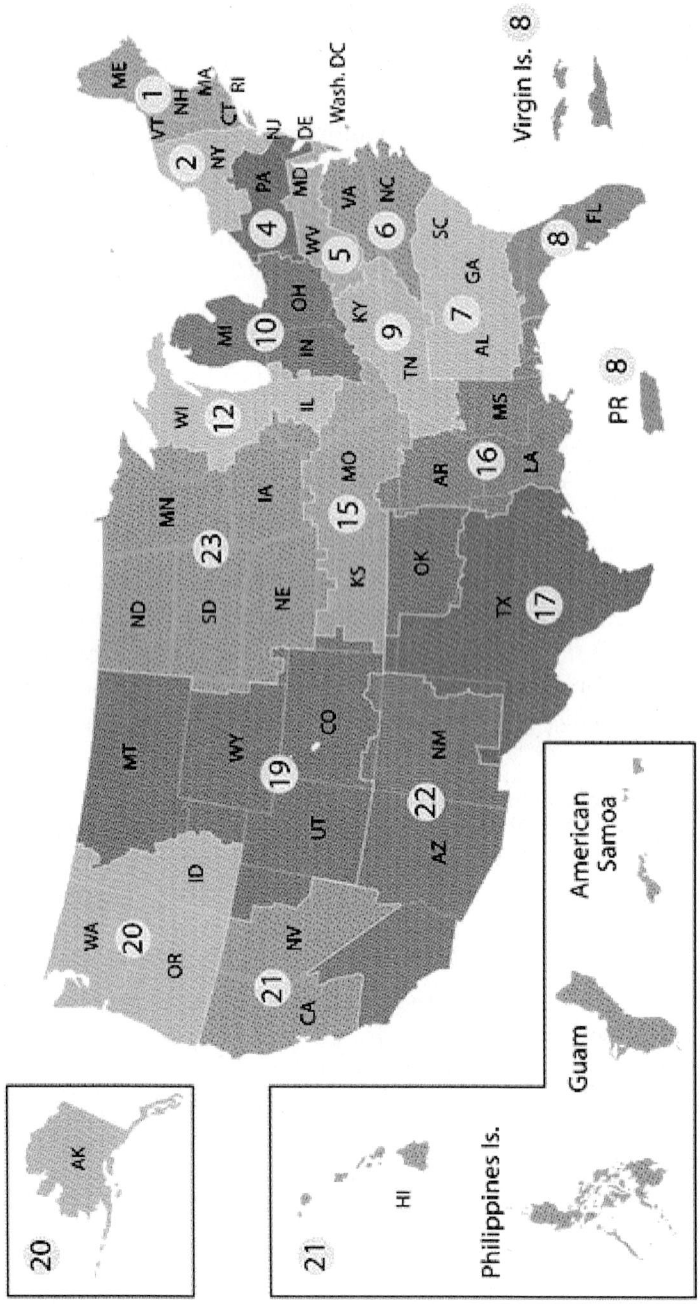

FIGURE 12–1. U.S. Department of Veterans Affairs Veterans Integrated Service Network (VISN) system, 2020.

To view this figure in color, see Plate 2 in Color Gallery.

Source. U.S. Department of Veterans Affairs 2021b. Facilities included in each VISN are available at this reference.

cialized recovery-focused outpatient programs and team-based outpatient care (including mental health services integrated within primary care), as well as education and outreach for veterans residing in the community. Similar efforts in primary care allowed for the transition of many veterans receiving specialty care to newly established community-based outpatient clinics (CBOCs) (Fortney et al. 2002). As a result of these and other factors, including the greater number of effective mental health treatments, fewer veterans now require psychiatric hospitalization, and the chronic inpatient psychiatric units of the past have largely become extinct. However, despite savings realized from deinstitutionalization and other cost containment measures, overall VA health care costs continue to rise at a rate that exceeds the rate at which U.S. health care costs as a whole are rising (Centers for Medicare & Medicaid Services 2022), likely due to a complex mix of factors, including increasingly broad health care coverage offered by VA (Congressional Budget Office 2014).

VA is currently both the largest health care provider in the nation and the largest employer of medical specialists. According to the U.S. Office of Personnel Management (2020), as of June 2019 there were 396,000 VA employees nationwide, of whom 22,000 had doctoral or postdoctoral degrees. VA is also the largest provider of health care training in the United States, sponsoring programs for all levels of medical and mental health training, as well as nursing, and dentistry and ancillary technologies—accommodating more than 100,000 trainees annually. It has been estimated that well over half of all U.S. physicians working today received some part of their training at a VA site.

VA funds extensive research within its own facilities and in collaboration with affiliated universities. Combined with non-VA funding sources, millions of dollars annually are invested in VA research activity. The VA nationwide network makes possible large-scale, multicenter trials that would be daunting if not impossible in smaller systems. Accomplishments in mental health attributed to VA research and development initiatives include advances in the genetic underpinnings of schizophrenia and the dementias; chronic pain; trauma disorders; biomarkers for PTSD and TBI (traumatic brain injury) and other conditions; and precision medical care (genomics).

The vast VA system is organized and undergirded by its information technology (IT) systems. VA was a pioneer in electronic health record (EHR) development, with its earliest forerunners in the 1970s. In 1996 VA successfully integrated computer technology into routine clinical care with the Computerized Patient Record System (CPRS), a nationwide information network storing clinical information back to 1995. CPRS is consistently ranked by physicians among the best EHRs available, public or private.

CPRS facilitates daily tasks such as entering diagnostic test orders, requesting consultations, and monitoring results. The system alerts physicians before they can make potentially fatal errors, such as ordering medication for a veteran allergic to it or requesting an incorrect dose. CPRS enhances preventive care by posting reminders for routine annual screenings. Through its remote access feature, known as the Joint Legacy Viewer, or JLV, clinicians in one VA facility can retrieve a veteran's clinical information from anywhere across the nationwide system. This capability has proved invaluable for clinical tasks such as gathering or verifying medical history, reviewing prior medication trials, and monitoring chronic illness by tracking laboratory or imaging results.

In 2005, VA established an electronic interface linking individual veterans to VA known as MyHealtheVet ("My Healthy Vet"). Veterans can enroll in this service at www.myhealth.va.gov. Among its many features, this program enables veterans to refill prescriptions online, check scheduled appointments, view copay balances, review some parts of their electronic medical record, and send secure messages to health care providers. They also can record and track their personal health data such as blood pressure and weight. MyHealtheVet is popular among veterans, who appreciate the autonomy, convenience, and self-care it affords.

An ambitious and expensive EHR project is under way to fully integrate military/DoD and VA patient record systems. Implementation of the new system began in 2020 in a phased approach that is expected to take up most of the next decade. During this time VA will be operating two medical record systems, creating both internal and external (with DoD) interoperability challenges. Once fully operational, it will be possible for a clinician sitting at one terminal to review a veteran's entire medical history, from entrance physical through military career and into the VA system.

The VA Medical Center

Like many hospitals in the private sector, the VAMC[3] is the hub of a clinical care system designed to provide an array of high-quality services to meet veterans' needs in a timely manner. Viewing the system of care through the veteran's eyes, VA is committed to provide care according to the following principles:

- Providing the right care at the right time
- Promoting timely and effective treatment at the least intensive level of care appropriate to meet veterans' needs in the moment and as needs change
- Being proactive, flexibly delivered, and veteran-centric

Medical services provided in VAMCs are similar to what would be seen in the private sector and are defined in VA's comprehensive Medical Benefits Package; in addition, these core services are augmented with an array of ancillary supports, including information on benefits, legal assistance, and employment and housing opportunities. These services are often provided within the VAMC so the veteran can "one stop shop." With rare exceptions, family members are not eligible for VA services—a situation that can create difficulties in coordination, as when a pregnant veteran receives prenatal care at VA but her child must be delivered and cared for elsewhere.

There is considerable variation among VAMCs due to size, complexity of services offered, market considerations (including demand for services, competition, and state law), age of the physical plant, workforce training, and leadership quality and stability. Many facilities are new and have state-of-the-art features, but others are in need of renovation and may be in locations serving a diminishing veteran population or at risk from weather-related disasters. All VAMCs must conform to Joint Commis-

[3]Historically, the term *Veterans Hospital* has been in general usage, but as VA has expanded its health care services beyond the traditional bricks and mortar with CBOCs, Readjustment Counseling Centers (also called Vet Centers), mobile treatment services, and telehealth, the term *VA Medical Center* (or VAMC) is now the standard.

sion standards and other requirements of hospital building codes. Of note, VA's "4th Mission" is to provide care to non-VA populations in times of crisis, and newer facilities have been built with this capability in mind. Like private and academic medical centers, VAMCs provide emergency services, but these are limited to use by eligible veterans. It is worth noting that VAMCs (and their associated outpatient clinics) are federal property and not subject to state jurisdiction—they have their own police force that may act freely within but not outside the facility grounds.

Variation also occurs in VAMC's ability to maintain the full number of trained staff needed to carry out its essential mission. Some facilities find it difficult to attract or retain qualified personnel due to location, bureaucratic issues, and, in some markets, challenges in competing with private sector salaries. Nevertheless, VA's mission compels it to provide timely access to services, and this has contributed to the recent growth of telehealth capabilities to meet the growing demand. Concerns about access have also been the basis for recent federal legislation enabling veterans to obtain services in the community (at VA expense) if necessary (Veterans' Access to Care through Choice, Accountability, and Transparency Act of 2014; VA MISSION Act of 2018).

The Mental Health Service Line

Psychiatric services within the VAMC are arranged within the interprofessional mental health service line. Often, but not always, the clinical leader of this service line is a physician/psychiatrist and functions as an associate chief of staff. Similarly, inpatient psychiatric units are usually overseen by an inpatient medical director, with attending psychiatrists responsible for admissions, clinical care, and discharge planning in collaboration with other mental health professionals (e.g., advanced practice nurses), some of whom are empowered by VA policy (and federal supremacy) to function independently regardless of their state of licensure. At times, this team-based model, which requires clinical care responsibilities to be shared by the team and members to adopt new roles and functions, may be challenging during initial implementation; however, it can be an advantage when there is an insufficient supply of psychiatrists to manage all the care that is needed. Collaborative care agreements assist teams in determining the optimal configuration(s) needed to provide high quality care to their panel of patients. The mental health service line also provides staffing for emergency department, outpatient, residential, outreach, and consultation-liaison services. When a facility is associated with an academic affiliate, the service line takes on the added mission of training students and preprofessionals in all mental health disciplines, many of whom remain in VA when they make their first career choices. Of note, even nonaffiliated sites may attract new mental health professionals through utilization of VA's generous Education Debt Reduction Program.

The VA Inpatient Psychiatric Unit

As mentioned previously, inpatient psychiatric units[4] in VAMCs must adhere to Joint Commission accreditation standards in order to operate. Staffing is heavily dependent

---

[4]Although *mental health* is now the preferred term to *psychiatric* when describing VA inpatient units (as it suggests an interdisciplinary team-oriented approach), we have chosen to maintain the more widely prevalent use of *psychiatric* largely to align with the aims and vision of this book.

on sufficient nursing resources to ramp up availability to meet demand at times of peak acuity (e.g., patients with comorbid medical conditions requiring care, need for staff to provide one-to-one levels of observation for suicidal or unstable patients). The staffing methodology formulas utilized by nursing do not carry over to the remainder of the clinical team, however. Each facility must provide adequate physician staffing to ensure that admission, discharge, and daily review of medical necessity occur and adequate staffing of other mental health professionals (i.e., psychologists, social workers, licensed professional mental health counselors, marriage and family therapists) to ensure that minimum programming requirements are met and that recovery-oriented principles (e.g., shared decision-making, utilization of psychiatric advance directives) are followed.

As in civilian facilities, legal proceedings to retain a patient involuntarily and involving the state administrative legal offices may occur on hospital grounds. A key point here is that the federal government does not have the authority to forcibly hospitalize a patient, whereas each state does (using similar but varying criteria). This means that the requirements of the state where the VAMC is located must be followed from the initial evaluation phase to involuntary admission (and medication administration if deemed clinically necessary) to the timeline for case review and appeal.

Not surprisingly, some necessary clinical care occurs outside the inpatient psychiatry unit. Essential medical services (e.g., specialized diagnostic/therapeutic services, physical rehabilitation, wound care, dialysis) may need to be provided elsewhere, and safety concerns usually require clear protocols for observing the patient and ensuring the safety of all involved. Similarly, psychiatric treatments such as electroconvulsive therapy, repetitive transcranial magnetic stimulation, or ketamine/esketamine are typically administered elsewhere in the medical center than in the inpatient mental health setting.

To maximize safety on the VA inpatient psychiatric unit, there are strict environmental requirements enshrined in the Mental Health Environment of Care Checklist that every unit must adhere to. A multiprogram team that includes engineering, patient safety, nursing, and mental health leadership conducts a structured review every 6 months and records any environment features that might pose risk to patients. Identified items must be reported to the VA Central Office National Center for Patient Safety and corrected as soon as possible with a temporary mitigation plan. As a result of this protocol, inpatient suicides on VA psychiatric units have decreased from approximately 3–5 per year to 0–1 per year over the last decade (Mills et al. 2021).

Although patient safety is the highest priority, ensuring a therapeutic milieu that encourages recovery-oriented care is an essential feature of VA inpatient psychiatric units. Accordingly, VA has taken great pains to incorporate human-centered design principles to optimize the inpatient experience for patients, visitors, and staff alike by producing an inpatient mental health design guide (U.S. Department of Veterans Affairs 2021a). Examples include requirements for clear lines of sight, natural light, and nursing stations that are not fully enclosed, allowing for more patient and nurse interaction (while preserving safety). This document aims to anticipate patient and staff needs years into the future and maintain accordingly flexible requirements and undergoes revision every few years.

An indispensable feature of high-quality inpatient mental health care is the provision of safe care with minimal coercion, threats, and violence. Violence by patients and use of seclusion and restraints by staff (including intramuscular injection of sedating medications) often reflect a failure to implement adequate therapeutic strategies aimed at anticipating and preventing harm. Through its Prevention and Management of Disruptive Behavior program, VA has instituted a mechanism whereby all employees in high-risk workplaces as designated by the annual Workplace Behavioral Risk Assessment must be trained in all levels of responding to behavioral emergencies, including the manual restraint of patients. The only exceptions to this are if the facility opts to use an "in-place" behavioral emergency response team to provide manual restraint of patients, further de-escalation, and medical intervention when needed. Through a careful review of incidents as they occur, the prevention and intervention models employed in VA training have become more refined and specific, with the result that seclusion and restraint incidents on a majority of VA inpatient psychiatric units have approached zero per year.

Clinical Challenges in Veteran Inpatient Mental Health Care

It is important to note that VA inpatient psychiatric units and their community counterparts serve similar needs. Both VA and non-VA units treat acute mental health crises and aim for short stays in the least restrictive environment, with a focus on aftercare planning. Admitted patients typically have suicidal or homicidal ideation, psychoses, mood disorders, and/or substance abuse. Inpatient management of these conditions does not differ between sectors. Beyond that, differences appear.[5]

VA acute psychiatric units differ from most civilian units in their admission of a considerable number of veterans with trauma-related conditions, and it can be challenging to determine whether a veteran's condition is related to military service. For example, among the diagnoses to consider for new-onset psychosis in a combat veteran are combat stress, sequelae to a military (or nonmilitary) traumatic incident, sequelae to mild TBI (mTBI, commonly referred to as a "concussion"), substance-related psychosis, and the onset of major mental illness. The presence of concurrent diagnoses heightens the complexity of diagnosis and treatment. After psychiatric stabilization, these veterans may be referred for specialized treatment. It is noteworthy that psychiatric and behavioral exclusions to military service—conditions preventing enlistment—limit in theory the likelihood of a veteran being admitted with a diagnosis that predates their entry into military service. However, several variables affect actual enlistment of those with a mental health history, including the urgency of recruitment efforts (and flexible adherence to standards when the need is high), denial of preexisting conditions by potential enlistees, evidence that childhood and/or adolescent conditions have resolved, and, perhaps most important, the candidate's option to request a waiver for any impairment. A full discussion of these conditions and their significance to VA clinicians is beyond the scope of this chapter, but lists of current

---

[5]Most veterans do not receive care from VA; therefore, the information provided here regarding the optimal care of veterans with mental health conditions is vital knowledge for non-VA as well as VA providers to acquire.

exclusionary criteria to enlistment are publicly available (U.S. Department of Defense 2020, 2021).

Another significant difference between VA and most nonpublic acute inpatient psychiatric units is the percentage of patients with severe psychosocial impairments such as homelessness, lack of social supports, and unemployment. Because psychosocial problems create barriers to discharge, admission of a veteran with one or more of these issues can make aftercare planning especially challenging. In response, VA has developed a multifaceted system to meet veterans' psychosocial care needs, including referral to a variety of specialized programs along the continuum of care; examples include residential mental health, homeless domiciliaries, psychosocial rehabilitation and recovery centers, outpatient mental health care, and wrap-around supportive services, including various housing options and vocational rehabilitation).

Homelessness

It is not uncommon for a homeless veteran to be admitted to a VA inpatient psychiatric unit. Staff are trained to work supportively and respectfully with homeless veterans during the admission process, which may be especially difficult for the veterans to tolerate. Upon identification of their homeless status, steps are immediately taken to connect these veterans with services that will permit discharge into a supportive and safe environment. By contrast, non-VA hospitals do not offer a similarly comprehensive system, and their links to state and local homeless services are variable. This poses a special problem when a veteran enrolled in VA is admitted to a non-VA facility and efforts are often made to transfer the veteran to a VA facility to continue their treatment plan and ensure access care to the full array of services they are entitled to.

A significant question for a VA psychiatrist (and other mental health providers) is whether (and how) a homeless veteran admitted to the inpatient unit might differ clinically from their nonhomeless counterpart. Historically, factors implicated in veteran homelessness mirror those in the general population, including unemployment, mental health conditions, and substance abuse (Tsai and Rosenheck 2015). However, some risk factors for homelessness are found more commonly in the veteran population. For example, lower socioeconomic status may predispose to homelessness when military benefits such as competitive pay, financial support for education, and the opportunity for travel (all of which may be a motivator to join the military) are no longer available. Clinical conditions experienced by veterans at higher rates than nonveterans that predispose to homelessness include trauma-related conditions (Duan-Porter et al. 2018). One study found that 40% of homeless female veterans had a history of military sexual trauma (MST) (Pavao et al. 2013). Challenges with reintegration into society after discharge are another veteran-specific risk factor for homelessness. This group includes veterans who become distant from family and other supports while in the military and/or following discharge. Those particularly at risk include service members who suffered long and/or repeated deployments and those who were severely traumatized during their service (Rosenheck and Fontana 1994).

VA addresses homelessness with a number of programs intended to provide a safety net for veterans unable to afford or maintain shelter. In 1987, the VA Homeless Program was initiated, creating locally based medical care programs, residential programs, outreach, subsidized community shelter beds for veterans, and long-term recovery programs for homeless veterans with substance abuse. VA's Grant and Per Diem

Program supports community-based agencies with outreach, housing, and other programs for homeless veterans and their families.

In 2009, VA announced its goal of *ending* veteran homelessness. Innovative programs were initiated to support this goal, including the Veterans Justice Outreach (VJO) program. Its goal

> is to avoid the unnecessary criminalization of mental illness and extended incarceration among Veterans by ensuring that eligible justice-involved Veterans have timely access to [VA services]....VJO specialists provide direct outreach, assessment and case management for justice-involved veterans in local courts and jails and liaison with local justice system partners. (U.S. Department of Veterans Affairs 2019c)

Each of these programs contributes to the effort to end veteran homelessness, but likely the largest contributor to VA's success is the collaboration started in the early 1990s between the U.S. Department of Housing and Urban Development (HUD) and VA Supported Housing (VASH), creating the HUD-VASH program. HUD-VASH provides HUD rental assistance vouchers to qualifying homeless veterans and their families, along with VA case management and clinical services designed to support enrollees' continued ability to remain housed. From its small-scale beginning, the program grew to major proportions; by the end of FY18, more than 85,000 veterans had vouchers.

VA appears to be succeeding at its goal to end veteran homelessness. Since 2010, veteran homelessness has decreased by 46%. In January 2015, New Orleans became the first major city to announce that it had ended veteran homelessness. As of September 2019, three states (Connecticut, Massachusetts, Virgina) and 78 communities had announced an end to veteran homelessness. On a national scale, veteran homelessness has decreased such that it is nearly on par with homelessness among the general population: one 2019 report estimated that veterans make up 8.5% of the general population and only 9.2% of all homeless (Miller 2019).

Unemployment

Veterans with psychiatric issues, substance abuse, and/or homelessness face serious barriers to stable employment. Many who have been admitted to an inpatient psychiatric unit will have recently lost a job or been unable to find one. Similar to the approach taken for admitted patients who are identified as homeless, patients without stable employment are directed immediately on admission to a variety of opportunities available on discharge.

From a clinical standpoint, employment instability can be a significant barrier to recovery and result in prolonged inpatient stays. Some of these factors cannot be reversed or mitigated easily; for example, some veterans without premilitary employment may find that the military skills and training they acquired are not readily transferable to civilian trades. Recognizing these barriers, VA instituted employment assistance, education, and vocational rehabilitation programs that now are important components of VA care and benefits. A description and brief history of these programs follows.

Education benefits were introduced in 1944 to assist World War II veterans. Known as the GI Bill of Rights, these benefits made higher education accessible to veterans for whom it might not otherwise have been affordable; in 1949 a remarkable 70% of college admissions were veterans and were considered "the best class the country has ever produced" (Olson 1973). (Legislation enacted in 2009 updated veteran benefits. Known as the Post-9/11 GI Bill, it set new terms for education subsidies for service members and veterans who served on or after September 11, 2001. The Post-9/11 GI Bill provides a subsidy for tuition and fees up to 100% for qualifying programs, a stipend for books and supplies, and a housing allowance for qualifying veterans with an honorable discharge. Veterans can use this money for undergraduate and graduate degrees, vocational training, technical training, licensing programs, and other educational activities.

VA's current vocational rehabilitation program for SC veterans is the Veteran Readiness and Employment (formerly Vocational Rehabilitation and Employment) program (VR&E). It has evolved into a complex assessment and treatment network interfacing extensively with community businesses. Veterans are assisted with resume development, vocational coaching, job training, and sheltered employment. VR&E participation can facilitate a veteran's transition to mainstream community work. The Homeless Veterans Reintegration Program under the U.S. Department of Labor and Office of Personnel Management also offers vocational programs to assist veterans with employment skills and job searches.

VR&E services are available for veterans in outpatient and residential mental health care, and on some psychiatric inpatient units. Incentive therapy through work assignments provides structure to daily activity and some financial compensation. Veterans in outpatient or residential care who are ready to work part-time can apply to VA's Compensated Work Therapy programs, which prepare veterans for community employment or further rehabilitation.

VA has achieved dramatic success in reducing veteran unemployment. In 2011, the veteran unemployment rate was 12.5%. By early 2018 the veteran unemployment rate had dropped below the nonveteran unemployment rate, and it has remained low; as of October 2019, the veteran unemployment rate was 3.2% compared with the nonveteran unemployment rate of 3.5% (U.S. Department of Labor 2019).

Substance Abuse

Substance abuse is a significant problem in the United States at large and for veterans. Approximately 11% of veterans presenting initially for VA care have an established substance use disorders (SUD) diagnosis (Teeters et al. 2017). However, these data are probably an underestimate due to increasing SUD prevalence (especially among younger veterans), the reluctance to self-report, and the lack of any universal substance use screening in VA. In the VA inpatient setting, "high utilizers" (commonly defined as the top 10% of generators of total bed days) with SUD and a co-occurring psychiatric diagnosis (largely serious mental illness, but other diagnoses as well) account for nearly all the high utilizer bed days of care, mostly on psychiatric units (Painter et al. 2018). This finding suggests the need to carefully coordinate care of this population in order to prevent continued frequent readmissions. SUDs are treated similarly in VA and non-VA sectors.

Fortunately, VA has a comprehensive set of treatment options for veterans seeking treatment for substance use disorders not usually seen in the private sector. VA inpatient psychiatric hospitalization for substance abuse (for high and low utilizers alike) largely is reserved for those with comorbid acute psychiatric and/or psychosocial needs. Although some VAMCs provide medically uncomplicated detoxification on the inpatient psychiatric units, most have shifted detox to medical units or outpatient levels of care similar to non-VA hospitals. Examples of specific treatment settings include residential programs and intensive outpatient programs (including opioid treatment programs). Evidence-based SUD treatments arie provided, including cognitive-behavioral therapy and other psychotherapies, 12-step and peer support programs, motivational enhancement therapy, and contingency management. Pharmacological treatments are state of the art and include disulfiram, acamprosate, topiramate, gabapentin, and naltrexone for alcohol use disorder and methadone, buprenorphine, and naltrexone for opioid use disorder. These approaches and supporting evidence are extensively reviewed in the most recent revision of the VA/DoD clinical practice guideline for the management of substance use disorders (U.S. Department of Veterans Affairs and U.S. Department of Defense 2021b).

From a clinical perspective, understanding how a veteran's military experiences intersect with their substance abuse history can lead to improved treatment outcomes. Consider alcohol—the primary drug of abuse among active service members and veterans alike. Alcohol use can begin or become entrenched at any age or stage (e.g., premilitary, military, or postmilitary) in a soldier's life, and the severity may wax and wane. Self-reports of alcohol (and other substance) use are notoriously unreliable, but the best available data regarding recent and current use among active and reserve service members derive from DoD's Health Related Behaviors Survey (HBRS), which is scheduled for every 3 years. The 2018 HRBS measured binge drinking (consuming five or more drinks on the same occasion for men and four or more drinks for women at least once in the past 30 days) and heavy drinking (binge drinking at least one day each week in the past 30 days) and found that among active service members, 34.0% reported binge drinking and 9.8% reporting heavy drinking (Meadows et al. 2021). The same survey also noted that 28.2% of active service respondents attributed a permissive attitude toward drinking to leadership. A number of beneficial effects of alcohol in the military setting have been suggested, including stress relief, fortification for battle, group bonding, psychological respite, and entertainment. Despite the negative effects of alcohol abuse on mission readiness, an association of abuse with an elevated risk of attrition has been noted in female service members only (Porter et al. 2020).

Marijuana is the most frequently used illegal substance among service members and veterans, and its use among veterans continues to climb (as does use of amphetamines). Heroin and cocaine rarely are used prior to military service or by active-duty personnel but are more prevalent in the population of veterans served by VA. While the frequency of both heroin and cocaine abuse among VA enrollees has stabilized in recent years, it is the use of pharmacologically similar substances (e.g., prescription pain medications and illicit compounds containing opioids, and prescription and nonprescription stimulants) alone or in combination that is increasing and of grave concern. One unfortunate consequence of this broadened availability of opioids has been a marked increase in opioid-related overdoses and deaths among veterans and nonveterans despite the decrease in numbers of opioid prescriptions being written as a result of stringent state and federal restrictions (some of which have been relaxed as a result of the COVID pandemic) in recent years. Trending data show that U.S. opioid overdose deaths continue to rise rapidly and are estimated to have surpassed 100,000 (Ahmad et al. 2021).

Chronic pain, a frequent complication of military service, can be a contributing factor to veterans' substance abuse and psychiatric impairment as may be a clinical focus of inpatient psychiatric care, regardless of the reason for admission. The combination of chronic pain, substance abuse, and psychiatric preexisting conditions (or sequelae) can at times evolve synergistically to crisis proportions, necessitating inpatient psychiatric treatment. Historically, many VA and non-VA physicians alike prescribed opioids liberally for chronic pain, and these were often continued when veterans using these medications were admitted to inpatient psychiatry units. In recent years, responding to increasing rates of opioid abuse and a lack of effectiveness data, VA and DoD revised their joint clinical practice guideline for opioid therapy for chronic pain (U.S. Department of Veterans Affairs and U.S. Department of Defense 2017b) to encourage prescription of opioids only for short-term use to treat acute pain. Extinction of the practice of long-term opioid treatment was hastened by research advances indicating that this approach generally fails to reduce pain, improve function, or increase quality of life for those with chronic pain. Pharmacological treatment of chronic pain in the VA now mostly relies on nonsteroidal anti-inflammatory drugs, antidepressants and antiepileptic agents, and a variety of nonpharmacological treatments, including psychoeducation, individual and group therapy, physical therapy, exercise, and complementary and integrative approaches such as acupuncture, meditation, and tai chi. While cannabinoid products (touted by some as effective for treatment of chronic pain) are a subject of VA research efforts, they are not permitted by federal law to be used for clinical purposes.

On a positive note, tobacco use among veterans has been decreasing steadily in association with overall societal efforts to curb the practice and with VA promotion of tobacco cessation tools, including nicotine replacement therapy and various coaching programs. Impressively, veterans enrolled in VA health care who identified as smokers dropped from 15.9% in 2017 to 12.9% in 2021, which is lower than the prevalence of smokers in the general U.S. population (14.2%) (U.S. Department of Veterans Affairs 2021c). This development allows for improved focus on therapeutic goals when veterans who smoke are hospitalized and additionally facilitates institutional compliance with VA's blanket no-smoking policy.

Geriatric Psychiatry

The majority of the more than 8 million veterans enrolled in VA care are over the age of 55, and the median age for this group continues to increase. VA is becoming de facto a geriatric service organization. For the VA inpatient psychiatrist (and other inpatient mental health providers), this development poses a dilemma because many of them lack any formal training in geriatric psychiatry. Since 1989, a 1- or 2-year fellowship after residency is required to become eligible for board certification in geriatric psychiatry. However, the number of formally trained psychiatrists being produced cannot keep up with demand, and most psychiatrists with an interest in the field must learn from self-study, generous colleagues, and continuing medical education opportunities.

Psychiatric conditions typically manifesting in older veterans include the various neurocognitive disorders (including the conditions more commonly known as dementia), neurotrauma (such as TBI and mTBI), alcohol and other substance abuse (including long-term psychiatric sequelae), mood disorders, psychoses, and trauma-related conditions. Older inpatient veterans may present with more severe and difficult-to-treat psychiatric conditions than their private sector counterparts because of their higher incidence of trauma-related diagnoses, comorbid substance abuse, and psychosocial challenges. For example, VA researchers found almost double the incidence of dementia in Vietnam War veterans with PTSD compared with those without PTSD, differences thought to be due to PTSD-induced cognitive impairment (Yaffe et al. 2010). Similarly, TBI also seems to increase the risk and lower the age at onset of Alzheimer's disease and other neurodegenerative disorders (Mendez 2017).

It is noteworthy that psychiatric hospitalization itself can create added difficulties in attempting to stabilize older veterans in acute distress, especially when a neurocognitive disorder is involved. The loss of familiar support and the introduction of rigid treatment protocols in an institutionalized environment may worsen the symptoms that were originally of concern (e.g., verbal and physical expressions of agitation) and may directly interfere with treatment and lead to overreliance on restraints and medications with poorly tolerated side effects. Often these veterans will have extended stays because they are not considered safe for transfers to a less restrictive level of care. Previously, such patients were able to move to long-term psychiatric units within VA. But the gradual discontinuation of these long-term units coupled with the downsizing of acute psychiatric units in recent decades has led to efforts to create and support alternative pathways for safe and stable care transitions.

For example, some of these veterans may receive appropriate psychiatric care in one of VA's Community Living Centers (CLCs, equivalent to private sector nursing homes) provided they meet the medical eligibility requirements. Typically, this care is provided by a geriatric treatment team with an embedded mental health provider who has access to further consultation. Because of the added burden on staff and due to safety considerations, CLCs have become adept more at caring for veterans with challenging behaviors through specialized trainings. STAR-VA is a training program that helps staff understand and respond to challenging, disruptive, and dangerous behaviors by searching for antecedents to the behavior so they can be modified and the behavior eliminated or reduced (Karel et al. 2016). This model of nonpharmacological intervention may have broader applicability in both high-intensity environments (e.g., inpatient settings) and low-intensity ones (e.g., home).

Other challenges in care transitions include discharges delayed by veterans with impaired decision-making capacity who lack a health care agent or guardian. Only the states can make decisions regarding guardianship, which means that VA cannot lawfully discharge (or make other decisions on a veteran's behalf) until the process is completed. This may take an extended period of time (in some states waitlists exceed a year), resulting in the veteran being stuck at a higher level of care than is appropriate. This in turn results in a lack of resources for those needing them (e.g., an inpatient bed), financial waste, and higher risk of adverse events (e.g., disorientation, infection).

While veterans of all ages are at elevated suicide risk after discharge from a hospital inpatient unit, especially if suicidal ideation or behavior was part of the reason for admission (McCarthy et al. 2015), the elderly may be at special risk. For generational reasons, they may exhibit an increased reluctance to discuss such issues, and they may be prone to more distress when discharged into an environment with few social supports and new medical and other challenges to face. Careful screening for re-emerging symptoms prior to discharge and close follow-up are warranted for these patients.

Trauma: A Universal Military Experience

Traumatic experiences—both intentional and incidental—are woven inexorably into military service. New service members may bring a history of personal trauma with them. Some candidates face initial stress in achieving enlistment requirements (such as significant weight loss). All recruits must complete basic training—a rite of passage that includes arduous physical training, strict obedience to authority figures, live-fire exercises, and realistic prisoner-of-war simulations. Once on active duty, service members face other but equally formidable risks, especially when in specialized combat training and when deployed into high-risk operations.

In considering the effects of trauma in the military, it is noteworthy that combatants trained by the U.S. military were exclusively male until 1990, when Congress began authorizing women to serve in combat zones, initially on combat ships and aviation missions. Incremental policy shifts continued; in 1994 women were admitted as members of ground combat units, specifically to participate in raids when women and children might be encountered. Since then, women have been offered progressively greater roles and assignments. In 2015, all military units and occupations were opened to women, achieving full gender integration (Moore 2020). However, this has also meant that men and women are now equally vulnerable to combat traumas, and women veterans may be affected in ways that we are only just beginning to understand.

While a history of trauma alone is rarely the chief complaint for an inpatient psychiatric admission, that history may both fuel and provide a filter for the presenting complaint, findings on initial assessment and subsequent presentation. Familiarity with the specifics of military trauma improves a psychiatrist's skill at treating those suffering from the effects of trauma, whether the trauma occurred recently or remotely. A brief review of four military/veteran specific traumas—moral injury, psychiatric combat/war trauma, MST, and mTBI/blast neurotrauma—follows.

Moral Injury

Moral injury is a specific psychological trauma resulting from (but not limited to) participation in certain combat and other war situations. The injury is to the individual's conscience. Moral injury is a phenomenon as old as war itself and is recorded in ancient texts such as Homer's *Iliad* but has only become a topic of general and academic discussion in recent decades. Because it has no associated flesh-and-blood injury, moral injury is one of the "hidden wounds of war." It may be a veteran's sole mental health affliction and can occur independently of other psychiatric trauma. Circumstances that might lead to moral injury are described by Maguen and Litz (2015) and others and include the following:

- Directly participating in acts of combat such as killing
- Causing or witnessing deaths of civilians, particularly women and children
- Making unintentional errors leading to deaths
- Experiencing survivor's guilt
- Failing to prevent immoral acts of others
- Participating in or witnessing war crimes
- Participating in immoral wars, causing unnecessary deaths

- Participating in war itself (by conscientious objectors and others who see war as a gross moral violation) (U.S. conscientious objectors can apply for exemption from military service.)

Some types of warfare may result in higher rates of moral injury (e.g., battle conditions requiring "close combat" fighting). It is common for soldiers and veterans to carry the burden of moral injury for years, perhaps never addressing the associated psychological trauma. For some, there may be no outward sign of distress. But for others, the psychological pressure of moral injury may lead to social withdrawal, addiction, feelings of anxiety, anger, rage, and even aggressive behavior toward self or others (Shay 1994), which at times may require psychiatric admission for stabilization. Questions about war experiences and about feelings of guilt, and a high index of suspicion, aid in identifying combat veterans with moral injury. Once moral injury is identified and the veteran's acute crisis is stabilized, the veteran can be referred for specialized therapy.

Treatment of moral injury is a psychotherapeutic process that has been termed "soul repair" (Brock et al. 2012). Ironically, though sharing with others is critical to recovery and healing, the war experiences leading to moral injury are exceedingly difficult to talk about, and overcoming the barrier of silence is the first step toward healing. Therapeutic avenues include group therapy, individual therapy, and chaplain counseling. Group therapy is particularly effective for treatment of moral injury (Shay 1994, p. 4). Groups should be composed of carefully selected members who are grappling with similar questions. Skilled, empathic participation by the therapist—who need not be a combat veteran—is crucial to group effectiveness. A chaplain may be particularly helpful for those sufferers who feel the need for forgiveness for their actions. A potentially complicating factor (that may affect all veterans regardless of their mental health status) is that group therapy may not be an option if the veteran was engaged in a highly classified operation that does not allow sharing of self-identifying information or mission details.

Psychiatric Combat/War Trauma

Some traumatic experiences in war and combat are so profound that they can overwhelm even the strongest psychological defenses and mental resilience. Combat trauma is not a uniform syndrome and in fact manifests differently in every war depending on the precipitating events, degree of popular support, whether the war was fought at home or on foreign soil, voluntary or draft recruitment, types of combat, duration, and ultimate conclusion—victory or defeat? Each factor affects the stress reactions of the participants as a group and individually. Because this trauma affects not only combatants but also frontline medical and support personnel, "war trauma" is another commonly used descriptor.

The first cases of combat trauma during World War I occurred in apparently unwounded frontline soldiers with a novel set of symptoms: "They could neither see, smell nor taste properly. Some were unable to stand up, speak, urinate or defecate; some had lost their memories; others vomited uncontrollably" (Shapiro 2001, p. 1). Some military psychiatrists considered these symptoms psychological in origin, representing hysteria, conversion disorders, and/or repressed trauma; others considered them intentional, put on by malingerers or cowards (Jones 2012). Eventually, with the observation that many soldiers developed symptoms immediately following proximity to an exploding shell, combat trauma came to be called "shell shock," the signature injury of World War I (though toward the end of the war, the use of the term was officially discouraged because of its very popularity) (Jones and Wessely 2005).

The role of the military psychiatrist is complicated in every war by their responsibility to differentiate between soldiers who are capable of returning to the battlefield and those who are not. An entire book could be written about military psychiatrists' moral dilemmas as they face dual loyalties: soldier-patients and facilitation of the war effort. Identifying soldiers who are not capable can be complicated by the possibility that a soldier was not "powerless to help himself, but…using his medical symptoms as a weapon of resistance to military authority" (Shapiro 2001, p. xxi). Today's VA psychiatrists face the same challenges in assessing disabilities for SC benefits, differentiating malingering from psychiatric breakdown, combat trauma, MST, and/or neurological injury.

World War II warfare led to a different constellation of trauma symptoms. These deployments were long, and many battles were fought in extreme conditions, from scorching summers in Egypt's Sahara Desert to freezing winters in Russia (Shapiro 2001). Under these combat conditions, stress reactions commonly were a consequence of physical trauma and manifested with psychosis, panic, and severe depression (rarely as hysteria). World War II combat stress syndrome came to be called "battle fatigue" or "combat exhaustion" (nomenclature varied between American and British psychiatry), the signature injury of World War II. During the Korean War, the term "battle fatigue" remained in use for combat trauma. With very little media coverage in the United States, average citizens knew little about the war or the condition of the soldiers. Following the war, it was socially taboo to seek mental health care, but even a veteran who did seek help for combat trauma would have found little assistance from VA or the civilian sector, as the Korean War predated development of trauma-specific treatment. As a result, comparatively little is known about the war and postwar psychiatric status of Korean War veterans.

Domestic opposition to U.S. involvement in the Vietnam War—known as the "antiwar movement" (Zunes and Laird 2010)—negatively affected active-duty soldiers and Vietnam War veterans, in stark contrast to strong popular support during World War I and World War II, and the public's relative indifference during the Korean War. Demoralization among service members is reflected in their above-average rates of desertion, drug abuse, resistance to authority, and regrets about participation in the war. Shay (1994, p. xx) worked with Vietnam War veterans suffering from war trauma and identified key features of their trauma:

- Persistent mobilization of the body and the mind for lethal danger, with the potential for explosive violence
- Persistence and activation of combat survival skills in civilian life
- Chronic health problems stemming from chronic mobilization of the body for danger
- Persistent expectation of betrayal and exploitation, and destruction of the capacity for social trust
- Persistent preoccupation with both the enemy and the veteran's own military/governmental authorities
- Alcohol and drug abuse
- Suicidality, despair, isolation, and meaninglessness

The diagnostic construct of PTSD emerged in the postwar period following a period of mental health professional collaboration, personal testimonies by Vietnam veterans, public hearings, social pressure, and political interest (Scott 1990; Summerfield 2001). The diagnosis of PTSD entered the professional lexicon in the postwar era when it was included in DSM-III (American Psychiatric Association 1980), and its definition has been slightly modified in subsequent editions of DSM. PTSD became the signature injury of the Vietnam War.

VA trauma services range from outpatient counseling to long-term residential care. Currently the national VA system has specialized programs in residential and outpatient levels of care, including 135 PTSD Specialty Outpatient Treatment programs. The National Center for PTSD (NCPTSD) began in 1989, legislated by Congress to address the PTSD treatment needs of Vietnam veterans. Its current mandate is broader, addressing PTSD in all veterans and its effects on their support systems. NCPTSD also serves as a clearinghouse for new trauma research, provides education for veterans and families, and offers continuing education and consultation for professionals within VA and to community health care providers. Postdeployment transitional programs are designed to educate new veterans and their families about the signs and symptoms of PTSD and other sequelae of military service. It is hoped that these preventive efforts will lead to early treatment interventions and minimize comorbidities. Given continuous U.S. involvement in military conflicts since 1990, effective treatment of combat PTSD will remain a critically important VA mental health service.

Screening for PTSD is a requirement for all patients seen in the VA. Even when a screen is negative, the possibility of unreported PTSD requires a careful and systematic interview process that is sufficiently flexible to permit delays that may be due to the veteran's reluctance to share information or memory gaps. Treatment of PTSD is a multidisciplinary effort including therapists to provide individual and group therapy and therapists trained in trauma-specific modalities, including prolonged exposure, cognitive processing therapy, and eye movement desensitization and reprocessing. Psychopharmacological agents can be useful, particularly for severe anxiety/panic, depression, and sleep disturbances due to nightmares. These recommendations are to be found in the most recent VA/DoD clinical practice guideline for the management of posttraumatic stress disorder and acute stress disorder (U.S. Department of Veterans Affairs and U.S. Department of Defense 2017a).

Military Sexual Trauma

Although sexually related crimes can occur anywhere, they occur at an alarming frequency among service members. The term *military sexual trauma*, as used by VA, specifically applies to a wide range of offenses, including sexual harassment (e.g., comments, sexual advances, touching), coercion into sexual activity, and acts of sexual violence (e.g., sexual assault, rape, sexual attack by a group), that occur during a veteran's period of military service. (Note: the military does not use the term MST, referring rather to *sexual trauma*, which has minor definitional differences from MST.) and both men and women are affected. Among veterans who used VHA outpatient care in FY2021, 32.8% of female veterans (150,395) and 1.9% of male veterans (80,799) screened positive for MST (Military Sexual Trauma Support Team 2022a).

Conditions of military life intensify the potential shame, intimidation, and stigma of reporting sexual trauma within the survivor's chain of command (Wolfe et al.

1998). "Of women who reported a penetrative sexual assault, 59% were assaulted by someone with a higher rank than them, and 24% were assaulted by someone in their chain of command" (Protect Our Defenders 2019). Emotional trauma intensifies for survivors of MST when they must live and work alongside their assailants. Subordination to an attacker "often [leads] to an increased sense of feeling helpless, powerless, and at risk for additional victimization.... [MST] that occurs in this setting often means that victims are relying on their perpetrators (or associates of the perpetrator) to provide for basic needs including medical and psychological care" (Street and Stafford 2019).

Per U.S. military justice system policy, commanders are responsible for prosecuting sex crimes within their ranks, but MST survivors may decline to report a crime when the perpetrator is in their chain of command. Although requests have been made to the Pentagon to remove sexual trauma cases from the military hierarchy and direct them through an independent prosecutorial process, legislative efforts with this goal to date have thus far failed.

The MST reporting rate has quadrupled over the past 10 years, reflecting the reduced social stigma for reporting these crimes, yet *most* events still go unreported (Kirby 2019). Presumably, screening requirements within VA contributed to this increase as well. Some survivors do not report sexual trauma because they fear that nothing will come of their report, a realistic concern given the low conviction rate for these crimes. Other deterrents include potential retaliation for reporting, which could result in geographical relocation and/or assignment of the trauma survivor to undesirable or more dangerous duties, damaging their career plans or promotion trajectory. Military discharge is the ultimate retaliation for sexual trauma reporting. Retaliatory discharges are even more egregious when service members are denied honorable discharges: "24% of MST survivors are separated under less than fully honorable conditions compared to 15% of all service members" (Protect Our Defenders 2019).

Every VA medical center now has an MST coordinator to provide information and treatment coordination for veterans and staff, and screening for MST is a requirement for all veterans. VA offers a full spectrum of care for MST, including standard inpatient and residential care and outpatient services at VHA clinics and Vet Centers. In addition, veterans can be referred for admission to specialized inpatient and residential coed and single-sex MST programs nationwide. In FY2021, VHA provided over 2 million MST-related outpatient visits to veterans who experienced MST (Military Sexual Trauma Support Team 2022b).

While not a diagnosis, MST is an experience that is associated with mental health conditions that command attention and may lead to inpatient psychiatric admission. Even under the close observation afforded by an inpatient admission, a history of MST may be overlooked, often because of a reluctance of the MST survivor to share this information. A careful and respectful assessment should occur with consideration for the veteran's preference for a provider of a specific gender and sensitivity to the common practice of asking inpatients to repeat their story for the benefit of trainees or cross-covering staff. Symptoms span the psychopathology spectrum, including depression, anxiety, and substance abuse, and may develop immediately after an attack or other precipitating event, or they may not surface until years later. Estimates vary, but about a third of all MST survivors develop PTSD, with a lesser but significant percentage developing a depressive disorder (Gilmore et al. 2016). MST survivors are also at increased risk of homelessness and suicide (Kimerling et al. 2016). Treatments for these conditions include the same psychotherapies and psychopharmacological and other somatic therapies that are indicated for these conditions without the presence of MST.

Neuropsychiatric Trauma: Mild Traumatic Brain Injury

Neurological and psychiatric sequelae of mTBI follow physical trauma to the brain. Veterans who have experienced neurotrauma with psychiatric sequelae may be admitted to VA inpatient psychiatric units and, in fact, will be some of the most challenging cases a VA inpatient psychiatrist will treat.

Military service members throughout their careers, from basic training through combat, are at increased risk of mTBI compared with civilians. Classification of TBI severity ranges from mild (a concussion; following at most a brief loss of consciousness and brief disorientation), through moderate, to severe (following extended loss of consciousness, penetrating brain injury, or coma). Most TBIs are mild, but neurotrauma from even an apparently mild TBI can persist and can lead to progressive neurodegeneration.

Military vulnerability to mTBI is associated with high-intensity training, regular exposure to weaponry, motor vehicle accidents, assaults, falls, and high-risk off-duty activities enjoyed by many service members (Defense and Veterans Brain Injury Center 2019). Falls, followed by motor vehicle accidents, are the most common cause of TBI in older adults (both military and civilian) (Thompson et al. 2006). Substance abuse increases the risk of mTBI.

Soldiers with post-9/11 deployments to Iraq and Afghanistan conflicts must contend with counter-insurgency operations using a new form of warfare—improvised explosive devices (IEDs). IEDs concealed by the enemy put all ground forces (combatants and support services) operating in a war zone under constant threat of sudden death from an IED explosion. Proximity to an IED explosion, if not resulting in death, commonly results in mTBI. mTBI has become the signature injury of post-9/11 conflicts.

The increased incidence of TBI from 2000 through 2011 in the four branches of the military is illustrated in Figure 12–2.

Legislation in 2008 authorized the Polytrauma[6]/TBI System of Care for service members and veterans, creating an integrated national network and continuum of care. Those most severely affected by TBI can be referred for consideration for admission to one of the network's five Polytrauma Rehabilitation Centers (which provide the highest level of care). Those with less-critical needs can be referred to an abundance of Network Sites, Support Clinics, and Points of Contact. The Polytrauma/TBI System of Care provides clinical evaluation and management, family support and education, and locations for cutting-edge research.

A history of mTBI can be difficult to elicit from a veteran when they present years after the index injury; they may never have known, or may have forgotten, that they

---

[6]*Polytrauma* is defined as mTBI with a significant secondary physical injury or psychiatric condition.

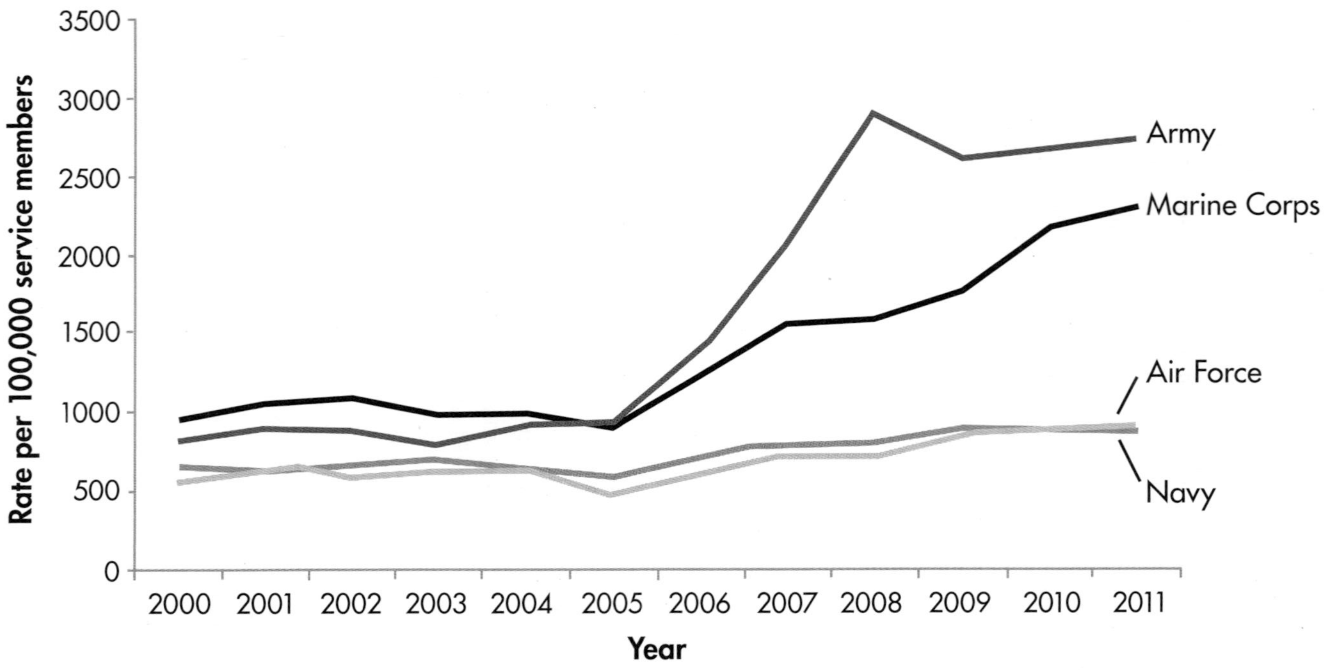

FIGURE 12–2. Estimated overall annual incidence rates of traumatic brain injury among active-duty U.S. military service members by service branch, 2000–2011.

Source. Centers for Disease Control and Prevention: *Report to Congress on Traumatic Brain Injury in the United States: Understanding the Public Health Problem Among Current and Former Military Personnel* (online). Atlanta, GA, Centers for Disease Control and Prevention, 2016. Available at: www.cdc.gov/traumaticbraininjury/pubs/congress_military.html. Accessed November 18, 2019.

suffered a wartime head injury. Even with a known history of TBI during active duty, information about the circumstances or severity of the injury may be incomplete in the veteran's medical record or in their memory. (It is hoped this information gap will be eliminated after DoD and VA electronic medical records are merged.)

Psychiatric sequelae of neurotrauma span the breadth of psychopathology. Veterans may manifest memory, attention, and other cognitive impairments. TBI symptoms include chronic pain and chronic fatigue, mood symptoms, psychoses, personality changes, impulsivity/apathy, behavioral disturbances, executive function deficits, and even nonspecific observations of "unusual behavior." Physical symptoms such as tinnitus, visual changes, or balance problems can be clues to an underlying TBI. Because psychiatric symptoms due to an underlying TBI are indistinguishable from primary psychiatric symptoms, TBI should be in the differential diagnosis of every veteran presenting for mental health care. Key diagnostic tools include brain imaging and neuropsychological testing. Uncovering and addressing previously undiagnosed mTBI may lead to life-altering improvements in an affected veteran's life.

The approach to the hospitalized veteran with mTBI includes environmentally supportive treatment including assessment of the head-injured patient's need for low light and noise, low-key approaches by staff, and increased rest. Pharmacotherapy, psychotherapy, speech therapy, occupational therapy, vocational rehabilitation, and physical therapy typically are components of an mTBI treatment plan. Family involvement is important for education and to address damaged family relationships (Rao et al. 2015). Psychopharmacological intervention to address the mTBI patient's psychiatric symptoms requires close attention to the veteran's responses to medication following the maxim "Start low and go slow." Given the high rate of substance abuse in the mTBI population, treatment with potentially addicting substances such as benzodiazepines for anxiety should be avoided. For similar reasons, caffeine is preferable to stimulants to address attentional and concentration deficits.

A full review of these and related treatment recommendations can be found in the VA/DoD clinical practice guideline for the management and rehabilitation of postacute mild traumatic brain injury (U.S. Department of Veterans Affairs and U.S. Department of Defense 2021a).

Vet Centers

Vet Centers, also known as Readjustment Counseling Centers, are a unique VA resource for eligible veterans in need of treatment for trauma-related conditions. Vet Centers are community-based counseling centers established to provide services apart from the VAMC and outpatient clinics and focused on providing a wide range of social and psychological services, including professional readjustment counseling. Eligibility for Vet Center treatment includes active-duty service in any combat theater or area of hostility, MST, military emergency medical personnel (e.g., medics, physicians), and mortuary service to the casualties of war. Individual, group, marriage, and family counseling are offered in addition to referral and connection to other VA or community benefits and services. Vet Center counselors and outreach staff, many of whom are veterans themselves, are experienced and prepared to discuss the tragedies of war, loss, grief, and transition after trauma (U.S. Department of Veterans Affairs

2019b). Of note, the medical records of veterans treated at Vet Centers are not accessible to other VA providers without the veteran's permission.

Conclusion

The VA health care system is the largest U.S. provider of medical care and the largest provider of medical training. As a result, all the nation's hospitals benefit from VA education, training, and research progress. State-of-the-art IT, including an electronic patient record, improves efficiency and effectiveness. VA inpatient hospital psychiatry today is a unique blend of mainstream and veteran-specific treatments. Veterans benefit from multidisciplinary collaboration and a full continuum of clinical services (as well as assistance with homelessness, legal involvement, and unemployment issues) to an extent largely unavailable in the private sector. The full spectrum of invisible injuries of war (including moral injury, combat trauma, MST, and mTBI) remains a distinctive and prominent focus of interest in VA. As a result of its unique combination of clinical, education, and research opportunities, psychiatrists may find that VA offers one of the most compelling and potentially satisfying experiences in U.S. hospital psychiatry today. However, optimal veteran care can be provided in any setting by psychiatrists and other mental health providers who are willing to learn (often via VA resources) about the unique elements of military experience and its enduring effects on the human psyche, nervous system, and body. Long after Lincoln's call for care of veterans, VA continues to carry on the mission.

References

Ahmad FB, Rossen LM, Sutton P: Provisional Drug Overdose Death Counts. Hyattsville, MD, National Center for Health Statistics, 2021

American Psychiatric Association: Diagnostic and Statistical Manual of Mental Disorders, 3rd Edition. Washington, DC, American Psychiatric Association, 1980

Brock RN, Keizer H, Lettini G: Moral injury: the crucial missing piece in understanding soldier suicides. Huffpost, July 23, 2012 (updated September 22, 2012). Available at: www.huffpost.com/entry/moral-injury-the-crucial-missing-piece-in-understanding-soldier-suicides_b_1686674. Accessed November 14, 2019.

Centers for Medicare & Medicaid Services: National Health Expenditure Accounts: Historical. 2022. Available at: www.cms.gov/Research-Statistics-Data-and-Systems/Statistics-Trends-and-Reports/NationalHealthExpendData/NationalHealthAccountsHistorical. Accessed March 26, 2022.

Congressional Budget Office: Comparing the Costs of the Veterans' Health Care System With Private-Sector Costs. December 10, 2014. Available at: www.cbo.gov/publication/49763. Accessed March 26, 2022.

Curyto KJ, McCurry SM, Luci K, et al: Managing challenging behaviors of dementia in veterans: identifying and changing activators and consequences using STAR-VA. J Gerontol Nurs 43(2):33–43, 2017 27711931

Defense and Veterans Brain Injury Center: Traumatic brain injury awareness: concussion/mild traumatic brain injury. Traumatic Brain Injury Fact Sheet, February 2019. Available at: https://dvbic.dcoe.mil/material/traumatic-brain-injury-awareness-fact-sheet. Accessed November 18, 2019.

Duan-Porter W, Martinson BC, Greer N, et al: Evidence review: social determinants of health for veterans. J Gen Intern Med 33(10):1785–1795, 2018 30030735

Fortney JC, Borowsky SJ, Hedeen AN, et al: VA community-based outpatient clinics: access and utilization performance measures. Medical Care 40(7):561–569, 2002 12142771

Gilmore AK, Brignone E, Painter JM, et al: Military sexual trauma and co-occurring posttraumatic stress disorder, depressive disorders, and substance use disorders among returning Afghanistan and Iraq veterans. Womens Health Issues 26(5):546–554, 2016 27528358

Jones E: Shell shocked. Monitor on Psychology 43(6):18, 2012. Available at: www.apa.org/monitor/2012/06/shell-shocked. Accessed January 7, 2020.

Jones E, Wessely S: Shell Shock to PTSD: Military Psychiatry from 1900 to the Gulf War. London, Psychology Press, 2005

Karel MJ, Teri L, McConnell E, et al: Effectiveness of expanded implementation of STAR-VA for managing dementia-related behaviors among veterans. Gerontologist 56(1):126–134, 2016 26185155

Kimerling R, Makin-Byrd K, Louzon S, et al: Military sexual trauma and suicide mortality. Am J Prev Med 50(6):684–691, 2016 26699249

Kirby J: Pentagon report shows sharp rise in military sexual assaults. Vox, May 3, 2019. Available at: www.vox.com/world/2019/5/3/18528148/pentagon-military-sexual-assault-report-shanahan. Accessed November 13, 2019.

Lincoln A: Second inaugural address. Saturday, March 4, 1865 (online). Bartleby.com, 1989. Available at: www.bartleby.com/124/pres32.html. Accessed November 29, 2019.

Maguen S, Litz B: Moral Injury in the Context of War. Washington, DC, National Center for PTSD, 2015

McCarthy JF, Bossarte RM, Katz IR, et al: Predictive modeling and concentration of the risk of suicide: implications for preventive interventions in the US Department of Veterans Affairs. Am J Public Health 105(9):1935–1942, 2015 26066914

Meadows SO, Engel CC, Collins RL, et al: 2018 Health Related Behaviors Survey: Substance Use Among the Active Component. Santa Monica, CA, RAND Corporation, 2021. Available at: www.rand.org/pubs/research_briefs/RB10116z3.html. Accessed March 26, 2022.

Mendez MF: What is the relationship of traumatic brain injury to dementia? J Alzheimers Dis 57(3):667–681, 2017 28269777

Military Sexual Trauma Support Team: Military Sexual Trauma Screening Report, Fiscal Year 2021. Washington, DC, Department of Veterans Affairs, Office of Mental Health and Suicide Prevention, 2022a

Military Sexual Trauma Support Team: Summary of Military Sexual Trauma–Related Outpatient Care, Fiscal Year 2021. Washington, DC, Department of Veterans Affairs, Office of Mental Health and Suicide Prevention, 2022b

Miller S: Homeless Veterans Committee Update: January/February 2019. Silver Spring, MD, Vietnam Veterans of America, February 21, 2019. Available at: https://vva.org/programs/homeless-veterans/homeless-veterans-committee-update-januaryfebruary-2019. Accessed October 23, 2019.

Mills PD, Watts BV, Hemphill RR: Suicide and suicide attempts on hospital grounds and clinic areas. J Patient Saf 17(5):e423–e428, 2021 28230577

Moore E: Women in Combat: Five-Year Status Update. Washington, DC, Center for a New American Security, March 31, 2020. Available at: www.cnas.org/publications/commentary/women-in-combat-five-year-status-update. Accessed March 26, 2022.

Olson KW: The G. I. Bill and higher education: success and surprise. American Quarterly 25(5):596–610, 1973

Painter JM, Malte CA, Rubinsky AD, et al: High inpatient utilization among Veterans Health Administration patients with substance-use disorders and co-occurring mental health conditions. Am J Drug Alcohol Abuse 44(3):386–394, 2018 29095057

Pavao J, Turchik JA, Hyun JK, et al: Military sexual trauma among homeless veterans. J Gen Intern Med 28 (suppl 2):S536–S541, 2013 23807062

Porter B, Rodriguez LM, Woodall KA, et al: Alcohol misuse and separation from military service: a dyadic perspective. Addict Behav 110:106512, 2020 32623237

Protect Our Defenders: Facts on United States Military Sexual Violence. Alexandria, VA, Protect Our Defenders, December 2019. Available at: www.protectourdefenders.com/factsheet. Accessed January 23, 2020.

Rao V, Koliatsos V, Ahmed F, Lyketsos C, et al: Neuropsychiatric disturbances associated with traumatic brain injury: a practical approach to evaluation and management. Semin Neurol 35(1):64–82, 2015 25714869

Rosenheck R, Fontana A: A model of homelessness among male veterans of the Vietnam War generation. Am J Psychiatry 151(3):421–427, 1994 8109652

Scott C: Veterans Affairs: Historical Budget Authority, FY1940–FY2012. Washington, DC, Congressional Research Service, June 13, 2012. Available at: https://fas.org/sgp/crs/misc/RS22897.pdf. Accessed October 11, 2019.

Scott WJ: PTSD in DSM-III: a case in the politics of diagnosis and disease. Social Problems 37(3):294–310, 1990

Shapiro B: A War of Nerves: Soldiers and Psychiatrists in the Twentieth Century. Cambridge, MA, Harvard University Press, 2001

Shay J: Achilles in Vietnam: Combat Trauma and the Undoing of Character. New York, Simon & Schuster, 1994

Street A, Stafford J: Military Sexual Trauma: Issues in Caring for Veterans. Washington, DC, National Center for PTSD, U.S. Department of Veterans Affairs, 2019. Available at: www.ptsd.va.gov/professional/treat/type/sexual_trauma_military.asp. Accessed September 26, 2019.

Summerfield D: The invention of post-traumatic stress disorder and the social usefulness of a psychiatric category. BMJ 322(7278):95–98, 2001 11154627

Teeters JB, Lancaster CL, Brown DG, Back SE: Substance use disorders in military veterans: prevalence and treatment challenges. Subst Abuse Rehabil 30(8):69–77, 2017 28919834

Thompson HJ, McCormick WC, Kagan SH: Traumatic brain injury in older adults: epidemiology, outcomes, and future implications. J Am Geriatr Soc 54(10):1590–1595, 2006 17038079

Tsai J, Rosenheck RA: Risk factors for homelessness among US veterans. Epidemiol Rev 37:177–195, 2015 25595171

U.S. Department of Defense: DoD Instruction 6130.03, Vol 2: Medical Standards for Military Service: Retention. September, 4, 2020

U.S. Department of Defense: DoD Instruction 6130.03, Vol 1: Medical Standards for Military Service: Appointment, Enlistment, or Induction. April 30, 2021

U.S. Department of Labor: Veterans' Employment and Training Service: latest unemployment numbers: October jobs report. Washington, DC, U.S. Department of Labor, 2019. Available at: www.dol.gov/agencies/vets/latest-numbers. Accessed December 2, 2019.

U.S. Department of Veterans Affairs: Compensation. Washington, DC, U.S. Department of Veterans Affairs, 2019a. Available at: www.benefits.va.gov/compensation/types-compensation.asp. Accessed October 2, 2019.

U.S. Department of Veterans Affairs: Vet Centers (Readjustment Counseling) (online). Washington, DC, U.S. Department of Veterans Affairs, 2019b. Available at: www.vetcenter.va.gov. Accessed October 2, 2019.

U.S. Department of Veterans Affairs: VA Homeless Programs: Veterans Justice Outreach Program. Washington, DC, U.S. Department of Veterans Affairs, 2019c. Available at: www.va.gov/homeless/vjo.asp. Accessed October 23, 2019.

U.S. Department of Veterans Affairs: Design Guide for Inpatient Mental Health and Residential Rehabilitation Treatment Program Facilities. Washington, DC, U.S. Department of Veterans Affairs, January 2021a. Available at: www.cfm.va.gov/til/dGuide/dgMH.pdf. Accessed May 3, 2021.

U.S. Department of Veterans Affairs: Locations: Interactive US Map (online). 2021b. Available at: www.va.gov/directory/guide/map.asp?dnum=1. Accessed November 1, 2019.

U.S. Department of Veterans Affairs: 2021 Survey of Veteran Enrollees' Health and Use of Health Care. September 24, 2021c. Available at: www.va.gov/VHASTRATEGY/SOE2021/2021_Enrollee_Data_Findings_Report-508_Compliant.pdf. Accessed March 26, 2022.

U.S. Department of Veterans Affairs, Advisory Committee on Women Veterans: 2012 Report: Honoring Women Veterans—Yesterday, Today, and Tomorrow. Washington, DC, U.S. Department of Veterans Affairs, September 2012. Available at: www.va.gov/womenvet/docs/acwv/Final_Advisory_Committee_on_Women_2012_Report.pdf. Accessed October 28, 2019.

U.S. Department of Veterans Affairs, National Center for Veterans Analysis and Statistics: VETPOP2016 living veterans by age group, gender, 2015–2045. Washington, DC, U.S. Department of Veterans Affairs, 2016. Available at: www.va.gov/vetdata/docs/Demographics/New_Vetpop_Model/1L_VetPop2016_National.xlsx. Accessed September 30, 2019.

U.S. Department of Veterans Affairs, U.S. Department of Defense: VA/DoD Clinical Practice Guideline: Management of Posttraumatic Stress Disorder and Acute Stress Reaction. Washington, DC, U.S. Department of Veterans Affairs, 2017a. Available at: www.healthquality.va.gov/guidelines/MH/ptsd. Accessed March 26, 2022.

U.S. Department of Veterans Affairs, U.S. Department of Defense: VA/DoD Clinical Practice Guideline: Opioid Therapy for Chronic Pain, Washington, DC, U.S. Department of Veterans Affairs, 2017b. Available at: www.healthquality.va.gov/guidelines/Pain/cot. Accessed March 26, 2022.

U.S. Department of Veterans Affairs, U.S. Department of Defense: VA/DoD Clinical Practice Guideline: Management and Rehabilitation of Post-Acute Mild Traumatic Brain Injury. Washington, DC, U.S. Department of Veterans Affairs, 2021a. Available at: www.healthquality.va.gov/guidelines/Rehab/mtbi. Accessed March 26, 2022.

U.S. Department of Veterans Affairs, U.S. Department of Defense: VA/DoD Clinical Practice Guideline: Management of Substance Use Disorders. Washington, DC, U.S. Department of Veterans Affairs, 2021b. Available at: www.healthquality.va.gov/guidelines/MH/sud. Accessed March 26, 2022.

U.S. General Accounting Office: Female active-duty personnel guidance and plans needed for recruitment and retention efforts. Report to Congressional Committees. GAO-20-61. May 2020. Available at: www.gao.gov/assets/710/707037.pdf. Accessed July 8, 2020.

U.S. Office of Personnel Management: Federal workforce data. Fedscope, 2020. Available at: https://www.fedscope.opm.gov. Accessed January 24, 2020.

Wolfe J, Sharkansky EJ, Read JP, et al: Sexual harassment and assault as predictors of PTSD symptomatology among U.S. female Persian Gulf War military personnel. J Interpers Violence 13(1):40–57, 1998

Yaffe K, Vittinghoff E, Lindquist K, et al: Posttraumatic stress disorder and risk of dementia among US veterans. Arch Gen Psychiatry 67(6):608–613, 2010 20530010

Zunes S, Laird J: The US Anti-Vietnam War Movement (1964–1973) (online). Washington, DC, International Center on Nonviolent Conflict, January 2010. Available at: www.nonviolent-conflict.org/us-anti-vietnam-war-movement-1964-1973. Accessed January 15, 2020.

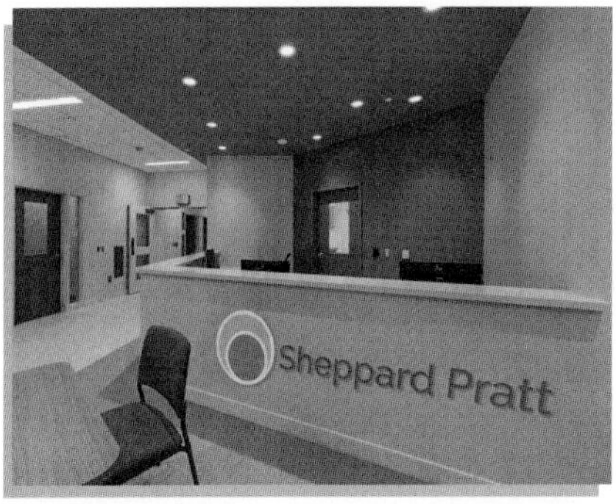

PART 2

The Continuum of Care

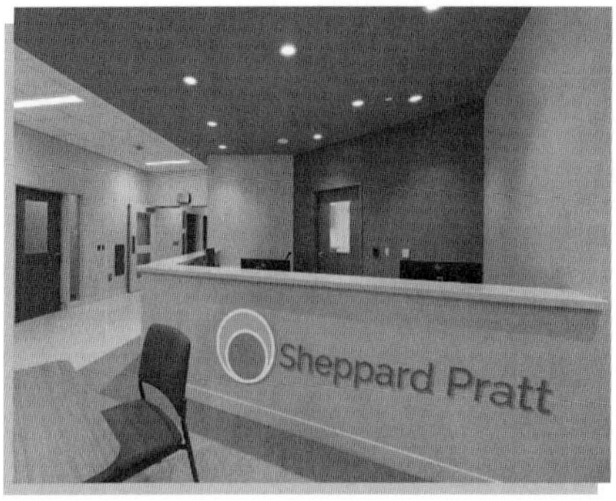

CHAPTER 13

Community Mental Health and Hospital-Based Outpatient Services

Deepak Prabhakar, M.D., M.P.H.
Manan Shah, M.D.
Jason Addison, M.D.
Jeff Richardson, M.S.W., M.B.A.

History of Community Mental Health

As access to psychiatric care and efficacious treatment modalities have expanded, treatment settings have gradually shifted from an overwhelming number of inpatient settings to outpatient care. In the United States, this change was also accelerated by societal factors. First, in the late twentieth century, there was a general consensus and public outcry against the use of large institutions as points of care for those with mental illness; second, with the advent of Medicare, Medicaid, and Social Security Disability Insurance, states moved away from primarily funding large state hospitals and started relying on federal entitlement programs for alternatives; third, with the advent of effective medications such as antipsychotics, an increasing number of patients achieved symptomatic remission, reducing the reliance on inpatient psychiatric facilities for long-term care (Bloche and Cournos 1990; Shore and Cohen 1994; Talbott 1982).

With the growing attention being afforded community options for care, Congress enacted the Mental Health Study Act of 1955, leading to the creation of the Joint Commission on Mental Illness and Health. The commission's report ultimately led to the Community Mental Health Act of 1963. The 1963 act authorized grants to states for local mental health centers, thereby accelerating the movement toward community-based care as an alternative to institutionalization (Sharfstein 2000). However, the program was poorly actualized, and even though it did lead to significant reduction in inpatient beds across the United States, the expected growth in community-based programs never followed. In the 1980s, federal funding was converted to block grants for states, further accelerating the change while reducing the federal role to one of advisement and technical assistance (Sharfstein 2000).

Hospital-Based Outpatient Services

As provision of care came under attention, it was clear that ambulatory services needed to be delivered in a variety of settings to help meet the growing needs of populations. Hospital-based outpatient settings provide one such opportunity for care in close-to-community settings (Cournos and LeMelle 2009). These settings vary depending on whether they are established in general medical hospitals or specialty psychiatric facilities. Hospital-based clinics further vary based on the available community resources, the hospital's primary mission, and the host institution's majority funding source. Broadly, these clinical services are integrated into a hospital; therefore, hospital-based clinics are better suited to offer high-quality, seamless coordinated care. To meet patient care needs, hospital-based outpatient clinics offer programs closely aligned with other hospital programs, often utilizing cross-coverage of staff. Since hospitals and health systems are well organized to provide support with fiscal management, legal framework, centralized recruitment of staff, and regulatory requirements, hospital-based outpatient programs are generally well situated to take advantage of these preexisting systems (Cournos and LeMelle 2009). These programs often provide all levels of outpatient care, while some hospital-based clinics may offer only the ones more appropriate to their local needs. Hospital-based outpatient services can be organized in any number of ways, one of which is by levels of care.

Levels of Care

Scheduled Outpatient Assessments and Follow-Up

Generally, patients who are relatively stable and higher functioning and can benefit from less intense interventions utilize regularly scheduled appointments in an outpatient program. Patients are typically assigned a therapist and a medication provider, who in most cases is a psychiatrist but, depending upon applicable local state regulations, can also be an advanced practice practitioner (Blackwell and Neff 2015; Hudspeth and Klein 2019). Ideally, medication providers are also able to carry a caseload of patients for combined medication management and psychotherapy. Similarly, therapists also assume case management roles for a number of their patients. Given the case complexity and psychosocial needs of the patient panel, this clinical model can also include a separate case manager. In addition to administrative support staff, staff may include medical assistants and nurses to help facilitate care for complex cases needing ongoing care coordination.

Case Management

In an effort to improve overall health outcomes, hospitals and other stakeholders are increasingly acknowledging the role of social, economic, and environmental factors that influence health (Shim and Compton 2018). Taken together as social determinants of health, these include factors like socioeconomic status, education, physical environment, social support networks, employment, and access to health care (Allen et al. 2014; Forchuk et al. 2016). Case management services help patients address social determinants of health impacting their individual-level health outcomes (Dieterich et al. 2017; Kahan et al. 2016; Leutwyler et al. 2017). Typically, case management services include baseline assessment, planning, and coordination of services to help meet an individual's specific needs. Hospital-based outpatient case management services provide assistance with general health care needs, transportation, school or work, food security, and housing (Dieterich et al. 2017; Kahan et al. 2016). Since hospitals care for patients from all walks of life and a significant number of these patients may have social determinants negatively impacting their clinical outcomes, case management services should be an integral part of any outpatient service.

Walk-in Assessments and Follow-Up

For a variety of psychosocial and clinical reasons, some patients are not able to take advantage of regularly scheduled appointments, leading to a high no-show and cancellation rate. This leads to treatment disruption and potential worsening of clinical conditions. Clinics also miss an opportunity to utilize a high-value resource in the form of non-utilized clinical time. Walk-in clinical appointments offer an opportunity to maintain such patients in regular clinical care (Cullen 2018; Kroll et al. 2016, 2019). These appointments can be staffed by clinical therapists and medication providers rotating from a bigger outpatient pool, thereby helping improve patient adherence and retention for ongoing treatment while also providing a balanced clinical exposure, limiting chances of clinician burnout.

Same-Day Crisis Clinics

Hospital-based outpatient clinics also serve as point of entry for patients who may be in crisis but not necessarily needing inpatient care. Same-day crisis clinics offer an opportunity to conduct psychiatric evaluation and connect patients to appropriate resources, including ongoing care. These clinics are uniquely situated to provide immediate psychiatric triage. Generally, those receiving services from same-day crisis clinics are otherwise medically stable, are free of drug intoxication, and are able to wait safely for an evaluation in an outpatient clinic setting. These clinics are generally not equipped to manage highly unstable conditions more appropriate for an emergency room setting. Psychiatrists, advanced practice practitioners, and licensed therapists generally staff these clinics. Nursing staff and clinic administrators help with care coordination and securing disposition for ongoing care.

Intensive Outpatient Programs

Intensive outpatient programs (IOPs) offer a combination of group treatments and individual consultations for an average of 3–5 days a week. An IOP is generally considered an intermediate level of outpatient care, offering a step-down level of care for patients transitioning from an inpatient or residential facility, as well as a step-up level of care for patients requiring more than the traditional outpatient treatment setting. An IOP may also serve as an entry point for patients with specific mental health and substance use disorders. Groups are generally organized around diagnostic and therapeutic focus (Breland et al. 2016; Cook et al. 2014; Kennard et al. 2019; Shaffer et al. 2019). For example, a general mental health IOP may be structured to address general needs of the patients in groups, such as psychoeducation, medication management, and skills training, while a mental health IOP organized for patients with high-risk self-injurious behaviors may include groups emphasizing dialectical behavior therapy (DBT). Similarly, an IOP focusing on substance use disorders may include groups emphasizing psychoeducation, motivation to change, treatment engagement, early recovery, and maintenance toward transition to outpatient treatment.

Partial Hospital Programs

Partial hospital programs (PHPs) or day treatment programs have clinical activities that generally run 5 days per week. The value of PHPs in the care continuum is well established in various settings and for a wide variety of clinical conditions (Brown et al. 2018; Lande and Pourzand 2016). These clinical programs offer step-up opportunities for patients who need more intensive treatment than other general outpatient treatment programs or an IOP. A PHP also offers step-down options for patients who are in the process of stabilization after an acute crisis right after inpatient psychiatric hospitalization. These programs offer flexibility, and patients can stay in the program for a duration considered clinically appropriate while attending activities consistent with their treatment plan. PHPs offer a good balance of autonomy and a structured environment, thereby providing a valuable option for patients who may still not be at their baseline functioning and need more support with gradual tapering toward an outpatient discharge. PHPs also offer a mix of individual consultation and group programming to patients. Typically, group treatments include psychoeducation, social skills training, dialectical behavior skills, medication management, and, in some instances, a vocational skills group. Individual consultation time is utilized for specific medication management as well as individual therapy and case management on an as-needed basis. Since these programs are geared toward rehabilitation, PHPs are staffed at a higher staff-to-patient ratio (Cournos and LeMelle 2009) compared with IOPs. Typically, the PHP staff consists of psychiatrists, psychiatric nurse practitioners, mental health workers, registered nurses, psychologists, and licensed therapists. In general, patients referred to a PHP should be able to maintain their safety in the community. Further, patients should be motivated to attend group therapy, be able to attend regularly, and be stable from any acute medical and psychiatric perspective in order to engage in and benefit from therapeutic interventions. Achievable, attainable, and time-limited treatment goals need to be identified at the time of admission to a PHP. For patients with chronic conditions in need of longer-term supportive care, other treatment programs, such as rehabilitation programs, should be considered. For patients with personality disorders, day treatment settings can be particularly helpful due to the intensive, structured, and group-oriented approach.

Integration With Other Hospital Programs

When patients enter treatment, it is pertinent that the level be appropriate to their needs, with provisions for more intense step-up and less intense step-down services available. For care to be effectively integrated across different levels of severity, transfer of patients must account for efficient transfer of health records along with adherence to relatively similar treatment goals (Cournos and LeMelle 2009). For example, if the goal is to keep patients in an outpatient setting where they are able to participate in their daily life with minimal disruption to routines, all hospital care environments, such as emergency settings and inpatient units, should work systematically together coordinating care and helping patients move through each transition point. Hospital-based settings provide unique opportunities for effective care coordination, especially for those suffering from severe and persistent mental illness. In addition to more intense residential and inpatient settings, hospital-based outpatient programs can offer typical individual and group management settings along with step-up options such as relatively regular care in an IOP or PHP. This care continuum offers a platform where recovery-oriented approaches can be implemented. For example, during the more subacute phase of illness, patients can engage in combined individual and group treatments, including regular medication management and psychotherapeutics in IOP or PHP settings. Treatment can then be tapered to regular individual sessions appropriate to response.

The patient population primarily served by the hospital also impacts the delivery-of-care continuum. For example, patients with severe and persistent mental illness are often in programs funded primarily by Medicare and Medicaid, because hospitals rely on these funding mechanisms. Many outpatient programs focus on this population to help alleviate the disease burden by interlinking broader community services. Further, specialty programs such as those that provide care for children with intellectual developmental disorder and elderly persons with dementia often benefit from closely aligned inpatient and outpatient services. These specialty programs are often staffed by the same clinicians in split-day fashion, thereby enhancing the the quality of the care continuum. Some of these care continua may also include community settings such as schools and patient homes, and although labor intensive, this offers an opportunity to keep patients closer to settings that offer optimal psychosocial functioning.

Patients with acute and serious psychiatric illness often present in emergency psychiatric settings, requiring timely screening and evaluation. Hospital-based outpatient programs rely on these settings as an avenue for patients in crisis as well as for after-hours crisis care. In integrated health care systems, these settings are often located in the emergency department, while other systems rely on stand-alone crisis centers or integrated crisis walk-in clinics. When patients need inpatient psychiatric hospitalization from these emergency settings, some systems are able to offer beds, whereas others may have to refer out. Final disposition for the day is also often impacted by bed availability as well as patients' insurance coverage. At times, in-network options for patients to receive care might be at a different site from where the patient initially presented for emergency psychiatric needs. Since these decisions are primarily driven by insurance coverage, outpatient settings may not be able to control the final disposition-related outcomes; hence, it is pertinent to ensure that handoffs are attended to not only at the point of admission but also at discharge. This again underscores the importance of hospital-based outpatient programs working actively and coordinating care with local emergency departments and inpatient psychiatric units. Since during acute psychiatric crises a patient may have difficulty reporting important treatment history and psychosocial factors pertinent to their active management, it is generally advantageous to keep patients in one continuum of care (Cournos and LeMelle 2009). In all other scenarios, care must be taken that appropriate medical records follow the patient. Because outpatient treatment teams are most likely to have consistent contact with patients through their life span, every effort should be made to coordinate care while the patient is admitted. The input, especially about the patient's normal baseline, can be of great value to the inpatient psychiatric team. This kind of coordination not only helps stabilize the acute episode but also can go a long way in improving long-term outcomes and adherence to treatment protocols. Lack of coordination can lead to conflicting treatment goals and confusion for patients.

Residential and Housing Support

Though a typical outpatient program does not cater to housing and residential program needs, with the movement away from long-term hospitalization, hospitals and states have increasingly invested in housing options to help mitigate this gap for individuals with severe and persistent mental illness. Stable housing is a key factor leading to improved overall quality of life and clinical outcomes. Housing programs have been shown to decrease homelessness and readmissions. These programs can be organized to take care of specific clinical populations and may also have provisions to provide respite care for those who care for these patients. One such program, Crisis Residential, can be organized in a short-term framework for individuals having a mental health crisis to help avoid hospitalization (Fenton et al. 2002; Stroul and Goldman 1990). Crisis beds also help decrease the length of stay by allowing patients to transition from inpatient facilities to community-based care in a seamless fashion. Given the relatively intense clinical presentation, crisis residential services are operated by highly trained staff, with provisions for round-the-clock support, supervision, and clinical consultation as applicable. Patients in these programs are connected with their community support systems, including community providers, to aid gradual transition back to daily routines. Residential rehabilitation services offer individuals with severe and persistent mental illness housing assistance and coordinated support services (Jain et al. 2016; Meehan et al. 2017). These programs are unique in providing employment support and educational opportunities along with ongoing treatment for psychiatric disorders. Such services, given their comprehensive and integrated nature, help reduce the overall risk of homelessness while fostering community integration.

Diversity

It is pertinent that outpatient programs cater to the needs of increasingly diverse populations. Clinicians and support staff need to be sensitive to the cultural background of the patients they serve. Cultural background influences mental health by impacting an individual's understanding of health and illness as well as health-seeking behaviors (Soto et al. 2018; Watt et al. 2016). Similarly, the treatment team's attitudes toward patients from a different cultural background also directly impact health outcomes. Health and illness are perceived differently among individuals from different cultural backgrounds; therefore, cultural background directly impacts an individual's motivation to seek professional help. While some individuals may rely on their community support network in times of crisis, others may simply not seek help, considering a mental health crisis to be a personal failure. Stigma can also play a key role by influencing treatment-seeking behaviors. Stigma can cause individuals to feel ashamed of their symptoms to the point that they hide them and do not seek treatment until an acute crisis manifests; hence, staff must be adequately trained to address these issues (Corral et al. 2017; Mills et al. 2016). Language barriers can also directly impact treatment outcomes by negatively influencing development of a therapeutic alliance. A patient's primary language must also be considered in delivery of care. Since all programs at some point provide care to those who speak languages other than English, depending on the location of a clinical program and the population mix, hospital-based outpatient programs should invest in training and recruitment of diverse staff along with investing in on-site and off-site synchronous language interpretation services (Jacobs et al. 2018; Karliner et al. 2007).

Hospital-Based Virtual Care

Traditionally, outpatient psychiatric care has primarily been offered in resource-intensive in-person settings. Though such settings are valuable and in many cases clinically necessary, restriction of outpatient care to brick-and-mortar settings limits access for patients who may live far away. This is especially the case for rural areas, but patients in urban parts of the country with poor access to mental health care due to provider shortages are also impacted. Virtual care enables provision of health care from a distance utilizing technology (Deslich et al. 2013; Hilty et al. 2018). With recent advances, delivery of virtual care can be both synchronous and asynchronous. Synchronous care often utilizes videoconferencing, typically under the realm of telepsychiatry, with services that can include psychiatric evaluations, ongoing medication management, and group as well as individual psychotherapy. While synchronous care provides an opportunity for patients to ask questions and provide valuable updates to the treatment team, asynchronous care allows clinicians to utilize their time in a much more effective manner by addressing these clinical concerns on an ongoing basis during nonclinical administrative time instead of investing valuable face-to-face clinical time addressing nonurgent concerns (Dixon and Rao 2014).

Since hospital-based outpatient programs are centrally located, they offer a unique opportunity to serve as virtual care hubs for a variety of telepsychiatry services. These settings also offer recruitment centralization and support staff services, which free up resources that can then be utilized to reach patients in their homes or at distant clinical sites. There are several advantages to using virtual care and delivery of psychiatric services. First, virtual care helps improve access to psychiatric care that might not otherwise be available. Second, since care is delivered closer to a patient's primary location, virtual care is relatively less disruptive to an individual's daily life. Third, it helps improve continuity of care by providing opportunities for ongoing follow-up with relative ease. Lastly, virtual care presents additional opportunities for care integration with primary care clinics as well as in settings such as schools and correctional facilities (Deslich et al. 2013).

Despite all these advantages, crossover from in-person care to virtual care has its own challenges. For many patients as well as providers, the technology interface presents a challenge, leading to slower adaptation. Since patients are at a distant site, safety-related concerns also limit application in some instances. Licensure requirements and insurance reimbursement pose potential roadblocks as well. Providers must be licensed in states where the patients are located. Further, since the patient is not at the hospital-based clinic site, these programs may not collect facility fees and have to primarily rely on professional fees for services. Notwithstanding some of these disadvantages, virtual care has the potential to link hospital-based clinicians to patients at distant sites and in settings such as primary care, schools, emergency rooms, correctional facilities, and other specialty clinics, thereby improving access at a fraction of the cost compared with what would be a significant investment in recruitment and retention of clinical teams in all these settings.

Despite all the resources and availability of programs, at times, because of the nature of psychiatric illness, patients may benefit from additional provisions to help ensure access to much needed services. Outpatient civil commitment is one such recourse that providers and hospital-based outpatient teams need to be aware of.

Outpatient Civil Commitment

Outpatient civil commitment (OCC), sometimes called *assisted outpatient treatment*, is a legal intervention designed to benefit people with severe mental illness who need ongoing psychiatric treatment, rehabilitation, and community supports to prevent hospital readmission and re-incarceration, as a mechanism for community safety, and to prevent homelessness. From a legal perspective, outpatient commitment represents an extension of states' civil commitment authority into the community. Conceptually, a community treatment order commits the patient to a treatment plan, but more importantly it commits the mental health authority to serving the high-need patient, as a priority, creating an extra layer of system accountability (Substance Abuse and Mental Health Services Administration 2019).

At present, 47 states utilize a legal structure to allow some form of outpatient commitment. There is enormous variability in state and local jurisdictions' OCC laws and their actual implementation (Substance Abuse and Mental Health Services Administration 2019). As a practical matter, outpatient commitment laws have sometimes been used to leverage or prioritize outreach and often-scarce intensive community-based services to individuals who are difficult to engage in treatment, just as inpatient commitment laws have been used to prioritize access to beds for those who may be acutely ill. In addition to OCC, the following three court-directed alternatives are also often applicable:

1. *Conditional release*, where release from an inpatient facility is subject to the right of the hospital to return the patient to inpatient care. The patient is under direct su-

pervision of the hospital during this time. Conditional releases are usually limited to previously hospitalized, involuntarily committed patients or patients who have been adjudicated by the justice system.

2. *Guardianship*, a legal procedure in which the court determines if a person's ability to make health and safety decisions for themselves is significantly diminished. In most cases, the court appoints a guardian to act as a substitute decision-maker.
3. *Psychiatric advance directive*, a legal tool that allows a person with a mental illness to state prior to an onset of a mental crisis a plan for treatment. A psychiatric advance directive can serve as a legal and clinical mechanism to preserve and protect an individual's right to choose their specific course of treatment (Appelbaum 2004).

OCC is intended for adults diagnosed with a serious mental illness who are unlikely to live safely in the community without supervision and treatment and are less likely to voluntarily participate in treatment. The goal is to improve access and adherence to intensive behavioral health services in order to avert relapse, repeated hospitalizations, arrest, incarceration, suicide, property destruction, and violent behaviors. A wide range of services can be included in the treatment plan, such as case management, medication management, individual or group therapy, psychiatric rehabilitation, day programs, consumer-run drop-in centers, substance abuse testing and services, housing or housing support services, and urine or blood toxicology (to ensure adherence to medication). In many states, no court order goes into effect unless a treatment plan has been submitted to the court. The length of the court order can vary by individual. Typically, court orders may not last longer than 6 months unless they are renewed by the court (Substance Abuse and Mental Health Services Administration 2019). When the court order expires and it is not renewed, individuals continue receiving voluntary services. Noncompliance can lead to a temporary hold to evaluate for involuntary hospitalization.

Hospital-Based Care Teams

Typically, outpatient care has been delivered in 1:1 settings utilizing physician and licensed therapist time for the majority of care. Though valuable, this model tends not to be cost-effective and also limits access to patients desperately in need of care. Since hospitals cater to patients who tend to be complex, and since they also have access to wide array of clinical and nonclinical support staff, hospital-based outpatient programs offer an opportunity for innovation in delivery of care. Here we present a few scenarios to illustrate this further.

Team-Based Care for Treatment-Resistant Depression

Case Vignette

A 22-year-old was diagnosed with major depression 2 years ago. At the time of his initial presentation, the patient reported severe hopelessness, anhedonia, lack of sleep, and poor appetite. He also reported feeling guilty about letting his parents down by dropping out of college. Since then, the patient has made three separate suicide attempts, each leading to inpatient psychiatric hospitalization. Even after adhering to adequately dosed medications for an appropriate duration, the patient has not responded to three different antidepressants. He continues to report hopelessness and passive suicidal thoughts.

Patients who have undergone multiple failed trials of medication and therapy often struggle to establish care where they can access state-of-the-art therapeutic modalities. Further, since such expertise is not widely available in community settings, patients often suffer from ongoing symptoms and suboptimal functioning, leading to frequent relapses and readmissions. A hospital-based treatment team approach offers an opportunity to deliver care to such a highly complex patient panel.

Intakes

Since patients with treatment-resistant depression may be accessing care in community settings or in an acute care psychiatric setting, these teams can potentially serve as a step-up option for patients already in community care or as a step-down from an inpatient psychiatric unit. Patients can be referred from these settings to a central intake office. Licensed clinicians, preferably therapists, complete the intake by obtaining useful medical and psychosocial history. Some of these patients may come from community settings where their current providers may simply be seeking expert consultation or a second opinion. In such cases, after the intake, the team psychiatrist can complete second opinion consultations and refer the patient back to the community setting with treatment recommendations. In other cases, there may be a need to provide ongoing care to these patients until they are stabilized and reintegrated into community settings. For these patients, the treatment-resistant-depression treatment team provides an opportunity where patients can be closely monitored and treated utilizing best available therapeutic options.

Management

Since patients may have failed to respond to previous trials of first- and second-line medications, a treatment-resistant-depression team must offer expert psychopharmacology as well as have provisions for evidence-based psychotherapy and interventions such as brain stimulation. Hospital settings already have access to milieus where medically complex patients can be managed in a safe and effective manner. A hospital-based outpatient treatment-resistant-depression team is uniquely positioned to monitor patients receiving complex psychopharmacology such as ketamine and esketamine. Further, staffing resources such as pharmacy and nursing support can be colocated to offer brain stimulation services such as electroconvulsive therapy, vagal nerve stimulation, and repetitive transcranial magnetic stimulation in addition to specialty pharmacological options.

Clinical Programming

In a treatment-resistant-depression team, clinical and nonclinical staff closely coordinate ongoing care of a complex patient panel. Expert physicians are primarily responsible for providing ongoing consultation to the direct care teams. Beyond initial consultation, they may also offer ongoing evaluations to patients who may not be responding to treatment. Consultations are best handled in a treatment team setting for group cohesion and advancement of knowledge related to therapeutic principles. Team settings also help improve the competence of all clinical and nonclinical staff while providing an opportunity for ongoing supervision. Since the team is handling a panel of patients with fairly complex presentations, these teams also provide an opportunity for ongoing support to the members. Direct care can be handled in an individual as well as group setting. Individual monitoring can be handled by advanced practice practitioners and licensed therapists. Clinical pharmacists can play an important role by providing psychoeducation and medication monitoring groups (Tallian et al. 2012; Tewksbury et al. 2018). Since patients are likely to also have case management needs, licensed social workers can serve the dual role of therapist and case manager. Nursing staff can assist with clinical tasks such as medication reconciliation and ongoing monitoring of vitals, including primarily staffing the observation period required for specific therapeutic agents such as esketamine.

Once the course of treatment is completed, the majority of the patients can be referred back to the primary clinical setting, while some patients may continue to access maintenance treatment in close collaboration with their primary treating psychiatrist.

Clozapine and Long-Acting Injection Clinics for Psychotic Disorders

Vignette

A clinic completed chart reviews as a quality assurance measure on patients receiving care for schizophrenia. This retrospective chart review revealed about 40% of the patients were receiving first-generation antipsychotic medications, while the rest were receiving second-generation antipsychotics. Only 30% of the patients receiving second-generation antipsychotics had baseline glucose and lipid profile reviewed prior to the initiation of the medication, while 25% of the charts revealed movement monitoring in the previous year. This exercise also revealed that even after poor response to an adequate dose trial of two to three antipsychotic medications, only 15% of patients were considered for clozapine treatment. Readmission rates were also found to be high.

Severely and persistently ill patients primarily suffering from psychotic disorders often need long-term treatment with antipsychotic medications. Additionally, because of clinical factors such as treatment failure and psychosocial factors impacting adherence, many need therapeutic options such as long-acting injectable medication or clozapine and ongoing monitoring. Hospital-based high-fidelity psychotic disorders programs can help meet the needs of these patients. Just as with a treatment-resistant-depression team, a psychotic disorders program can benefit from close coordination with inpatient units and outpatient providers. Most outpatient programs do not have resources to adequately manage and monitor patients with brittle psychotic disorders. Since hospital-based outpatient clinics have the advantage of centralized resources such as clinical pharmacy and nursing, these clinics are better suited to provide ongoing care for patients needing long-acting injectable medications and clozapine.

Clinical pharmacists collaboratively working with physicians and advanced practice practitioners can primarily staff clozapine and injection clinic appointments. Patients can be referred to such a program both from the inpatient setting and from outpatient settings. For clozapine, patients who have treatment-resistant schizophrenia, medication-induced tardive dyskinesia, or Parkinson's disease, or who exhibit suicidal behaviors with schizophrenia or schizoaffective disorders, can participate in group medication management settings with provision for simultaneous individual care on an as-needed basis. Clinical therapists can also run psychoeducation groups for patients as well as family psychoeducation groups. Because hospitals have on-site labs or collection agreements with off-site labs, these programs can run to coincide with the lab collection schedule to help facilitate ongoing absolute neutrophil count monitoring as required by clozapine treatment guidelines as well as testing indicated for metabolic screening. Patients receiving long-acting injectable medications can also benefit from a similarly structured program. In both instances, given the availability of nursing staff, clinical pharmacy, and a lab, patients can be closely monitored for metabolic side effects as well as movement disorders, thereby improving adherence, leading to improved clinical outcomes and overall quality of life. For the hospitals, these outpatient programs help to improve outcomes by increasing monitoring of patients receiving medications with serious side effects, improving care coordination with primary care, improving access to care by shifting care from resource-intensive individual models to clinically effective group treatment models, and, finally, improving the capacity to manage complex patients in an outpatient level of care, reducing readmissions and overreliance on inpatient psychiatric treatment.

Comprehensive Team-Based Dialectical Behavior Therapy

Case Vignette

A 30-year-old patient suffers from chronic emotional dysregulation, and during times of acute crisis, the patient experiences extreme mood swings and thoughts of self-harm. He frequently engages in self-injurious behavior as a way to "cope with pain." The patient has been admitted to an inpatient psychiatric facility multiple times in his life span. He receives outpatient care in a private practice clinic, where he sees a psychiatrist for medication management and a therapist for ongoing supportive psychotherapy. The clinic is unable to manage the patient's long-standing self-injurious behaviors, which lead to frequent emergency room visits and ultimately result in inpatient psychiatric admission.

Patients who suffer from mood dysregulation and exhibit chronic suicidal and nonsuicidal self-injurious behaviors often present to emergency room settings. Because of their safety risk, these patients often get admitted for inpatient psychiatric care. Given the chronic nature of their presentation, a short-term hospital stay on its own does not necessarily change the prognosis for a majority of these patients. Hospital-based outpatient clinics are situated right at the interface of emergency crisis settings and inpatient psychiatric units; hence, they present an ideal setting for ongoing management of patients with chronic risk to self. DBT is an evidence-based modality for the treatment of individuals with chronic risk to self, such as in borderline personality disorder. The treatment involves individual as well as group therapy sessions. Given the high-stakes nature of this clinical population, along with after-hours need for crisis support, a group of trained therapists participates in these programs. Ideally, the program should also have access to an on-site medical provider to help address any medication-related needs. Since the treatment team is actively involved in patient care and provides ongoing crisis support, this program is highly valuable in reducing clinical morbidity and improving psychosocial functioning. Patients participating in comprehensive DBT are more likely to stay in community settings and are at a lower risk for readmissions.

Peer Support Services

Peer support workers are individuals who have been impacted by mental illness or substance use disorders and are further along in their individual recovery. Given the unique shared experience, peers are uniquely situated to help others experiencing similar problems. Peers bring hope to those struggling and help remove stigma associated with mental illness. With the help of a shared understanding and trust, peer support workers help drive engagement in treatment, thereby reducing the risk of relapse or clinical worsening. Peers are involved with advocacy, skill development, leading supportive interventions, resource development, education, mentoring, and goal setting, and play a role in administration of programs. Many states have outlined requirements to become peer support specialists; generally, a high school diploma or GED is required in addition to specific numbers of hours of volunteer work and training (Center for Substance Abuse Treatment 2009).

Future Directions

As hospitals and health systems adapt to the changing health care landscape, hospital-based ambulatory settings are likely to play an ever-increasing important role. Patients, families, employers, and insurance carriers are all advocating transition from a fee-for-service to a value-based care model. An emphasis on cost reduction and delivery of quality outcomes is facilitating the move of health care delivery to outpatient settings across health care, and mental health is not an exception. With the advent of efficacious treatments and increasing awareness related to the negative impact of untreated mental illness, more and more individuals are in psychiatric care while maintaining optimal psychosocial functioning. Taken together, these factors are expediting the transition of mental health care delivery to hospital-based and community outpatient settings. As technology advances, evolving into a user-friendly health care interface, the outward movement of health care from hospitals to patient homes is only expected to be realized in the near future. This, however, should not mean that all health care will move away from hospitals. Some patients, such as those with certain complex clinical disorders, will continue to be treated in tertiary care settings; however, the share of outpatient care in the overall health enterprise is only expected to grow.

Conclusion

Hospital-based outpatient services continue to play an important role in the care continuum for patients with mental illness. These services are uniquely situated to cater to the needs of patients being discharged from inpatient psychiatric facilities as well as those who seek care during a crisis. With their integrated patient services along with access to well-trained staff, hospital-based outpatient services are uniquely positioned to provide team-based care for highly complex conditions as well as function as a hub for services to patients at distant sites.

References

Allen J, Balfour R, Bell R, Marmot M: Social determinants of mental health. Int Rev Psychiatry 26(4):392–407, 2014

Appelbaum PS: Law and psychiatry: psychiatric advance directives and the treatment of committed patients. Psychiatr Serv 55(7):751–752, 763, 2004 15232012

Blackwell CW, Neff DF: Certification and education as determinants of nurse practitioner scope of practice: an investigation of the rules and regulations defining NP scope of practice in the United States. J Am Assoc Nurse Pract 27(10):552–557, 2015 25939736

Bloche MG, Cournos F: Mental health policy for the 1990s: tinkering in the interstices. J Health Polit Policy Law 15(2):387–411, 1990 2212530

Breland JY, Asch SM, Slightam C, et al: Key ingredients for implementing intensive outpatient programs within patient-centered medical homes: a literature review and qualitative analysis. Healthc (Amst) 4(1):22–29, 2016 27001095

Brown TA, Cusack A, Anderson LK, et al: Efficacy of a partial hospital programme for adults with eating disorders. Eur Eat Disord Rev 26(3):241–252, 2018 29542211

Center for Substance Abuse Treatment: What Are Peer Recovery Support Services? (HHS Publ No SMA 09-4454). Rockville, MD, Substance Abuse and Mental Health Services Administration, U.S. Department of Health and Human Services, 2009

Cook MN, Crisostomo PS, Simpson TS, et al: Effectiveness of an intensive outpatient program for disruptive children: initial findings. Community Ment Health J 50(2):164–171, 2014 23299227

Corral I, Johnson TL, Shelton PG, Glass O: Psychiatry resident training in cultural competence: an educator's toolkit. Psychiatr Q 88(2):295–306, 2017 27815802

Cournos F, LeMelle S: Outpatient community mental health services, in Textbook of Hospital Psychiatry. Edited by Sharfstein SS, Dickerson FB, Oldham JM. Washington, DC, American Psychiatric Publishing, 2009, pp 327–338

Cullen BA: Altering the attendance rate successfully for new patients at an outpatient mental health clinic. Psychiatr Serv 69(12):1212–1214, 2018 30152272

Deslich SA, Thistlethwaite T, Coustasse A: Telepsychiatry in correctional facilities: using technology to improve access and decrease costs of mental health care in underserved populations. Perm J 17(3):80–86, 2013 24355894

Dieterich M, Irving CB, Bergman H, et al: Intensive case management for severe mental illness. Schizophr Bull 43(4):698–700, 2017 20927766

Dixon RF, Rao L: Asynchronous virtual visits for the follow-up of chronic conditions. Telemed J E Health 20(7):669–672, 2014

Fenton WS, Hoch JS, Herrell JM, et al: Cost and cost-effectiveness of hospital vs residential crisis care for patients who have serious mental illness. Arch Gen Psychiatry 59(4):357–364, 2002 11926936

Forchuk C, Dickins K, Corring DJ: Social determinants of health: housing and income. Healthc Q 18(spec no):27–31, 2016 26854545

Hilty DM, Sunderji N, Suo S, et al: Telepsychiatry and other technologies for integrated care: evidence base, best practice models and competencies. Int Rev Psychiatry 30(6):292–309, 2018 30821540

Hudspeth RS, Klein TA: Understanding nurse practitioner scope of practice: regulatory, practice, and employment perspectives now and for the future. J Am Assoc Nurse Pract 31(8):468–473, 2019 31348141

Jacobs B, Ryan AM, Henrichs KS, Weiss BD: Medical interpreters in outpatient practice. Ann Fam Med 16(1):70–76, 2018 29311179

Jain S, McLean C, Adler EP, Rosen CS: Peer support and outcome for veterans with posttraumatic stress disorder (PTSD) in a residential rehabilitation program. Community Ment Health J 52(8):1089–1092, 2016 26839108

Kahan D, Poremski D, Wise-Harris D, et al: Perceived case management needs and service preferences of frequent emergency department users: lessons learned in a large urban centre. PLoS One 11(12):e0168782, 2016 28002491

Karliner LS, Jacobs EA, Chen AH, Mutha S: Do professional interpreters improve clinical care for patients with limited English proficiency? A systematic review of the literature. Health Serv Res 42(2):727–754, 2007 17362215

Kennard B, Mayes T, King J, et al: The development and feasibility outcomes of a youth suicide prevention intensive outpatient program. J Adolesc Health 64(3):362–369, 2019 30502117

Kroll DS, Chakravartti A, Gasparrini K, et al: The walk-in clinic model improves access to psychiatry in primary care. J Psychosom Res 89:11–15, 2016 27663104

Kroll DS, Wrenn K, Grimaldi JA, et al: Longitudinal urgent care psychiatry as a unique access point for underserved patients. Psychiatr Serv 70(9):837–839, 2019 31084294

Lande RG, Pourzand M: Components and characteristics of a psychiatric partial hospital military program. Mil Med 181(3):213–218, 2016 26926745

Leutwyler H, Hubbard E, Zahnd E: Case management helps prevent criminal justice recidivism for people with serious mental illness. Int J Prison Health 13(3–4):168–172, 2017 28914124

Meehan T, Stedman T, Parker S, et al: Comparing clinical and demographic characteristics of people with mental illness in hospital- and community-based residential rehabilitation units in Queensland. Aust Health Rev 41(2):139–143, 2017 27119964

Mills S, Wolitzky-Taylor K, Xiao AQ, et al: Training on the DSM-5 Cultural Formulation Interview improves cultural competence in general psychiatry residents: a multi-site study. Acad Psychiatry 40(5):829–834, 2016 27093964

Shaffer RC, Wink LK, Ruberg J, et al: Emotion regulation intensive outpatient programming: development, feasibility, and acceptability. J Autism Dev Disord 49(2):495–508, 2019 30143951

Sharfstein SS: Whatever happened to community mental health? Psychiatr Serv 51(5):616–620, 2000 10783179

Shim RS, Compton MT: Addressing the social determinants of mental health: If not now, when? If not us, who? Psychiatr Serv 69(8):844–846, 2018 29852822

Shore MF, Cohen MD: Providing treatment to persons with mental illness. Milbank Q 72(1):31–35, 1994 8164610

Soto A, Smith TB, Griner D, et al: Cultural adaptations and therapist multicultural competence: two meta-analytic reviews. J Clin Psychol 74(11):1907–1923, 2018 30091201

Stroul BA, Goldman SK: Study of community-based services for children and adolescents who are severely emotionally disturbed. J Ment Health Adm 17(1):61–77, 1990 10106571

Substance Abuse and Mental Health Services Administration: Civil Commitment and the Mental Health Care Continuum: Historical Trends and Principles for Law and Practice. Rockville, MD, Office of the Chief Medical Officer, Substance Abuse and Mental Health Services Administration, 2019

Talbott JA: Twentieth-century developments in American psychiatry. Psychiatr Q 54(4):207–219, 1982 7187509

Tallian KB, Hirsch JD, Kuo GM, et al: Development of a pharmacist-psychiatrist collaborative medication therapy management clinic. J Am Pharm Assoc (2003) 52(6):e252–e258, 2012 23229987

Tewksbury A, Bozymski KM, Ruekert L, et al: Development of collaborative drug therapy management and clinical pharmacy services in an outpatient psychiatric clinic. J Pharm Pract 31(3):272–278, 2018 28539104

Watt K, Abbott P, Reath J: Developing cultural competence in general practitioners: an integrative review of the literature. BMC Fam Pract 17(1):158, 2016 27846805

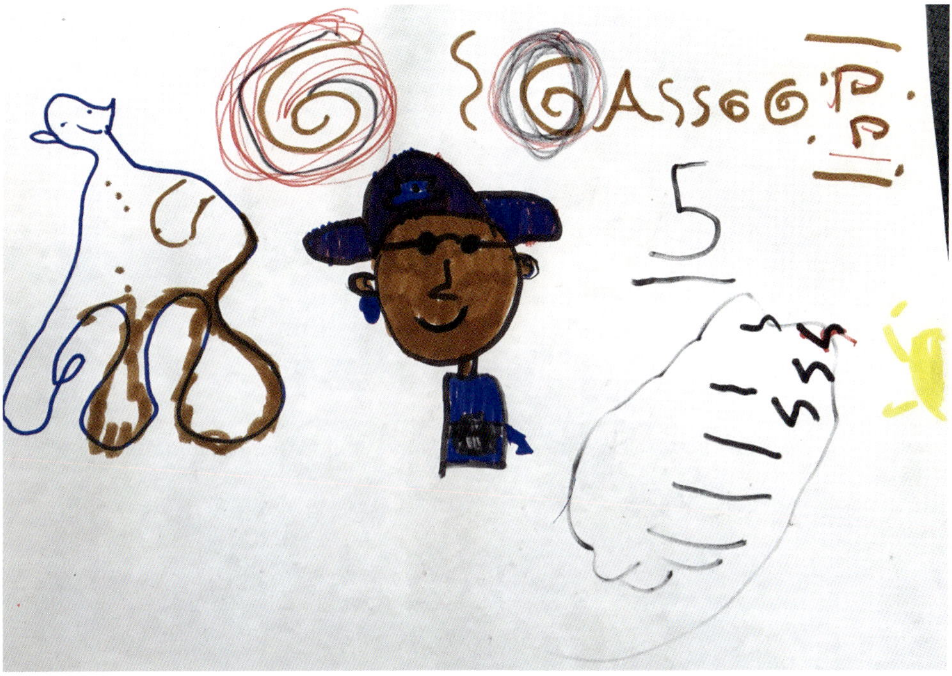

PLATE 1. *(Figure 2–1)* Picture drawn by Sam, an 8-year-old boy living in foster care after being removed from his mother's care for abuse and neglect.

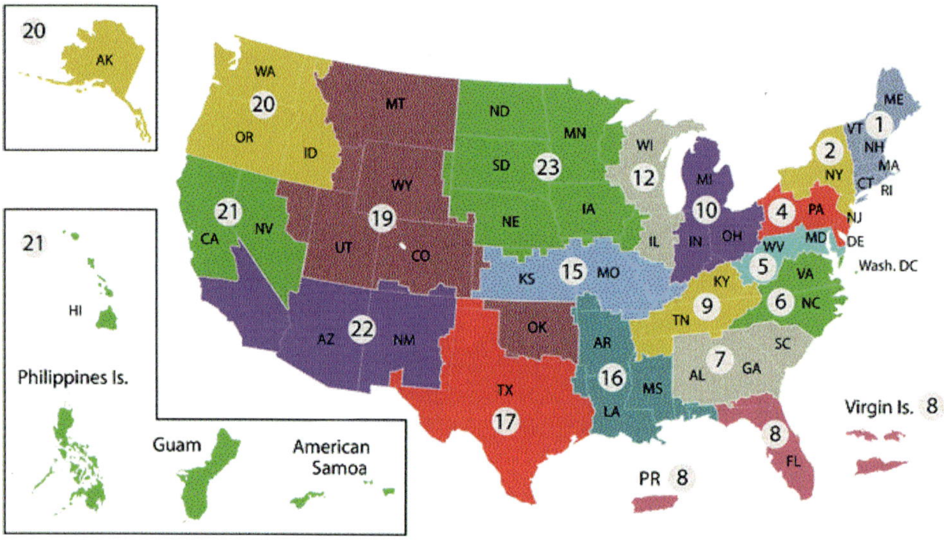

PLATE 2. *(Figure 12–1)* U.S. Department of Veterans Affairs Veterans Integrated Service Network (VISN) system, 2020.

Source. U.S. Department of Veterans Affairs 2021b. Facilities included in each VISN are available at this reference.

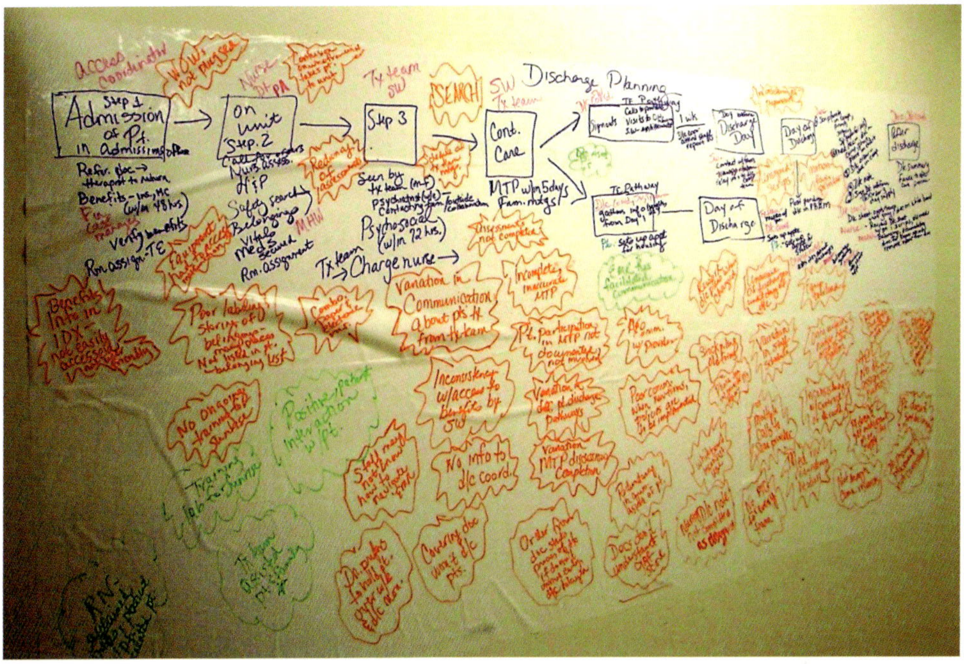

Plate 3. *(Figure 22–1)* Process map of the journey of a patient from admission to discharge.

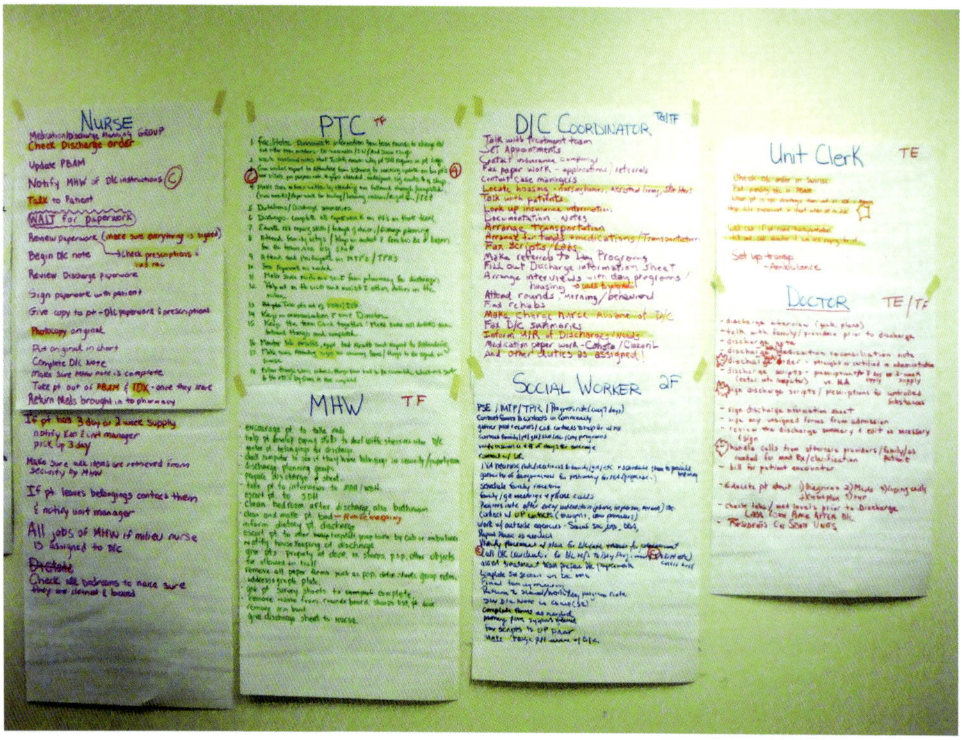
NURSE
Check Discharge order
Update PBAM
Talk to Patient
WAIT for paperwork
Review Discharge paperwork
Sign paperwork with patient
Photocopy original
Put original in chart
Complete D/C Note
Return Meds brought in to pharmacy
PTC
D/C COORDINATOR
Talk with treatment team
Set Appointments
Contact case managers
Look up insurance information
Documentation Notes
Arrange Transportation
Fax Scripts/Labs
Fill out Discharge information sheet
Attend rounds
Find rehabs
Fax D/C summaries
Unit Clerk
TE
Set up transp
DOCTOR
TE/TF
MHW
TF
SOCIAL WORKER
2F

PLATE 4. *(Figure 22–3)* Role clarification of various disciplines in order to reduce ambiguity and increase role clarity.

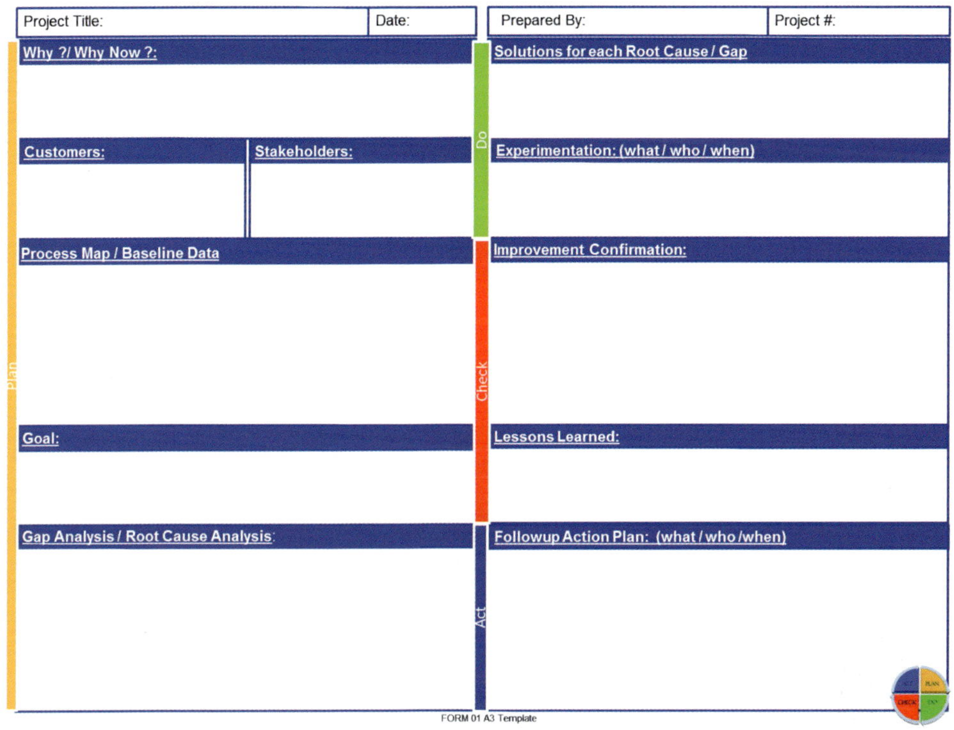

PLATE 5. *(Figure 22–4)* The standardized A3 template.

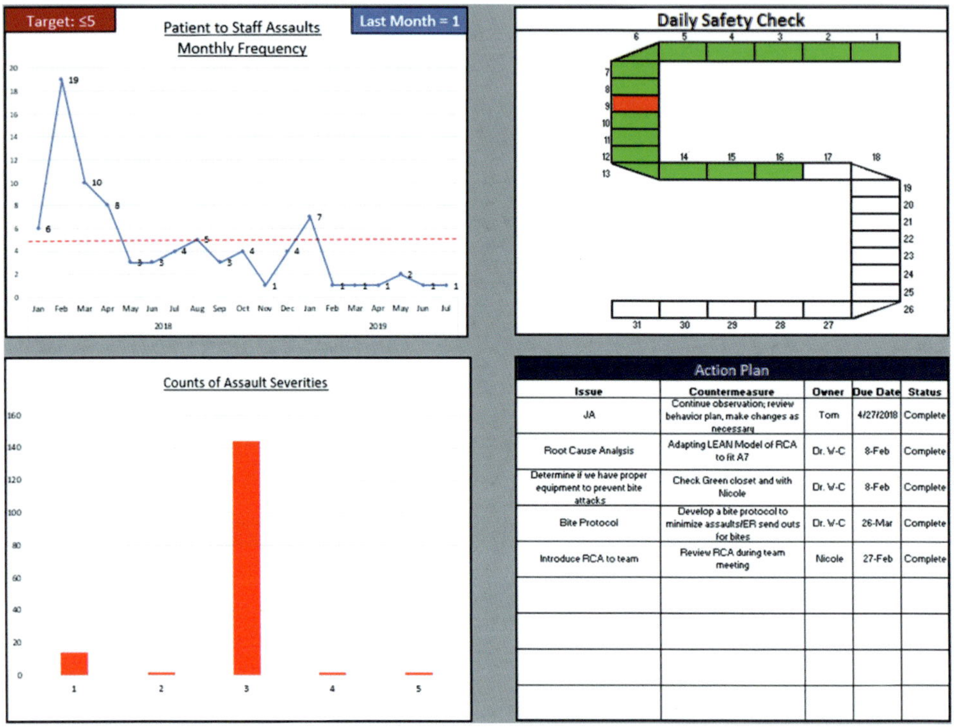

Target: ≤5
Patient to Staff Assaults Monthly Frequency
Last Month = 1
Jan Feb Mar Apr May Jun Jul Aug Sep Oct Nov Dec Jan Feb Mar Apr May Jun Jul
2018
2019
Daily Safety Check
Counts of Assault Severities
Action Plan
Issue | Countermeasure | Owner | Due Date | Status
JA | Continue observation; review behavior plan, make changes as necessary | Tom | 4/27/2018 | Complete
Root Cause Analysis | Adapting LEAN Model of RCA to fit A7 | Dr. W-C | 8-Feb | Complete
Determine if we have proper equipment to prevent bite attacks | Check Green closet and with Nicole | Dr. W-C | 8-Feb | Complete
Bite Protocol | Develop a bite protocol to minimize assaults/ER send outs for bites | Dr. W-C | 26-Mar | Complete
Introduce RCA to team | Review RCA during team meeting | Nicole | 27-Feb | Complete

PLATE 6. *(Figure 22–5)* The four-block daily huddle board.

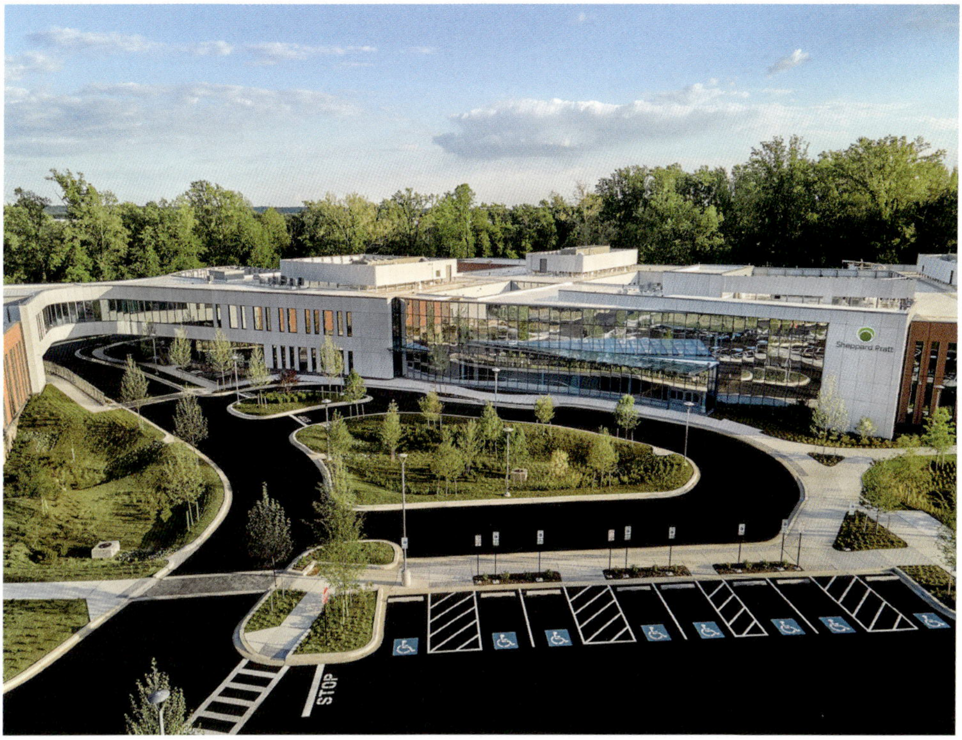

PLATE 7. *(Figure 23–1)* **Sheppard Pratt Baltimore/Washington campus.**
New state-of-the-art behavioral health facilities incorporate thoughtful design and set the standard for psychiatric and behavioral health care.

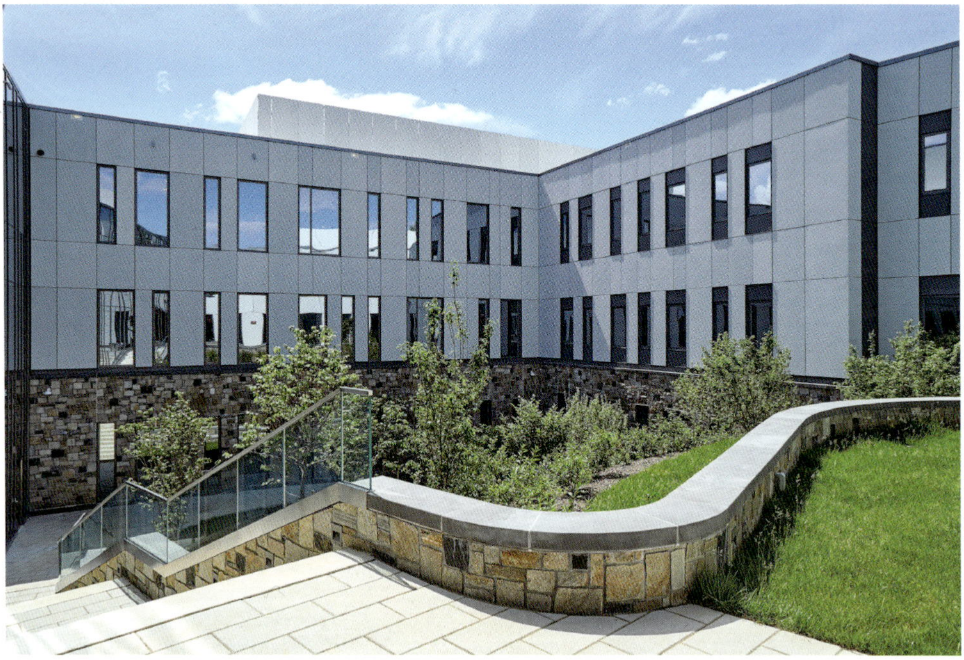

Plate 8. *(Figure 23–2)* Interior courtyard.

Patient rooms and units that face wooded areas or interior courtyards offer well-lit spaces and capitalize on the healing effects of nature.

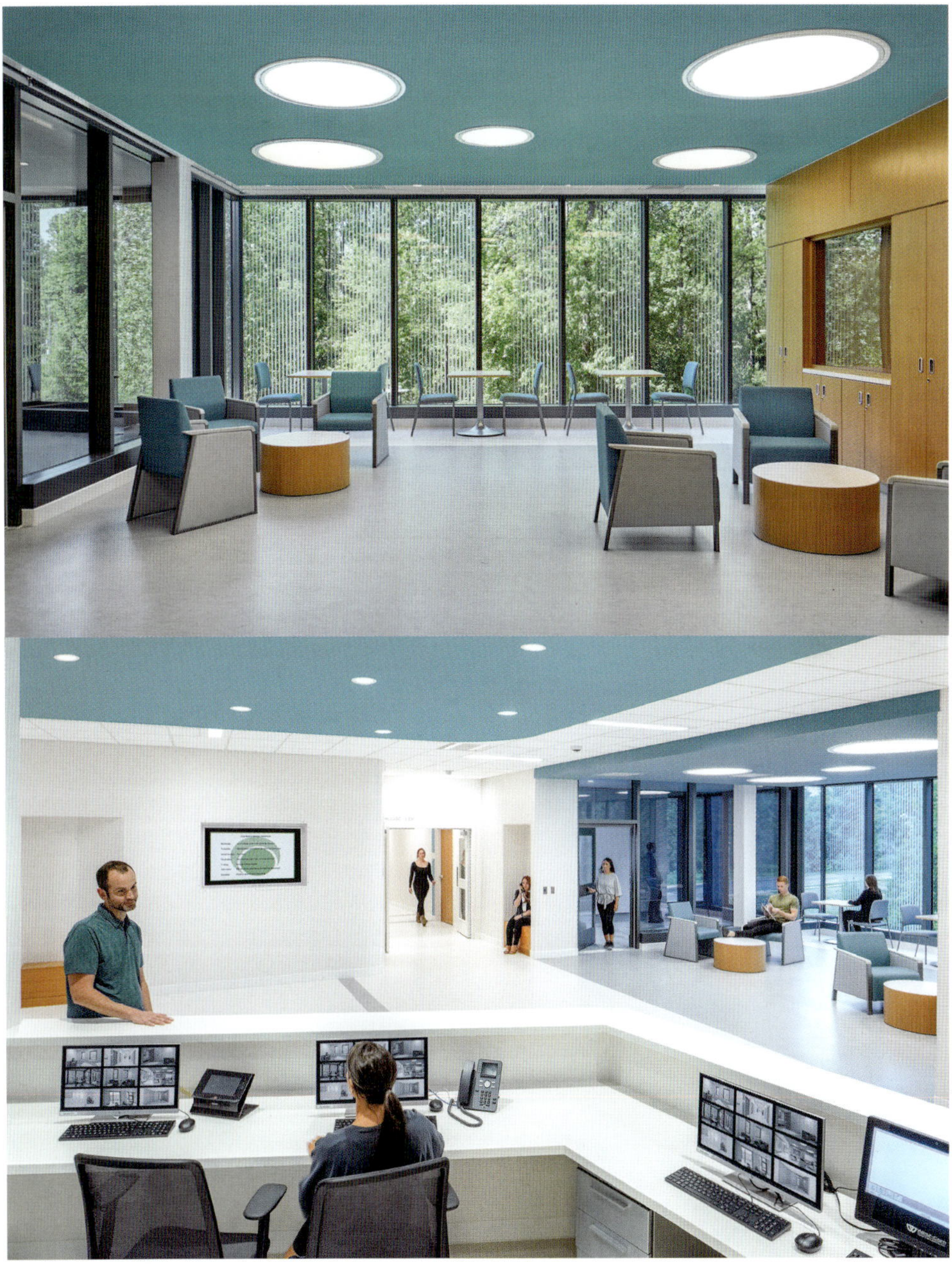

PLATE 9. *(Figure 23–3)* Patient care area.

Patient care areas offer contemplative and restorative spaces where patients can learn skills to help them succeed in the long term.

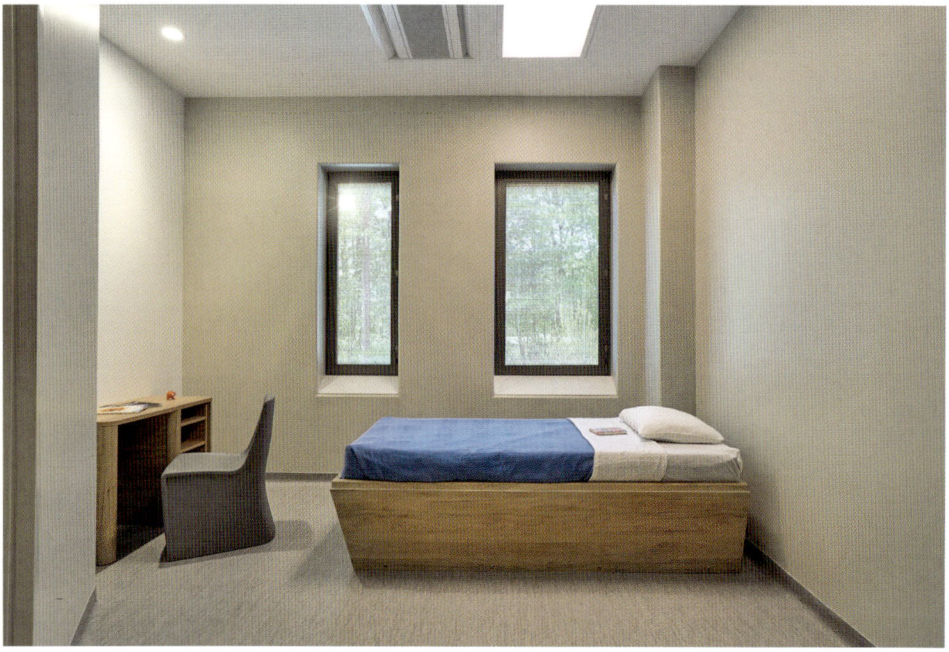

PLATE 10. *(Figure 23–4)* Patient bedroom.

Single-occupant patient rooms with private bathrooms are the single most important feature in reducing aggression and stress in patients.

LIGATURE RISK PHASE I COMPLETION DASHBAORD

AREA	RM #	STATUS	AREA	RM #	STATUS	AREA	RM #	STATUS	AREA	RM #	STATUS
	1	100%		1	91%		1	100%		1	82%
	2	91%		2	82%		2	91%		2	91%
	3	100%		3	91%		3	91%		3	73%
	4	100%		4	100%		4	100%		4	82%
A	5	91%	E	5	82%	I	5	91%	M	5	73%
	6	100%		6	100%		6	100%		6	91%
	7	100%		7	91%		7	91%		7	73%
	8	100%		8	100%		8	100%		8	91%
	9	91%		9	91%		9	91%		9	91%
	1	91%		1	100%		1	100%		1	91%
	2	91%		2	91%		2	82%		2	100%
	3	91%		3	91%		3	100%		3	91%
	4	100%		4	91%		4	100%		4	100%
B	5	91%	F	5	91%	J	5	100%	N	5	73%
	6	100%		6	100%		6	91%		6	100%
	7	91%		7	91%		7	100%		7	100%
	8	91%		8	100%		8	91%		8	73%
	9	100%		9	82%		9	100%		9	91%
	1	100%		1	100%		1	91%		1	91%
	2	100%		2	82%		2	91%		2	64%
	3	91%		3	100%		3	91%		3	
	4	100%		4	91%		4	91%		4	
C	5	100%	G	5	73%	K	5	100%	O	5	100%
	6	100%		6	91%		6	100%		6	91%
	7	100%		7	100%		7	100%		7	100%
	8	100%		8	82%		8	100%		8	82%
	9	100%		9	100%		9	100%		9	82%
	1	100%		1	82%		1	100%		1	91%
	2	100%		2	100%		2	100%		2	82%
	3	100%		3	91%		3	100%		3	91%
	4	100%		4	91%		4	100%		4	82%
D	5	100%	H	5	91%	L	5	100%	P	5	100%
	6	100%		6	100%		6	100%		6	100%
	7	91%		7	91%		7	100%		7	82%
	8	100%		8	100%		8	100%		8	91%
	9	91%		9	91%		9	91%		9	100%

STATUS BY TYPE	Door Handle	Roton Hinge	Sink Pipe Cover	Toilet Pipe Cover	Faucet	Bed	Shower Head	Dresser/ Wardrobe	Tub	PTAC Bar
% Complete	73%	93%	90%	76%	99%	100%	99%	100%	100%	100%

PLATE 11. *(Figure 23–5)* Visual dashboard for completion of Phase I of Sheppard Pratt Health System project to reduce ligature risk.

LIGATURE RISK PHASE II COMPLETION DASHBAORD

Area \ STATUS BY TYPE	Door Handle	Roton Hinge	Sink Pipe Cover	Toilet Pipe Cover	Faucet	Shower Head	Shower Diverter	Tub Diverter	Other
A	100%	100%	97%	50%	97%	100%	100%	100%	100%
B	100%	100%	100%	55%	100%	100%	100%	100%	100%
C	100%	100%	94%	50%	94%	100%	100%	100%	100%
D	100%	100%	100%	55%	100%	100%	100%	100%	100%
E	100%	100%	100%	50%	100%	100%	100%	100%	100%
F	100%	100%	100%	50%	100%	100%	100%	100%	100%
G	100%	100%	95%	50%	95%	100%	100%	100%	100%
H	80%	80%	65%	25%	65%	100%	100%	100%	100%
I	50%	0%	50%	50%	50%	100%	100%	100%	100%
J	53%	50%	53%	53%	53%	100%	100%	100%	100%
K	50%	0%	100%	50%	100%	100%	100%	100%	100%
L	0%	0%	33%	33%	100%	100%	100%	100%	100%
M	0%	0%	93%	100%	93%	80%	100%	100%	100%
N	0%	0%	100%	78%	100%	100%	100%	100%	67%
O	0%	10%	57%	100%	52%	57%	100%	100%	100%
P	0%	0%	43%	64%	43%	57%	100%	100%	100%
TOTALS									

PHASE II PERCENT COMPLETE	79%

PLATE 12. *(Figure 23–6)* Visual dashboard for completion of Phase II of Sheppard Pratt Health System project to reduce ligature risk.

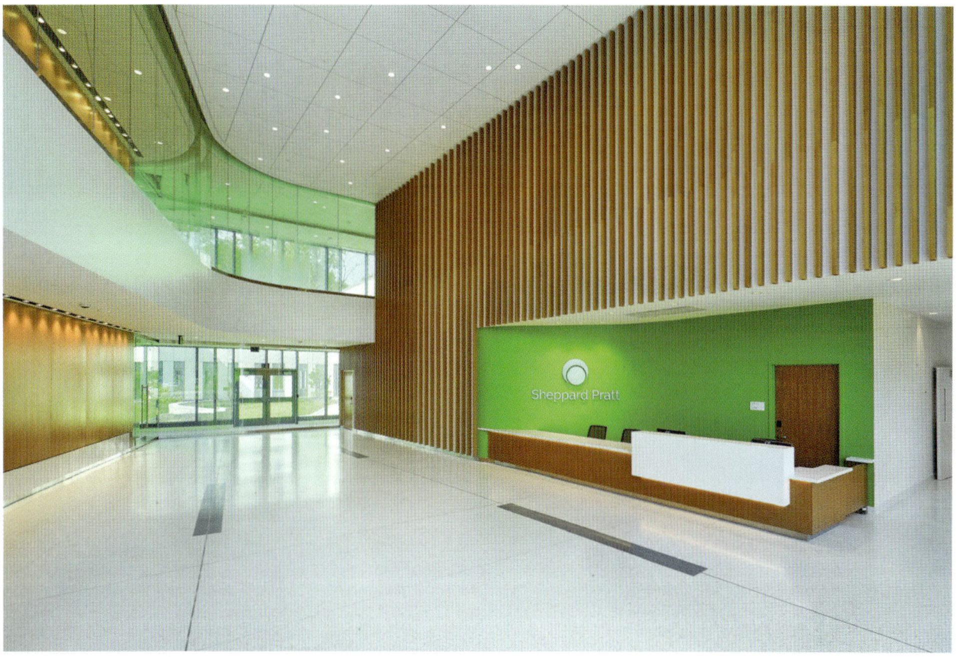

Plate 13. *(Figure 23–7)* Lobby.

The need for mental health treatment spaces is rising, and modern, well-designed spaces can contribute to the healing and therapeutic benefit of the patient.

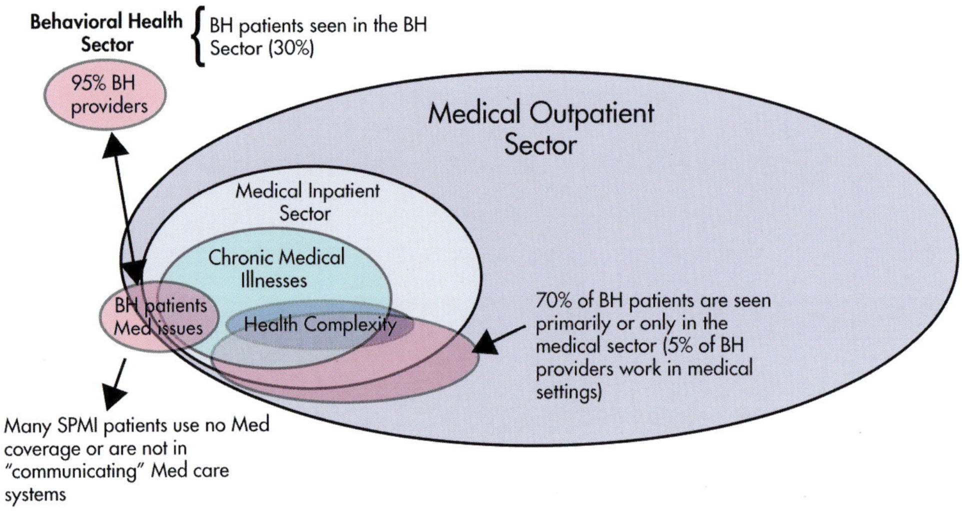

PLATE 14. *(Figure 29–2)* Where patients go for care.

BH=behavioral health; SPMI=severe and persistent mental illness. (Cartesian Solutions Inc. ©)

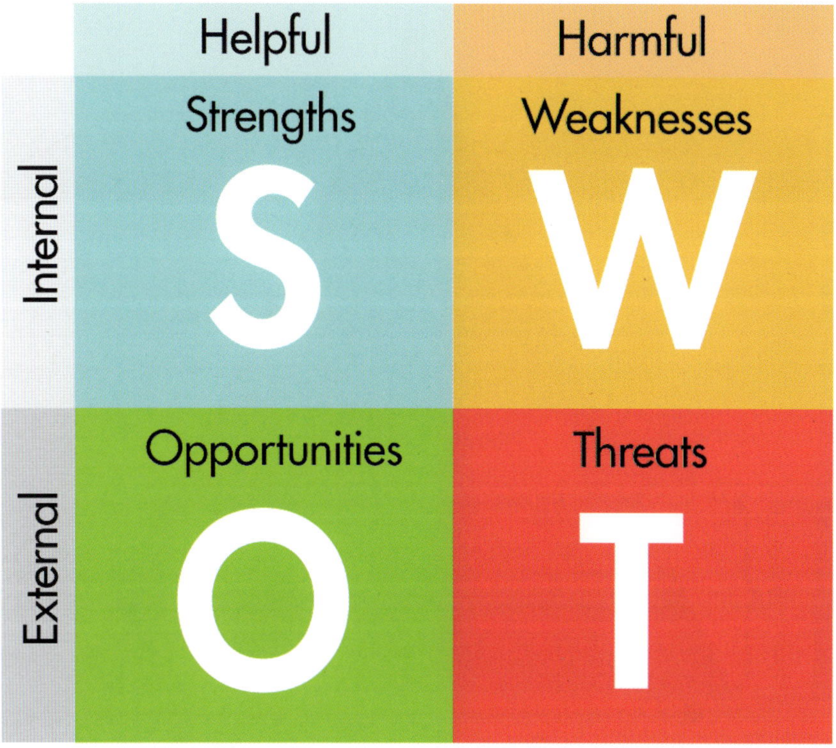

PLATE 15. *(Figure 29–4)* Components of a strengths-weaknesses-opportunities-threats (SWOT) analysis.

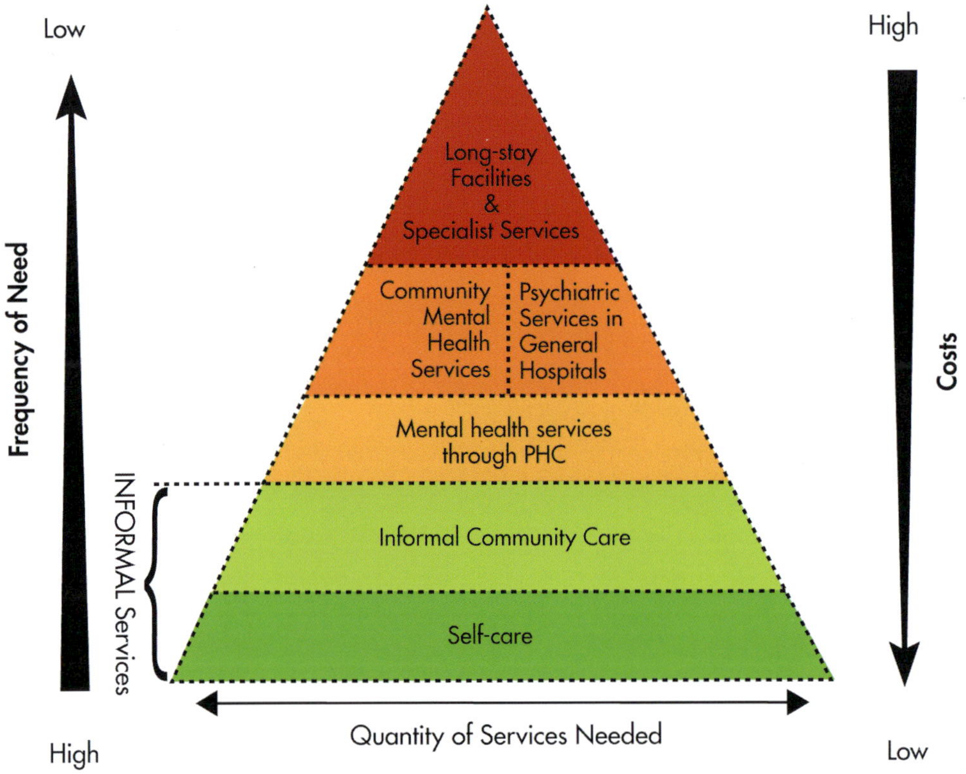

PLATE 16. *(Figure 29–5)* World Health Organization's optimal mix of services pyramid.
PHC=primary health care.

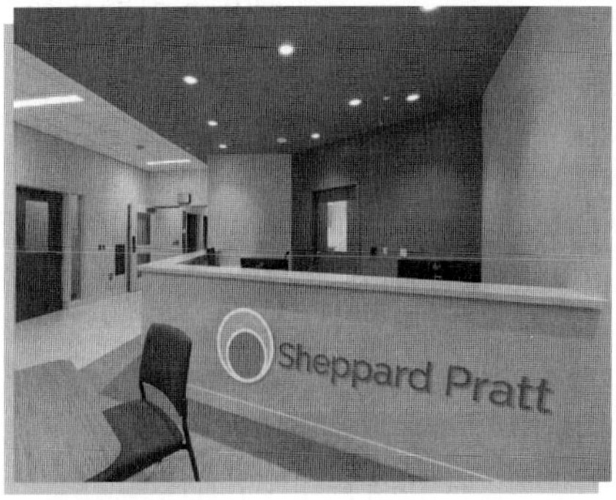

CHAPTER 14

Residential Treatment for Children and Adolescents

Virginia Susan Villani, M.D.

Residential treatment centers (RTCs) currently provide care for children and adolescents who have severe and persistent mental health needs that cannot be met in a less restrictive setting, yet do not meet medical necessity criteria used for inpatient hospitalization. RTC level of care is necessary because outpatient treatment has failed and lesser levels of care have not been sufficient to ensure the security and safety of the child or adolescent. Beyond these two simplistic statements, there is not a standard definition of what constitutes an RTC, with programs varying from state to state.

RTCs are also considered in the child welfare continuum of services, which includes all out-of-home care. In 2014, there were 415,129 youth in out-of-home care, with 23,233 (6%) placed in group homes and 32,955 (8%) placed in residential treatment facilities or other institutional settings (Pecora and English 2016). Within this system, RTCs have become a tertiary level of care, with the child needing to "fail up" to gain access (Bellonci 2010).

RTCs have evolved to this level over the past 30 years because of two trends in the provision of psychiatric care for children: 1) the medicalization of inpatient child psychiatry with the advent of managed care and application of medical necessity criteria for admission and discharge and 2) the closing of state hospitals. Prior to this current era of managed care in inpatient psychiatry, children and adolescents received thorough diagnostic assessments over weeks and sometimes months. Inpatient units had schools that the patients attended, and educational assessments were a part of the complete evaluation process.

Inpatient psychiatric hospitalization of children and adolescents has evolved to a model of acute stabilization, with length of stay on an inpatient unit now a few days, and at most 2–3 weeks. There are no schools on inpatient units; at most, they may have a classroom where a child in the hospital might spend a few hours a day. Medications are added quickly, and a discharge plan is hastily put together.

As inpatient child psychiatry changed and state hospitals closed, RTCs became the de facto level of care for children with complex mental health needs. RTCs are now considered a part of the medical system of care when less restrictive services have failed. A child or adolescent admitted to an RTC often had many brief inpatient stays and multiple short trials of medications. Day hospital and intensive outpatient services have failed. Wraparound services, therapeutic foster care, and group homes have also been unsuccessful, and the symptoms that led to hospitalization have returned. After several cycles of failed treatment the child is referred for residential treatment.

This chapter is both administrative and clinical in nature. The first two sections focus on administrative aspects of running RTCs, including outlining regulation and oversight of RTCs and the types of RTCs. The next two sections have a clinical focus and describe the population of children being served and the process of clinical care. The chapters ends with a discussion about outcome studies and future needs.

Regulation and Oversight

Regulation of RTCs and oversight of compliance with regulations vary from state to state and are often lumped together with the regulation of nonhospital, out-of-home placement facilities and programs, such as therapeutic group homes. The regulations distinguish RTCs from therapeutic group homes by regulating the amount of medical and psychiatric care that must be provided in order for the program to qualify as an RTC. A survey fielded by the U.S. Department of Health and Human Services in 2003 in 38 states revealed 71 types of facilities, 3,628 facilities, and 50,507 beds (Ireys et al. 2006). The regulatory methods, which differed from state to state, included on-site inspection, documentation of staff turnover, record reviews, resident interviews, critical incident reports, standards for resident-to-staff ratios, and education level of the facility director. Furthermore, there were oversight and regulatory differences depending on the funding agency and the different missions involved, with many programs (47%) answering to more than one agency. The Substance Abuse and Mental Health Services Administration cited the increased number of facilities in the previous two decades as a function of the closing of long-term psychiatric hospitals and inpatient units (Manderscheid et al. 2001).

The National Mental Health Services Survey of mental health treatment facilities used a more restrictive definition of *residential treatment center* and identified 601 RTCs for children in the United States, with 143 identified as for profit, 439 private nonprofit, 143 private for profit, and 19 public-funded regional facilities (Substance Abuse and Mental Health Services Administration 2017). The survey included information about the treatment approaches being offered at the RTCs, such as individual therapy, cognitive-behavioral therapy, dialectical behavior therapy, behavior modification, trauma treatment, and psychotropic medication management, but it did not address oversight and regulation.

The American Academy of Child and Adolescent Psychiatry (AACAP), in its *Principles of Care for Treatment of Children and Adolescents With Mental Illnesses in Residential Treatment Centers*, described a number of standards for residential facilities, in addition to state licensing and oversight through national quality programs (e.g., Joint Commission, URAC, CARF), insurance companies, and federal governmental agencies (TRICARE/Centers for Medicare & Medicaid Services) (American Academy of Child and Adolescent Psychiatry 2010). It noted that there are no federal laws that regulate residential treatment programs and that adoption of national standards is voluntary. The AACAP endorsed the adoption of the national Joint Commission standards for certification of residential facilities; however, the academy felt the standards were not complete and thus published their guideline document as a supplement to the Joint Commission standards. The guideline specifically made recommendations for leadership structure and staffing (Table 14–1) as well as giving guidance in other areas, such as the admission process, treatment planning and discharge planning, prevention of aggressive and dangerous behavior, and therapeutic services standards.

The International Work Group for Therapeutic Residential Care (Whittaker et al. 2016) has provided overarching principles for all residential programs:

1. First do not harm (*primum non nocere*)—ensure child safety and focus on prevention of abuse and "deviancy training."
2. Strive to constantly forge and maintain strong and vital family linkages.
3. Be fully anchored in the community, culture, and web of social relationships that define and inform the children and families served.
4. Be informed by a culture that stresses learning through living, where teaching occurs in a series of deeply personal human relationships.
5. View as an ultimate goal the identification of evidence-based models or strategies that are effective for youth and families, replicable, and to scale.

Types of Programs

Programs can be defined in different ways. However, for the purposes of this chapter, level of security (unlocked and locked) and program type (general versus specialty) will be described.

Level of Security

There are two types of RTCs by level of security: unlocked and locked. Unlocked RTCs are most often in a campus-like setting that may or may not have a secure perimeter. Children move around without the need for locked doors, but it is made clear that if they leave the campus, they will be brought back to complete their treatment. There is a school on the grounds that the residents attend, often a short walk from the buildings or cottages where they live. Recreational space is provided in the form of a gymnasium and fields to allow for much-needed exercise. Some group homes have clusters of cottages on a campus and may even have a school; however, they do not provide the

TABLE 14–1. American Academy of Child and Adolescent Psychiatry recommendations for leadership structure and staffing of residential treatment centers (RTCs)

RTC program should
Be appropriate for all acuity levels.
Be multidisciplinary and culturally competent.
Have sufficient staffing for the number of patients.
Include a child and adolescent psychiatrist or, in the case of an adolescent program, an adult psychiatrist with training in treating that age group.
Include on-site nursing care and supervision for one shift a day, with on-call availability for other shifts.
Provide medical care (ill and preventive care) by a qualified primary care provider who is available 24 hours a day, with hospital resources identified when necessary.
Include leadership provided by professionals with graduate-level training and appropriate licensure and credentials who demonstrate expertise in the treatment of youth.
Ensure that ancillary staff have appropriate training and licensure.
Require all staff to be screened with finger printing on a national level, driver's license and criminal record reviews, and a face-to-face interview to minimize the possibility of employing a predator who could endanger a child.
RTC staff should
Be trained in evidence-based/research-based psychosocial and other interventions.
Be trained in use of family-centered care within the facility.
Be of an appropriate gender for daily hygiene and activities of daily living needs.

Source. American Academy of Child and Adolescent Psychiatry 2010.

range of services offered in an RTC. RTCs treat children with higher acuity and have more psychiatric and nursing services as compared with group homes.

Locked programs vary in their level of security from complete containment and highly secure to ones that are less secure. For the most secure, the school is within the locked space and outdoor spaces are made secure with fencing to prohibit running away. Secure, locked RTCs can look institutional; this is by necessity, given the dangerousness of the population being served. Many secure settings treat adjudicated youth who have been identified by the courts as having a treatable mental illness. RTCs that treat adjudicated youth are different from boot camps, ranch/wilderness camps, and training programs, which do not offer diagnostic and counseling services. The Office of Juvenile Justice and Delinquency Prevention, in a biennial survey, found more than 900 facilities that housed and treated juvenile offenders, with 35% self reporting to be RTCs (Hockenberry et al. 2009).

General vs. Specialty Programs

Residential treatment programs that treat children with a variety of diagnoses are best termed *general* RTCs. There are concerns about mixing populations with widely different levels of behavioral difficulties, with some citing the risk of deviancy training for those with less severe behaviors who are housed and treated with youth whose behaviors are more severe. General programs, however, are common because of the need to accept all referrals to maintain high bed occupancy.

Other programs specialize in specific diagnoses, with programs tailored to meet the needs of an identified diagnostic group: eating disorders; substance use disorders; reactive attachment disorder; autism/pervasive developmental disorders; oppositional, defiant, and conduct disorders; and sexual perpetrators. Specialty programs vary in the level of security provided and may use self-injurious behaviors or aggression toward others as admission exclusion criteria.

The Casey Foundation research brief on the elements of effective practice for children in therapeutic residential care (Pecora and English 2016) identified seven program models and indicated whether they were supported by evidence-based research (Table 14–2). In addition to program models, the brief described 39 interventions and described the problem each was designed to treat and the level of evidence-based research available. The specifics of the evidence-based research regarding age, problem, and treatment duration were also provided in the brief. For example, trauma-focused cognitive-behavioral therapy is designed to treat anxiety, depression, and PTSD for children ages 4–18, with one 60- to 90-minute session per week for a treatment duration of 12–16 weeks. Dialectical behavior therapy is effective for borderline personality disorder and substance abuse for ages 18–25, with a treatment duration of about 6 months. The brief raised concerns about general programs, which are not specific in matching the type of intervention with the child's needs.

Most residential programs are designed to safely contain children who have severe aggressive outbursts directed toward themselves, others, or the environment. The ability to safely physically restrain and the presence of seclusion rooms are a part of RTCs, and further distinguish them from group homes and necessitate the need for psychiatric and nursing management.

All residential treatment programs face the challenge of being a safe environment that does not look or feel institutional and does not create institutionalization in the residents. The daily activities for children—meals, showers, homework, playtime—all have to be provided for, in addition to the vast array of therapeutic services. And all of this must happen 24 hours a day, 7 days a week, 365 days a year.

Clinical Description of Children in Residential Treatment Centers

It is important to highlight the severity of illness in youth being treated in RTCs, whether general or specialty programs, while also acknowledging the lack of accurate data currently available on diagnoses and risk factors. In the case of specialty programs, diagnostic data are skewed by the lack of rigor and the need for the facility to diagnose on the basis of who they have been designed to treat. Records are also notoriously incomplete and inconsistent from facility to facility, obscuring the discernment of national trends over time. The National Child Traumatic Stress Network data set of more than 11,000 youth (Briggs et al. 2012) does, however, provide a description of youth in RTC at the time of the survey. In this data set, youth in RTCs were significantly more likely to have suffered all eight trauma types: physical abuse, sexual abuse, emotional abuse, domestic violence, traumatic loss/bereavement, school violence, community violence, and impairment in caregivers. They also had greater functional impairment in behavior, more difficulties with academics, more attachment issues, and

TABLE 14–2. Evidence-based program models

Boys Town Family Home Program and Teaching Family Model*
Menninger Clinic Residential Treatment Program*
Multifunctional Treatment in Residential and Community Settings (MultifunC)[NR]
Positive Peer Culture (PPC)**
Re-ED (originally called Re-Education of Children with Emotional Disturbance)[NR]
Sanctuary model of a trauma-informed treatment culture*
Stop Gap Model*

Level of evidence-based research: *promising; **supported by some research evidence; ***well supported by research evidence; [NR]not rated for level of research evidence.

higher rates of running away, substance abuse, self-injury, suicidality, and criminal activity.

Use of the Child and Adolescent Needs and Strengths (CANS; Anxderson et al. 2003) has become more prevalent, with some states, New Jersey and Illinois, adopting it more vigorously (Chor et al. 2012; Lyons 2009). As an instrument, CANS is reliable and valid at the item level (Anderson et al. 2002) such that one can track improvement of symptoms from admission to discharge. For example, in a sample of 5,268 youth treated in residential treatment care in Illinois, anger control was identified as a presenting problem in 60.2% of admissions, with less than 50% reporting it resolved at discharge, yet 56.1% reporting it improved.

Survey data do not, however, capture the tragic lives of many youth or the complex, dangerous trajectory of other youth who may have had no trauma but have severe mental illness. The commonality is the severity and intensity of the illness. The diagnoses vary, and the youth come from diverse socioeconomic backgrounds, but all have severe illness. Comorbidity is often present such that a child with early childhood trauma presents with severe depression, labile mood, aggressive outbursts, and substance abuse.

While generalities are beset with exceptions, there are five common clusters of problems present for children who need residential treatment that, although discussed below as distinct clusters, frequently overlap.

Early-Onset Aggression and Defiance of Social Norms

Children who have early onset of aggression, before age 5, accompanied by defiance of social norms, may require residential treatment as they become older and their behaviors more dangerous. The early life experiences of these children are often as witness to abuse and/or as victim of abuse. Intrauterine exposure to substances is also commonly a part of the child's history. The home environment is chaotic and unstable, and the child enters either a group care setting or early childhood education without basic social skills. Behavior problems begin with aggression toward other children and caregivers. There is a complex interplay of genetic vulnerability inherited from the biological parents, intrauterine insult, the effects of early childhood stress, impoverished nurturing, and lack of appropriate behavioral consequences. Short hospitalizations that target behaviors with medications are often inadequate for these children. If the child's behaviors are severe and persistent, the child may need residential treatment prior to adolescence. There is also a subgroup of children who receive residential treatment prior to adolescence, yet their behaviors reemerge when they leave. Failed placement in foster homes, therapeutic foster homes, and group homes with brief hospital stays in between creates an additional pattern of instability.

Severe Depression or Psychosis With Danger to Self or Community

Children with severe early-onset depression or psychosis can be the product of normal pregnancies and have relatively uncomplicated childhoods. Their illnesses erupt gradually over time, often beginning with social isolation and the inability to get along with peers. Early school years are buffered by small elementary schools where teachers know them and adjust to their needs. In middle school, the child's moods become more labile as the child struggles to fit into the world.

The clinical picture becomes more complicated if the preteen or teen begins to use marijuana in an attempt to self-medicate sleep problems or social anxiety. This unfortunately makes the child's depression worse and can cause underlying psychosis to become full blown with paranoia and aggression. Similarly, social media and violent video games are cultural phenomena readily available to youth, and their excessive use and play are further risk factors that enhance the symptoms of the underlying disorder. RTCs are unique in their ability to create an environment that is free of social media, video games, and other cultural phenomena that may worsen a child's underlying psychiatric illness.

Severe Anxiety That Impacts School and Interferes With Outpatient Treatment

The child with severe anxiety may have suffered with social anxiety as a young child and school refusal. Over time, the school refusal becomes more severe, and the child refuses to leave the house. In-home services are tried but are not successful. Similarly, medication trials are not successful, often because of noncompliance. The school may order in-home or online teaching, but the child is unable to complete work, with this inability attributable to overwhelming anxiety, depression, or both. If the parent gets the child to go to school, the child either cowers in a corner unable to function or externalize their fear or commits a dangerous act to get out of the situation that to them is catastrophically overwhelming. A brief hospital stay cannot ameliorate what has become a pattern of months, and sometimes years, of severe anxiety and maladaptive behaviors, which have become intertwined around the child and family.

Substance Abuse With Anxiety, Depression, or Psychosis

Substance use disorder is highly prevalent in adolescents receiving residential treatment, with the most commonly used substance currently being cannabis. The reason for the need for residential treatment is straightforward: the youth must be removed from their environment so that they can be drug-free in order for treatment providers to understand and treat whatever underlying psychiatric condition is present. It is folly for outpatient providers to prescribe psychotropic medications to a youth who is actively using marijuana on a frequent basis, especially when the youth is using during the school week and going to school high.

With marijuana legal in many states, its use has become normalized in both urban and suburban communities, with parents and guardians largely unaware of its potential risks for preteens and teens. The precipitation of psychosis with aggression as a side effect of use followed by psychiatric hospitalization is a common history for teens in RTCs. Youth referred to an RTC from the courts because of their involvement in illegal activities often have an extensive history of early-onset cannabis use, at ages 10–12.

Developmental Delay, Autism Spectrum Disorder, and Aggression

Children who have developmental delays or autism spectrum disorder with accompanying aggression that renders them unsafe at home or at school may need residential treatment. Programs that specialize in treating children with these disorders most commonly use behavior modification programs and techniques in order to shape the child's behavior away from aggression and toward a more adaptive, prosocial way of handling frustrations and challenges. The scenarios that lead toward residential treatment for these children follow two paths: parental support is inadequate to the needs of the child; or the child's behaviors are such that, despite the best efforts of supportive parents working with a skilled treatment team, they cannot ensure the safety of the child or community. This latter path represents the experience of a subset of children with autism spectrum disorder who have extreme challenges and require comprehensive care.

The Clinical Process of Residential Treatment: Seven Components of Care

The clinical process described in the seven components of care below operationalizes the principles of care outlined in the International Work Group's consensus paper and the AACAP Principles of Care for Treatment. Just as the previous clinical section sought to bring to life the clinical picture of the children being served, this section details the process of treatment within an RTC.

Complete Array of Services

A complete array of services is necessary because of the complexity of the children being served in RTCs. RTCs must offer clinical services, residential care services (frequently referred to as *milieu treatment*), educational services, and medical and psychiatric services, as well as supplemental services on a case-by-case basis as necessary. RTCs that seek to distinguish themselves beyond this offer recreational therapy and occupational therapy. Clinical services encompass individual, group, and family therapy, with their treatment approach tailored to the need of the child. Social workers, licensed counselors, and psychologists work as clinicians in RTCs and hone their skills for the populations they are treating. For example, the child with a history of trauma may need trauma-informed therapy, whereas the adolescent with self-injurious behavior may need dialectical behavior therapy. Clinicians in RTCs adapt the treatment to both diagnoses and intellectual ability, utilizing a variety of techniques and therapeutic approaches. Clinicians also lead group therapy sessions to address such issues as peer interactions, substance abuse, and the development of prosocial skills.

Milieu-based treatment involves a structured day, which includes attention to hygiene (including sleep hygiene), leisure activities, care of personal belongings and personal space, and setting routines. The core premise of milieu treatment is that treatment occurs not only in therapy but also across all 24 hours of the day (Redl 1959; Trieschman et al. 1969). Residential staff model appropriate behaviors, help children to de-escalate at times of stress, intervene when maladaptive behaviors erupt, and help the children with the development of healthy peer relationships.

RTCs also must have a school attached in order to provide educational services. The school has to be designed and approved by the local department of education to serve the children whom the RTC accepts. The ability of the school to educate children with specific federal handicapping codes as defined under the Individuals with Disabilities Education Act (IDEA) and specified in a child's individualized education plan (IEP) may actually drive the decision about whether to accept a child into the RTC, because schools do not typically serve all federal handicapping codes. For example, the school must be approved by the state department of education to serve children who have a federal handicapping code of autism if that is what the child's IEP designates. The RTC would therefore not accept a referral for a child coded with autism because the attached school would not be able to educate the child. In addition, for adolescents, class credits for graduation, preparation for standardized tests under No Child Left Behind, and in some states volunteer service learning hours must all be a part of the education provided to RTC high school students/residents.

Medical and psychiatric services are also a necessary part of the array of services for RTC residents. Usually a pediatrician comes weekly, or at a greater frequency if necessary, to perform initial physical exams when a resident is admitted and to provide ongoing medical care as necessary. A child psychiatrist must also be a part of the RTCs to provide initial evaluations, diagnostic services, and psychopharmacological treatment. Some programs have child psychiatrists as leaders, with some states mandating that an RTC have a medical director. The shortage of child psychiatrists nationwide has made staffing RTCs challenging, and some programs are using telepsychiatry.

In addition to this wide but basic array of services, specialty programs may also need other services. An RTC that serves children with autism and/or developmental disabilities will need a behavior specialist to develop behavior modification plans to be used in the residence. The school will need its own psychologist to do functional behavioral analyses and develop behavior intervention plans consistent with educational practices.

Family Engagement From the Beginning

Welcoming the family at the beginning of the child's stay is essential to engaging them in their child's treatment. The process that families undergo en route to an RTC is often long, and they can even feel blamed for their child's difficulties. In cases where there has been abuse and neglect, it is all too easy for the RTC to not be welcoming, and indeed safety has to be a part of assessing the degree to which a parent or parents can have contact with their child. Ideally this should be done prior to admission by the social services agency, with the RTC given clear information about who the parent/guardian is that should be involved in the child's stay. For all parents/guardians, hearing their story, listening to the details about what has happened, and giving them the time to talk and share their pain constitute a crucial first step in engagement.

Family engagement can be particularly challenging for residents who have juvenile justice involvement and may have committed crimes involving their families. Keeping these families involved may require victim impact work and restitution in order to repair damage incurred secondary to the youth's behaviors.

Families may also live a considerable distance from the RTC, and this creates a barrier to visiting and participating in family therapy. In addition, lower-socioeconomic-status families often do not own cars, and this lack of access to a car, combined with the lack of public transportation near an RTC, makes regular visiting and family meetings difficult. Programs that prioritize family engagement find ways to overcome these barriers by helping with transportation for families, using conference calling for treatment review meetings, and increasingly using secure-line videoconferencing for family therapy sessions.

There are a myriad of other small ways that RTCs can be family friendly and demonstrate the high priority the program places on engaging families, from offering family-friendly visiting rooms, to providing handbooks and welcome brochures that clearly describe program rules in simple friendly language, to creating outdoor spaces for walks and activities that can be done together on visits, as well as allowing ample time for phone calls, to name a few.

The most important aspect of family engagement, however, is the attitude of staff as they deal with family members. Staff need to embrace the principle that families are essential for the child's success and make all their interactions with family members positive. Each interaction, from the manner in which families are greeted each time they visit to the tone of the voice on the phone when they call, should convey dignity and respect. This not only helps to engage families, it simultaneously models for the family and the child the importance of dignity and respect for all interpersonal interactions.

Holistic Diagnostic Approach

As noted before, children who are admitted to an RTC most often have had multiple failed inpatient stays, failed outpatient treatment attempts, and multiple placements. Children arrive with thick packets of referral information that can be overwhelming to assimilate. It is incumbent, however, for the treaters not only to thoroughly review the referral information on each child but also to do their own diagnostic assessment. One cannot assume the information provided is accurate. Information is frequently repeated from report to report in a cut-and-paste manner, which can lead to mistakes being repeated without anyone checking with the parent, guardian, or agency as to their accuracy.

The child's life should be carefully reconstructed year by year, through each phase of development, such that the clinicians involved have a thorough and complete understanding of the child's life story. Gaps need to be filled in with information from either the parent, the child, or agency personnel who may have access to additional reports and data. Significant life events, especially adverse life events, need to be demarcated as to when they occurred, where the child was, and what follow-up was provided. Each school year should be reviewed, with school attended, problems that may have arisen, and success or failure of educational goals noted. A thorough medical history must be taken, with review of past medical problems, diagnostic workups, and hospitalizations.

The process of taking the history creates an important bond between the resident and clinician and between the parent/guardian and clinician. The small details one learns that may have been easily missed in a more rushed history gathered during an inpatient stay or in an outpatient clinic can be elaborated and understood in the slower-paced environment of the RTC.

This kind of holistic diagnostic approach extends to integrating information across treatment domains. An evaluation generated in one setting may not have been thoroughly reviewed with a parent/guardian because the child was discharged or moved abruptly to another setting. It also may not have been shared with the school for the purpose of better designing the child's educational program. For example, a neuropsychological testing report ordered by the court and done at a detention facility for a teenager may not have been reviewed with the parent. And unless the parent is counseled to request an IEP meeting to share it with the educators, the testing results will not make it to the child's educational record. The MRI recommended by the evaluator may have fallen by the wayside and never been ordered and done. Similarly, discharge recommendations from a prior hospital stay for follow-up labs or X-rays may have never been completed.

The treatment plan developed using this holistic approach provides a road-map guiding and informing the treatment in the weeks and months to come.

Multidisciplinary Team Meetings With Strong Case Management

The backbone of treatment in an RTC is the regular meeting of and review of the child's treatment by a multidisciplinary treatment team. Most often the team is led by the child's therapist, who also functions as a case manager. The clinician's job is to coordinate all the treatments the child is receiving and to work with the family or guardian in family therapy. The members of the treatment team depend on the services offered at the RTC; however, there should always be representation from the residential staff on the unit where the child is residing, medical staff (usually nursing), psychiatry, and the school. Additional team members may include an occupational therapist who is working with the child or a recreational therapist on staff who does regular groups and activities with the children.

There are two basic types of team meetings: regularly scheduled treatment team reviews without child and family and treatment team reviews with child and family. Usually the team meetings without the child and family occur frequently, often weekly. During these meetings, the team comes together to discuss issues the child might be having in various areas of the program—which could include at the residence, in school, or on outings. Academic progress and school behavior are also reviewed. Upcoming important events such as family meetings, court dates, and medical appointments are noted and planned for. Diagnostic issues that may have been identified are tracked and the results followed up on and integrated into the child's treatment plan.

The second type of meeting is a treatment review meeting that includes the child, family, and any outside agency representatives involved with the child. The initial meeting occurs a short time after admission—anywhere from 1 week to 1 month. During this meeting the events that led to admission are summarized, the goals for treatment outlined, and the master treatment plan developed. The support network for the child is identified, and there is an opportunity to expand the necessary supports. The goals and objectives are developed, and the treatment plan is signed by all present and sent to those not in the room. Following the development of the master treatment plan, the treatment team meets periodically with the child and whoever can attend, either in person or on the phone, for the purpose of continuing to align goals and expectations, review what progress has been made since the previous meeting, and think together about what needs to happen for the child to be ready for discharge to a less restrictive setting. Discussion in these meetings is wide ranging and can cover topics such as concerns about stalled treatment, readiness for sign-outs home, academic progress or lack thereof, planning for academic needs, and the need for medication changes and/or the effects of changes. As the child becomes free of the behaviors that led to placement, the focus naturally shifts to celebrating the child's successes and discharge planning.

Regulations about the frequency of treatment review meetings and who attends, as well as the type of documentation required, vary from state to state and agency to agency. Oversight agencies and funders look closely at the documentation to ensure that there is active treatment with regular reviews and adjustments to treatment in order to continue to ensure that active treatment is occurring.

Psychopharmacological Management

Increasingly with the advent of psychopharmacological interventions, children who need residential treatment fall into three categories: those who were nonresponders to standard, basic psychopharmacology; those who did not have an adequate response but who might have needed higher-than-expected doses; and those whose compliance with medications was complicated by external factors. It is important that the diagnostic phase of care as outlined above include a review of previous medications that were tried, what the doses were, and whether they were taken with regularity for a sufficient period of time to allow them to work or were stopped because of side effects or lack of efficacy. External factors that may have interfered with efficacy, such as active drug use or a co-occurring substance use disorder, must also be taken into account. An adolescent or preteen who is no longer using substances might respond well to the medications that were attempted as an outpatient and failed. The security of the RTC and the length of stay allow for psychopharmacological management that can be thoughtful and thorough, with efficacy tracked over time in a controlled environment.

Children frequently arrive at an RTC taking four or more medications. Polypharmacy with children and adolescents has become widespread, with psychiatrists prescribing medication for target symptoms, adding medications as different symptoms arise, and yet being reluctant to discontinue previously existing medications. The RTC is a setting where everything can and should be assessed. Simplifying a medication regimen to arrive at the least number of medications needed at the appropriate doses is the goal, and fortunately there is time to do this.

The psychopharmacological outliers are also a part of medication management in an RTC. Children with severe and persistent aggression or self-injurious behaviors may actually need more than three medications in order to keep them and others safe.

Judiciously adding a second mood stabilizer, and augmenting the treatment of depression with an atypical antipsychotic or lithium in addition to a selective serotonin reuptake inhibitor, are examples of adjustments that can be done safely in an RTC. Treatments such as use of clozpine for severely aggressive patients, naltrexone for self-injurious patients, and even electroconvulsive therapy for severely depressed patients are extraordinary treatments that may be necessary for children who need an RTC level of care. While child psychiatrists often feel boxed in to making these decisions for outpatients because of a lack of resources, these treatments are more safely done in the structured treatment setting of an RTC, where all relevant variables can be examined and controlled.

Staff Training and Support

The backbone of treatment is the staff who spend the most time with the children, the residential staff. While the administrative staff and clinical staff are essential, it is those who provide the day-to-day, hour-to-hour, minute-to-minute care for the children who are the backbone of treatment. The concept of "the other 23 hours" has been recognized for decades and is best described in the rich literature on therapeutic milieu (Redl 1959; Trieschman et al. 1969). These seminal works emphasize the importance of the other 23 hours for teaching and learning social competence and behavioral control.

RTCs are prone to limit staff training to the regulatorily defined areas of needed competence such as cultural sensitivity, proper documentation, and so forth. Although training on these topics is necessary, it is insufficient and will leave staff woefully unprepared to manage the children currently in RTCs.

With this in mind, there are three areas that deserve heightened attention to training: child development, behavior management, and understanding and managing boundaries. While all staff who work with children in a treatment setting need training in these areas, children in residential treatment are among the most vulnerable by nature of their diagnoses and histories, the length of time in residence, and often the absence of parents, with only agencies as guardians. The quality of care provided to the children is a direct function of the training, both initial and ongoing, that staff receive.

It cannot be assumed that staff have basic knowledge about normal child development. Educational requirements for residential staff are not comprehensive and in some programs may only be a high school education. While staff training cannot and should not attempt to make staff experts in child development, it should include an overview of the tasks for the age and stage of development of the children under supervision. Staff must have a basic understanding of what is reasonable for a child to be able to do, how an adolescent thinks, and the appropriate range of social interactions between children during play and sports. Staff training about normal development must also be adapted to the population of children being served, their age, and the type of disability.

Behavior management training is the second core area that warrants special attention. RTCs typically serve children with a wide range of behavioral difficulties, with many RTCs needing to provide safety in the form of restraint and/or seclusion. Given that the regulations for their use vary from state to state and guide what the RTC can and cannot do, staff must receive training that is consistent with where they are located. If the RTC is licensed to use restraint and/or seclusion, the RTC will need to have chosen from a variety of training approaches and provide training for all staff, most especially in the residence, where the events that lead to restraint commonly occur. The types of training programs available include, but are not limited to, the Mandt System (www.mandtsystem.com), Crisis Prevention Institute (www.crisisprevention.com), Therapeutic Crisis Intervention (TCI; https://rccp.cornell.edu/TCI_LevelOne.html), and Professional Crisis Management (PCM; https://crisisintervention.com). Each has specific modules on working with children with behavioral regulation problems, understanding the escalation cycle, and learning safe hands-on techniques for restraint when absolutely necessary to prevent harm to self or others. Thorough staff training and periodic retraining constitute a core component of RTC treatment.

The third training area is comprehensive boundary training. RTC residential staff spend large amounts of time with the child over weeks and months in intimate settings. They become a part of that child's life as they guide them regarding activities of daily living such as daily hygiene, homework, playtime or sports, phone calls to friends and relatives, and even the development of love interests with peers. It is natural, given the proximity to the child and amount of time spent together, that residential staff become confidants and develop an understanding of the child and their struggles. Staff cannot, however, cross the boundary of treating any one child as special or become overly familiar with the resident in a sexualized manner. While this might seem obvious, one has to remember that children who are in an RTC may well have been victims of physical and/or sexual abuse. Their interpretation of simple interactions can be complicated by intrusive memories from the past, which can lead to misinterpretation of a staff member's behavior. A simple well-intended touch for support can lead to an allegation of abuse. Similarly, physical restraint can be misinterpreted as abuse by a resident. And unfortunately, staff who are not well trained and supervised can become overwhelmed with demands and managing aggressive youth and retaliate with force. Ongoing refresher trainings, debriefings after aggressive incidents, and supervision of staff that focuses on coaching them to do a better job are essential aspects of ensuring safe, therapeutic care for residents.

The administrative leadership team needs to invest heavily in all aspects of staff training in order to create a culture that is safe, therapeutic, and nonpunitive.

Discharge Planning

Discharge planning for a child leaving an RTC is considerably different from discharge planning for a child leaving an inpatient hospitalization. There are three phases of discharge planning: the assessment phase, to determine where the child will discharge to; the treatment planning phase, to plan for the provision of necessary aftercare services; and the transition phase, to facilitate the child's adjustment from the structure of the RTC to the less structured non-RTC environment.

The assessment phase includes determining whether where the child came from is where the child will return to. A careful history about the events that led to an RTC admission must be taken, with the relevant adults allowed to speak openly and candidly without the child present. For some cases, this will be the biological family telling their story of the fear engendered in their home for themselves and other children. For other cases, it will be agency staff relaying information from a group home, or grandparents who because of age and illness can no longer provide care. This kind of meeting must occur without the child present to provide adults with an opportunity to honestly share their pain and feel understood. It is important that the treatment team member hearing this listen in a nonjudgmental manner to build trust and, where possible, build a bridge back for the child should that be the best outcome for everyone. By and large, families are amazingly resilient; however, when they have reached their limit, whatever that limit may be, it must be respected and an alternative plan developed. It is also not uncommon for family members who were exhausted with caring for a child to catch their breath during the RTC stay and, with family work and observation that the child has improved, decide to have the child return home. These issues require adroit family therapy that supports both the child and the family.

Once it has been determined where the child will be living, necessary aftercare services, including outpatient therapy, medication management, and school, can be addressed. Locating and securing outpatient therapy and medication management are more complicated than simply calling and making an appointment, given the complex nature of the problems faced by children who require an RTC. The standard protocol for an outpatient clinic often requires a clinic-based therapist to do an intake, and then an appointment with a psychiatrist can be set up. This may create too large a gap in care for a child exiting an RTC. Similarly, because of the shortage of child psychiatrists nationwide, it may be difficult to locate one with the time and expertise to manage a complex medication regimen. When the discharge is to a group home, the frequency of care provided by the consulting psychiatrist can be an issue, as well as the expertise of the staff in dealing with a child who may have medication compliance issues.

The third component, school, is often the most difficult to address because of the complicated interface between mental health care and state departments of education. Schools attached to RTCs have small classroom sizes and are therapeutic in nature with behavior management that does not exist in non–special educational settings. Therefore, children in an RTC receive a different level of educational service even if they do not have an IEP when they enter the program. It is not uncommon for the child to have been receiving inadequate educational services prior to an RTC admission and to need an IEP meeting and their educational plan rewritten to address issues that have become better defined during their stay.

Also, with the current national trend of standardized testing, the requirements for the attainment of a high school diploma are more stringent. Adolescents who enter high school unprepared because they failed in middle school, or they deviated off track because of their mental illness or substance abuse, can find themselves behind and frustrated, and this further contributes to their hopelessness and increases their behavior problems. Treatment in an RTC is a time to get the child educationally back on track and then to find them a school that can address their individualized needs.

The last phase of discharge planning is the transition phase. One of the unique aspects of residential treatment is the ability to send children on sign-outs. This allows the treatment team to assess whether the gains the child has made are solid enough to withstand the stresses and strains of a less structured environment. The RTC by its very nature is a contained, highly structured living environment with school close by or even physically connected to the living space. There are staff everywhere ready to intervene at the first sign of behavioral escalation. There are quiet rooms and rooms that can be locked for safety, and dangerous objects are not readily available. It is not a normal space for a child to grow up. It is instead a safe therapeutic space for treatment. Sign-outs outside of the therapeutic space usually begin gradually, with visiting in unlocked areas, then on grounds, followed by off grounds. If safety has been maintained, home sign-outs begin with day passes and then progress to overnight stays. Most programs have a limit on how long the resident can be home, with these limits ranging from 24 hours to 72 hours. Longer overnight sign-outs test both the family's readiness to reintegrate the child into family life and the resident's ability to be safe in the less structured normal environment of a home. When children return from sign-outs, families are encouraged to discuss challenges that occurred and how they were handled, with the goal of improving management strategies and communication. The child's individual therapy similarly focuses on how they were able to use the coping skills and strategies they have been learning in their therapy. The transition from an RTC to home is successful when everyone is feeling comfortable that treatment goals not only have been met within the RTC but have been transferred to home and community. A successful transition phase enhances the probability of success after discharge.

Conclusion

RTCs are an essential component of the system of care for children with major mental illness, yet research on effective treatment and aftercare for this population of children is scant. The reasons for this are both practical and philosophical. On the practical side, most programs fit into the category of general RTCs and accept children with a variety of diagnoses and adapt the treatment they provide to the child's needs. The naturally occurring comorbidity and the variable socioeconomic backgrounds of children in residential treatment conflict with the methodology of research underlying evidence-based practices that align a specific treatment with a specific well-defined diagnosis. Because of their need to stay financially afloat, programs cannot restrict admissions to fit a particular diagnosis. Programs must accept a child who is in need of care, versus excluding or denying admission to a child who falls into an exclusion category for a research paradigm that is being tested.

Specialty programs do have the ability to limit who they accept and are a better fit with testing and utilizing evidence-based research. Specialty programs such as eating disorder programs, autism programs, and programs for youth with conduct disorder—all of which use strict admission criteria—are able to adopt evidence-based treatment approaches. The Boys Town Family Home Program, with its admission criteria restricted to boys with conduct disorder, is an example. Specialty programs often have specific funding streams that they have developed over time, including foundations and private grants.

For both general and specialty programs, however, what one learns about a program in one state may not apply to another state because of the extremely varied aftercare resources available depending on geographical locale. Sustaining the success a child has achieved with residential treatment is closely tied to the aftercare resources available. A child successfully treated and doing well on a complex combination of medications will almost certainly relapse and be rehospitalized if medications are not monitored and refilled. Similarly, a child who has a well-developed, functional behavioral plan that requires aftercare with professionals with applied behavioral analysis training may not be able to find this treatment if discharge is to return to living in a rural area.

Promising research has evolved with a collaborative approach focused on outcomes data utilizing the CANS (Lyons 2009). As noted earlier, the CANS has been utilized to identify children who need residential treatment and also to look at improvement at discharge from care. Two states, Illinois and New Jersey, have used it extensively, while its use is sporadic in other states.

Whittaker et al. (2015) emphasize the development of residential treatment into a "cogent and complete intervention strategy" within a system of care. Emphasized as a last-resort treatment, residential treatment serves the most challenging youth in the United States and is the "optimal intervention for very high-risk, multi-need youth." They make the distinction, however, that if the youth do not have someone in the community to return to, there is a great risk of institutionalization. Their research has also shown that youth who are at lower risk are in danger of learning high-risk behaviors from peers if residential treatment is utilized for them when other less restrictive and equally effective interventions could have worked.

Two practical areas of concern regarding research are the meager nature of funding for residential care and the lack of academic affiliation. The population of children served in RTCs is heavily weighted toward those children from lower socioeconomic backgrounds. Neither they nor their parents have a voice that might shine a light on the quality-of-care issues that exist in programs or the need for research. Bleak residential care facilities are not uncommon, while shiny state-of-the-art cancer treatment centers are the norm. The stigma of mental illness combined with the disproportionate number of lower-socioeconomic-status youth affected keeps RTCs in the shadows. While there has been a tradition in American medicine for academic institutions to provide research and training, few RTCs are academically affiliated. Many child psychiatrists will train in a program without an RTC, thus creating a knowledge deficit for this crucial component of the system of care for children. Also, without academic affiliation, RTCs lack the infrastructure necessary for research.

Perhaps the most concerning area in the United States is the lack of political will to provide a comprehensive, well thought out system of care for children with serious mental illness. While child welfare organizations like the Casey Foundation and others continue to advocate on behalf of children, it has been 40 years since therapeutic residential care has received federal grant funding to develop model programs in the United States. It remains to be seen whether the current trend toward a universal health care system will include a comprehensive approach to treating children and adolescents with severe mental health needs.

References

American Academy of Child and Adolescent Psychiatry: Principles of Care for Treatment of Children and Adolescents With Mental Illnesses in Residential Treatment Centers. Washington, DC, Work Group on Healthcare Access and Economics, 2010

Anderson RL, Lyons JS, Giles DM, et al: Reliability of the Child and Adolescent Needs and Strengths-Mental Health (CANS-MH) Scale. Journal of Child and Family Studies 12(3):279–289, 2003

Bellonci C: Physician leadership in residential treatment for children and adolescents. Child Adolesc Psychiatr Clin N Am 19(1):21–30, 2010 19951804

Briggs EC, Greeson JKP, Layne CM, et al: Trauma exposure, psychosocial functioning, and treatment needs of youth in residential care: preliminary findings from the NCTSN Core Data Set. J Child Adolesc Trauma 5:1–15, 2012

Chor BKH, McClelland GM, Weiner DA, Lyons JS: Predicting outcomes of children in residential treatment: a comparison of a decision support algorithm and a multidisciplinary team decision model. Child Youth Serv Rev 34(11):2345–2352, 2012

Hockenberry S, Sickmund M, Sladky A: Juvenile Residential Facility Census, 2006: Selected Findings. Washington, DC, U.S. Department of Justice, Office of Justice Programs, Bureau of Justice Statistics, 2009

Ireys H, Achman L, Takyi A: State Regulation of Residential Facilities for Children With Mental Illness (DHHS Publ No [SMA] 06-4167). Rockville, MD, Center for Mental Health Services, Substance Abuse and Mental Health Services Administration, 2006

Lyons JS: Knowledge creation through total clinical outcomes management: a practice-based evidence solution to address some of the challenges of knowledge translation. J Can Acad Child Adolesc Psychiatry 18(1):38–45, 2009 19270847

Manderscheid R, Atay J, Mernandes-Cartagena M, et al: Highlights of organized mental health services in 1998 and major national and state trends, in Mental Health, United States, 2000 (DHHS Publ No [SMA] 01-2527). Edited by Manderscheid RW, Henderson MJ. Washington, DC, Superintendent of Documents, U.S. Government Printing Office, 2001, pp 135–172

Pecora PJ, English DJ: Elements of Effective Practice for Children and Youth Served by Therapeutic Residential Care. Seattle, WA, Casey Family Programs, 2016. Available at: www.casey.org/media/Group-Care-Exec-summ-complete.pdf.

Redl F: The concept of a "therapeutic milieu." Am J Orthopsychiatry 29:721–736, 1959 14436829

Substance Abuse and Mental Health Services Administration: National Mental Health Services Survey (N-MHSS): 2016, Data on Mental Health Treatment Facilities. Rockville, MD, Substance Abuse and Mental Health Services Administration, 2017

Trieschman AE, Whittaker JK, Brendtro LK: The Other 23 Hours. Chicago, IL, Aldine, 1969

Whittaker JK, del Valle JF, Holmes L: Therapeutic Residential Care for Youth: Developing Evidence-Based International Practice. London, Jessica Kingsley, 2015

Whittaker JK, Holmes L, del Valle JF, et al: Therapeutic residential care for children and youth: a consensus statement of the International Work Group on Therapeutic Residential Care. Resid Treat Child Youth 33(2):89–106, 2016

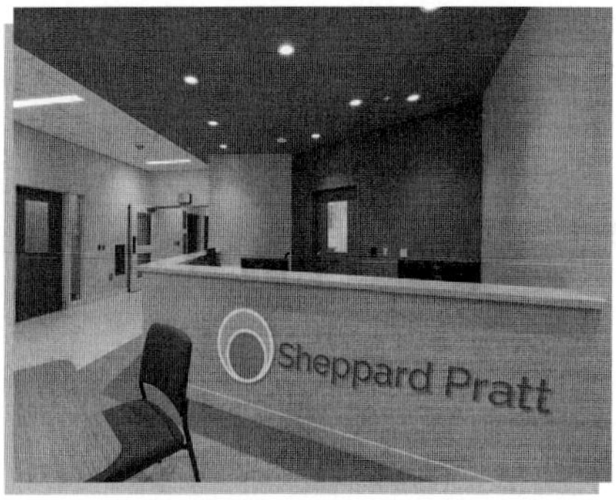

CHAPTER 15

Residential Intensive Psychodynamic Psychotherapy for Adults

Eric M. Plakun, M.D.
Edward R. Shapiro, M.D.

Pursuit of Recovery Within a Continuum of Care

The generally accepted overall goal of treatment for patients with mental health and substance use disorders is the achievement of "recovery." *Recovery* is defined by the Substance Abuse and Mental Health Services Administration (2014) as "a process of change through which individuals improve their health and wellness, live a self-directed life, and strive to reach their full potential." For most patients, pursuit of recovery may be achieved in an outpatient setting. For outpatient treatment to be effective, though, a patient must have two capacities. The first is the capacity to use the sessions: getting to them; engaging in the process whether it be medication management, psychotherapy, or something else; tolerating whatever affects arise during the session; and leaving when the session ends. The second essential capacity is functioning adaptively between sessions, including functioning in relationships, instrumental functioning (e.g., work or school), and managing affects between sessions (Plakun 2018a).

When an individual struggles with one or both of these capacities, we add treatment components. We may add medications if the treatment was psychotherapy, or add psychotherapy if treatment was medications. We also may add support groups, skills training, substance use disorder treatment, family therapy, or more frequent sessions. For a subset of patients, adding services does not adequately help them use the sessions or manage between them as they pursue recovery. For many of these patients, crises lead to brief inpatient treatment with a focus on crisis stabilization and prompt return to outpatient treatment.

For another group of patients struggling as outpatients, a pattern of recurrent crises or enduring impasses mitigates against the achievement of recovery as outpatients. For these patients, appropriate treatment requires so-called intermediate levels of care (e.g., residential treatment or intensive outpatient programs [IOPs]). These offer additional support for a long enough period so that a patient can address underlying issues (e.g., trauma or early adversity) or comorbid disorders that interfere with successful use of outpatient treatment to achieve recovery.

Emergence of Residential Treatment

The transformation of both the delivery and funding of health care in the last part of the twentieth and early twenty-first centuries had a dramatic impact on the treatment of mental health disorders and hospital psychiatry. Escalating health care costs in the 1980s and 1990s led to the dramatic expansion of managed care in the 1990s. Managed care operates with the same moral imperative as the environmental movement in that limited resources must be managed responsibly. However, in order to contain and manage costs, insurance entities refocused psychiatric treatment away from pursuit of recovery and toward more limited goals of crisis stabilization and symptom remission. They shortened the duration of outpatient treatment, often severely limiting the number of sessions allowed annually and expecting a focus on symptom remission through prescription of medication. They dramatically shortened the inpatient length of stay, from weeks, months, or more to days or perhaps weeks, again with a goal of crisis stabilization followed by prompt discharge. In response to these changes, a number of high-quality, long-term hospitals that had been focused on recovery closed their doors or became short-term crisis stabilization centers. Patient readmissions to inpatient hospitals increased and the doctor-patient relationship continued its transformation from an intimate encounter to a bureaucratically structured negotiation of the need for and terms of treatment with third-party payers (Geller 2006; Plakun 1999, 2018a; Shapiro 2001b).

Though clinicians recognized that the ultimate goal of treatment was the achievement of recovery, there was little they could do in the face of these changes. A few long-term hospitals, most notably the Austen Riggs Center, recognized that pursuit of recovery would sometimes require longer-term immersion in a 24/7 treatment setting. In response, these hospitals shifted their identity to become residential treatment centers. Of necessity this shift meant largely operating outside the world of insurance.

Since the expansion of managed care in the 1990s, top-down legislation and bottom-up litigation have begun to reshape the landscape of care for mental and substance use disorders. Among the top-down legislative influences was the 2008 Mental

Health Parity and Addiction Equity Act (MHPAEA or mental health parity law), which required that if an insurance entity provided mental and substance use disorder benefits, obstacles to access these benefits could not be substantially more stringent than those for medical and surgical care. The 2014 "final rules" of MHPAEA clarified that parity applied to all levels of care, including so-called intermediate levels of care, specified as partial hospital programs, residential treatment centers, and IOPs.

In 2011, the Affordable Care Act (ACA), in addition to providing insurance access to millions of previously uninsured citizens, reinforced the terms of the mental health parity law, requiring that mental and substance use disorders be covered as part of the essential benefit package of ACA exchange plans and that previously secret criteria for access to care be disclosed to those denied treatment. However, 11 years after passage of the mental health parity law, implementation is still incomplete. In 2020, the bipartisan Mental Health Parity Compliance Act, which requires insurance companies to disclose their degree of compliance with the terms of the mental health parity law, was passed into law as part of the 2020 Consolidated Appropriations Act.

Bottom-up actions impacting managed care include class action lawsuits against insurance companies, alleging that they had breached their fiduciary duty by substituting crisis stabilization for the broader recovery-oriented focus that is the generally accepted standard among clinicians. In *Wit v. United Behavioral Health/Optum*, the class of plaintiffs alleged a systematic breach of fiduciary duty as demonstrated in UBH's access-to-care criteria for outpatient, intensive outpatient, and residential treatment (Appelbaum and Parks 2020). In his landmark verdict for the plaintiffs, Chief Magistrate Judge Joseph Spero faulted United Behavioral Health/Optum for focusing treatment too narrowly on crisis stabilization rather than on addressing underlying issues and co-occurring disorders, and for putting profits above fiduciary duty to patients.

In their summary of Judge Spero's 106-page verdict in the liability phase of the trial, Appelbaum and Parks (2020, p. 204) cite eight central principles of accepted standards of care (*emphasis ours*):

1. Effective treatment requires treatment of the individual's underlying condition and *is not limited to alleviation of the individual's current symptoms.*
2. *Effective treatment requires treatment of co-occurring mental health and substance use disorders and/or medical conditions in a coordinated manner* that considers the interactions of the disorders when determining the appropriate level of care.
3. *Patients should receive treatment for mental health and substance use disorders at the least intensive and restrictive level of care that is safe and effective.* [The least restrictive setting for treatment that will not only address the patient's safety, but also promote improvement in the patient's condition. The fact that a lower level of care is less restrictive or intensive does not justify selecting that level if it is also expected to be less effective. Placement in a less restrictive environment is appropriate only if it is likely to be safe and just as effective as treatment at a higher level of care in addressing a patient's overall condition, including underlying and co-occurring conditions.]
4. *When there is ambiguity as to the appropriate level of care, the practitioner should err on the side of caution by placing the patient in a higher level of care.*
5. Effective treatment of mental health and substance use disorders includes services needed to maintain functioning or prevent deterioration. [Treatment services should continue if there is a reasonable expectation that if treatment services were withdrawn the patient's condition would deteriorate, relapse further, or require hospitalization.]

6. *The appropriate duration of treatment for mental health and substance use disorders is based on the individual needs of the patient; there is no specific limit on the duration of such treatment.*
7. *The unique needs of children and adolescents must be taken into account* when making decisions regarding the level of care involving their treatment for mental health or substance use disorders.
8. *The determination of the appropriate level of care for patients with mental health and/or substance use disorders should be made on the basis of a multidimensional assessment* that takes into account a wide variety of information about the patient.

Recognition in federal court that generally accepted standards for treatment of mental disorders must focus beyond mere crisis stabilization is relevant to all levels of care but especially for residential treatment centers. These top-down pieces of legislation and bottom-up litigation victories should require managed care entities to support the pursuit of recovery and increase access to all levels of care, including residential treatment when indicated.

Indications for Residential Treatment

As noted above, residential treatment may be indicated for patients who are unable to pursue recovery as outpatients because they lack one or both of the essential skills necessary to achieve recovery through outpatient treatment. Patients lacking these skills are often those who become known as "treatment resistant," though it is likely that the resistance lies in the limits of our treatment offerings for them, or in our own limits, rather than in the patients themselves.

Although many of our treatments—medication and psychotherapy—are evidence based and efficacious, these findings are generally established through randomized controlled trials (RCTs) that carefully select only those patients with one disorder. Although this may be a rigorous methodology for testing the efficacy of a treatment for a given disorder, most patients—as they present for treatment in the real world—do not present with just one disorder. For example, the large, multisite STAR*D study indicated that fully 78% of those presenting for treatment with a diagnosis of depression also have the kind of comorbid disorders or suicidal ideation that would exclude them from RCTs (Wisniewski et al. 2009). Further, these patients with comorbid conditions or suicidal ideation have significantly lower response rates to the treatments tested and remission rates.

Comorbidity is widely recognized as the rule rather than the exception among patients, especially those with treatment-resistant disorders. In addition, researchers have discovered that there are no specific genes for the Kraepelinian categories of mental disorders described in DSM-5 (American Psychiatric Association 2013), but instead dozens to hundreds of single nucleotide polymorphisms associated with one or more disorders (Plakun 2015, 2018b). This recognition has led to the delineation of a single underlying psychopathology factor ("p") that predicts the presence of one or more mental and substance use disorders (Caspi and Moffitt 2018; Caspi et al. 2014), and to the emergence of alternative diagnostic systems such as the National Institute of Mental Health Research Domain Criteria (RDoC) and the Hierarchical Taxonomy of Psychopathology (HiTOP) (Cuthbert 2015; Kotov et al. 2017). These findings are congruent with our experience at Austen Riggs, where we found, using reliable measures of diagnosis, that the average patient had six DSM-IV Axis I and II disorders at the time of admission (American Psychiatric Association 1994; Perry et al. 2009; Plakun 2003, 2006).

Comorbidity is one factor that appears to contribute to the now widely recognized phenomenon of treatment resistance (Plakun 2006, 2011b). There is evidence that personality disorder comorbidity, in particular borderline personality disorder (BPD), plays an especially important role. Data from the Collaborative Longitudinal Personality Disorders Study (CLPS) suggest that personality disorders adversely affect the prognosis of major depressive disorder and are associated with persistent functional impairment, extensive treatment utilization, and significant risk of suicide in depressed patients (Bender et al. 2006; Skodol et al. 2005). Skodol et al. (2014) report that the presence of BPD "robustly predicts" the persistence of major depressive episodes. BPD appears to increase the likelihood that depression and other disorders will be treatment resistant (Plakun 2015, 2018b).

Although mood disorders serve as a useful illustration of the complexity of treatment-resistant disorders, the problem is not limited to that diagnosis. Nearly 75% of patients in the Clinical Antipsychotic Trials of Intervention Effectiveness (CATIE) study of patients with schizophrenia discontinued the study medication regimen before 18 months of treatment (Lieberman et al. 2005). Mintz and Belnap (2011) noted that in a 20-year period from 1998 to 2008, while overall citations in psychiatry increased by 25%, citations on treatment resistance increased 800%.

In addition to the contribution of comorbidity to treatment resistance, there is also evidence suggesting the impact of adverse childhood experiences (ACEs) on treatment outcome. For example, among the subset of patients with chronic major depressive disorders and histories of serious childhood trauma or abuse, psychotherapy alone appeared to be more effective than medication alone, and the combination superior to either modality alone (Nemeroff et al. 2003). Increased exposure to ACEs predicts an increasing likelihood of the presence of one or more mental health, substance use, and/or medical disorders, and even early death (Plakun 2018b).

ACEs not infrequently involve the failure or absence of early caretakers. Such experiences predispose the child to cautious and mistrusting attitudes toward authority. Rather than anticipating good treatment from authorities like parents or clinicians, such individuals have learned to mistrust, complicating the formation of therapeutic alliances, the most robust predictor of response to treatment. This is an issue not only in the alliances associated with psychotherapy but also in the alliance that is part of a prescribing relationship. Mintz (2002) reports the impact of nocebo (negative placebo) phenomena associated with expectation of harm, affecting both medication adherence and medication response.

Taken together, the presence of comorbidity, especially personality disorder comorbidity and ACEs, increases the likelihood that patients will be unresponsive to our best evidence-based treatments and will tend toward treatment resistance. Among this group of patients, some will be unable to use outpatient treatment successfully to pursue recovery. Therefore, even if not in a crisis requiring inpatient treatment, they might be candidates for residential treatment that addresses the presence of comorbid disorders and the impact of underlying issues, like the impact of adversity, on their capacity to form a treatment alliance that supports recovery.

Varieties of Residential Treatment

The *sine qua non* of residential treatment is a period of immersion in a setting with a milieu treatment program or therapeutic community combined with other forms of treatment. Milieu treatment may include an expectation of participation in shared work, in community meetings or other groups or roles, thus implicitly recognizing that patients are both individuals and citizens of a community. With some exceptions, residential settings are unlocked. Patients are intentionally offered more freedom than in locked inpatient settings because the intent of residential treatment centers is to give patients the opportunity to improve through practice and trial and error their ability to balance freedom with responsibility, which they will need to do in order to function better in or between sessions when they return to outpatient treatment (Belnap et al. 2004; Biel and Plakun 2015, 2019). Hence, the 24/7 containing structure or "supervision" of residential treatment is generally more "available" than "imposed," while the opposite is true of locked inpatient settings, where the containing structure is imposed.

Some residential treatment centers for mental disorders focus primarily on treatment of a particular diagnosis, though comorbidity remains the rule and not the exception. This is true in residential treatment programs for eating disorders or for those struggling with comorbid active mental and substance use disorders, as in dual diagnosis residential treatment centers (Biel and Plakun 2015, 2019).

A subset of residential treatment centers offers a relatively brief alternative to inpatient treatment for those patients struggling with suicidal or other crises that do not absolutely require an inpatient level of care. This subset of short-term residential programs focuses on crisis stabilization followed by return to outpatient treatment, with lengths of stay generally measured in weeks to a month. As managed care and insurance entities came to recognize their obligation to provide access to intermediate levels of care under the 2014 "final rules" of the mental health parity law, it was this kind of "crisis" or "short-term residential" treatment for which they developed access-to-care criteria. These criteria were essentially the same as those that had to be met to gain access to or continue treatment in acute inpatient hospitals, requiring a high degree of acuity, such as the continuing presence of "significant risk of suicide." All residential treatment was thus reduced to crisis residential in a way that was inconsistent with the intent of the mental health parity law final rules.

Indeed, the website of America's Health Insurance Plans (AHIP), an insurance industry group with close to 200 insurance plan providers as members, included a link to a white paper, authored by a nonpsychiatrist physician, that falsely argued that achievement of parity in access to intermediate levels of care in the treatment of mental disorders is not possible because "such treatment is primarily focused on stabilizing acute crises" while, in the rest of medicine and surgery, the intermediate care focus is on improving functional capacity (Yohanan 2017; see Plakun 2018a). It was this kind of misrepresentation of the generally accepted goals of residential and other forms of treatment that led to the allegation of breach of fiduciary duty in the *Wit v. United Behavioral Health/Optum* class action and to the verdict cited above.

Longer-term, "noncrisis" residential treatment centers offer treatment to address comorbidity, including underlying issues, like the impact of trauma and adversity and the chronicity and the risk of recurrence of disorders, with lengths of stay measured in months to a year or more (Sowers 2016). In addition to offering milieu treatment and/or a therapeutic community, they provide access to medications, varying degrees of nursing care, and case management, and many offer group, family, and individual psychotherapy. Some, notably Skyland Trails, may use a cognitive-behavioral orientation to individual therapy, while others, most notably the now over 100-year-old Austen Riggs Center, work from a psychodynamic perspective that shapes the intensive individual psychotherapy as well as group and family work, and even the prescription of medications, into an integrated psychodynamic system of care (Biel and Plakun 2015, 2019; Plakun 2019; Shapiro 2020). Some residential programs may offer only one residential level of care or, like Riggs, offer a continuum of care through which patients progress as they move from the greatest-intensity immersion in a 24/7 setting through less intensively staffed programs as they approach returning to outpatient care.

Psychodynamic Systems of Care: The Austen Riggs Center

There is evidence that for patients with severe personality disorders as the principal or comorbid diagnosis, an extended residential treatment program with a psychodynamic focus and a continuum of care promotes social adaptation, reduces symptoms—including the frequency of self-harm and suicide attempts—and decreases the length and frequency of readmission (Chiesa et al. 2004). In addition, data from Austen Riggs (Fowler et al. 2004; Plakun 2003, 2011b) suggest that longer-term, psychodynamic residential treatment with step-down programs can be useful for that subset of patients with treatment-resistant disorders and severe personality disorders, especially when there is a history of prominent early adversity or chronic significant risk of suicide (Perry et al. 2009).

For this group of patients, treatment resistance is often a phenomenon related to personality pathology, ordinarily manifested in disturbances in interpersonal relatedness. Organizing treatment around these personality resistances offers a focused and precise intervention to overcome the chronic risk of suicide, achieve delayed age-appropriate role functioning, and help patients take charge of their lives in a way that breaks the cycle of crisis and despair. The integrative set of specialized and intensive individual, family, group, and milieu psychotherapeutic and psychosocial treatment components (Plakun 2003, 2006, 2011b; Shapiro 2011, 2020) helps patients to learn from and better tolerate their affective experiences, allowing them to manage their lives more adaptively between sessions and ultimately return to outpatient treatment to pursue recovery.

The Patients

Who are these patients? The prospective, naturalistic, longitudinal Austen Riggs Center Follow-Along Study followed 226 patients every 6–8 months during and after treatment at Riggs for a mean of 9 years. Our data indicate complex diagnostic comorbidity, with a mean of six Axis I and II disorders (Perry et al. 2009; Plakun 2003). Fully 80% have treatment-resistant mood disorders that have failed to respond to standard interventions in inpatient and outpatient settings. Over 80% also have presentations that meet criteria for one or more personality disorders, most commonly BPD. Two-thirds have histories suggesting significant early adverse experiences of abuse, trauma, neglect, loss, or deprivation, and one-third have symptoms that meet criteria for PTSD. Nearly half have substance use disorders complicating their clinical picture, and about a quarter have symptoms of an eating disorder. About 15% present with psychotic spectrum disorders.

Beyond diagnosis, these patients typically have not been able to benefit from treatments of lesser intensity and have been unable to sustain functioning between outpatient sessions. They often demonstrate repeated struggles with authority deriving from early family dynamics, presenting histories of family conflict around the management of relationships and generational role boundaries (Berkowitz et al. 1974; Schwartz 2011; Shapiro 1982, 1982–1983; Shapiro et al. 1975). In response to problematic family dynamics, their struggles with authority contribute to considerable and frequently unconscious rage at clinicians who represent authority. While this aggression can be a useful element for patients to learn about during the course of treatment, many outpatient clinicians do not have the specialized training or experience to notice, focus on, withstand, or productively engage these patients' rage at authority (Kernberg 1984; Plakun 2006, 2011c; Shapiro 1982, 1982–1983, 2004; Winnicott 1949).

These patients often use actions rather than words for communication of intense and unbearable affect states; many have histories of recurrent self-injury and/or suicidal behavior. They have regularly been unable to adhere to prescribed medication regimens, are exquisitely sensitive to side effects, or induce countertransference reactions in the prescribers that confound treatment efforts (Mintz 2002; Mintz and Belnap 2011). On admission to Riggs, half have made at least one potentially lethal suicide attempt; over 40% have had six or more episodes of self-destructive behavior; 60% had three or more previous hospitalizations. A period preceding admission involving a downward spiral into chronic crisis management is typical, with repeated maladaptive patterns in relationships and behavior and multiple treatment failures involving medication trials and inpatient and outpatient treatment.

Nevertheless, these are also individuals with strengths. Many have had earlier life trajectories with academic, athletic, or artistic promise that have collapsed as their symptom picture has unfolded—often beginning during the period of late adolescence and early adulthood. Either the task of moving from the child role in the family to the adult role in the world has been unmanageable during this developmental transition, in what has come to be known as "failure to launch" (Erikson 1964a, 1964b; Shapiro et al. 1975), or later in life a previously good-enough equilibrium becomes destabilized when a long-standing adaptation crumbles in the face of a loss or life transition (e.g., parental death, the end of a long-term relationship, an empty nest, repetition of abuse). These patients appear to have the capacity—though usually not the experience—to learn how to use words to describe their feelings while tolerating the associated affects. They indicate a readiness to learn how to delay acting on their impulses. Often, they are at a point in their lives where they are poised between increasing desperation and readiness to change.

Basic Dilemmas in Constructing Treatment

Patients presenting with treatment-resistant disorders who are appropriate for the kind of residential treatment described in this chapter raise three central dilemmas for treatment:

1. **Alliance:** Because of difficult past experiences with caregivers, these patients fear and resist a treatment alliance. To engage them in an atmosphere that maximizes interdependency and engagement in the task of treatment requires an unremitting focus on their own authority and the importance of relationships.
2. **Limits:** In response to efforts by others (e.g., family, society, treaters) to set reasonable external behavioral limits and controls, these patients, because of their adverse early experiences, inevitably experience limits as arbitrary, unempathic, corrupt, and rigid. In response, they may attempt to defeat limits and blame treaters for their own self-destructive behavior. To construct a treatment environment that puts them in charge and offers opportunities to gain perspective on their anger and the developmental context for their attack on limits—while helping them to remain safe—is a formidable task. When the patient's strengths allow it, treatment is optimally carried out in a completely open setting that requires careful negotiation and ongoing maintenance of a therapeutic alliance (Knight 1953; Plakun 2011b), with differential authority for patients and staff. The staff's recognition of patient authority and the responsibility that goes with it creates the basis for a therapeutic community. Interdependent and clearly defined role relationships in such a community emphasize the centrality of the commitment by both patients and staff to the treatment process (Kubie 1960; Shapiro 2011, 2020).
3. **Behavior:** These patients tend to use actions rather than words to communicate. To construct a treatment where they have the opportunity to recognize and acknowledge the meaning of their behavioral communications, translate their experience into language, bear the associated feelings, and put their feelings into historical perspective requires a therapeutic community with a focused task. If such a community can focus on "examined living"—that is, providing feedback about the meaning and impact of behavior—individual patients can begin to develop a language for experience to bring into their individual psychotherapy and family work (Belnap et al. 2004; Elmendorf and Parish 2011; Fonagy et al. 2002; Shapiro 2011; Stern et al. 1986).

Suitability for Residential Care in an Open Setting

Since the program at Riggs is predicated on these core notions, the admission consultation explores them in detail in the service of negotiating a treatment alliance that can support work in an open setting (Plakun 2011a). The prospective patient's capacity to take up their own authority in the admission negotiation, use the relationship with the admissions officer for learning, and open the possibility of finding meaning in symptoms determines the patient's suitability for treatment. Admission requires an explicit offer from the admissions officer after a 2-hour consultation with the patient alone and with relevant family members. The patient's interest in accepting the offer, however ambivalently, with acknowledgment of the anxiety that must inevitably accompany the freedom of the setting, indicates the beginning of an alliance. Similarly, any third party who may be supporting the treatment financially, such as a relative, must also agree to the conditions of treatment.

A central aspect of the admission consultation is a negotiation with the prospective patient and family (if available) about managing the risks of the open setting. When the patient's treatment-resistant disorder is organized around rebellion against authority, the patient may take a passive stance of abdication of responsibility with the expectation that those in authority will take over (and fail). This becomes apparent at admission when a patient's presentation seems to insist that it is the institution's job to keep them alive.

Admission is dependent on patients beginning to recognize that it is their responsibility to manage their safety (or commit to inform staff if they become unsafe), while staff members take responsibility for overseeing the treatment process. Inevitably, engaging in and maintaining this negotiation is not possible for some, and 15%–20% of those admitted are ultimately not able to tolerate the responsibility sufficiently to sustain their treatment. Nonetheless, such an initial alliance—while often shaky and requiring ongoing vigilance—offers the best chance for a treatment process that patients can own as the first step in taking charge of their lives.

Although understanding and agreeing to the basic terms of such an alliance are preconditions for beginning treatment, patients may lack the capacity to fully enter such an alliance. This is to be expected when treating those who have experienced failure from caretakers. In many ways, achievement of a reliable, mutually trusting alliance is a goal of treatment rather than simply a precondition. As Bach (1998) notes, each rupture followed by repair and each enactment untangled and sorted out offer an opportunity for incremental increases in the capacity for mutual trust and, ultimately, the formation of the kind of alliance that will allow outpatient treatment to be more successful in the future. This kind of opening discussion with patients and their families also helps put family anxieties and unrealistic expectations in perspective and begins the process of more clearly defining roles in treatment.

The following vignette illustrates some of these points. The case and treatment principles related to it are described in more detail elsewhere (Plakun 2003).

Case Vignette

Ms. A was a widowed woman in her 40s with treatment-resistant depression and BPD who was referred to the Center because of recurrent suicidal ideation and behavior that kept her outpatient treatment chronically in crisis. Her insurance company agreed to support longer-term treatment because of the high cost to them of multiple previous short-term hospitalizations and recognition of her high suicide risk. In the admission consultation, Ms. A was able to engage with the admissions officer about the rage and despair beneath her recurrent suicidal threats, their link to an early history of sexual abuse and fears of abandonment, exacerbated by her husband's death several years earlier. She found the discussion of these issues and the tentative connections drawn between her symptoms and life history helpful and surprisingly calming, noting that she and her outpatient psychiatrist had rarely had the opportunity to explore anything but her response to medications and the level of her suicide risk. She felt able to contain her suicidal behavior if admitted, and admission was offered. Although the patient's insurance company was willing to support treatment a week at a time, it would not commit in advance to the minimum stay of 6 weeks. As a result, the patient, who had the resources, was asked to make the usual prepayment to secure the initial period of evaluation and treatment. On the day before admission the patient called to indicate her refusal to make the required prepayment, stating that if she were not admitted, she would carry out her suicide plan. The admissions officer noted her use of a suicide threat to get her way and reminded her of the work they had done to achieve an initial perspective on her struggles. He reminded her of her competence and determination in negotiating coverage with her insurance carrier and said it would be too bad if she threw away the chance for a treatment that might work. He then told her that he would not allow her to come in any way other than the one they had negotiated, which was the same for all patients admitted. Although initially enraged, Ms. A was also reassured by the holding of limits, made the prepayment, and was admitted.

Treatments

Many of the patients presenting for treatment at Austen Riggs come from multiple short-term inpatient hospitalizations in locked settings in major cities. The Austen Riggs Center presents a striking contrast. A completely open residential treatment center in stately white buildings on the main street of the small New England village of Stockbridge, Riggs offers a semirural setting for voluntary treatment. There are no privilege systems, no locked doors, and no explicit requirements to attend any treatments, though a lack of attendance inevitably leads to review of the patient's interest in treatment (Plakun 2011b).

Patients are admitted for an initial 6-week period of intensive evaluation and treatment, though most stay longer. The median length of treatment in the Riggs continuum of care (from highest-level residential programs through step-down programs to intensive outpatient care) is 6 months, with a range from 6 weeks to several years. In general, the effort is to interrupt the cycle of thwarted treatments by helping patients develop the capacity to express experience in language. This capacity increases the likelihood that after discharge patients will be able to manage outpatient psychotherapy without self-destructive behavior or other recurring crises interrupting the work, and with new abilities to engage in adaptive social role functioning.

While a brief voluntary inpatient level of care is available for patients whose treatment alliance is breached during the course of treatment, patients enter treatment at one of two residential levels of care depending on whether they are candidates for a more group-intensive or nursing-intensive initial phase of treatment. The nursing-intensive residential program offers daily individual nursing care (often used with patients struggling to contain impulses to harm themselves or to use substances), while the group-intensive residential program has less intensive nursing and relies more on peer-group support. Having been screened at admission for their capacity to engage in verbal psychotherapy, all patients begin and continue throughout their Riggs stay in four-times-weekly psychodynamic psychotherapy with a doctoral-level therapist (M.D. or Ph.D.). In addition, skill-based and symptom-focused groups are available in the community program. Those patients in psychotherapy with a psychologist also work with a psychiatrist in the limited role of psychopharmacologist who prescribes medication for sufficient symptom relief to allow the patient to participate fully in the range of treatments. Social workers, often with the individual therapist as family cotherapist, work with their families. The same interdisciplinary team that includes these clinicians and others follows the patient in transitions through various residences throughout the continuum of care. The team works together over time to integrate a coherent view of the patient from the perspectives of different disciplines (Krikorian and Fowler 2011).

Case Vignette

In a treatment team review of John, a 30-year-old man with major depressive disorder, narcissistic personality disorder, and substance use disorder, team members presented differing views of him. Nursing staff found him aloof and arrogant, challenging hospital policy and avoiding their efforts to engage him. Therapeutic community staff noted John's efforts to help younger female patients in distress, often encouraging them to speak up in community meetings. The female therapist reported John's deepening engagement in therapy and his increasing recognition of his defensive devaluation of her in the context of his beginning exploration of his vulnerability and anxiety about potential abandonment by women he depended on. The social worker reminded the team of John's younger sister's suicide in his youth—in the context of his parents' divorce—and his mother's worsening breast cancer. The discussion put John's confusing combination of defensively arrogant devaluation of older women and his caretaking efforts toward younger women in perspective, helping nursing staff to persist in their efforts to engage John and to help him see the defensive nature of his withdrawal. John began to recognize the historical determinants for his problematic relationships and the repetition of these patterns in his relationship with community members and his therapist.

There is an activities program, described by Riggs staff as a nonclinical "interpretation-free zone," where patients take up the role of "student," working in visual media, ceramics, woodworking, fiber arts, and a greenhouse. The program includes a preschool for children from the local community, where patients may serve as volunteers or paid aides. There is also a community theater, where patients collaborate with members of the outside community and a professional theater director to perform plays open to the local Berkshire community.

Case Vignette

Fran, a 36-year-old woman with an extensive history of childhood sexual abuse and multiple abusive adult relationships, was reading through a script for a planned play with a group of patients, Stockbridge residents, and the Riggs theater director. Fran was to take the role of the wife of an army officer. In one scene, the woman dies and is carried offstage in the arms of the officer. As Fran read the stage directions, she gasped, saying, "I could never let a man touch me!" The theater director responded, "But you are dead!" Fran said, "Oh, that's right," and went on to do the play with great success, bringing her struggle around her experience into her psychotherapy.

The evaluation phase culminates in the fifth week with a 2-hour case conference involving the entire clinical staff. This conference includes a 15- to 20-minute interview with the patient, in which they are invited to bring their own treatment focus and questions into a public conversation with a senior clinician. Often the patient's questions dovetail with the issues raised in the evaluation, so that the group can reach a formulation and treatment plan relevant to the patient's stated goals.

The Impact of the Setting

The open setting and the staff's reliance on patient authority meet and legitimize both autonomous functioning and dependency needs, including the need to belong (Shapiro 2013). The structures of the program support patients' strengths instead of focusing relentlessly on psychopathology:

- The open setting leans on patients' capacities to manage themselves and, in a version of free association, gives patients room for and invites them to notice the choices they make each day.
- The therapeutic community authorizes patients' leadership capacities in elected positions.

- The activities program, which formally removes them for periods of time from the patient role, offers these "students" a space for creative expression and the mobilization of strengths and capacities, conceptualized as separate from treatment.
- The culture of the Center is organized around patients developing the potential to take charge of their treatment and their lives.
- The staff is organized around the understanding that patient resistance—their "acting out"—is a form of communication that requires translation and that often is in reaction to something the staff has a role in.

All of these supportive and progressive structures serve to counterbalance the inevitable regressive pulls that are an aspect of intensive and deepening individual psychotherapy.

The treatment focuses on three sustaining values: *patient authority*, the *pursuit of meaning*, and the *importance of relationships* (Plakun 2011b). These patients communicate through projective identification and enactment the meaning of their painful life experience. In other settings, where staff authority is exercised to ensure treatment compliance, the patient may only be able to take up a passive role. This may unwittingly and paradoxically foster "treatment resistance," when resistance to treatment is the only way left for a patient to exercise authority (Plakun 2006, 2011b). Riggs, through its freedom and structured examination of relationships, is designed to engage this difficulty through individual psychotherapy, family treatment, and the way individual transferences are enacted through relationships with other patients and staff (Shapiro and Carr 1987; Kayatekin and Plakun 2011; Shapiro 2020). In a therapeutic community of examined living, the resources are available to unpack these transferences, help patients tolerate them, and provide perspective (Muller 1999).

The community is constructed as a kind of theater-in-the-round, a public opportunity for patients to live out—and begin to see—their difficulties with others. Managed by patients with staff consultation, the effort is to provide a structure for the translation of behavioral communication into words. Patient-led groups and a culture of ongoing interpersonal feedback communicate in different ways the impact that individual and group behavior have on others. For example, if a patient begins to get involved in an exclusive relationship with another patient, other patients inevitably feel envious and rejected. Public discussion of these reactions can illuminate how "pairing" is a group phenomenon (Bion 1961). If a patient is involved in self-destructive behavior, others inevitably become frightened, guilty, and worried. Discussion of these responses helps the particular patient feel less isolated and desperate. Characteristic individual defenses, ordinarily invisible to the individual, become powerfully visible in community life. Individuals—beginning to see themselves through the eyes of others—have the opportunity to take up authority and responsibility with others in a kind of participatory democracy (Elmendorf and Parish 2011; Stern et al. 1986).

Individual Psychodynamic Psychotherapy

Individual psychotherapy focuses on listening, making sense of transference and countertransference, and ensuring an unfolding receptiveness to the patient's newly formulated experience (Shapiro 1982, 1982–1983). Many patients with severe personality disorders manage their unbearable experience through the creation of painful and anger-filled relationships. Using the psychological mechanism of projective identification (Kernberg 1975, 1984; Klein 1946; Shapiro and Carr 1991) to protect themselves from their internal experience, patients unwittingly transform their internal self-critical torment into stormy and provocative behavior with others.

These patients have acute sensitivity to vulnerabilities and blind spots in their therapist's character that they unconsciously use to evoke intense countertransferences. Detection and careful unpacking of the countertransference enactments in staff discussions (Kayatekin and Plakun 2011; Kernberg 1984; Plakun 2001, 2007; Shapiro and Carr 1987) and eventually in individual psychotherapy are a frequent part of the unfolding of the treatment. This process helps patients to see the role of their self-hatred, rage, guilt, and shame in producing desperate acts of self-abuse (cutting, burning, parasuicidal and suicidal behaviors) and angry, provocative interpersonal behaviors.

The treatment environment at Riggs helps contain the impact of this behavior, translating it into a language that allows patients to gain perspective on their own unconscious motivations. However, the work proceeds with the evolving recognition that there are two fallible human beings in the consulting room when a therapist and patient meet. The therapy staff have opportunities to consult with colleagues (both on and off the treatment team) to help bear the intense countertransference of the work and find their own contribution to some of the struggles.

Psychodynamic psychotherapy in such a program focuses on character issues, paying particular attention to repeated maladaptive patterns of behavior. These are assumed to be behavioral communications ("acting out") of inarticulate and painful early experiences. Interpretive work attempts to make sense of the problematic, usually negative, transferences that for many of these patients interfere with deepening relationships. The effort in psychodynamic treatment is to help patients put feelings into words, focusing on the contexts that evoke these behavioral patterns.

Family Treatment

A central context for the development of their difficulties for many of these patients is their families. Although parents do their best to love and support their children, they may also unwittingly bring into the family system powerful unconscious issues that can contribute to treatment resistance. Riggs invites families to participate in the treatment both to help the patient and the clinicians grasp the family's perceptions of the patient's development and to begin to understand the family dynamics in which the patient's symptoms are embedded (Schwartz 2011; Shapiro and Freedman 1987). These patients often have irrational roles in their families in which they are covertly invited through projective identification to carry problematic aspects of their parents' past experiences (Berkowitz et al. 1974; Fromm 2004, 2006, 2011; Shapiro et al. 1975). Family work aimed at unpacking these relationships places each member's history in perspective, freeing the individual patient to consider their own life without the pressures of family needs (Schwartz 2011; Shapiro 1982–1983; Shapiro and Carr 1991; Shapiro et al. 1977).

Case Vignette

Bill, a brilliant and obsessive 32-year-old man, had failed at multiple attempts to complete his education. Unable to sustain a job because of frequent arguments with his male superiors, he had remained at home for years, isolated in his bedroom. Filled with hatred for his "cold, uncaring, and abusive" father, Bill insisted that he remained home in order to protect his mother. On one occasion, confronted with his own inability to motivate his son, father had said angrily to Bill, "I wish you'd never been born." These family tensions and Bill's periodic impulsive outbursts of rage led him to a potentially lethal suicide attempt that he survived by accident.

After Bill was admitted to Riggs, the therapist and social worker convened a family meeting. A rageful argument between father and son erupted, requiring the therapist to intervene. Turning to the silent mother, the therapist asked, "How do you stand this?" Mother responded, "I've given up." Both clinicians remarked to mother that given the potentially lethal outcome, she could not afford to withdraw. Recognizing how overwhelmed she was, they offered to assist her efforts to help her men discover their softer sides. This intervention opened for father and son the possibility of revealing their shared vulnerabilities and the ways they had deeply hurt each other. Their underlying love for one another, and the relationship of father's angry withdrawal to his own painful relationship with his father, slowly emerged over months of work, allowing Bill some perspective on his family experience. Mother's increasing competence in engaging this discussion helped Bill to recognize her strength, allowing him to begin to separate his needs from hers.

Psychopharmacology

Treatment resistance is often manifested in the patient's failure to respond to multiple medication trials. In work with treatment-resistant patients, the meaning of medication often plays a role in failure to respond to it (Mintz 2002; Mintz and Belnap 2011). Mintz (2002) describes the practice of "psychodynamic psychopharmacology" with these patients, exploring the meaning that medications—and their side effects—have, and the way these meanings may be part of a nocebo (negative placebo) effect. These patients regularly experience caretakers as people likely to cause harm and react to prescribed medication as potentially harmful. This may interfere with medication adherence or may manifest as side effects that have more to do with the meaning of the medication than with their pharmacokinetic effects, as in immediate side effects in response to even small doses. These adverse reactions evoke countertransference in the psychopharmacologist, contributing to the possibility of reactive irrational prescribing that adds multiple medications to respond to what is essentially a psychological problem. An interpretive treatment that includes team discussions about the meaning of medication in this patient's intrapsychic world helps uncover such patterns; translating them into words can lead to a patient's improved capacity to adhere to and tolerate potentially helpful medication regimens and engage more fully in treatment.

A second group of patients uses medications to replace relationships. Patients in this group experience their affects as "symptoms" and may use their clinical diagnoses and medications to reduce their responsibility for and engagement in life. Though patients in this group find medication helpful and necessary, they often do not appear to get better with them. Such patients at Riggs often find engagement in the therapeutic community to be an important stimulus for recognizing their own reactivity and responsiveness to others, opening the possibility of recognizing their affects as crucial instead of pathological (Mintz and Belnap 2011).

Management of Financial Resources

In the traditional medical model, others—clinicians, managed care representatives, family members—ordinarily manage the financing of treatment on behalf of the patient. Given the relevant issues for treatment of patients with mental disorders, this leaves patients in an unfortunate dependent position and creates an incentive to do poorly to prove that treatment is needed. The wish to provide patients medically necessary treatment in the face of resource limitations outside their control can lead clinicians to join patients in experiencing the "resource managers" in a shared projective way as bad, withholding, and unempathic (Shapiro 1997). Such collusion can both displace negative transference feelings from the therapy and interfere with rational collaboration around effective and appropriate use of inevitably limited resources.

Helping patients deal effectively with reality is an aspect of treatment. Facing the cost of treatment and the limitations of financial resources helps construct a mature and reliable treatment framework. Patients and families regularly have irrational emotional reactions to financial limitations, experiencing them through the filter of other limitations in life (emotional, security, health), making it difficult to think clearly. At Riggs, a group of clinicians and business staff work with patients and families around resource limitations in order to help them grasp the actual financial facts and face the often-conflicted feelings involved in using these funds (college funds, retirement assets, home equity loans) for treatment. When patients who value their Riggs treatment participate actively in discussions about the utilization of genuinely limited resources, they can emerge from a passive position and discover an incentive to manage themselves better so they can step down to a less expensive level of care to extend their treatment. Facing the limitations of resources provides opportunities for both patients and families to come to terms with anger, guilt, and grief about painful reality (Plakun 1996, 2002; Shapiro 1997, 2020).

Suicidal and Aggressive Behaviors in Treatment

The open setting at Austen Riggs allows a broad range of freedom and maintains a clear distinction between behaviors that are potentially lethal and those that are not (Plakun 1994, 2001, 2011a). Patients may well engage in non-life-threatening superficial cutting and burning and eating behaviors as inarticulate ways of managing (and expressing) their feelings or defining their boundaries (Elmendorf 2007; Gunderson 2001; Sacksteder 1989a, 1989b). These are ordinarily managed by nursing staff's bandaging or the local hospital's suturing when needed. Clinical staff members work with patients to understand the feelings, fantasies, and relationship events that lie behind these acts—and their impact on others—but recognize the futility of trying to take on the task of preventing them. These efforts over time begin to communicate to the patient that behavior is in fact communication, and often communication about unbearably painful feelings.

When self-destructive behaviors threaten the patient's life and the continuity of the treatment, the therapist immediately addresses the issue in relation to the alliance. Among other things, a suicide plan is a decision on the patient's part to end the treatment. It therefore reflects problems in the treatment relationship that must be explored, including, potentially, the therapist's unwitting contribution to that decision (Clarkin et al. 2001, 2006; Kernberg 1984; Plakun 1994, 2001, 2011a). Should a patient act with actual suicidal intent, the clinician assumes, in keeping with the clearly negotiated terms of admission, that the patient has chosen to end treatment at Riggs. The patient is ordinarily then transferred to a locked setting for emergency medical and psychiatric management. Often the patient returns to Riggs when safe, at which point a 2-week period of formal reevaluation is set in motion during which the focus of the work of the patient, therapist, and treatment team is on carrying out a consultation over the next couple of weeks to determine why the patient chose to end treatment by trying to end their life, how the therapist may have unwittingly played a role in that choice, what the patient has learned in the event, whether the patient wishes to and is able to return to the kind of alliance needed to do the work, and whether the treatment can continue or has been damaged beyond repair. This process is often a powerful intervention that, when successful, has been associated with good outcome (Plakun 1991, 2011a).

If patients engage in dangerous behaviors that suggest they are unable to keep the terms of the negotiated treatment alliance by keeping themselves safe, but they have not endangered their lives, they may briefly step up to a higher level of care for more support or, when the alliance has been ruptured in a way that does not warrant transfer to a locked setting elsewhere, to a fully voluntary inpatient setting in the principal residential setting building. Depending on which level of care they have entered, during this time they negotiate with nursing staff about the limits of their freedom (for example, turning in car keys and/or not leaving the hospital grounds) that make clinical sense while their treatment focuses intensively on monitoring their safety and determining whether they can repair the ruptured treatment alliance or need treatment elsewhere. The Center does not use any restraint or seclusion, unless acute psychotic or impulsive suicidal behavior requires temporary restraint prior to transfer. In such circumstances the police are called to help staff manage the situation. This happens rarely, since the culture of the community ordinarily helps patients turn to staff or to one another before they lose control.

Research

Wallerstein (1986) and Gabbard et al. (2000) have presented cohort studies of patients treated at the Menninger Clinic suggesting the value of extended treatment for similar patients. Chiesa et al. (2004) provided evidence that extended psychodynamic residential treatment within a continuum of care is an effective treatment for patients with severe personality disorders comorbid with other disorders.

The Austen Riggs Center has studied this patient population since the 1950s, when Robert Knight (1954) wrote the seminal paper on borderline patients. Psychoanalytic theoreticians, including Erik Erikson, David Rapaport, and Roy Shafer, developed the field of ego psychology at Riggs in the 1950s by working with this patient population (Erikson 1956, 1964a; Rapaport 1959, 1967; Shafer 1999). Otto Will (1980) deepened his studies of psychotic disorders at Riggs, while several studies in the 1970s and 1980s focused on the outcomes of patients in treatment at the Center (Blatt and Ford 1994; Plakun 1991); Plakun et al. 1985).

Recognizing that Riggs had an opportunity to study this group of patients more intensively and in more depth than colleagues could in other settings—and that the clinical data included the family and social context—the institution decided that it had an obligation to the larger field. In 1994, Riggs created the Erikson Institute for Education and Research to continue this learning and apply the concepts emerging from this work to other settings. For the next decade or more, Riggs was engaged in the follow-along study described above, examining the progression of 226 patients (51% of the available sample) at 6-month intervals for 6–10 years. The hope was to learn about the natural progression of this difficult-to-treat group of patients.

In a 2009 publication from this study, Perry et al. (2009) reported on outcomes with patients with previous suicide attempts and continuing struggles with suicide. Results showed that 75% of these suicidal patients were recovered from suicide as an active issue in their lives at an average of 7 years after admission. Using a more recent sample of similarly suicidal patients, Tillman (2019) also reports, from unpublished data, that 70%–75% moved from suicidal behavior to suicidal ideation without associated behavior at a mean of 7 years after admission.

In a 2021 publication from the above-referenced study of 226 Riggs patients, Perry and Fowler (2021) report on a subset of 54 patients who were followed at regular intervals for up to 14 years to determine the time required to achieve full recovery, not mere symptom remission. The patients were followed using measures of symptoms, psychopathology, global functioning, and psychodynamic measures of conflicts and adaptive functioning. Consistent with the role of intermediate levels of care as focused on improving patients' capacity to use outpatient treatment to pursue recovery, almost all patients continued outpatient therapy following a mean 10-month period of treatment in the Riggs continuum of care. As predicted, change in the other measures used converged with measures of psychodynamic change. Using the assumption that rates of recovery would continue after the last follow-up data point, Perry and Fowler identified four groups in terms of recovery:

- Those who were judged recovered or on a trajectory to recovery in 11.63 years (28, or 52%).
- Those who were likely to recover before 20 years (8, or 15%).
- Those who were more unlikely than likely to recover (11, or 20%).
- Those who deteriorated (7, or 13%).

Overall, 36 of 54, or 66.67%, were judged likely to achieve full recovery before 20 years. It is sobering that achievement of full recovery took over a decade, but improvement in symptoms and functional capacity preceded achievement of full recovery. It is hopeful that true recovery was possible for two-thirds of this group of treatment resistant patients.

In addition, the Erikson Institute has begun to apply the learning from Riggs to some of the problems of the larger society, ranging from administration (Shapiro 2001a, 2001c), to the transgenerational transmission of trauma (Fromm 2004, 2011), to citizenship (Shapiro 2003, 2005, 2020; Shapiro and Carr 2006).

Conclusion

There is a subset of patients with treatment-resistant disorders, often patients with ACEs and comorbid mood and personality disorders plus other comorbid disorders, for whom "resistance" to treatment is organized around unconsciously determined difficulty engaging in a treatment alliance in which they can find their own authentic voice and authority. Recognizing that the alliance is the foundation that supports treatment, the Austen Riggs Center has constructed a focused residential approach to these patients. The Center places patients in charge of themselves in an open setting in which authority is negotiated between staff and patients rather than exclusively assumed by staff. The negotiated agreement is to explore the patient's mind and the meaning of behavior and relationships. The patient's deviations from that agreement and related acting-out behavior—when not threatening the patient's life or the treatment of others—are seen as opportunities for learning, since these patients tend to communicate their difficulties through behavior.

In this residential setting, attention to both the meaning of medication and its pharmacological effects helps maximize its optimal utilization. Individual psychodynamic psychotherapy is designed to help patients focus on a deepening intimate relationship in which aspects of the past are reexperienced and translated into language. Since these patients tend to split their transferences—often by idealizing one relationship and devaluing another—the capacity of the staff to sustain and examine the patient's relationships with all members of the treatment team allows the possibility of showing the patient how this phenomenon occurs, while offering the possibility of reintegrating these split relationships within the individual therapy. At the same time, the experience of examined living, with continual feedback from a therapeutic community, helps patients translate their behavior into language and meaningful experience. Concurrent family work gives patients perspective on the developmental context of disturbance and helps to mobilize family relationships and resources for the treatment.

The constellation of resources available at Riggs adds to contemporary general psychiatric treatment a diverse range of psychosocial treatments integrated by a psychodynamic understanding of personality functioning. These patients with treatment-resistant disorders may also be conceived of as delegates of their families and social contexts who are carrying potential learning about the unbearable difficulties of the interpersonal world and the larger society. The evidence indicates that far from being doomed to chronic crisis management, such patients are treatable in a residential setting and capable of finding their voices and a role in society, as well as returning to outpatient treatment better able to use it, and to function adaptively between sessions as they pursue recovery. Further, many of the insights developed from the intensive clinical work in this national referral center are applicable to other settings, including outpatient settings.

Given the substantial problem of treatment resistance, it is important that this center and similar comprehensive, integrative, psychodynamically based residential treatment centers remain available as part of the generally accepted provision of care for these patients, who have much to offer and from whom we have so much to learn. It is reassuring the legislative and judicial action appear to be confirming the value of residential treatment and other intermediate levels of care, while reclaiming the generally accepted goal of treatment as pursuing recovery rather than mere crisis stabilization.

Patients with treatment-resistant disorders emerge from our increasingly complex and stressful social contexts. Successful treatment of these illnesses requires a serious clinical commitment from the profession both to recognize how these struggles develop and to provide a sufficient biopsychosocial treatment space so that these patients might find their way to rejoin the larger society.

References

American Psychiatric Association: Diagnostic and Statistical Manual of Mental Disorders, 4th Edition. Washington, DC, American Psychiatric Association, 1994

American Psychiatric Association: Diagnostic and Statistical Manual of Mental Disorders, 5th Edition. Arlington, VA, American Psychiatric Association, 2013

Appelbaum PS, Parks J: Holding insurers accountable for parity in coverage of mental health treatment. Psychiatr Serv 71(2):202–204, 2020
Bach S: On treating the difficult patient, in The Modern Freudians: Contemporary Psychoanalytic Technique. Edited by Ellman CS, Grand S, Silvan M, Ellman SF. Lanham, MD, Jason Aronson, 1998, pp 185–195
Belnap BA, Iscan C, Plakun EM: Residential treatment of personality disorders: the containing function, in Handbook of Personality Disorders: Theory and Practice. Edited by Magnavita JJ. New York, Wiley, 2004, pp 379–397
Bender DS, Skodol AE, Pagano ME, et al: Prospective assessment of treatment use by patients with personality disorders. Psychiatr Serv 57(2):254–257, 2006 16452705
Berkowitz DA, Shapiro RL, Zinner J, Shapiro ER: Family contributions to narcissistic disturbances in adolescents. Int Rev Psychoanal 1:353–362, 1974
Biel S, Plakun EM: Psychodynamic systems of residential treatment: another view from Riggs. Psychodyn Psychiatry 43(1):91–116, 2015 25734876
Biel S, Plakun EM: Therapeutic community then and now. Psychiatry 82(1):18–23, 2019 30870108
Bion WR: Experiences in Groups. London, Tavistock, 1961
Blatt SJ, Ford RQ: Therapeutic Change: An Object Relations Perspective. New York, Plenum, 1994
Caspi A, Moffitt TE: All for one and one for all: mental disorders in one dimension. Am J Psychiatry 175(9):831–844, 2018 29621902
Caspi A, Houts RM, Belsky DW, et al: The p factor: one general psychopathology factor in the structure of psychiatric disorders? Clin Psychol Sci 2(2):119–137, 2014 25360393
Chiesa M, Fonagy P, Holmes J, Drahorad C: Residential versus community treatment of personality disorders: a comparative study of three treatment programs. Am J Psychiatry 161(8):1463–1470, 2004 15285974
Clarkin JF, Foelsch PA, Levy KN, et al: The development of a psychodynamic treatment for patients with borderline personality disorder: a preliminary study of behavioral change. J Pers Disord 15(6):487–495, 2001 11778390
Clarkin JF, Yoemans F, Kernberg OF: Psychotherapy of Borderline Personality: Focusing on Object Relations. Washington, DC, American Psychiatric Publishing, 2006
Cuthbert BN: Research Domain Criteria: toward future psychiatric nosologies. Dialogues Clin Neurosci 17(1):89–97, 2015 25987867
Elmendorf DM: Containment and the use of the skin, in The Embodied Subject: Minding the Body in Psychoanalysis. Edited by Muller JP, Tillman JG. New York, Rowman & Littlefield, 2007
Elmendorf DM, Parish M: Silencing the messenger: the social dynamics of treatment resistance, in Treatment Resistance and Patient Authority: The Austen Riggs Reader. Edited by Plakun EM. New York, WW Norton, 2011, pp 204–223
Erikson EH: The problem of ego identity. J Am Psychoanal Assoc 4(1):56–121, 1956 13286157
Erikson E: Identity: Youth and Crisis (Austen Riggs Monograph No 7). New York, WW Norton, 1964a
Erikson E: The nature of clinical evidence, in Insight and Responsibility: Lectures on the Ethical Implications of Psychoanalytic Insight. New York, WW Norton, 1964b, pp 47–80
Fonagy P, Gergely G, Jurist E, et al: Affect Regulation, Mentalization and the Development of the Self. New York, Other Press, 2002
Fowler JC, Ackerman SJ, Speanburg S, et al: Personality and symptom change in treatment-refractory inpatients: evaluation of the phase model of change using Rorschach, TAT, and DSM-IV Axis V. J Pers Assess 83(3):306–322, 2004 15548467
Fromm M: Psychoanalysis and trauma: September 11 revisited. Diogenes 51(3):3–14, 2004
Fromm MG: Transmission of trauma and treatment resistance, in Treatment Resistance and Patient Authority: The Austen Riggs Reader. Edited by Plakun EM. New York, WW Norton, 2011, pp 80–96
Gabbard GO, Coyne L, Allen JG, et al: Evaluation of intensive inpatient treatment of patients with severe personality disorders. Psychiatr Serv 51(7):893–898, 2000 10875954

Geller JL: Avoiding extinction: successful private psychiatric hospitals in the opening decade of the twenty-first century. Psychiatr Q 77(2):189–201, 2006 16779684
Gunderson JG: Borderline Personality Disorder: A Clinical Guide. Washington, DC, American Psychiatric Publishing, 2001
Kayatekin MS, Plakun EM: From acting out to enactment in treatment-resistant disorders, in Treatment Resistance and Patient Authority: The Austen Riggs Reader. Edited by Plakun EM. New York, WW Norton, 2011, pp 24–41
Kernberg OF: Borderline Conditions and Pathological Narcissism. New York, Jason Aronson, 1975
Kernberg OF: Severe Personality Disorders: Psychotherapeutic Strategies. New Haven, CT, Yale University Press, 1984
Klein M: Notes on some schizoid mechanisms. Int J Psychoanal 27 (Pt 3–4):99–110, 1946 20261821
Knight RP: Management and psychotherapy of the borderline schizophrenic patient. Bull Menninger Clin 17(4):139–150, 1953 13066875
Knight RP: Borderline states, in Psychoanalytic Psychiatry and Psychology: Clinical and Theoretical Papers (Austen Riggs Monograph No 1). Edited by Knight RP, Friedman CR. New York, International Universities Press, 1954, pp 97–122
Kotov R, Krueger RF, Watson D, et al: The Hierarchical Taxonomy of Psychopathology (HiTOP): A dimensional alternative to traditional nosologies. J Abnorm Psychol 126(4):454–477, 2017 28333488
Krikorian SE, Fowler JC: A team approach to treatment resistance, in Treatment Resistance and Patient Authority: The Austen Riggs Reader. Edited by Plakun EM. New York, WW Norton, 2011, pp 245–268
Kubie LS: The Riggs Story: The Development of the Austen Riggs Center or the Study and Treatment of the Psychoneuroses. New York, Paul B Hoeber, 1960
Lieberman JA, Stroup TS, McEvoy JP, et al: Effectiveness of antipsychotic drugs in patients with chronic schizophrenia. N Engl J Med 353(12):1209–1223, 2005 16172203
Mintz D: Meaning and medication in the care of treatment-resistant patients. Am J Psychother 56(3):322–337, 2002 12400200
Mintz D, Belnap B: What is psychodynamic psychopharmacology? An approach to pharmacologic treatment resistance, in Treatment Resistance and Patient Authority: The Austen Riggs Reader. Edited by Plakun EM. New York, WW Norton, 2011, pp 42–65
Muller J: The Third as holding the dyad. Psychoanal Dialogues 9:471–480, 1999
Nemeroff CB, Heim CM, Thase ME, et al: Differential responses to psychotherapy versus pharmacotherapy in patients with chronic forms of major depression and childhood trauma. Proc Natl Acad Sci USA 100(24):14293–14296, 2003 14615578
Perry JC, Fowler JC: A naturalistic study of time to recovery in adults with treatment-refractory disorders. Psychiatry 84:260–275, 2021 34346828
Perry JC, Fowler JC, Bailey A, et al: Improvement and recovery from suicidal and self-destructive phenomena in treatment-refractory disorders. J Nerv Ment Dis 197(1):28–34, 2009 19155807
Plakun EM: Prediction of outcome in borderline personality disorder. J Pers Disord 5:93–101, 1991
Plakun EM: Principles in the psychotherapy of self-destructive borderline patients. J Psychother Pract Res 3(2):138–148, 1994 22700187
Plakun EM: Economic grand rounds: treatment of personality disorders in an era of resource limitation. Psychol Serv 47:128–130, 1996
Plakun EM: Managed care discovers the talking cure, in Psychoanalytic Therapy as Health Care: Effectiveness and Economics in the 21st Century. Edited by Haley H, Eagle M, Wolitsky D. Hillsdale, NJ, Analytic Press, 1999, pp 239–255
Plakun EM: Making the alliance and taking the transference in work with suicidal patients. J Psychother Pract Res 10(4):269–276, 2001 11696654
Plakun EM: Jihad, McWorld and enactment in the postmodern mental health world. J Am Acad Psychoanal 30(3):341–353, discussion 355–360, 2002 12389511

Plakun EM: Treatment-refractory mood disorders: a psychodynamic perspective. J Psychiatr Pract 9(3):209–218, 2003 15985933
Plakun EM: A view from Riggs—treatment resistance and patient authority, I: a psychodynamic perspective on treatment resistance. J Am Acad Psychoanal Dyn Psychiatry 34(2):349–366, 2006 16780414
Plakun EM: Perspectives on embodiment: from symptom to enactment and from enactment to sexual misconduct, in The Embodied Subject: Minding the Body in Psychoanalysis. Edited by Muller JP, Tillman JG. Lanham, MD, Rowman & Littlefield, 2007, pp 103–116
Plakun EM: An alliance-based intervention for suicide, in Treatment Resistance and Patient Authority: The Austen Riggs Reader. Edited by Plakun EM. New York, WW Norton, 2011a, pp 136–159
Plakun EM (ed): Treatment Resistance and Patient Authority: The Austen Riggs Reader. New York, WW Norton, 2011b
Plakun EM: Working with the negative transference, in Treatment Resistance and Patient Authority: The Austen Riggs Reader. Edited by Plakun EM. New York, WW Norton, 2011c, pp 66–79
Plakun EM: Psychotherapy and Psychosocial Treatment: Recent Advances and Future Directions. Psychiatr Clin North Am 38(3):405–418, 2015 26300031
Plakun EM: Clinical and insurance perspectives on intermediate levels of care in psychiatry. J Psychiatr Pract 24(2):111–116, 2018a 29509181
Plakun EM: Psychodynamic psychiatry, the biopsychosocial model, and the difficult patient. Psychiatr Clin North Am 41(2):237–248, 2018b 29739523
Plakun EM: One hundred years of Austen Riggs. J Psychiatr Pract 25(4):298–302, 2019 31291210
Plakun EM, Burkhardt PE, Muller JP: 14-year follow-up of borderline and schizotypal personality disorders. Compr Psychiatry 26(5):448–455, 1985 4028695
Rapaport D: A historical survey of psychoanalytic ego psychology. Psychol Issues 1:5–17, 1959
Rapaport D: The theory of ego autonomy, in Collected Papers of David Rapaport. New York, Basic Books, 1967, pp 722–741
Sacksteder JL: Psychosomatic dissociation and false self development in anorexia nervosa, in The Facilitating Environment: Clinical Applications of Winnicott's Theories. Edited by Smith BL, Fromm MG. New York, International Universities Press, 1989a
Sacksteder JL: Sadomasochistic relatedness to the body in anorexia nervosa, in Masochism: The Treatment of Self-Inflicted Suffering. Edited by Montgomery JD, Greif AC. New York, International Universities Press, 1989b
Schwartz A: Working with family resistance to treatment, in Treatment Resistance and Patient Authority: The Austen Riggs Reader. Edited by Plakun EM. New York, WW Norton, 2011, pp 224–244
Shafer R: Recentering psychoanalysis from Heinz Hartmann to the contemporary British Kleinians. Psychoanal Psychol 16(3):339–354, 1999
Shapiro ER: On curiosity: intrapsychic and interpersonal boundary formation in family life. International Journal of Family Psychiatry 3:69–89, 1982
Shapiro ER: The holding environment and family therapy with acting out adolescents. Int J Psychoanal Psychother 9:209–226, 1982–1983 7152815
Shapiro ER: The boundaries are shifting: renegotiating the therapeutic frame, in The Inner World in the Outer World. Edited by Shapiro E. New Haven, CT, Yale University Press, 1997
Shapiro ER: The changing role of the CEO. Organisational and Social Dynamics 1(1):130–142, 2001a
Shapiro ER: The effect of social changes on the doctor-patient relationship. Organisational and Social Dynamics 2:1–11, 2001b
Shapiro ER: Institutional learning as chief executive, in The Systems Psychodynamics of Organizations: Integrating the Group Relations Approach, Psychoanalytic, and Open Systems Perspectives. Edited by Gould L, Stapley L, Stein M. New York, Karnac, 2001c
Shapiro ER: The maturation of American identity: a study of the elections of 1996 and 2000 and the war against terrorism. Organisational and Social Dynamics 3(1):121–133, 2003

Shapiro ER: Discussion of Ernst Prelinger's "Thoughts on Hate and Aggression." Psychoanal Study Child 59:44–51, 2004
Shapiro ER: Joining a group's task: the discovery of hope and respect. Int J Group Psychother 55(2):211–227, 2005 15899760
Shapiro ER: Studying the process: a psychodynamic treatment system for patients with treatment-resistant disorders, in Treatment Resistance and Patient Authority: The Austen Riggs Reader. Edited by Plakun EM. New York, WW Norton, 2011, pp 269–284
Shapiro ER: Derailment in organizational development: consultations to the Austen Riggs Center. Organisational and Social Dynamics 13(1):41–54, 2013
Shapiro ER: Finding a Place to Stand: Developing Self-Reflective Institutions, Leaders and Citizens. London, Phoenix, 2020
Shapiro ER, Carr AW: Disguised countertransference in institutions. Psychiatry 50:72–82, 1987
Shapiro ER, Carr AW: Lost in Familiar Places: Creating New Connections Between the Individual and Society. New Haven, CT, Yale University Press, 1991
Shapiro ER, Carr AW: "Those people were some kind of solution": Can society in any sense be understood? Organisational and Social Dynamics 6(2):241–257, 2006
Shapiro ER, Freedman J: Family dynamics of adolescent suicide. Adolesc Psychiatry 14:191–207, 1987 3618917
Shapiro ER, Zinner J, Shapiro RL, Berkowitz DA: The influence of family experience on borderline personality development. Int Rev Psychoanal 2:399–411, 1975
Shapiro ER, Shapiro RL, Zinner J, Berkowitz DA: The borderline ego and the working alliance: indications for family and individual treatment in adolescence. Int J Psychoanal 58(1):77–87, 1977 838547
Skodol AE, Gunderson JG, Shea MT, et al: The Collaborative Longitudinal Personality Disorders Study (CLPS): overview and implications. J Pers Disord 19(5):487–504, 2005 16274278
Skodol AE, Geier T, Grant BF, Hasin DS: Personality disorders and the persistence of anxiety disorders in a nationally representative sample. Depress Anxiety 31(9):721–728, 2014 24995387
Sowers W: Level of Care Utilization System for Psychiatric and Addiction Services, Adult Version 20. Dallas, TX, American Association of Community Psychiatrists, December 2016
Stern DA, Fromm MG, Sacksteder JL: From coercion to collaboration: two weeks in the life of a therapeutic community. Psychiatry 49(1):18–32, 1986 3704021
Substance Abuse and Mental Health Services Administration: Recovery: National and Regional Resources. Rockville, MD, Substance Abuse and Mental Health Services Administration, 2014. Available at: www.samhsa.gov/sites/default/files/samhsa-recovery-5-6-14.pdf. Accessed November 11, 2019.
Tillman JG: Four R's that protect against suicide: relationships, resilience, reasons for living, and restriction of lethal means. Presented at Austen Riggs Center Centennial Conference: The Mental Health Crisis in America: Recognizing Problems, Working Toward Solutions, Lenox, MA, September 21, 2019
Wallerstein RS: Forty-Two Lives in Treatment: A Study of Psychoanalysis and Psychotherapy. New York, Guilford, 1986
Will O: Schizophrenia: psychological treatment, in Comprehensive Textbook of Psychiatry III. Edited by Kaplan HI, Freedman AM, Saddock BJ. Baltimore, MD, Williams & Wilkins, 1980, pp 1217–1240
Winnicott DW: Hate in the countertransference. Int J Psychoanal 30:69–74, 1949
Wisniewski SR, Rush AJ, Nierenberg AA, et al: Can phase III trial results of antidepressant medications be generalized to clinical practice? A STAR*D report. Am J Psychiatry 166(5):599–607, 2009 19339358
Yohanan M: Mental health parity: Where have we come from? Where are we now? MCG, June 2017. Available at: www.ahip.org/wp-content/uploads/2017/06/MCG-White-Paper-Mental-Health-Parity.pdf. Accessed December 27, 2017.

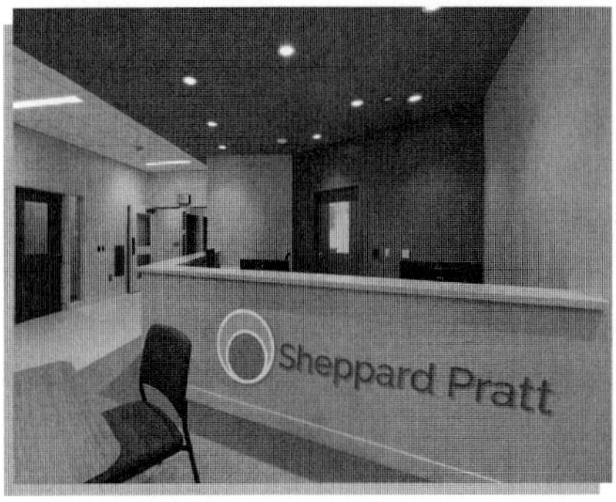

CHAPTER 16

Psychiatric Emergency Services and Interface With the General Hospital

Deepak Prabhakar, M.D., M.P.H.
Benedicto Borja, M.D.
Aaron Winkler, M.D.
Rachna Raisinghani, M.D.

Across the nation, general hospitals and emergency departments (EDs) play an important role on the frontlines of managing emergency psychiatric needs. In communities urban and rural, the emergency room is the place of last resort for a person in mental health crisis. EDs with multiple patients awaiting psychiatric evaluation or boarding while waiting for an inpatient bed are often a sign of a behavioral health system of care that is under-resourced and underfunded. Patients are unable to access care at earlier stages and prevent a crisis situation from occurring. Because of phantom networks and network inadequacy within health plans, even those individuals with commercial insurance have difficulty accessing care. For many, the ED is the only place to reliably see a physician for their mental health concern in a timely fashion. And as such, more and more hospitals identify mental health as a top concern in their community health needs assessments.

The Emergency Medical Treatment and Active Labor Act is a federal law that requires anyone coming to an ED to be stabilized and treated, regardless of their insurance status or ability to pay (American College of Emergency Physicians 2021). Of the 6,000 hospitals in the United States, only 2,500 have access to any mental health provider in the emergency room setting. In the absence of an informed psychiatric consultation and without the presence of viable options for patient referral to the most appropriate level of care, the ED physician is faced with only two stark options: admit or discharge. All too often, as the patient's condition has not sufficiently stabilized for discharge, the decision is made to admit and the wait begins for an available inpatient psychiatric bed. Increasing lengths of stay (LOSs) in the ED due to boarding are a cause of concern for general hospitals.

Hospitals have developed various models to help meet the emergency care needs of those with psychiatric and substance use disorders. Dedicated psychiatric emergency services can help provide competent compassionate care while helping divert patients away from the main ED. Hospital-based urgent care and other crisis-oriented outpatient services can help alleviate the use of EDs for primary psychiatric triage. Within recent years, there has also been a greater emphasis placed within general hospitals on developing more robust ambulatory behavioral health services.

The Role of General Hospitals

Given the current suicide and opioid epidemics along with the high prevalence of mental illness, ED visits for psychiatric indications are increasingly common in the United States. With an often hectic pace, trauma cases accumulating and ambulance siren whirring, multiple medical services actively consulting, and a steady stream of patients arriving, the ED is rarely an ideal environment for those experiencing an acute psychiatric crisis. Throughout the ED's history, several competing factors have helped shape hospital emergency services (Borja and Sharfstein 2009). Hospital systems and free standing hospitals have all responded in different ways to help meet the needs of the community for emergency psychiatric care.

The first hospital-based psychiatric emergency clinic was established in 1952, when Maudsley in England began providing care for patients outside usual business hours utilizing dedicated room and a telephone to consult physicians (Brothwood 1965). In the United States, federal funding for psychiatric emergency services was first categorized in 1963's Community Mental Health Act (Borja and Sharfstein 2009). As the era of deinstitutionalization gained momentum, there was increasing use of the ED as the primary access point for acute psychiatric help (Pearlmutter et al. 2017). Just after the turn of the millennium, psychiatric crises and emergencies accounted for 7%–10% of ED visits nationally (Hazlett et al. 2004; Larkin et al. 2005; Weiss et al. 2012). Since that point, according to data from the U.S. Department of Health and Human Services, the rate of mental health– and substance use–related ED visits increased 44.1% from 2006 to 2014. The greatest increase in volume has been for suicide-related visits, growing by over 400% (Moore et al. 2017). While mental health ED visits for adults went up by 41% between 2009 and 2015, mental health ED visits for children increased 56.5% during the same period (Santillanes et al. 2018).

Even though the demand for psychiatric care and visitations to the ED have increased, the number of available psychiatric inpatient beds in the United States has stayed stagnant since 2000. The United States is ranked 32nd out of 36 developed nations in psychiatric inpatient beds, with only 0.21 per 1,000 people (OECD 2019). Beyond inpatient beds, most communities lack key resources in terms of the continuum of psychiatric services. The lack of follow-up care options and limited acute care disposition often lead to longer LOS and frequent ED visits. Patients arriving at the ED for psychiatric indications tend to have a longer LOS, about three times longer than for those presenting with nonpsychiatric indications (Nicks and Manthey 2012). From 2009 to 2015, ED LOS for patients receiving inpatient care increased by 32% (Santillanes et al. 2018). Further, many patients are admitted to the hospital in acute medical care settings—incurring higher-than-necessary costs within a care setting that is not optimal for a patient needing psychiatric care—because other care options are not available (Nolan et al. 2015; Zeller et al. 2014). Interestingly, from 2005 to 2014, the total number of hospital stays for all causes fell by 6.6%. One would surmise that excess bed capacity on medical and surgical units in general hospitals combined with increasing psychiatric boarding in EDs would naturally lead to a growth in availability of psychiatric inpatient beds in general hospitals. The primary trend, however, has been a decrease in bed capacity or even closure of psychiatric units, as the economics of building out any other medical service far outweighs maintaining a psychiatric unit. And as hospitals face decreasing margins and economic challenges, the psychiatric services are often the first to be cut.

Our health care system often utilizes the narrow lens of dangerousness to respond to psychiatric emergencies and in determining risk to self or others. According to the Substance Abuse and Mental Health Services Administration (2009) (SAMHSA), psychiatric emergencies or crises are conditions that include intense feelings of distress and changes in functioning, often accompanied by catastrophic life events. Only a portion of real-life crises may actually result in serious harm to self or others. A response that is activated only when physical safety becomes an issue is often too little, too late, or of no help at all in addressing the root of the crisis. And a response that does not meaningfully address the actual issues underlying a crisis may do more harm than good (Substance Abuse and Mental Health Services Administration 2009). Such an approach is not a scientific one, nor is it an ethical manner in which to provide psychiatric care; it is, unfortunately, prejudiced against those seeking care. To help alleviate this concern, SAMHSA put forward a set of essential values for patient care in the ED, with an emphasis on avoiding harm, sharing responsibility, ensuring safety, and addressing trauma to encourage the health care field to develop a patient-centered strength-based approach.

As mental health–related ED visits increase in number and ED LOS continues to rise, the cumulative effect of these multiple factors has led to overcrowding in the ED (Nicks and Manthey 2012; Zeller et al. 2014). Not only does this have a negative impact on hospital operations, but this has led to a stressful ED experience for patients already in a crisis state. There have also been sentinel events, caught on surveillance video and hitting the nightly news, in which psychiatric patients have died of medical issues while waiting to be seen. In this chapter, we describe some of the ways health systems and communities are organizing resources to help meet the emergency psychiatric needs of patients they serve. Given the wide variability in state regulations and business strategies, we will not address specific revenue-related outcomes and regulatory mechanisms. The issues of reimbursement for psychiatric care, difficulty creating financially sustainable models of psychiatric care, and inability of patients to access health benefits due to discriminatory practices or barriers to accessing care by health plans are key drivers covered in other chapters of this textbook.

Models of Emergency Psychiatric Care

Dedicated Psychiatric Emergency Services

In England, The Maudsley Emergency Clinic opened in 1952, treating all comers regardless of catchment area. In the 1970s it offered 24/7 walk-in services open to all. The Maudsley experience demonstrated the need for 24-hour psychiatric crisis care in the community, given that many patients arrived after regular hours, and the decreased need for admission after a short stay (Lim 1983). An important concept from the Maudsley is the detachment of the ability to provide care from the concept of catchment area. Throughout the United States, crisis service planning and funding remain stuck with hyperlocal catchment area–based behavioral health authorities. Originally developed as a core tenet of community psychiatry over 50 years ago (Zusman 1969), a focus on regional or statewide solutions to mirror what has occurred in the hospital field may allow for better care, at scale and with financial sustainability.

In 1989, and with various statutory updates since, New York State created the Comprehensive Psychiatric Emergency Program (CPEP) model. Broadly, it included a psychiatric emergency room that operated 24/7 and had extended-observation beds for a 72-hour stay, crisis outreach services to provide assessment and intervention in the community; and crisis residence services where patients may stay for up to 5 days. The novelty of this model is the ability to stabilize and treat patients for up to 72 hours in the CPEP setting, a dedicated space for such care. Likewise, the ability to build relief valves for those who need additional time, such as the crisis residence, provides a necessary option and alternative to directing all patients for psychiatric hospitalization. Lastly, the ability to go upstream and provide crisis outreach services in the community also means fewer CPEP admissions, fewer inpatient hospitalizations, and, most importantly, better care for people who need care. As of 2018, New York State had licensed 22 CPEPs. Sixteen of these were in the city of New York. During the 2017 calendar year, approximately 25% of those evaluated were admitted for acute psychiatric stabilization and care (New York State Office of Mental Health 2012, 2017).

Emergency Psychiatric Assessment, Treatment, and Healing (EmPATH) Service

For many communities, personnel-related resources are scarce and the cost to help support dedicated psychiatric emergency services is prohibitive. EmPATH offers a valuable alternative. This service is an independently run program that operates in close coordination with a primary ED. Since the program is colocated, initial triage is completed in the ED and then patients with mental health or substance use disorders are provided rapid access to mental health experts in a calming environment. The layout itself is conducive to medical interventions with a thoughtful, patient-centered approach. Patients are observed, evaluated, and treated in a spacious common milieu. Staff are interspersed and rotate for constant observation and support. Beyond acute management and stabilization, patients are linked to next-step disposition right from EmPATH. In addition to psychiatric hospitalization, patients and families are supported with referrals to outpatient programs. Overall, the programs have led to a positive impact on ED LOS, revenue, patient satisfaction, and boarding time (Stamy et al. 2021).

Crisis Now

Another, more recent model gaining traction is termed "Crisis Now," which combines mobile crisis teams, crisis facilities, and a call center hub. Maricopa County in Phoenix, Arizona, is developing the model. At this time, there are insufficient outcome data to draw conclusions about its long-term efficacy.

Hub and Spoke

This model is particularly useful when the population served is relatively spread out and the emergency psychiatric care needs around the outposts may not be as significant as would be required to have a dedicated resource at each site. For example, the Banner Psychiatric Center, in Arizona, is a private, voluntary-only, all-hours facility, opened in 2010, that provides both centralized and remote assessment and stabilization services to hospitals in Phoenix and the surrounding area within the Banner private health care network. The centralized facility triages an average of 17 patients daily: 11 transferred from other Banner network hospitals and 6 walk-ins. Before it opened, ED "hold times" averaged 15 hours and 75% of patients were admitted. Subsequently, hold times fell to 9 hours and 50% were admitted (Little-Upah et al. 2013).

Alameda County in California includes Oakland, Berkeley, and other East Bay population centers—a catchment area of 1.5 million. All psychiatric patients medically cleared in the field or at a hospital are transferred to a single central psychiatric facility for assessment and management. In the community, patients being placed under 72-hour observation hold are assessed by emergency medical technicians and are often diverted to the psychiatric facility rather than the ED. Patients accepted for transfer from area hospitals are transported immediately, regardless of bed availability, in order to speed bed turnover in area EDs. The psychiatric facility provides crisis assessment, observation, and admission. The ED of the main psychiatric facility has no beds; rather, there are 48 reclining chairs in one large room. Taken as a whole, this combination of field assessment, rapid transport, and reclining-chair observation "beds" that can reduce the need for full admission is referred to as the "Alameda Model" (Zeller et al. 2014). The important takeaway point from the Alameda Model story is a common one in mental health. Although it is an excellent model, substantial difficulties were experienced when resources and funding did not keep up with the volume of demand for access.

A main lesson from such models relates to who funds the model and who receives the benefit. Innovative public programs, which are well intentioned and deliver necessary care, often become the provider for all patients. In a community where access does not exist, patients will seek care wherever it is available. As such, while many public programs are created focusing on Medicaid or uninsured recipients, it is important to have buy-in, both figuratively and literally, from all insurance payers to share in the costs to ensure the success of the program.

Brief-Stay Observation Units

Brief-stay observation units are often aligned closely with an ED or, in some cases, may operate semi-independently. The primary goal is to provide much-needed support in the immediate aftermath of a psychiatric crisis without having to admit patients to a more restrictive and resource-intensive inpatient setting. In New Haven, Connecticut, an observation unit was opened at a tertiary care academic hospital in December 2013. Patients were to be observed for up to 48 hours, with the goal of reducing admissions to the inpatient units. In the 11 months prior to opening, 42% of 3,501 patients seen in the adult ED by urgent psychiatric assessment staff were admitted, whereas in the 7 months following, 25.4% of 3,798 patients were admitted (Parwani et al. 2018).

Mobile Crisis Intervention

This model leans on the useful components of New York's CPEP (New York State Office of Mental Health 2012, 2017). Services typically cover a designated geographical area and include a crisis call center, mobile crisis teams, crisis housing units, and resources for addressing and treating substance use. Services are generally self-initiated. Patients or their families and friends call in for crisis support and, after a brief phone screening, are picked up in the community and brought directly to the crisis housing or, in some cases, when medically indicated, are taken to an emergency room. These services are able to provide interventions in the community and help divert a majority of individuals in crisis away from the local ED.

The catchment areas created in the 1970s are rife with inefficiency when it comes to providing such services. In some cases, the local catchment area may not have the funds to set up and sustain a 24/7 mobile crisis service. In others, the hyperlocal focus may not lead to best practices in selecting the best provider for the service and/or holding a provider accountable for subpar performance. In a local municipality bidding process, these contracts may simply go to the lowest bidder, regardless of ability to deliver reliable services. When mobile crisis providers are unable to meet the service demand, they may fall back on referring people to the emergency room—which defeats the purpose of having a mobile crisis intervention.

Psychiatric Urgent Care/Walk-in Clinics

Same-day crisis clinic appointments serve an important role in helping assess patients during a relatively urgent psychiatric presentation. Psychiatric urgent care (PUC) is a relatively new concept where services are organized in a way to offer broader assessments and some crisis-oriented short-term interventions. These services offer immediate psychiatric triage. Patients are generally referred to these settings by their outpatient providers, at times by their families, and many are self-referred; further, with careful planning, these programs also serve as a short-term step-down from more intensive inpatient settings. It is important for a PUC clinic to have a well-defined access pathway for services such as short-term urgent-care-based therapeutic management, outpatient services, crisis housing, intensive outpatient programs, a partial hospitalization program, and inpatient beds. Since a PUC clinic resembles and aligns closely with an outpatient model for care, it is imperative that patients be screened initially and rapidly for medical stability. Given the setting, a PUC clinic can potentially offer a more appealing and comfortable space for families and patients who present in a challenging crisis state. In a select few cases, if the patient is medically unstable or if acute psychiatric stabilization is needed but is unavailable because of a lack of beds, patients are referred to an ED.

Integrated Emergency Department Care

Integrated care has been a success story in chronic disease management in mental health care in primary care settings (Unutzer et al. 2008). This model builds on and improves the capability and timely access for psychiatric consultations in the ED. A care manager or a behavioral health specialist is available in the ED setting to work closely with the primary ED team; these integrated care specialists are supported by a consulting psychiatrist. The integrated care team not only assists with initial consultations but also helps with improving ED providers' skills in general behavioral observation and screening. Given the nature of this work and the available expertise, this model can also potentially help with institution of programs specifically designed to address high ED utilization (Elanouari et al. 2018).

Psychiatric Consultations

One model still being utilized in EDs is that of psychiatric consultation. These consultations tend to follow the general framework of consultation-liaison psychiatric practice (Leentjens et al. 2011). In this model, there is no separate area for the treatment of psychiatric patients. Once medically cleared for an initial psychiatric assessment, the patient remains in a bed in the medical ED. Even though psychiatric emergencies are medical emergencies, the general ED, with its multiple, smaller, tight quarters, is not an ideal setting for patients in a crisis state. These settings are extremely disruptive for patients with severe anxiety and those who may be suffering an acute psychotic episode. When this setting is utilized as the primary site for psychiatric emergency services, clinical processes should be carefully planned to help move patients as swiftly as possible. Process-flow bottlenecks in a crowded, somewhat claustrophobic setting may inadvertently lead to worsening of clinical condition. Timely consultations and disposition planning are integral to ensuring that patients are in these settings for only the minimum required period.

Future Directions

As health care transitions from a fee-for-service to a value-based care model, provision of psychiatric emergency services is likely to come under increasing scrutiny. This is an important level of care for individuals in acute psychiatric crisis. With careful placement and organization, these services can serve as an integral part of the continuum, rather than duplicating or merely shifting care episodes from one environment to another. With the increasing use of virtual health technology, models such as hub and spoke and integrated care are becoming more feasible for communities with limited resources. These models, when built on effective electronic medical platforms utilizing local or regional pooled data–sharing resources such as prescription monitoring, can also help improve patient safety outcomes.

Conclusion

Psychiatric emergency services are an integral part of the care continuum. With the growing utilization of hospital EDs for psychiatric care, hospitals and communities should consider providing psychiatric emergency and crisis services in alternative settings that are more conducive for patients, their families, and general hospital operations. Doing so has the potential not only to bring much needed evidence-based compassionate acute psychiatric care to our communities but also to improve the overall patient experience in a general hospital ED.

References

American College of Emergency Physicians: EMTALA Fact Sheet (online). Irving, TX, American College of Emergency Physicians, 2021. Available at: www.acep.org/life-as-a-physician/ethics--legal/emtala/emtala-fact-sheet. Accessed January 13, 2021.

Borja B, Sharfstein SS: The role of emergency care, in Disparities in Psychiatric Care: Clinical and Cross-Cultural Perspectives. Edited by Ruiz P, Primm A. Riverwoods, IL, Wolters Kluwer Health Adis (ESP), 2009, pp 248–256

Brothwood J: The work of a psychiatric emergency clinic. Br J Psychiatry 111(476):631–634, 1965 14344927

Elanouari A, England S, Hartoch A: Addressing mental health in the emergency department: the development of a complex care manager role. Collaborative Case Management 65:3–6, 2018

Hazlett SB, McCarthy ML, Londner MS, Onyike CU: Epidemiology of adult psychiatric visits to US emergency departments. Acad Emerg Med 11(2):193–195, 2004 14759965

Larkin GL, Claassen CA, Emond JA, et al: Trends in U.S. emergency department visits for mental health conditions, 1992 to 2001. Psychiatr Serv 56(6):671–677, 2005 15939942

Leentjens AFG, Rundell JR, Diefenbacher A, et al: Psychosomatic medicine and consultation-liaison psychiatry: scope of practice, processes, and competencies for psychiatrists or psychosomatic medicine specialists: a consensus statement of the European Association of Consultation-Liaison Psychiatry and the Academy of Psychosomatic Medicine. Psychosomatics 52(1):19–25, 2011 21300191

Lim MH: A psychiatric emergency clinic: a study of attendances over six months. Br J Psychiatry 143:460–466, 1983 6640214

Little-Upah P, Carson C, Williamson R, et al: The Banner psychiatric center: a model for providing psychiatric crisis care to the community while easing behavioral health holds in emergency departments. Perm J 17(1):45–49, 2013 23596368

Moore BJ, Stocks C, Owens PL: Statistical brief: trends in emergency department visits, 2006–2014. Healthcare Cost and Utilization Project, September 2017

New York State Office of Mental Health: 2012 Annual Report to the Governor and Legislature of New York State on Comprehensive Psychiatric Emergency Programs. Albany, New York State Office of Mental Health, 2012. Available at: www.omh.ny.gov/omhweb/statistics/cpep_annual_report/2012.pdf. Accessed November 28, 2019.

New York State Office of Mental Health: Appendix F: Comprehensive Psychiatric Emergency Program 2017 Annual Summary, in 2017 Interim Report to the OMH Statewide Comprehensive Plan. Albany, New York State Office of Mental Health, 2017, pp 63–64. Available at: www.omh.ny.gov/omhweb/planning/docs/2017interimreportappendixf.pdf. Accessed November 28, 2019.

Nicks BA, Manthey DM: The impact of psychiatric patient boarding in emergency departments. Emerg Med Int 2012:360308, 2012 22888437

Nolan JM, Fee C, Cooper BA, et al: Psychiatric boarding incidence, duration, and associated factors in United States emergency departments. J Emerg Nurs 41(1):57–64, 2015 25034663

OECD: Hospital beds (indicator) (online). OECD iLibrary, 2019. Available at: www.oecd-ilibrary.org/social-issues-migration-health/hospital-beds/indicator/english_0191328e-en. Accessed October 28, 2019.

Parwani V, Tinloy B, Ulrich A, et al: Opening of psychiatric observation unit eases boarding crisis. Acad Emerg Med 25(4):456–460, 2018 29266537

Pearlmutter MD, Dwyer KH, Burke LG, et al: Analysis of emergency department length of stay for mental health patients at ten Massachusetts emergency departments. Ann Emerg Med 70(2):193–202.e16, 2017 28063614

Santillanes G, Lam CN, Axeen S, Menchine MD: Trends in emergency department mental health visits from 2009–2015. Ann Emerg Med 72(4 suppl):S21, 2018

Stamy C, Shane DM, Kannedy L, et al: Economic evaluation of the emergency department after implementation of an emergency psychiatric assessment, treatment, and healing unit. Acad Emerg Med 28(1):82–91, 2021 32869891

Substance Abuse and Mental Health Services Administration: Practice Guidelines: Core Elements for Responding to Mental Health Crises (HHS Publ No SMA-09–4427). Rockville, MD, Center for Mental Health Services, 2009

Unutzer J, Katon WJ, Fan MY, et al: Long-term cost effects of collaborative care for late-life depression. Am J Manag Care 14(2):95–100, 2008 18269305

Weiss AP, Chang G, Rauch SL, et al: Patient- and practice-related determinants of emergency department length of stay for patients with psychiatric illness. Ann Emerg Med 60(2):162–171, 2012 22555337

Zeller S, Calma N, Stone A: Effects of a dedicated regional psychiatric emergency service on boarding of psychiatric patients in area emergency departments. West J Emerg Med 15(1):1–6, 2014 24578760

Zusman J: Design of catchment areas for community mental health services. Arch Gen Psychiatry 21(5):568–573, 1969 5823479

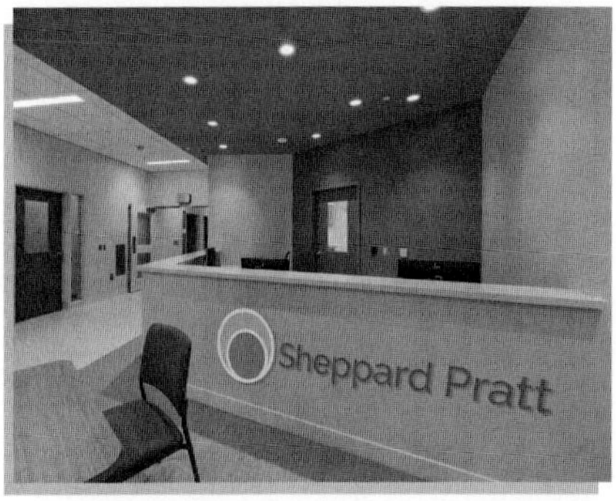

PART 3

Hardwiring Excellence

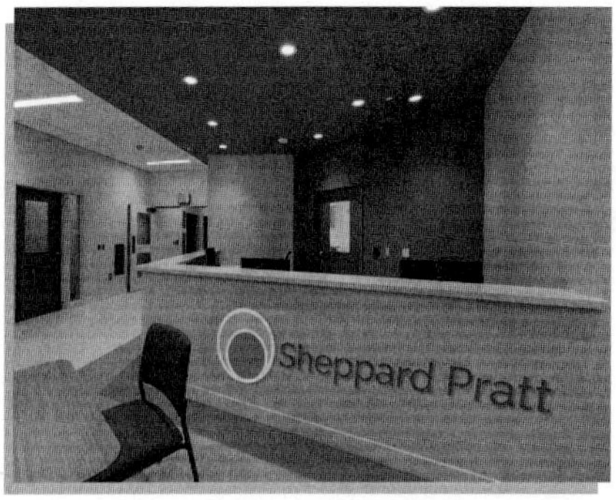

CHAPTER 17

Administration and Leadership

Gregory Gattman, FACHE
Kelly Savoca, CPA, M.B.A.
Harsh K. Trivedi, M.D., M.B.A.

Achieving optimal performance from any team is no easy task. As the scale of services grows, the complexity of aligning teams to row in the same direction increases. At the level of a complete hospital or health system, strategic execution requires leadership, structure, and operational excellence. To do so with resource constraints and still build a highly reliable system of care requires a high-functioning executive team. This chapter provides a primer on administration and leadership. It cannot replace formal education and years of executive-level experience, but it can highlight key concepts to form a solid foundation.

Corporate Structure

Inpatient psychiatric care comes in many forms. Starting with ownership, facilities can be owned by government (U.S. Department of Veterans Affairs [VA], state hospitals, county hospitals), by a community-led board, by corporations, or by individuals (Substance Abuse and Mental Health Services Administration 2019). Facilities can be operated as for-profit enterprises or hold not-for-profit status. The key difference here is what happens with earnings: for-profit facilities return their earnings to the owners or investors, who then decide how those earnings will be spent, whereas nonprofit organizations use their earnings to improve facilities and services for their patients. Psychiatric facilities may be freestanding, independent enterprises or have multiple locations providing similar services. Numerous multihospital systems provide psychiatric services exclusively, operate medical/surgical and psychiatric hospitals, or run psychiatric units within medical/surgical hospitals. Psychiatric facilities within a larger system may be operated by their owners or managed by a contractor who specializes in these services (Culhane and Hadley 1992).

Ownership typically determines the population targeted for care. VA cares for veterans; state hospitals provide services to the citizens of a specific state; county-sponsored hospitals target residents of their home county and may or may not limit care to this geographical area. Hospitals operated by a community board tend to give priority to their home community but typically will accept patients from surrounding areas; some offer highly specialized services that draw patients from across the country. Facilities owned by corporations or individuals show a similar pattern, with the highest percentage of their patients being those who live closest to the facility, and the percentages lowering as distance from the facility increases. Similar patterns will be found for most health care facilities because utilization is heavily influenced by proximity (Figure 17–1). Given the shortage of inpatient psychiatric services in the United States, facilities draw from a larger geographical region because patients and families are willing to travel farther to receive needed services.

The for-profit/nonprofit distinction is important in psychiatric care because profit motives can heavily influence facility goals and operations (McCue and Clement 1993). Although facilities of all types must maintain financial viability, for-profit organizations place a greater emphasis on financial performance. Earnings in for-profit organizations are returned to investors or shareholders, whereas earnings in nonprofit organizations are used to reinvest in plant/property/equipment, to support services that do not cover expenses yet are important to the organization's mission, and to grow reserves. For-profit organizations tend to emphasize operating efficiency, utilize less-costly staffing patterns, and pay closer attention to payer sources and insurance coverage. Leaders are often heavily incentivized to achieve financial goals. They may be more selective with admissions, although they are still subject to government regulations such as the Emergency Medical Treatment and Labor Act (Horwitz 2005). For-profit organizations often have well-developed marketing divisions, advertise their services, and have staff dedicated to creating awareness of their services among referral sources.

Nonprofit organizations pursue similar goals—a positive financial return, operational efficiency, outreach for service awareness—while prioritizing community health care needs and serving patients regardless of financial means (Sloan 2000). These distinctions can be blurred; today's challenging reimbursement environment has forced nonprofit providers to give more attention to the efficiency of their operations and reduce or eliminate unprofitable services to ensure financial viability. Additionally, nonprofits have realized the need to diversify revenue sources beyond Medicaid, Medicare, and commercial insurance, opting to include private pay services and at-risk arrangements as well. Interestingly, research in the early 2000s showed

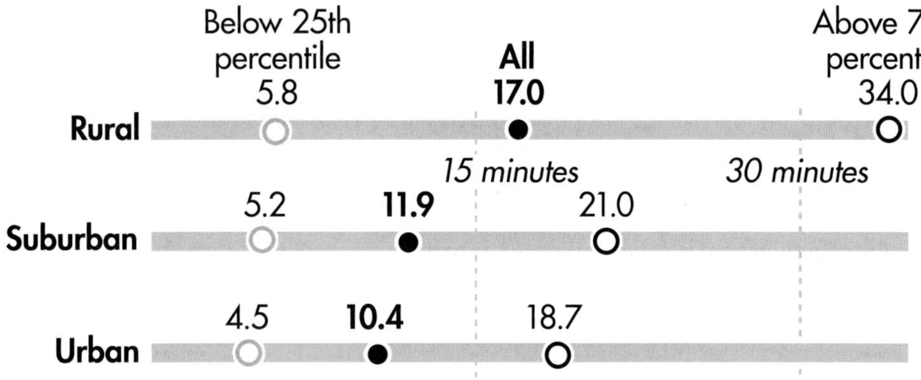

FIGURE 17–1. The influence of proximity on hospital utilization: average minutes of car travel time to nearest hospital by community type.

Source. Pew Research Center: Survey of U.S. Adults Conducted Sept. 24–Oct. 7, 2018, and Homeland Infrastructure Foundation-Level Data. Reprinted from Lam O, Broderick B, Toor S: "How Far Americans Live From the Closest Hospital Differs by Community Type." Washington, DC, Pew Research Center, December 12, 2018. Used with permission.

that nonprofit psychiatric facilities performed better than for-profits in nearly all measures (Rosenau and Linder 2003).

Freestanding/Independent and Multihospital Systems

Another distinction within the psychiatric hospital field is that of independent versus system ownership. The number of independent psychiatric hospitals has shrunk significantly over the past two decades, a reflection of poor reimbursement, increased regulatory burden, managed care, and advancements in clinical treatment. It is difficult to successfully operate an independent facility in the current business environment. Those facilities that are successful have built and maintained reputations based on clinical excellence, offer specialized services not widely available, and have positioned themselves as essential providers. Mergers between hospitals and systems have become more common since 2010, when the Patient Protection and Affordable Care Act (PPACA) was signed into law. Reimbursements by government payers have decreased and, combined with PPACA, are encouraging collaboration and better use of limited capital. As freestanding facilities have declined, multihospital psychiatric health systems have grown. The benefits of a system come from shared services. Financial systems, electronic medical records (EMRs), quality and regulatory compliance, planning, marketing, human resources, and other common corporate services are managed at the system level and support all facilities. This consolidation typically yields efficiency and ensures consistency through uniformity. A larger system also has greater leverage negotiating contracts with payers.

Trends in Psychiatric Bed Availability

In a public facility, the government owns the facility, and that, along with the patient care, is supported with public funding. Inpatient psychiatric beds have declined by more than 500,000 since the 1950s because of the closure of many state-run psychiatric hospitals. Between the 1950s and 1980s, many of those in state-run beds were patients age 65 and older with a brain disorder or patients with intellectual and developmental disabilities. Since then, there has been a change in approach by the state mental health and VA systems to community-based mental health in programs, such as the assertive community treatment model (Lutterman et al. 2017). Expansion of coverage for Medicaid and Medicare allows for patients to be treated in nursing homes or in their own homes. Over time, the capacity of private psychiatric hospitals and the number of psychiatric beds at general acute care hospitals have increased some, but the patient population is very different from that of state-run psychiatric hospitals. Options for patients with intellectual and developmental disabilities remain limited, however, and patients often get stuck in the general hospital emergency department (ED) without many options for long-term care (Fisher et al. 2009).

Regulatory Oversight

Although the ownership, geographical coverage, and populations targeted for services vary widely, nearly all facilities are subject to the same regulatory requirements nationally and at the state level. The Centers for Medicare & Medicaid Services (CMS) have established conditions of participation for hospitals who want to receive Medicaid and Medicare reimbursement. These standards are enforced through surveys and site visits. Agencies such as The Joint Commission have earned "deemed status" and are allowed to survey facilities and enforce government standards on behalf of CMS. The federal government also requires extensive data reporting on cost and quality metrics, comparing hospitals against each other. Poor performance on these measures can lead to reduced reimbursement. Many nonhospital organizations have chosen to be accredited by the Commission on Accreditation of Rehabilitation Facilities (CARF). Both The Joint Commission and CARF measure organizations against a set of operating standards to determine whether they meet best practices for safety, clinical care delivery, facility maintenance, quality improvement, and staff competency. States also enforce their own regulations and licensure standards.

The Value of Behavioral Health Services

Psychiatric beds have declined in medical/surgical systems primarily because of poor financial results. Reimbursement for services does not support the costs of care, and as hospitals and health systems face shrinking returns, many make the decision to reduce or eliminate psychiatric services. A broader view of value offers a different perspective on psychiatry's contributions. One of the most pressing issues in general hospital EDs is the boarding of psychiatric patients. EDs have become the primary source of urgent/emergent care for behavioral health patients, and most are poorly prepared to care for these patients' needs. Although many EDs have created holding areas and have some staff dedicated to assessment and management, the setting does not support restorative care. Models exist (Farley et al. 2015) for ED-based care that combine assessment/evaluation and interventions for stabilizing patients in crisis, which avoids unnecessary hospitalizations.

With studies suggesting that ≥21% of all hospitalized patients have a primary or secondary mental health diagnosis (Saba et al. 2008), consultation-liaison services provide psychiatric expertise for managing patients' mental illness within a medical/surgical setting and teach unit nursing staff how to work more effectively with patients. Although these services rarely cover their direct expenses, the reductions in sitter use and lengths of stay more than offset their costs. Similarly, efforts to target high-cost patients, such as those with multiple chronic diseases, have shown that these patients often have a psychiatric illness that impacts their ability to comply with care plans. Efforts to reduce their cost of care will be ineffective without appropriate psychiatric care. This becomes important as more health systems look to take on risk and become responsible for the total cost of care. Behavioral health leaders within general health care systems or those looking for opportunities to partner with such systems would do well to highlight areas in which an investment in psychiatric care will yield broader benefits.

Corporate Governance

Regardless of the type of hospital—nonprofit, for-profit, or government—increasing complexities and regulations make the role of a board and management more important than ever, particularly for nonprofit boards. For successful governance, boards must have effective decision-making and oversight. *Oversight* is a critically important board function but must be distinguished from *management*. The board selects the chief executive officer (CEO) and guides the overall direction of the organization. The CEO serves as the only corporate position accountable to the board. Management of the organization is outside of board scope, and board interference with management can cause disruption to the organization (Arnwine 2002). Despite this, boards have general oversight for all activities within hospitals. Decisions made by boards are significant and strategic, such as setting the mission, vision, and values of the enterprise (Table 17–1) and approving major corporate changes. Management teams create the strategic plan, but boards approve and guide direction.

Another important function of the board is ownership of the system's strategic plan, a collection of major objectives to be achieved over multiple years (typically 3–5 years) that drive annual goal setting. Yearly goals represent the steps required to achieve a strategic objective in the desired time frame. Done effectively, strategic planning lets the board set the broad objectives that support the mission. These are broken down into annual operating goals under the key performance categories or pillars. Executive leadership cascades strategic and operating goals down through the organization. This creates "line of sight" from the boardroom to the bedside, connecting employees directly with the strategic activities of the organization, which fuels their passion for purpose and their connection to the mission.

Beyond developing the strategic plan, throughout the year the board can be helpful in the decision-making process. Effective boards have a mix of industry and functional expertise that support oversight of the corporation. Trustees with skill sets in finance, legal, and risk management are helpful given the overall board fiduciary responsibility. As a fiduciary, one must act in the organization's best interest, ignoring personal interest of the fiduciary. This creates a heightened responsibility and good faith effort on the part of the fiduciary; its absence can lead to conflicts of interest.

One key fiduciary obligation of a board is ensuring that charitable tax-exempt status is preserved. This is timely because an incredible amount of scrutiny has been placed on hospitals' nonprofit status in recent years. Nonprofit charitable tax-exempt status is a valuable distinction and one that hospitals defend annually with community benefit reporting and other reporting on the nonprofit tax return (IRS Form 990) (Hazen

TABLE 17–1. Mission, vision, values, and strategy defined

Mission/Purpose	A statement of why the organization exists, at the most meaningful level. It is aspirational, in that it can never be fully achieved. In this way, the purpose states why the organization does the work it does but does not define how that work is to be done.
Vision	A clear, specific, compelling picture of what the organization will look like at a specific time in the future (1, 2, or 5 years), including those few key metrics that define success. It defines key results achieved and yet to be accomplished, the expected impact to the clients, and specific behaviors that the organization must display to be successful. A clear vision delimits potential strategies; it helps define what is within or outside the organization's bounds.
Values	The boundaries within which the organization will operate in pursuit of its vision. It is critical to distinguish between *core values* (those the organization will never compromise on and is willing to pay a price to uphold) and *aspirational values* (those that the organization espouses but has yet to live up to in day-to-day operations). To be meaningful, values must be described in clear behavioral terms.
Strategy	A clear, time- and market-based plan that describes the path by which an organization intends to reach its vision. Strategy determines such things as resource priorities, organization structure, and what issues get daily organizational attention.

and Hazen 2011). Hospitals have a significant burden for reporting information; they are required to share specific patient information (protected health information), quality reporting metrics required by the state and other payers, claims information to payers, and provider information to license and enroll providers in insurance plans. This reporting is varied in detail, and the information is duplicative. The following section offers a high-level description of some of the most significant financial reporting for hospitals, but discussion of all reporting requirements is outside the scope of this chapter (Moody-Williams 2020).

Required Hospital Reporting

Nonprofit Required Reporting, IRS Form 990

Stemming from the debate that hospitals are simply for-profit organizations dressed to appear as charities, Congress enacted the PPACA section 501(r), which places additional requirements on hospitals with 501(c)(3) tax-exempt status. Hospitals must complete a community health needs assessment and have a published financial assistance policy. Nonprofit hospitals must post their 990s publicly, and interested parties can review the extent of the hospital's charitable activities.

Medicare Cost Reports

Another annual filing for hospitals who care for Medicare patients is the Medicare Cost Report, which is the only national repository that exists for detailed hospital accounting data. As such, it is used to set standards for future reimbursement and reviewed for statistics.

Audited Financial Statements

Although hospitals must obtain annual audited financial statements, they are not required to make this information public. Audited financial statements are one of the best sources of information on a hospital or health system. There are rigorous standards for reporting balances in accounts, and audited financial statements ensure a level of accuracy. From an audit, one could view the hospital's financial position over time and operational performance, and from the financial statement notes, one can learn about the hospital's payer mix, reimbursement, debt financing, and outlook into the future.

Funding Challenges of Psychiatric Services

Outside of philanthropic efforts, payment for psychiatric services comes from insurance, which has historically been more limited than for general medicine. In recent years, expansion of mental health benefits has increased coverage for patients, but reimbursement can be a challenge for some payers. This is particularly an issue for patients with chronic mental illness. Medicaid has an enormous impact on financial outcome, and this is largely dependent on location because Medicaid is a state-administered program, and reimbursement for services varies widely by state.

In 2006, Medicare transitioned to a prospective payment system for psychiatric units. For acute-care hospitals, Medicare payment is a predetermined amount based on diagnosis-related groups. For psychiatric hospitals, however, such groups would not clearly capture costs. Both the positive outcomes and the challenges that go along with Medicare's prospective payment system have been well documented in journal articles throughout the years and are beyond the scope of this text.

Institutions for Mental Diseases

Another factor that influences reimbursement for psychiatric services is whether the care delivery occurred at an institutions for mental diseases (IMD). IMDs are hospitals, nursing homes, or other institutions that have more than 16 beds and primarily provide diagnosis, treatment, or care of persons with mental diseases aside from dementia or intellectual disabilities. In a Medicaid policy that dates back to the original 1965 law, an exclusion prohibits federal Medicaid payments for services delivered to individuals ages 22–64 who are treated in an IMD. This means that the state must provide all of the Medicaid funding for these services. The IMD exclusion has come under scrutiny for targeting psychiatric hospitals, which already have funding challenges; however, although minor modifications have been made, this exclusion remains largely in place (Mitchell 2019).

Translating Strategy Into Action

A strong organization delivers clinical services of high quality (patient engagement indicates satisfaction with services, clinical outcomes are strong compared with other organizations) and efficiency (cost/unit of service, costs less than collected revenues) to fulfill its mission. The leadership team recognizes that these results are achieved when all parts of the organization are engaged, clearly understand their roles and how they contribute to the organization's success, have the resources (personnel, supplies and equipment) and training to perform their roles effectively, and understand how each department/service relates to the others. There is a shared sense of purpose and recognition of individual/group contributions, and goal achievement occurs often. These outcomes do not occur by chance; they are the result of deliberate planning, goal setting, and performance monitoring against stated objectives. Success requires clear communication of expectations in ways understood by all levels of the organization and a strong connection to individual and organizational purpose. Combine clarity and purpose with leadership that ensures employees have the training, tools, and equipment to do their jobs well, and the organization will be positioned well for success.

In health care, examples of inspiring mission statements and compelling vision statements are everywhere. The St. Jude's Children's Hospital vision statement is "To accelerate progress against catastrophic disease at a global level." Mayo Clinic's mission statement is "To inspire hope and contribute to health and well-being by providing the best care to every patient through integrated clinical practice, education and research." Operating in a health-focused service organization is a natural source of purpose, the core of any mission statement. Health care naturally draws employees who want to serve others. Harnessing and directing their energy is the role of leadership. Quint Studer, author and founder of Studer Group (now part of Huron Consulting), developed a framework to show how mission, vision, and values support the creation of more tangible operating goals that move an organization forward on its desired path (Studer 2003) (Figure 17–2). The mission and values form the foundation of the organization (aspiration/purpose and the behavioral expectations for employees). The vision forms the roof (a compelling picture of where the organization wants to be in 3–5 years) and is supported by five columns, each representing an area of operational performance: people, service, quality, finance, and growth. Some organizations add other columns, such as community or research, to better match their priorities. These "pillars of performance" help organizations organize, balance, and communicate their goals internally and externally.

As noted earlier, the organization's board sets the mission, vision, and values of the enterprise and takes ownership of the strategic plan, a collection of major objectives to be achieved over multiple years (typically 3–5 years) that drive annual goal setting. Yearly goals represent the steps required to achieve a strategic objective in the desired time frame. Executive leadership oversees operations to achieve those goals.

Looking at the five core columns, "People" represents the human resource goals of the organization. It focuses on the employees and providers who work for the organization. Goals under this pillar can include any objective the organization selects to advance relations with its employees, including retention, employee satisfaction and engagement, internal promotions, and recruitment. The "Service" pillar focuses on the clients/customers of the organization (for hospitals, their patients) and captures the goals chosen to improve service outcomes. Examples include patient satisfaction, engagement, and loyalty. The national Hospital Consumer Assessment of Healthcare Providers and Systems survey results are often used as a service goal. The "Quality" pillar represents the goals and tactics the organization will use to improve clinical care delivery. Examples include reduction in patient harm, such as infections, falls, surgical errors, and mortality. Several national metrics (i.e., average length of stay, re-

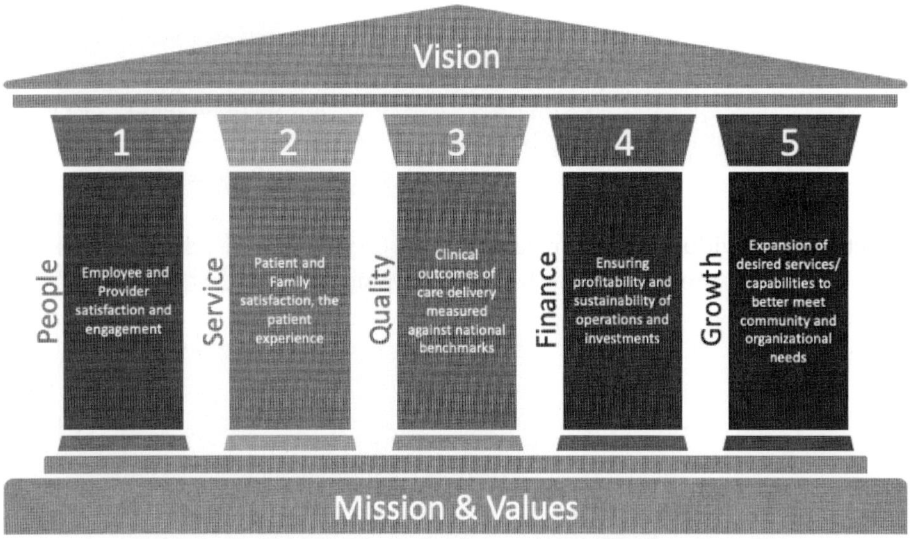

FIGURE 17–2. Operating goals within the context of mission, vision, and values: five key areas of performance for annual goals.

admissions within 30 days) can also be used. The "Finance" pillar captures expected financial performance, such as net operating income, operating margin, days in accounts receivables, or donations raised through philanthropy. The "Growth" pillar highlights areas of new business development or expansion of existing services, such as volume growth (*x* new admissions or procedures), opening new outpatient clinics, entering new geographic areas, or adding a new service. For organizations that include a "Community" pillar, these goals highlight efforts to improve access to care and impact broader measures of community health. Examples include health screenings for detection and early intervention, as well as the organization's social, behavioral, environmental, and economic impact.

Strategic planning and the establishment of annual operating goals set the desired direction for the organization, division, or business unit. Executing on those plans is ultimately the responsibility of leadership. Executives direct and ensure that the delivery of clinical, support, and administrative processes is aligned with the strategic direction of the organization. The departments determine if or how they can support each goal and identify tactics that will support goal achievement and share those with employees.

Organizational Structure

In most settings where behavioral health services are delivered, you will find supervisors, managers, and directors. Larger organizations may also have an administrator, vice president, or other executive-level leader. A sample organization chart (Figure 17–3) shows these levels and the hierarchy of leadership roles. Each level of leadership is important, and the focus of work changes as one moves through the hierarchy. Moving from supervisor to manager and upward, the leader shifts from the management of people and pro-

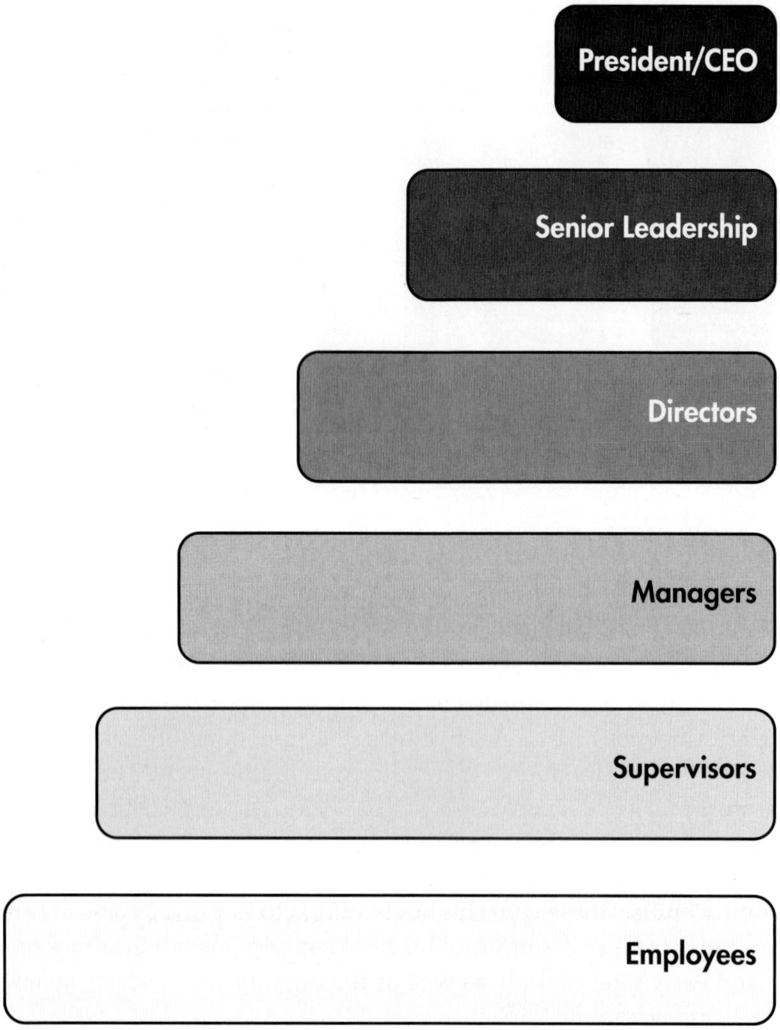

FIGURE 17–3. Sample organization chart showing levels and the hierarchy of leadership roles in settings where behavioral health services are delivered.

cesses to a more strategic/visionary focus on goals and resource allocation. Both skill sets are necessary for success, but the proportion varies at the different organizational levels.

Supervisors or their equivalents are the first level of leadership. They are responsible for the employees providing direct services (clinical, support, and administrative). Their duties include work assignments and schedules to ensure adequate staffing, training and orientation of employees, and management of resources (human and supplies/equipment). Supervisors are often involved in hiring/firing decisions, complete performance appraisals on each staff member, and counsel or discipline staff when required, so their people-related duties are significant. They also play an important role in communication, serving as an interpreter of messages from higher levels of leadership.

Supervisors report to managers, the next level of leadership. Managers typically have several supervisors reporting to them, such as a nurse manager with several charge nurses (supervisors) covering different shifts or an environmental services manager with supervisors responsible for different parts of the building. Managers also have a heavy focus on human resource responsibilities (hiring, firing, discipline, and coaching), with a stronger focus on the financial performance of their area. Control of overtime and control of supply spending are important metrics. Managers are concerned with other performance metrics, such as measures of quality, satisfaction, and safety. They work on interdepartmental processes, collaborating with other leaders to pursue broader organizational goals and initiatives.

Managers report to directors, who typically oversee organizational departments or units such as pharmacy, food services, social work, or patient care units. Directors own the performance of their unit, which usually has its own budget and performance metrics that align with broader organizational goals and targets. Communication is an important role at the director level: these leaders translate organizational policies, goals, and initiatives into meaningful actions at the unit level. For example, an organizational goal to reduce patient harm could be translated to a focus on reducing seclusion use on a patient care unit through more effective de-escalation techniques, reducing medication errors in the pharmacy, or installing ligature-resistant doors in patient bathrooms. Directors work with their peers across the organization to create, revise, and refine processes (process improvement) and lead initiatives related to organizational goals. They tend to be less involved in human resources issues unless disputes cannot be resolved by other leaders.

Directors report to an executive leader, who can carry many titles: administrator, vice president, chief, system director, and so forth. Executives are charged with achieving organizational objectives and goals. They are responsible for large sections or divisions of the organization—finance, operations, strategy, nursing/clinical services, quality—and important corporate services such as information technology, compliance, and legal affairs. Executives typically have numerous leaders reporting to them at the director level and above. Their focus is more strategic, that of working to achieve organizational goals.

Executive Leadership Positions

Hospital CEOs have an incredibly demanding role with responsibility for complex large organizations, and the stakes are high. Arguably, one of the most important tasks for the hospital CEO is selecting the right talent for roles in executive and program-level leadership. Core staff that report to the CEO and are considered essential for hospital oversight and structure are the chief financial officer (CFO), chief medical officer (CMO), and chief operating officer (COO). The CFO leads the hospital's or health system's finance team, is responsible for ensuring viability, and is involved in due diligence for mergers and acquisitions. The CMO is responsible for overseeing quality of care, establishing care delivery models, and managing the providers on staff. The role of the COO is broad, and often the hospital COO is involved in providing leadership to divisions/programs and ensuring operational efficiency and integration between programs and leadership. Other positions that are part of a hospital leadership team are the chief human resources officer, chief information officer, and chief compliance officer. Hospitals also typically have a chief nursing officer to manage nursing services throughout the hospital. All of these executive-level positions are responsible for operationalizing the strategic plan and the annual operating goals.

The hospital C-suite has evolved over time to include many new roles. The chief administrative officer has a role similar to that of the COO but is described as an intermediary between departments and the CEO. The chief business development officer and chief strategy officer positions have been created at many hospitals and health systems to manage growth and community partnerships. The chief development officer is concerned with managing the organization's fundraising or philanthropic efforts.

Some roles at large organizations have been developed to manage increasing complexity. The chief legal officer oversees legal management of the hospital or health system, which is particularly important given the recent rise in malpractice cases. The chief medical information officer is responsible for overseeing the data gathered within the EMR and other systems and is especially concerned with external reporting of protected health information. This role is important because the frequency of reportable data breaches is increasing, and the penalties are high. The chief of government relations assists in creating partnerships with government agencies and influencing legislation that impacts the health care industry.

Role of Physicians and Other Providers in Leadership

One characteristic of health care leadership is the participation of providers, especially physicians, in operations. Providers are responsible for the plan of care for each patient and direct the course of treatment—tests ordered, procedures performed, medications administered, the order and means by which health problems are addressed. The relationship between a provider and the health care facility is a partnership because each needs the other to provide the care and treatment patients require. Patients are also partners in their care and treatment, creating a three-way relationship unique to health care. Patient-centered care promotes a customized plan for patients based on their specific needs and those of their caregivers (Figure 17–4). It is a team approach to caring for patients that requires collaboration with a focus on overall well-being.

The growth of employed providers has changed this relationship, but only slightly. The employment relationship does not impact the provider's responsibility to direct patient care. Provider employment can help organizations through goal alignment, collaboration, and availability. When providers understand and share organizational goals, barriers to achievement are reduced. Employed providers have more incentive and opportunity to collaborate on process improvement. The stability of an employment model can improve retention and ties a provider to the facility more strongly than the connection created by medical staff membership. This availability allows the facility to better meet patient care needs by matching demand for care with provider staffing.

Within the organization, providers serve in many different roles (department medical directors, service chiefs, direct care, medical leadership functions/medical executive committee, pharmacy and therapeutics committee, board membership). Over the past decade, the number of providers in administrative roles has grown, especially at the executive level. Many health systems have chief-level positions designed for physicians: CMO and chief quality officer are commonly found. These executive-level roles give providers a voice within senior leadership and help organizations provide leadership to their employed providers and for quality improvement efforts.

More recently, providers have taken on more traditional administrative roles, such as CEO/president and operational leadership positions. Provider executives bridge

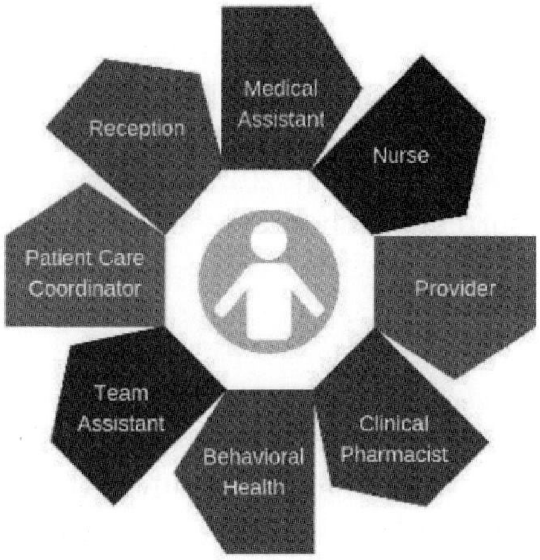

FIGURE 17–4. Patient care process: a team approach to care allows treatment to be customized to each patient.
Source. Virginia Garcia Memorial Health Center: Patient Centered Care (online). Available at: https://virginiagarcia.org/what-we-do/patient-centered-care. Graphic courtesy of Virginia Garcia Memorial Health Center. Used with permission.

the gap between traditional administration and clinical care. They are uniquely qualified to make decisions through the clinical care lens. This perspective is important as health care leaders balance the competing interests within operations.

Models of Leadership

> *Large healthcare institutions may be the most complex in human history, and even small healthcare organizations are barely manageable.*
>
> —Peter Drucker

Healthcare Leadership Alliance

Peter Drucker, one of the top business thinkers, was describing the complexity of health care in 2002, and not much has changed since then. Navigating a highly regulated industry that has decreasing reimbursement, workforce shortages, and calls for improved transparency requires a sophisticated skill set. Health care leaders are expected to have the educational requirements and lived experience and to be flexible enough to adapt to changing regulations. Much has been written on the subject of the ideal skill set for health care leaders. Some notable work has been produced by the Healthcare Leadership Alliance (HLA), a consortium of six major professional associations within the health care field. The HLA determined five common competency domains of health care leaders based on their membership (Stefl 2008):

1. Communication and relationship management
2. Leadership

3. Professionalism
4. Knowledge of the health care environment
5. Business skills and knowledge

The "Leadership" competency is considered central to performance. The other competencies feed and inform it (AONE/AONL 2015) (Figure 17–5). This provides insight into the shared skill set of current health care leaders, although it is somewhat generic and adaptable to most industries.

Dye and Garman

In their book *Exceptional Leadership: 16 Critical Competencies for Healthcare Executives,* Dye and Garman (2006) divided leadership fundamentals into four categories, called cornerstones, that build upon each other: well-cultivated self-awareness, compelling vision, a real way with people, and masterful execution. Sixteen competencies fall under these cornerstones, as shown in Figure 17–6. Dye and Garman's approach focuses on values and character as opposed to technical knowledge. They emphasized the servant nature of leadership and the need for leaders to develop and grow their skills throughout their careers. Their approach reinforces many of the HLA's domains but with a stronger focus on leadership skills that would be applicable in a health-related setting. Their focus on values and character is deliberate, because they see health care as more of a public trust requiring ethical leadership than as another category of industry (Dye and Garman 2006).

Cornerstone 1 focuses on leaders' self-awareness: Do they know what they value most? Are they emotionally intelligent, aware of their natural responses to different situations and thereby able to respond appropriately? Knowing what biases and tendencies they bring to the work setting helps leaders engage in an informed manner. Cornerstone 2 looks at vision and recognizes the power associated with a compelling purpose that is effectively communicated. Health care workers are drawn to the field because they want to help others to heal. Effective leaders connect tasks to that purpose and show how the work supports mission and vision. Cornerstone 3 highlights the skills needed to make strong connections with others: listening, giving honest feedback, mentoring, and developing and motivating the team. This cornerstone leans into servant leadership with an emphasis on supporting and developing the team, giving it priority over personal goals or ambition. Finally, Cornerstone 4 looks at six competencies targeting execution: translating plans into results. It emphasizes the need to build support for change, be adaptable and creative in problem solving, and stay focused on results.

Process Improvement

Health care delivery continues to evolve. To make progress on any number of initiatives, including patient safety, more efficient patient flow, and financial improvement plans, health care leaders need to operationalize information and use it to drive improvement. Process improvement has become an essential part of leadership. Application of process improvement techniques is required of most accrediting bodies, such as The Joint Commission, which expects to see examples of successful process improvement during site visits. Many health systems have created departments of experts in Lean and Six Sigma to help drive process improvement activities and train

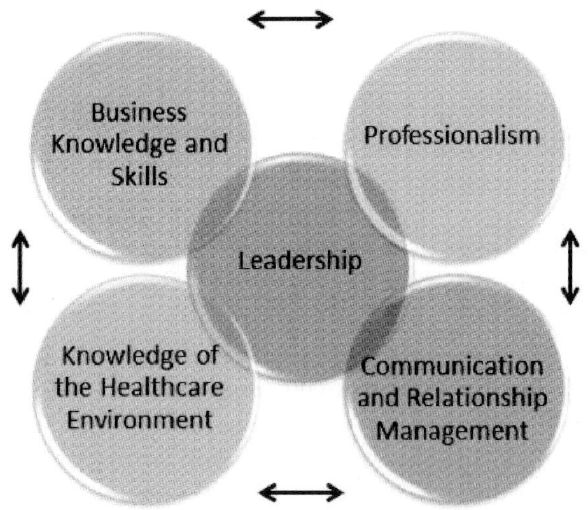

FIGURE 17–5. The Healthcare Leadership Alliance competency model.
Source. American Organization of Nurse Executives/American Organization for Nursing Leadership: Nurse Executive Competencies. Chicago, IL, AONE/AONL, 2015. Available at: http://www.aone.org/resources/nurse-leader-competencies.shtml. Accessed August 2020.

1. Self-Awareness • Leading with conviction • Using emotional intelligence	**2. A Compelling Vision** • Developing vision • Communicating vision • Earning trust and loyalty
3. Masterful Execution • Listening like you mean it • Giving great feedback • Mentoring • Developing high-performing teams • Energizing staff	**4. A Real Way With People** • Generating informal power • Building true consensus • Mindful decision-making • Driving results • Stimulating creativity • Cultivating adaptability

FIGURE 17–6. Healthcare leadership competencies according to Garman and Dye (Dye and Garman 2006).

leaders and staff in process improvement techniques. According to Health Catalyst, a top provider of health care data systems, leaders should master the following skills to facilitate process improvement (Hansmann 2016):

1. *Communication*—Communication is the number one skill of anyone in process improvement. Using data, along with active listening, is the path to helping a team identify a solution.
2. *Trust building*—Effectively articulating information and keeping people informed of what is happening helps to build trust within a team. Teams need to trust their leaders, think of them as part of the team, and believe that they will support the group regardless of challenges.
3. *Coaching*—Health care leaders are also coaches, supportive but able to critique and help a group to change direction or make modifications to the plan.
4. *Understanding process management*—Understanding the work process is mandatory for enacting change. Leaders need to understand current state, communicate vision, and use data gathered to help determine how the process should happen.
5. *Understanding care management personnel*—Understanding the process is one part, but truly understanding the real environment, including the people involved, is also important. Leaders can provide the vision and provide direction, but involving the people who are working on the issues daily is imperative.
6. *Constructive accountability and conflict*—Many leaders hear the phrase "that's the way we have always done it." Challenging this notion and allowing the environment to be collaborative, as well as allowing for disagreement, will help move the team forward.
7. *Resilience and persistence*—Being in process improvement mode often feels like pushing a boulder up a hill. Leaders must have resilience and persistence or ideas never make it to action.
8. *Seeing the big picture*—What separates leaders from the rest of the team is the ability to have perspective on the entire system and keep focused on the goal to keep moving.

Health Care Operations

Within most hospital settings, many functions must occur consistently: floors cleaned, medications administered, patients admitted and discharged, meals prepared, care documented, and many more. In broad strokes, the fundamental operations fall into three categories: clinical service delivery, facility operations, and administrative functions. Each area is important; they are also interdependent. Weaknesses in any area impact the others, directly or indirectly. A facility that is not clean or well maintained is a hazard to staff and patients and can lead to higher hospital-acquired infection rates, falls, or other harm. If a special diet is not strictly followed, a patient may die of a food allergy. If bills are not paid in a timely way or revenues not collected to the fullest degree possible, the facility may not be able to purchase the supplies needed for patient care or to pay their employees. A facility with poor clinical outcomes or low patient satisfaction may receive reduced revenue from payers while their reputation suffers. Attaining and maintaining high performance in each category is important for long-term success. The job of leadership is to establish performance expectations in these key areas, communicate those standards to the responsible teams, monitor performance against those expectations, address performance gaps, and celebrate success.

Clinical care delivery in the psychiatric hospital consists of those activities that intentionally touch patients to address their mental illness. These include nursing services to monitor health status and maintain patient safety; therapeutic activities, such as educational and recreational groups; individual, family, and group process therapy; medication therapy through the selection and administration of medicines; behavioral interventions to help shape patient actions; and psychotherapy provided by a trained provider. Physicians may prescribe electroconvulsive therapy or transcranial magnetic stimulation for patients whose illness is treatment resistant and does not respond to traditional therapy and medications. Care is personalized to each patient, with the treatment team (the clinical personnel working with the patient) creating a plan that lists the reasons for admission, primary problems to be addressed, and interventions best suited to resolve these problems. Ideally, this plan is shared with the patient and updated regularly to reflect progress or changes in treatment approach.

Maintaining a safe environment is an important element of inpatient psychiatric care and has received intense scrutiny from accrediting and regulatory bodies due to data showing suicide as one of the top preventable causes of death in hospitals. Strategies to prevent suicides include making the physical environment safe by eliminating ligature risks, having sufficient staffing, and employing practices to monitor patients closely enough to prevent self-harm, such as 15-minute checks, line of sight, or one-to-one monitoring. Many facilities have given nursing staff the ability to increase precautions for patients without a physician order, allowing staff to use their clinical judgment to prevent harm.

The clinical care team on a psychiatric unit often includes one or more psychiatrists, registered nurses, mental health workers or assistants, social workers, adjunctive therapists often shared with other units or programs (e.g., recreation therapy, occupational therapy, music therapy, art therapy, movement therapy), and a unit secretary. Other clinical disciplines that are present in the hospital and cover multiple units or programs include pharmacy, laboratory, imaging, clinical dietetics, and internal medicine/pediatrics.

Facility operations refers to the hotel services present in the hospital: environmental services or housekeeping to clean the building; engineering or maintenance services to manage the physical plant and provide a safe, comfortable environment for care; food services to provide nutritious and safe meals for patients and employees; and security services to maintain physical safety for patients and staff. Each of these services impacts clinical care directly and indirectly, and their success is critical to patient safety and experience.

Administrative functions encompass a wide range of departments and services that are less visible to patients yet unquestionably important to organizational success. These include financial (billing and collections, accounts receivable and payable, audit, treasury and asset management, financial planning and analysis, payroll, purchasing and contract management), information technology (software including EMR and other major systems, data governance, security and help desk function), human resources (recruitment, compensation, benefits, employee relations), compliance and safety, risk management, strategy, marketing and communications, and development/fundraising. Functions such as admissions/registration, utilization review/management, quality, and health information management contain both clinical and administrative functions.

The depth and breadth of these functions and their interdependence demonstrates the accuracy of Peter Drucker's statement quoted at the start of this section. Leading a health care enterprise of any size, at any level, is challenging. With that challenge comes the reward of contributing to the care and well-being of others.

Essential Activities of Leadership

Patient Flow

On any day, a wide variety of actions must occur for a psychiatric facility to function well. The basic functions can be viewed through the clinical/support/administrative framework. Clinically, those seeking care must be identified and assessed to determine the most appropriate level of care. Patients must be admitted before care is provided. Delivery of care and a patient's response to treatment are documented in the medical record. When treatment goals are reached, patients are discharged or transferred to a lower level of care, with an arranged plan for continuing care. Support services provide a safe, clean, comfortable environment for care to be delivered, food for patients and staff, and the supplies and equipment caregivers need. Administrative services ensure that charges are entered, billed, and collected; medical records are completed and securely maintained; and many other essential functions are carried out.

Patient flow or throughput is an area that requires daily attention from leadership. For any service or level of care, the organization must balance the demand for services with the capacity to provide care. Capacity is defined by the physical space needed to deliver services, the human resources needed to provide treatment services, and the supplies/equipment required. An inpatient unit treating adolescents may have 20 beds—10 for boys, 10 for girls—in semiprivate rooms. Any demand that falls outside those limits (>20 total patients, >10 boys or girls) cannot be met. If staffing levels have fallen due to illness, planned absence, or attrition, the unit's capacity may be limited. A room requiring repairs will limit capacity. Discharges create capacity. Multiply these constantly changing dynamics for every program offered, and the complexity increases rapidly.

Monitoring demand for services is an important part of managing patient flow. Psychiatric hospitals receive patients from many sources—general hospital EDs, community providers (psychiatrists, counselors/therapists, other physicians), and self- or family referrals are the most common sources. Leaders must monitor demand to ensure patient volume matches the organization's ability to provide care as closely as possible.

Building Relationships and Visibility

One of the most important relationships employees have is that with their direct supervisor. No matter the organizational level, the one-up leader heavily influences the work environment for every employee (Gallup n.d.). Making this relationship strong and healthy is essential. Three key activities for leaders are 1) getting to know employees on a personal level—interests, hobbies, family, career goals; 2) seeking their input on decisions that impact the workplace; and 3) ensuring they have the training and resources to do their best work. The concept of servant leadership states that a leader's purpose is to ensure the well-being and success of their employees (De Pree 1989). One important tool is rounding—regular, planned meetings with each employee. Studer (2003) recommends using a few standard questions for these meetings, focusing on the positive ("What's going well today?"), checking on basic needs ("Do you have the tools and equipment to do your job?), identifying opportunities for improvement ("What can I be doing to better support you?"), and harvesting recognition opportunities ("Is there anyone I should be recognizing?"). These questions, along with inquiries about family, school, vacations, and so on, provide useful and actionable information while building common bonds that lead to stronger relationships.

Another style of rounding is executive rounds. These can be scheduled or ad hoc and should always be purposeful. Scheduled rounds utilize a standard set of information gathered in advance so that the leader is well informed about departmental performance, recent events, and recognition opportunities. These rounds are meant to generate goodwill while providing an opportunity for senior leaders to hear from caregivers and other line staff. Ad hoc rounds are not scheduled and can occur when the leader has time available. Although unplanned, ad hoc rounds should have a purpose. This can be as simple as recognizing a work unit or individual, checking on an incident or safety event, getting feedback on a process change or new equipment, or providing feedback from a previous visit. This last point is important; whenever leaders make a commitment for follow-up, they must follow through. Doing so builds trust and credibility. Failure to do so makes leaders appear unauthentic and unconcerned.

Rounding is an effective way for leaders to increase their visibility and make themselves more accessible to all levels of employees. If practiced routinely, it is invaluable in gaining a better sense of morale and learning issues of importance to employees. Other practices that create visibility are participating in recognition events, attending huddles and staff meetings, and holding open meetings to receive feedback. Visibility is especially important for senior leaders, who are often seen as distant by line employees. Bridging the gap between levels of the organization helps to humanize leaders while giving them a more accurate view of employee engagement, leading to better decision-making.

Lead by Example

Leaders guide and direct an organization, division, or department through their goal setting, decision-making and resource allocation, both human and other. They also influence their employees and others through their words and actions. What leaders say and how they act convey powerful messages, as does the consistency between their words and deeds. Leaders are constantly observed by those they lead, and their actions tell others what they really value. Are they kind and courteous? Do they listen intently and pay attention when others are speaking? Do they value precision or productivity? Do they praise publicly and give more difficult feedback privately? When workload is high, do they step in to help? If they say "I'll get back to you," do they? These actions combine to form a clear picture of leaders' values. The phrase "lead by example" summarizes this axiom well. Employees will trust the message of a leader's actions more readily than a spoken or written message, especially when those messages are inconsistent.

Leadership Development and Succession Planning

An important leadership responsibility is continuity. Organizations outlive those who lead them. Promotions, career changes, retirements, illnesses, transfers, and dismissals can affect leaders and team members alike, creating a vacancy. Vacations and other forms of personal time off and business travel create short-term absences during which interim leadership is needed. One of the first jobs of any leader is identifying their replacement, also known as succession planning. Many departments/units/services have several leaders (e.g., a director and several managers), providing a hierarchy for coverage. When one leader is unavailable, the next in line serves as a surrogate. Such practices provide the needed coverage to support ongoing operations. They do not necessarily prepare leaders to advance in their careers. In order to ensure the business unit has a well-prepared leader to step up when needed, gaps in skills and experience must be addressed.

Leaders with an interest in and potential for advancement are candidates for succession planning, which should occur at all levels of the organization. Succession planning is leadership development targeted at the skills needed to succeed at the next leadership level: a supervisor is developed to become a manager, a manager to become a director, and so on. Because each level of leadership requires different skills and abilities, the one-up leader works with the candidate to identify the gaps between their current capabilities and those needed in the next role. That gap analysis serves as the foundation of a development plan, which may be executed using internal and external training resources. Ideally, one-up leaders will identify opportunities for candidates to take the lead on projects or assign them additional duties to grow needed skills and give them practical leadership experience. Candidates can be assigned call coverage, represent the department on larger committees, and give updates at staff meetings as ways of gaining needed experience. As the candidates' skills grow, so can their responsibilities, making their progression to the next leadership level natural.

Succession planning is a targeted form of leadership development. Progressive organizations recognize the need for and benefits of providing ongoing training and education for their leaders. Many organizations have formed leadership institutes for this purpose and offer a range of classes and assessments to improve leadership skills. An important part of the relationship between a leader and their one-up should be the creation and maintenance of a development plan that addresses growth opportunities. That specific plan, along with broader training provided by the organization to all leaders, helps leaders continuously grow their skills so they can be more effective in their roles.

References

American Organization of Nurse Executives/American Organization for Nursing Leadership: Nurse Executive Competencies. Chicago, IL, AONE/AONL, 2015. Available at: www.aone.org/resources/nurse-leader-competencies.shtml. Accessed August 2020

Arnwine DL: Effective governance: the roles and responsibilities of board members. Proc (Bayl Univ Med Cent) 15(1):19–22, 2002 16333402

Culhane DP, Hadley TR: The discriminating characteristics of for-profit versus not-for-profit freestanding psychiatric inpatient facilities. Health Serv Res 27(2):177–194, 1992 1592604

De Pree M: Leadership Is an Art. New York, Doubleday, 1989

Dye CF, Garman AN: Exceptional Leadership: 16 Critical Competencies for Healthcare Executives. Chicago, IL Health Administration Press, 2006

Farley HL, Troutman GA, Brown A, et al: Practical Solutions to Boarding of Psychiatric Patients in the Emergency Department: Does Your Emergency Department Have a Psychiatric Boarding Problem? Irving, TX, American College of Emergency Physicians, October 2015

Fisher WH, Geller JL, Pandiani JA: Care continuum: the changing role of the state psychiatric hospital. Health Aff (Millwood) 28(3):676–684, 2009 19414875
Gallup: What is employee engagement and how do you improve it? n.d. Available at: www.gallup.com/workplace/285674/improve-employee-engagement-workplace.aspx. Accessed August 2020.
Hansmann J: The top 8 skills every healthcare process improvement leader must have (online). Health Catalyst, March 28, 2018. Available at: www.healthcatalyst.com/8-skills-needed-healthcare-process-improvement. Accessed August 2020.
Hazen T, Hazen L: Punctilios and Nonprofit Corporate Governance: A Comprehensive Look at Nonprofit Directors' Fiduciary Duties. UNC Legal Studies Research Paper No 1920467. Chapel Hill, NC, University of North Carolina, 2011
Horwitz J: Making profits and providing: comparing nonprofit, for-profit, and government hospitals. Health Aff (Millwood) 24(3):790–801, 2005 15886174
Lutterman T, Shaw R, Fisher W, Manderscheid R: Trend in Psychiatric Inpatient Capacity, United States and Each State, 1970 to 2014. Alexandria, VA, National Association of State Mental Health Program Directors, August 2017
McCue MJ, Clement JP: Relative performance of for-profit psychiatric hospitals in investor-owned systems and nonprofit psychiatric hospitals. Am J Psychiatry 150(1):77–82, 1993 8417585
Mitchell A: Medicaid's institutions for mental disease (IMD) exclusion. In Focus: Congressional Research Service, July 30, 2019
Moody-Williams J: Moving to Value: CMS Strategy for Improving the Quality of Care. Independence, MO, Centers for Medicare and Medicaid Services, January 2, 2020. Available at: https://assets.hcca-info.org/Portals/0/PDFs/Resources/Conference_Handouts/Regional_Conference/2020/Atlanta/01_CMS%20Update.pdf. Accessed August 2020.
Rosenau PV, Linder SH: A comparison of the performance of for-profit and nonprofit U.S. psychiatric inpatient care providers since 1980. Psychiatr Serv 54(2):183–187, 2003 12556598
Saba DK, Levit KR, Elixhauser A: Hospital Stays Related to Mental Health, 2006. HCUP Statistical Brief #62. Rockville, MD, Agency for Healthcare Research and Quality, October 2008. Available at: www.hcup-us.ahrq.gov/reports/statbriefs/sb62.pdf. Accessed August 2020.
Sloan FA: Not-for-profit ownership and hospital behavior, in Handbook of Health Economics, Vol 1B. Edited by Culyer AJ, Newhouse JP. Amsterdam, Elsevier, 2000, pp 1141–1174
Stefl M: Common competencies for all healthcare managers: the Healthcare Leadership Alliance model. J Healthc Manag 53(6):360–373, 2008 19070332
Studer Q: Hardwiring Excellence: Purpose, Worthwhile Work, Making a Difference. Gulf Breeze, FL, Fire Starter Publishing, 2003
Substance Abuse and Mental Health Services Administration: National Mental Health Services Survey (N-MHSS): 2018, Data on Mental Health Treatment Facilities. Rockville, MD, Substance Abuse and Mental Health Services Administration, 2019

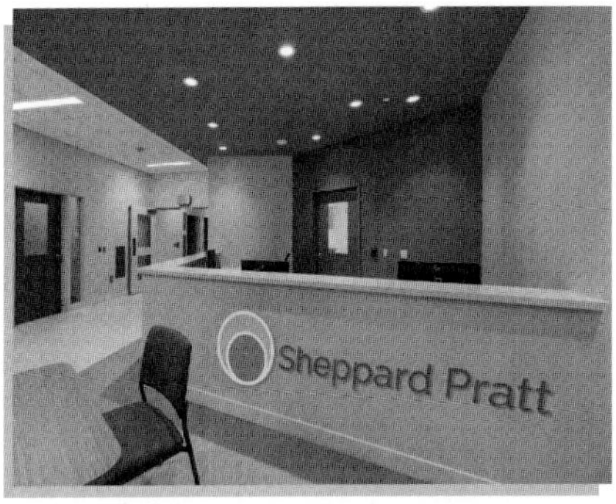

CHAPTER 18

Financing of Care

Paul Summergrad, M.D., FRCPsych (Hon)
Bruce J. Schwartz, M.D.
Peter Spyrou, M.D.

The mechanisms used to finance inpatient psychiatric services have a major impact on the availability, quality, and organization of care. The focus of this chapter is hospital psychiatry as it is practiced in the United States; therefore, financing mechanisms used in the United States are emphasized. However, other countries may have very different ways to finance care, and much can be learned from the differences among systems of care in other countries.

History

In the eighteenth century, people with mental illness were generally cared for by their families or social groups. Those persons who could not be cared for by family were confined to jails if they were deemed to be dangerous or to poorhouses if they were unable to care for themselves. According to Mora (1975), "the basic attitude of the general population toward the mentally ill was uncharitable and punitive." In contrast, the Quakers in Philadelphia had a more humanitarian approach to the mentally ill. The provincial Assembly of Pennsylvania established the first general hospital in America in 1751 to be a "Hospital for the Relief of the Sick Poor of this Province and for the Reception and Cure of Lunaticks" (Mora 1975). In 1770, the colonial legislature of Virginia established the first American asylum exclusively for the mentally ill in Williamsburg ("History of Eastern State" 2021).

Early in the nineteenth century, a number of private institutions were established on the basis of the experience of the York Retreat, a Quaker institution built under the leadership of Samuel Tuke in England. Although there were a number of charitably supported institutions, such as the McLean Asylum (established 1811), part of Massachusetts General Hospital; the Friends Asylum (1813) near Philadelphia, Pennsylvania; and the Bloomingdale Asylum (1821), under the auspices of the New York Hospital, the condition of mental patients in jails led reformers such as Dorothea Dix to push for the development of state-funded institutions (Summergrad 2015). From 1825 to 1865, other states, including Georgia, Kentucky, New York, and South Carolina, built public mental hospitals. Attempts to increase federal participation in the care of mentally ill persons via a federal land grant to establish asylums failed because of President Franklin Pierce's 1854 veto of a bill to support such asylums (Pierce 1854/1898).

For the next 100 years, patients with mental illness were treated in geographically separate institutions. Patients were cared for either in institutions funded by the state or in private institutions funded by their families or by the generous contributions of philanthropic individuals. In the second half of the nineteenth century, state institutions admitted large numbers of immigrants judged to be mentally ill and in need of confinement. Given the limitations of state funding, these institutions became overcrowded and were unable to provide a therapeutic milieu or deliver much in the way of treatment. Regardless of the exact form of financing, state psychiatric hospital care remained primarily a state rather than a federal responsibility, a circumstance that had ongoing implications for the current organization of care, even after the introduction of Medicare and Medicaid in the mid-1960s.

Psychiatric Units in General Hospitals

In the 1930s, a few academic medical centers developed inpatient psychiatric services funded in part by grants from the Rockefeller Foundation (Summergrad and Hackett 1987). That development also recognized that some patients with mental disorders have comorbid medical conditions that might require treatment and that medical or surgical patients treated at these institutions might require psychiatric inpatient care. At the time, no reliable source of funding was available for these units except subsidization by medical and surgical services and philanthropic support. When private health insurance was initiated in the mid-1930s with the establishment of Blue Cross organizations, coverage for mental illness was generally excluded or limited to several weeks of treatment in the belief that these services were already provided by state mental institutions, which were funded by state tax dollars.

The financing of psychiatric units in general hospitals changed dramatically with the enactment of Medicare and Medicaid when President Lyndon B. Johnson signed amendments to the Social Security Act on July 30, 1965. Medicare was developed as a federal program to provide universal health insurance coverage for persons older than 65 years but was later expanded to include younger persons who were disabled. Medicare initially paid for care in psychiatric units in general hospitals using the same cost-based reimbursement method used for other general hospital services. Title XIX, which became Medicaid, provided states with federal matching funds for the health care of individuals qualifying for, or close to qualifying for, public assistance. To receive federal funds, states could not reduce their health expenditures, most of which went to state psychiatric hospitals.

At the time Medicare and Medicaid were enacted, the inclusion of mental health coverage was considered progressive, given that many private health insurance plans continued to exclude or severely limit such coverage. However, because of concerns that utilization would be difficult to control, both programs instituted special discriminatory limitations on psychiatric coverage. Medicare limited care to 190 lifetime days in both state and private institutions but not general hospitals, thus limiting payment for care, which had always been a state obligation. Outpatient coverage for "nervous and mental conditions" was limited to $250 per year and was subject to a 50% copayment instead of the 20% copayment used for other medical conditions. Medicaid coverage to institutions for mental disease (IMDs; e.g., hospitals in which >50% of discharges involved psychiatric patients) was limited to persons younger than 21 years and those 65 years or older, again limiting federal support for state hospitals.

The availability of Medicare and Medicaid and burgeoning private insurance funding led to a dramatic increase in the number of inpatient psychiatric beds in general hospitals. In 1970, there were 22,394 psychiatric beds in general hospitals with separate psychiatric services; by 1990, there were 53,479 (Center for Mental Health Services 2006). Annual admissions to these units increased as well, from 478,000 in 1969 to 959,893 in 1990. General hospitals increasingly replaced public mental hospitals as the primary institutions caring for publicly funded patients (Mechanic et al. 1998). This trend continued between 1995 and 2002, especially for patients with serious mental illness, whose discharge rates from general hospitals increased by 35% during this time (Watanabe-Galloway and Zhang 2007). The number of beds in state and county mental hospitals declined 96%, from 340 beds per 100,000 population in 1955 to 11.7 beds per 100,000 population in 2016. The number of admissions also declined, from 486,661 in 1969 to 109,269 in 2016.

These trends toward deinstitutionalization had begun in the 1950s because advocates criticized institutions for warehousing patients without providing treatment and state legislators saw an opportunity to reduce expenditures by closing state hospital beds. Funding for the care of patients with serious mental illness did not follow them into the community. The acute short-term inpatient care provided by general hospitals and the absence of programs and housing in the community led to many of these persons becoming reinstitutionalized in jails and prisons or becoming part of the homeless mentally ill in our larger cities.

The closure of state mental hospital beds has impacted the emergency departments (EDs) of general community hospitals. Approximately one out of every eight visits to EDs is now attributable to psychiatric conditions (Weiss et al. 2014). Whereas septicemia and congestive heart failure are the leading causes of admission for adults older than 45 years, "mood disorder" is the primary cause of admission from a general hospital ED for younger adults ages 18–45 years (Weiss et al. 2014). The rate of psychiatrically related general ED visits increased 44.1% between 2006 and 2014, with the number of visits related to suicidal ideation growing the most (Substance Abuse and Mental Health Services Administration 2018). The EDs in general hospitals have become the treatment of last resort for the mentally ill throughout the United States. Closure of state beds has led to homelessness, trans-institutionalization of psychiatric patients to nursing homes or jails, and cost shifting to either Medicaid or state and county budgets.

As noted, another trend that supported the development of units in general hospitals was the inclusion of psychiatric benefits in private health insurance coverage. By 1974, 95% of health insurance plans surveyed provided some coverage for hospital care of mental conditions (Reed 1975). This trend of increasing coverage under private health insurance led advocates in many states to successfully argue for "mandated coverage" of psychiatric care in all state-regulated insurance plans. In 2008, the Mental Health Parity and Addiction Equity Act (MHPAEA) was signed into law by President George W. Bush. MHPAEA mandated coverage for mental illness that was comparable to the insurance coverage for medical care, provided that the insurance plan had a mental health benefit. The Affordable Care Act (ACA), signed into law by President Barack H. Obama in March 2010, required that as of January 2014, plans include mental health and addiction treatment as an essential benefit. Unfortunately, permanent regulations governing benefits under MHPAEA for pre-ACA insurance plans did not go into effect until 2014.

Patients with mood disorders who often have comorbid medical and substance abuse illnesses or dementing illnesses might have never been cared for in the traditional state hospital system. General hospitals have significantly expanded the clinical range of patients treated in their psychiatric units. Among Medicare, Medicaid, and dually eligible populations, more than 50% of adults treated for a behavioral health disorder have four or more comorbid physical conditions (Thorpe et al. 2017). These co-occurring conditions dramatically increase the cost of care for these patients in an inpatient setting.

Private Psychiatric Hospitals

The enhanced availability of payment for inpatient care encouraged the development of investor-owned psychiatric hospitals in addition to the small number of private non-profit charitable institutions. The increasing demand for inpatient care and the availability of coverage under public and private health insurance led to an increase in the number of beds and annual admissions to private psychiatric hospitals, peaking in the early 1990s and then declining into the twenty-first century. In 1970, there were 14,295 beds; by 1990, this number had increased to 44,871, but by 2002 it had decreased to 25,095 beds. The overall number of private psychiatric hospitals peaked in 1992 at 475; by 2004, the number had shrunk to 264 because of managed care review and other economic shifts (Sharfstein and Dickstein 2009).

A few private psychiatric hospitals abused the enhanced insurance coverage available for psychiatric care. Medicaid and employer-based insurance often included coverage for adolescents, and admissions of adolescents to private psychiatric units increased fourfold between 1980 and 1986. This explosive growth in utilization did not go unnoticed and, in part, led to the development of managed mental health care and carve-out insurers (Frank and Garfield 2007).

Diagnosis-Related Groups

Throughout the 1970s, overall health expenditures under Medicare rose rapidly—faster than the original projections had predicted when the program was first enacted. Development of diagnosis-related groups (DRGs) was included in the Tax Equity and Fiscal Responsibility Act of 1982 (TEFRA) and was intended to curb hospital price inflation. Congress in 1983 passed Public Law 98-21, which mandated DRGs as a new approach to hospital reimbursement (Iglehart 1982). On October 1, 1983, reimbursement was determined using a classification system that categorized diagnoses into 468 DRGs. Institutions had little or no previous experience using this approach for psychiatric care; therefore, Congress granted an exemption from this prospective payment system (PPS) for psychiatric hospitals and permitted psychiatric units in general hospitals to apply for an exemption. Congress asked the U.S. Department of Health and Human Services to report by the end of 1985 on the feasibility of including these facilities and specialty units in the Medicare PPS. Numerous studies were done and concluded that available classification systems were poor predictors of resource use (Mitchell et al. 1987).

Instead of including psychiatric patients in the DRG system, Medicare continued to reimburse psychiatric hospitals and exempt units in general hospitals under TEFRA, which used complicated formulas and retrospective calculations to determine allowable costs and to set a target reimbursement rate per discharge, regardless of psychiatric diagnosis. This was in contradiction to the DRG-based system for medical-surgical care, which was mirrored by the private insurance system and reduced payments for medical-surgical care, making psychiatric units and hospitals relatively more profitable in the early years of DRGs. Many hospitals in subsequent years underwent a marked reduction in lengths of stay and a decrease in bed utilization for medical and surgical patients that were partially offset by additional admissions and complex outpatient care. The financial viability of many community hospitals, especially in rural areas and cities with a large number of surplus beds, led to hospital closures or the repurposing of those beds. For some hospitals, opening a psychiatric unit was a way to utilize empty beds. Originally, conversion to a psychiatric unit required little capital investment; given the increase in demand for those services, it made business sense for hospitals. TEFRA was modified by the Balanced Budget Act of 1997, which diminished many advantages of the DRG exemption for psychiatric units through payment caps, rate updates, and reduced graduate medical education payments on psychiatric units (Lave 2003).

Any fiscal incentive to open psychiatric units has now disappeared because of new costly regulations. In 2018, the Joint Commission and the Centers for Medicare & Medicaid Services (CMS) began to strictly interpret anti-ligature guidelines, which make conversion of units prohibitively expensive. Furthermore, the cost of compliance is leading to the closure of existing inpatient psychiatric units. A recent survey of 88 facilities in 34 states reported that 14 were reducing the number of psychiatric beds and 10 hospitals were closing psychiatric units altogether, specifically stating that modifications were too costly (Kristin Kroger, Chief, Policy, Program, and Partnerships, American Psychiatric Association, personal communication, 2019). These reductions have been happening even as insurance has expanded to the private sector and government programs, which has brought increased numbers of patients into psychiatric care in general hospitals.

Inpatient Prospective Payment System

The psychiatric cost-based reimbursement system remained in effect until the development of a PPS for psychiatric hospitals and exempt units mandated by the Balanced

Budget Refinement Act of 1999, with phase-in of the new reimbursement rules starting January 1, 2005. The new PPS system has a base payment rate, with adjusters for patient characteristics (e.g., age, psychiatric diagnosis, medical comorbidities) and facility characteristics (e.g., teaching status, presence of an ED, rural vs. urban location). Despite Medicare data showing higher costs per case, often due to greater acuity and medical comorbidity in general hospital patients, the Medicare PPS for inpatient psychiatry is generally more favorable to freestanding hospitals (Centers for Medicare and Medicaid Services 2004; Kelley 2011). However, the new PPS does not fully account for the costs of patients cared for in general hospitals who have significant medical comorbidities or problems with activities of daily living (Drozd et al. 2006).

Although, by statute, the initial version of the PPS for psychiatry must be budget neutral overall, cost containment will depend on annual adjustments to the base rate and the behavior of providers. A rate adjustment below the increase in costs may save Medicare money but will disadvantage hospitals, whose operating margins will shrink as costs rise faster than reimbursement. Since the development of the Inpatient Psychiatric Facility Prospective Payment System in 2004, there has been a relative growth particularly in for-profit freestanding psychiatric hospitals and some decrease in general hospital psychiatric units (Medicare Payment Advisory Commission 2010). In 2019, Medicare payments to inpatient psychiatric facilities, both freestanding hospitals and specialized hospital-based units, totaled approximately $3.6 billion (Medicare Payment Advisory Commission 2021). These payments are determined by adjusting a daily base rate ($833 per day in FY 2022) based on geographical differences in labor costs, costs of care related to specified conditions, the length of stay, and overall facility characteristics (Medicare Payment Advisory Commission 2021).

All inpatient psychiatric units in acute care hospitals or critical access hospitals that are paid under the new Medicare PPS have to meet Inpatient Psychiatric Facility Quality Reporting (IPFQR) requirements. The IPFQR program encourages facilities and clinicians to improve the quality of inpatient care by submitting quality data to CMS annually. As this is a pay-for-reporting program, eligible facilities are paid less by Medicare if they do not participate. Inpatient psychiatric facilities that do not take part in the IPFQR program or do not meet all of the reporting requirements are subject to a 2.0% reduction in the annual update to their standard federal rate for that year.

Managed Behavioral Health Care

In contrast to Medicare's approach to cost containment, beginning in the 1980s, health maintenance organizations (HMOs) and private health insurance providers turned to specialized managed behavioral health care organizations (MBHOs) for oversight and utilization management of their psychiatric benefits. These companies are often referred to as *carve-outs*. The growth of these companies occurred in response to rising expenditures as psychiatric care became less stigmatized and as psychiatric benefits were included or improved in private health insurance as a result of consumer demand or state mandates. In addition, many primary private insurers did not have expertise in the management of psychiatric care.

The carve-out companies responded to the complaints of HMOs, insurance companies that reimbursed providers, and employers who purchased insurance for their employees that psychiatric care was unstandardized and that costs were growing rapidly. Just as experience with Medicare had taught people that psychiatric diagnosis did not predict resource use, purchasers were concerned that patients with similar diagnoses could remain in the hospital for widely various lengths of stay or could avoid hospitalization altogether. For context, in 2013, total expenditures by all payers for treatment of mental health disorders reached $201 billion, surpassing spending for heart conditions by $54 billion and cancer by $79 billion in the same year (Roehrig 2016). The carve-out companies developed programs of preadmission review and continued-care certification to control the utilization of psychiatric services, particularly on inpatient units (Kihlstrom 1997). These review criteria were generally proprietary and kept secret from providers.

MBHOs evolved from initially only providing administrative services to insurers to accepting financial risk, with the potential of generating additional profits by managing the behavioral health costs for a defined population of insured persons. With the growth and expansion of MBHOs, nonphysician reviewers could telephonically apply review criteria to approve or disallow inpatient admissions and continued stays. Disallowals were supposed to involve a psychiatrist reviewer, and providers were permitted to appeal an adverse determination. These review organizations avoided legal liability for any adverse outcomes that resulted from denied admissions or premature discharges by arguing that *clinicians* had the legal responsibility for admitting or discharging patients, not the review organization, which was simply authorizing or denying payment.

In addition to reviewing admissions and continued care, these carve-out companies often negotiated reduced rates with individual hospitals. Unlike Medicare, which had contracts with every hospital that were often standardized by region, prevailing wage, and employment costs, these private for-profit companies could pick and choose which hospitals could have their contracts. As small carve-outs consolidated or were bought up by larger ones, these companies developed significant purchasing power. In many markets, their monopolies allowed them to dictate rates to hospitals. Hospitals frequently accepted rates below their costs because not obtaining a contract would mean a loss of so much volume that the unit would have to be downsized or closed.

The effects of these carve-out companies on quality of care and patient outcomes have been difficult to measure. However, the number of inpatient psychiatric beds in general hospitals decreased from 53,000 in 1990 to 30,864 by 2014 (Center for Behavioral Health Statistics and Quality 2019). The number of general hospitals providing psychiatric services also continued to decline, from 1,707 in 1998 to 1,285 in 2002 and 1,066 by 2018 (Center for Behavioral Health Statistics and Quality 2019). Despite the recent reductions in the number of psychiatric beds, the annual number of discharges with primary psychiatric diagnoses from general hospitals increased by approximately 35% between 1988 and 1994, from 1.4 to 1.9 million. Looking specifically at Medicare discharges, there were 305,041 discharges from psychiatric units in general hospitals and 128,888 discharges from freestanding psychiatric hospitals in 2008. In addition to these psychiatric discharges from distinct part units, there were another 249,840 psychiatric discharges from general medical-surgical floors, so-called scatter beds, suggesting that the volume of psychiatric inpatient care in general hospitals is actually greater than usually considered (Medicare Payment Advisory Commission 2010).

Patient and provider dissatisfaction with these programs generated many complaints to state insurance regulators and legislators. These abuses led to a movement in support of patient protection legislation and efforts to enact mental health and substance abuse parity. Because many people receive their insurance through their employers under the Employer Retirement Income Security Act (ERISA), federal legislation was required to seek legal remedy for abusive managed care practices and was included in the portion of MHPAEA that mandated oversight of ERISA plans by the U.S. Department of Labor. Another trend, in part as a result of complaints, was for insurers to bring the review of psychiatric care back into their core review activities rather than carving them out.

Another consideration included recognition of the high rates of medical and psychiatric comorbidity among patients with psychiatric illness. Patients with psychiatric illness often have undiagnosed or untreated medical illness and, among severely ill populations, die at higher rates from cardiovascular, pulmonary, and metabolic disorders than do age-matched control subjects (Summergrad and Kathol 2014). Furthermore, costs are 75% higher for people diagnosed with both behavioral health and other common chronic conditions than for those without a co-occurring mental health diagnosis. Substantial expenditures for psychopharmacological agents, often borne by the primary insurer rather than the carve-out payer, have also led insurers to reclaim internal management of psychiatric services.

Medicaid Reimbursement

In the 1990s, state Medicaid programs also began to contract with these carve-out companies to manage their psychiatric benefits under Section 1915b or Section 1115 waivers from the U.S. Department of Health and Human Services. Medicaid rules define which services are reimbursable and which hospitals can be reimbursed (e.g., by nonallowance of payment to IMDs for patients ages 21–64 years). States can request modifications in traditional Medicaid payments (e.g., ability to admit patients of all ages to IMDs, including private psychiatric hospitals, or payments for residential or nonhospital emergency or community-based care). Waivers vary among state programs, depending on the organization of the state mental health system, and can be based on regional, countywide, or statewide programs. Because utilization of psychiatric services is generally significantly higher in the Medicaid population (especially in those considered disabled by their psychiatric illness) than in commercial populations, the organization of the Medicaid system has important implications for the overall system of care.

In an important effort to address the opioid crisis in the United States, the 115th Congress overwhelmingly passed the Substance Use-Disorder Prevention that Promotes Opioid Recovery and Treatment for Patients and Communities Act (H.R. 6, P.L. 115-271) to improve medical treatment for opioid addiction and stop the opioid epidemic. President Trump signed the bill on October 24, 2018. The law requires coverage of medication-assisted treatment under Medicaid and allows states to receive federal payment under Medicaid for services provided to pregnant and postpartum women with substance use disorders who receive care at IMDs. Child health insurance plans must cover mental health and substance use disorder services. Because of the shortage of substance use disorder services in acute care hospitals, the law temporarily allows states to receive Medicaid payment for services provided in IMDs for enrollees (ages

21–64) with these disorders. However, services may only be covered for a total of up to 30 days in a 12-month period. An important feature of the law requires coverage to individuals with Medicare for services provided by certified opioid-treatment programs.

State Mental Health Systems

Because of the unique responsibilities that states bear for the direct provision of psychiatric services, the organization, budgeting, and interrelationship of state mental health systems with Medicaid and Medicare are unique components of hospital psychiatry. Prior to the 1930s, 96% of all psychiatric hospitalizations occurred in state or veterans hospitals. Large psychiatric hospitals, often set at some distance from major population centers, accounted for 25% of all hospital beds in the United States (Summergrad and Hackett 1987). There has been a precipitous decline in the number of available state psychiatric beds; between 1970 and 2016, this number declined more than 90%, from 413,066 to only 37,679.

State hospital systems vary greatly among states. In some, state hospitals care only for those patients who require long-term care on transfer from general or private hospitals, whereas in others, county-based systems provide acute psychiatric care in public hospitals. Some states run psychiatric emergency services in state facilities; other states have created mobile non-hospital-based emergency services. States have often modified their state-run systems in coordination with Medicaid waivers (often Section 1115) and used state and federal funding streams from both Medicare and Medicaid programs to create more comprehensive systems of care. Within state and county psychiatric hospitals, 46% of beds are occupied by forensic patients (National Association of State Mental Health Program Directors 2014).

Financial Effects of Changing Reimbursement

As a result of the changes in reimbursement and managed care, the number of inpatient psychiatric beds has declined dramatically since 1990. The number of beds in private psychiatric hospitals declined from 44,871 in 1990 to 24,804 in 2014. Beds on inpatient units in general hospitals decreased in number from 53,479 in 1990 to 30,864 in 2014. During the same time period, the number of available beds in state and county mental hospitals dwindled from 98,789 to 37,209 (Center for Behavioral Health Statistics and Quality 2019; Treatment Advocacy Center 2016a). These changes may have led to the evolution and transformation of approaches to treatment, as there was significantly increased reliance on outpatient, residential, or partial hospital services rather than inpatient programs with shortened lengths of stay for admitted patients. Shorter lengths of stay may have also led to more readmissions, because between 1990 and 2002 the total number of admissions increased in private psychiatric hospitals from 406,522 to 477,395 and in general hospital units from 959,893 to 1,094,715 (Center for Mental Health Services 2006). The greatest impact was felt by patients with serious mental illness, and as a consequence there was increased homelessness and incarceration in jails and prisons. In 2006, the U.S. Department of Justice found that "an estimated

10% of state prisoners...reported symptoms that met criteria for a psychotic disorder" (James and Glaze 2006). In some estimates, nearly 20% of inmates in jails and 15% of inmates in state prisons had a serious mental illness. For context, based on the total inmate population in 2014, this would indicate that approximately 383,000 individuals with severe psychiatric disease were behind bars in the United States (Treatment Advocacy Center 2016b). Further exacerbating the issue, repeated incarceration is common for those who lack access to behavioral health services.

Revenue Sources by Type of Hospital

As overall expenditures on mental health steadily increased, from $32 billion in 1986 to $186 billion in 2014, the percentage of mental health care dollars spent on inpatient care shifted, from 42% to 27% (Substance Abuse and Mental Health Services Administration 2016). An analysis of sources of revenue for different types of hospitals illuminates the financial challenges faced by various organizations. For private psychiatric hospitals, the proportion of total revenue that came from patient fees, including private health insurance, decreased from 61.3% in 1990 to 42.7% in 2002. For general hospitals during this same time period, the decrease was from 36.5% to 31.5%. In contrast, for private psychiatric hospitals, the proportion of total revenue from Medicaid increased dramatically, from 9.4% to 25.9%, and the increase for Medicare revenue went from 10.8% to 18.2%. For general hospitals, Medicaid revenue was essentially unchanged between 1990 and 2002 (24.2% vs. 24.0%), but Medicare total revenue increased from 24.2% to 36.9%.

The Future Financial Viability of Inpatient Psychiatric Services

Given the trend of reimbursement increases under the inpatient PPS, it remains unclear whether they will keep up with rising costs and the shift in revenue sources toward more publicly financed patients. The opioid and suicide epidemics, the incarceration of the mentally ill in jails and prisons, and the need for more adult, child, and adolescent psychiatric beds may lead to increased reimbursement as a means to reincentivize hospitals to reopen or increase the number of psychiatric beds. Commercial coverage for private patients is typically higher than for Medicare or Medicaid patients and remains a viable portion of the market. In strictly economic terms, further reduction in the number of available beds is risky. As the Medicare Payment Advisory Commission data have shown, beds in general hospitals may be at particular risk (Kelley 2011; Medicare Payment Advisory Commission 2010), whereas psychiatric units in general hospitals can be cross-subsidized by more profitable services in orthopedics, cardiology, oncology, or surgery. However, hospitals that need more beds for these profitable services may look to downsize, close, or move their inpatient psychiatric units to off-site locations.

In its review of behavioral health care needs, the American Hospital Association (2007) concluded, "As an important player in the continuum of care, hospitals that positively address behavioral health care needs will contribute to the more effective and efficient use of health care resources, while also helping to produce positive outcomes for patients and their communities." The United States now has 32 beds per 100,000 population. In comparison, Western European nations have substantially more psychiatric beds. France and Switzerland have approximately 90 beds per 100,000 population, and Germany has 128. The United Kingdom, under its National Health Service, has 46 per 100,000. The multiple mental health crises in the United States, including the increase in suicides, the opioid epidemic, the incarceration of the mentally ill, and the increase in homelessness, may lead to new investments in acute care services. Most recently, in 2019, CMS increased Medicaid reimbursement in New York State by 25% for acute child and adolescent psychiatric beds per New York State's request. The long-term underinvestment in services may be coming to an end. Parity enforcement by states and the federal government may also lead to improved reimbursement from commercial insurance plans, especially as understanding grows of the impact of medical psychiatric illness on cost, disability, and mortality in all of health care.

Historically, inpatient services generated the surpluses that allowed other, less-profitable services (e.g., emergency, consultation, and outpatient services) to survive. Given changes in reimbursement, general hospitals may be able to use their contractual relationships with primary health insurers to negotiate better rates for their psychiatric services, especially as the impact of behavioral health carve-outs shrinks because of parity. Psychiatric hospitals may increasingly partner with general hospitals to divert less costly patients who do not need significant medical services away from general hospitals and thereby increase their volumes. Psychiatric services are now participating in quality improvement programs that assure high quality in the process of care and improved patient care outcomes (Institute of Medicine Committee on Crossing the Quality Chasm 2006), which will result in enhanced reimbursement. Pay-for-performance systems could conceivably provide enhanced reimbursement to high-quality programs, and reduction in the discrimination associated with psychiatric illness and its treatment may increase demand for acute care resources.

References

American Hospital Association: Community hospitals: addressing behavioral health care needs. TrendWatch, February 2007. Washington, DC, American Hospital Association, 2007

Center for Behavioral Health Statistics and Quality: National Mental Health Services Survey (N-MHSS): 2018. Rockville, MD, Substance Abuse and Mental Health Services Administration, October 2019. Available at: www.samhsa.gov/data/sites/default/files/cbhsq-reports/NMHSS-2018.pdf. Accessed November 13, 2019.

Center for Mental Health Services: Mental Health, United States, 2004 (DHHS Publ No SMA-06–4195). Edited by Manderscheid RW, Berry JT. Rockville, MD, Substance Abuse and Mental Health Services Administration, 2006

Centers for Medicare and Medicaid Services: 42 CFR Parts 412 and 413: Medicare program; prospective payment system for inpatient psychiatric facilities; final rule. Fed Regist 69(219):66921–67015, 2004

Drozd EM, Cromwell J, Gage B, et al: Patient casemix classification for Medicare psychiatric prospective payment. Am J Psychiatry 163(4):724–732, 2006 16585450

Frank RG, Garfield RL: Managed behavioral health care carve-outs: past performance and future prospects. Annu Rev Public Health 28:303–320, 2007 17112340

"History of Eastern State Hospital." Available at: https://esh.dbhds.virginia.gov/History.html. Accessed October 26, 2021.

Iglehart JK: Health policy report: the new era of prospective payment for hospitals. N Engl J Med 307(20):1288–1292, 1982 6813735
Institute of Medicine Committee on Crossing the Quality Chasm: Adaptation to Mental Health and Addictive Disorders: Improving the Quality of Health Care for Mental and Substance-Use Conditions. Washington, DC, National Academies Press, 2006
James DJ, Glaze LE: Mental health problems of prison and jail inmates. Bureau of Justice Statistics Special Report (NCJ 213600). Washington, DC, Office of Justice Programs, U.S. Department of Justice, 2006. Available at: https://bjs.ojp.gov/content/pub/pdf/mhppji.pdf. Accessed December 15, 2021.
Kelley D: Improving Payment and Care Under Medicare's Inpatient Psychiatric Benefit. Washington, DC, Medicare Payment Advisory Commission, October 6, 2011. Available at: www.medpac.gov/docs/default-source/meeting-materials/october-2011-meeting-presentation-improving-payment-and-care-under-medicare-s-inpatient-psychiatric-.pdf?sfvrsn=0. Accessed November 11, 2019.
Kihlstrom LC: Characteristics and growth of managed behavioral health care firms. Health Aff (Millwood) 16(4):127–130, 1997 9248156
Lave JR: Developing a Medicare prospective payment system for inpatient psychiatric care. Health Aff (Millwood) 22(5):97–109, 2003 14515885
Mechanic D, McAlpine DD, Olfson M: Changing patterns of psychiatric inpatient care in the United States, 1988–1994. Arch Gen Psychiatry 55(9):785–791, 1998 9736004
Medicare Payment Advisory Commission: Report to the Congress: Aligning Incentives in Medicare. Washington, DC, Medicare Payment Advisory Commission, June 2010
Medicare Payment Advisory Commission (MEDPAC): Inpatient Psychiatric Facility Services Payment System. November 2021. Available at: www.medpac.gov/wp-content/uploads/2021/11/medpac_payment_basics_21_psych_final_sec.pdf. Accessed October 29, 2021.
Mitchell JB, Dickey B, Liptzin B, Sederer LI: Bringing psychiatric patients into the Medicare prospective payment system: alternatives to DRGs. Am J Psychiatry 144(5):610–615, 1987 3107408
Mora G: Historical and theoretical trends in psychiatry, in Comprehensive Textbook of Psychiatry, 2nd Edition. Edited by Freedman A, Kaplan HI, Sadock BJ. Baltimore, MD, Williams & Wilkins, 1975, pp 1–75
National Association of State Mental Health Program Directors, Medical Directors Council: The Vital Role of State Psychiatric Hospitals. Edited by Parks J, Radke AQ. July 2014. Available at: www.nasmhpd.org/sites/default/files/The%20Vital%20Role%20of%20State%20Psychiatric%20HospitalsTechnical%20Report_July_2014%282%29.pdf. Accessed October 29, 2021.
Pierce F: Veto message, May 3, 1854, in A Compilation of the Messages and Papers of the Presidents, 1789–1897. Edited by Richardson JD. Washington, DC, Published by the Authority of Congress, 1898, pp 247–256
Reed LS: Coverage and Utilization of Care for Mental Conditions Under Health Insurance—Various Studies, 1973–1974. Washington, DC, American Psychiatric Association, 1975
Roehrig C: Mental disorders top the list of the most costly conditions in the United States. Health Aff (Millwood) 35(6):1130–1135, 2016
Sharfstein SS, Dickerson FB: Hospital psychiatry for the twenty-first century. Health Aff (Millwood) 28(3):685–688, 2009 19414876
Substance Abuse and Mental Health Services Administration: Behavioral Health Spending & Use Accounts, 1986–2014. Rockville, MD, Substance Abuse and Mental Health Services Administration, 2016. Available at: https://store.samhsa.gov/sites/default/files/d7/priv/sma16-4975.pdf. Accessed October 28, 2021.
Substance Abuse and Mental Health Services Administration: Health Care and Health Systems Integration. Rockville, MD, Substance Abuse and Mental Health Services Administration, 2018. Available at: www.samhsa.gov/health-care-health-systems-integration. Accessed October 28, 2021.
Summergrad P: The long view. Am J Psychiatry 172(8):714–716, 2015 26234596
Summergrad P, Hackett TP: Alan Gregg and the rise of general hospital psychiatry. Gen Hosp Psychiatry 9(6):439–445, 1987 3319770

Summergrad P, Kathol R (eds): Integrated Care in Psychiatry: Redefining the Role of Mental Health Professionals in the Medical Setting. New York, Springer, 2014

Thorpe K, Jain S, Joski P: Prevalence and spending associated with patients who have a behavioral health disorder and other conditions. Health Aff (Millwood) 36(1):124–132, 2017 28069855

Treatment Advocacy Center: Psychiatric Bed Supply Need Per Capita (online). Arlington, VA, Treatment Advocacy Center, September 2016a. Available at: www.treatmentadvocacycenter.org/component/content/article/220-learn-more-about/3696-psychiatric-bed-supply-need-per-capita. Accessed November 13, 2019.

Treatment Advocacy Center: Serious Mental Illness Prevalence in Jails and Prisons (online). Arlington, VA, Treatment Advocacy Center, September 2016b. Available at: www.treatmentadvocacycenter.org/component/content/article/220-learn-more-about/3695-serious-mental-illness-prevalence-in-jails-and-prisons-. Accessed November 13, 2019.

Watanabe-Galloway S, Zhang W: Analysis of U.S. trends in discharges from general hospitals for episodes of serious mental illness, 1995–2002. Psychiatr Serv 58(4):496–502, 2007 17412851

Weiss AJ, Wier LM, Stocks C, Blanchard J: Overview of emergency department visits in the United States, 2011. Healthcare Cost and Utilization Project Statistical Brief #174, June 2014. Available at: www.hcup-us.ahrq.gov/reports/statbriefs/sb174-Emergency-Department-Visits-Overview.pdf. Accessed November 13, 2019.

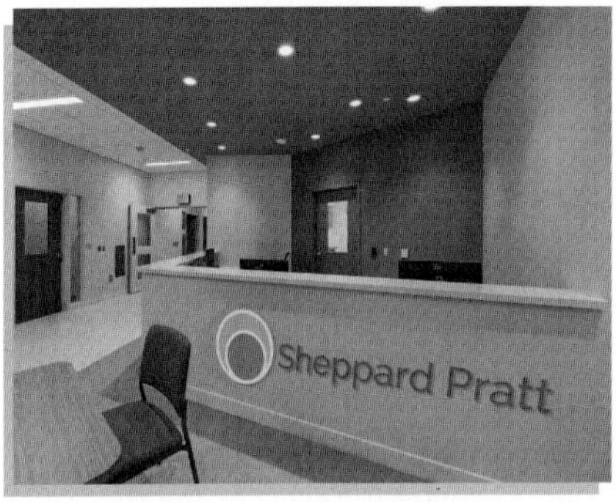

CHAPTER 19

Quality, Measurement-Based Care, and Outcomes

Robert J. Schloesser, M.D.

More than 2,500 years ago, Hippocrates codified two fundamental observations about health care quality (Katsambas and Marketos 2007): First, the practice of medicine, while intended to benefit patients, can also cause significant harm, and second, to avoid such harmful unintended consequences, best practices based on observation and evidence need to be followed. In today's complex health care systems, these observations seem more relevant than ever, and the topic of health care quality is receiving ever-increasing attention. Current estimates show that 1 out of 20 patients in the United States will experience preventable harm during treatment, with permanent disability or death resulting in 12% of these cases (Landrigan et al. 2010; Makary and Daniel 2016). Less-than-optimal treatment outcomes and exploding health care costs are increasingly attributed to an apparent gap between what is empirically proven to be efficient care and what is actually being delivered in routine practice. Efforts aimed at addressing health care quality problems are increasingly focusing on systematic implementation of quality measures (QMs) and their use in data-driven performance improvement programs.

In this chapter, we introduce QMs[1] for behavioral health care and review their use in current quality improvement programs. We also discuss impending changes to quality measurement, including efforts for the systematic implementation of measurement-based care (MBC) in routine psychiatric practice.

Health Care Quality

Health care quality has been defined as the assessment and provision of effective and safe care that results in the attainment of optimal or desired health. Good health care quality is considered to reflect a culture of excellence (Allen-Duck et al. 2017). The Institute of Medicine Committee on Quality of Health Care in America (2001) under the National Academy of Sciences defined six aims of high-quality health care:

1. *Safe*: Avoiding injuries to patients from the care that is intended to help them
2. *Effective*: Providing services based on scientific knowledge to all who could benefit and refraining from providing services to those not likely to benefit (avoiding underuse and overuse, respectively)
3. *Patient-centered*: Providing care that is respectful of and responsive to individual patient preferences, needs, and values and ensuring that patient values guide all clinical decisions
4. *Timely*: Reducing waits and sometimes harmful delays for both those who receive and those who give care
5. *Efficient*: Avoiding waste, including waste of equipment, supplies, ideas, and energy
6. *Equitable*: Providing care that does not vary in quality because of personal characteristics such as gender, ethnicity, geographical location, and socioeconomic status

Quality Improvement Efforts

There has been a growing appreciation for the fact that poor health care quality plays a key role not only in cases of preventable patient harm but also in the less-than-optimal treatment outcomes frequently observed in routine health care. In addition, the tremendous economic burden caused by suboptimal health care quality has been realized as a core component of exploding health care costs. A series of landmark reports issued by the Institute of Medicine highlighted issues with health care quality and increased public and political debate surrounding this topic. *To Err Is Human: Building a Safer Health System* and *Crossing the Quality Chasm*, published in 2000 and 2001, respectively, reviewed data on the negative impact of poor health care quality and reported estimates of the number of inpatient hospital deaths caused by medical errors (Institute of Medicine Committee on Quality of Health Care in America 2000, 2001), and in

---

[1]While the use of the term *quality measure* is fairly consistent, other terms are frequently used in this context. These include *performance measure* and *quality indicator*. While *performance measure* is practically synonymous, the term *quality indicator* is typically used to refer to subsets of QMs (e.g., QMs that meet specific criteria or are considered consensus standards) or refer to the specific construct of quality as opposed to the instrument (e.g., QM) used to measure the quality constructs.

2006, the report *Improving the Quality of Health Care for Mental and Substance-Use Conditions* specifically addressed problems due to poor health care quality in behavioral health (Institute of Medicine Committee on Crossing the Quality Chasm 2006).

Increasing political awareness resulted in numerous legislative efforts that fostered new laws and regulations aimed at improving health care quality. Whereas earlier laws and regulations focused on prevention of the most problematic incidences of quality and safety issues, modern programs aim to achieve the highest possible quality and most optimal outcomes throughout the entire health care system by facilitating implementation of continuous and systematic quality improvement strategies. A review of recent health care policy shows this noteworthy shift in the approach to health care quality improvement. In 1986, the Emergency Medical Treatment and Active Labor Act (EMTALA) was implemented. EMTALA requires hospitals to provide screening for and stabilization of emergency medical conditions regardless of patients' citizenship, legal status, or ability to pay. EMTALA is enforced through a complaint-driven process that involves investigations and surveys organized by the Centers for Medicare & Medicaid Services (CMS) in response to alleged violations. In 1997, CMS required public reporting of quantitative data on health care quality for several core areas. In 2005, implementation of the Patient Safety and Quality Improvement Act and initiation of the CMS "Hospital Compare" website established public reporting of quality data about adverse events and process measures for common conditions for Medicare beneficiaries aggregated at the hospital level (Centers for Medicare and Medicaid Services 2020). The Mental Health Parity and Addiction Equity Act of 2008 and the Affordable Care Act in 2010 included efforts to improve the quality of care through approaches to provider payment that are tied to QMs. In the Medicare Access and CHIP Reauthorization Act of 2015, these payment reform efforts were extended further. The ultimate goal of ongoing health care reimbursement reform efforts is to transition from fee-for-service to pay-for-performance reimbursement models. Such value-based health care models aim to directly incentivize best practices to achieve optimal quality and outcomes within the fiscal restraints of the system.

Quality Measures

QMs are statistical instruments designed to generate quantitative data about different constructs associated with health care quality. Quantitative data from QMs allow statistically sound comparisons of the levels of quality achieved between different groups or time points. For example, longitudinal QM data obtained before and after implementation of changes aimed at quality improvement can help administrators determine whether the implemented changes brought about the desired improvements. QMs allow the compilation of reference data sets that can be used as standards or to reference norms to assist with the interpretation of QM data. For example, modern, data-driven performance improvement programs use statistical benchmarking for performance comparisons across large numbers of providers or health care systems. Benchmarks provide a point of reference for the best achievable performance for a QM, typically based on the data from the best 10% performers in a group.

Compared with other metrics, such as means and averages, the ability to compare against the best achievable performance has been shown to increase the effectiveness of performance data feedback and the resulting degree of performance improvement. Many factors challenge the ability to make fair comparisons across different groups or approaches to care, which is a common problem encountered in programs that rely on comparisons of QM data. It is often important to employ methods for risk adjustment to address factors such as differences in case mix. Age, gender, and legal status are the most common factors contributing to significant differences between groups, but many other factors can confound a "fair" comparison of QM data. *Risk adjustment* is defined as "a means of statistically controlling for group differences when comparing non-equivalent groups on the outcomes that are of interest" (Schacht and Hines 2003, p. 220).

Three types of QMs distinguish different measurement approaches depending on whether the target of observation is an outcome, a process, or a structural factor. Examples of outcome measurements include instruments that quantify the proportion of patients who improve with therapy (positive outcomes) and instruments that quantify the degree of treatment-associated complications (negative outcomes). Outcome measures are considered the gold standard because they assess the results of health care most directly. However, in routine clinical care, it is often difficult or impossible to obtain direct measures of outcomes, and interpretation of outcome measure comparisons is frequently complicated by confounding variables. To overcome some of these limitations, systems or providers frequently employ process measures instead of outcome measures. Process measures assess how well the different steps of a process known to lead to a desired outcome are carried out, but these measures are only as valid as the relationship between the measured process and the desired outcome. Finally, structural measures can be used in cases in which specific features or parameters of infrastructure and policies are known to determine the level of quality. Most structural measures quantify features related to infrastructure and policies. They are often utilized when measurement of an outcome or process is not feasible or practical. Similar to process measures, the validity of structural measures depends on the strength of the association between the measured structural features and the provision of optimal health care.

QMs are composed of several elements that specify the data sources and algorithms used. The most basic elements of QMs are the denominator and numerator. The denominator defines the population being measured, while the numerator describes the target process, condition, event, or outcome being measured. Additional components to further specify exclusions and exceptions to the denominator and numerator are also included in most QMs (see Table 19–1 for examples of the basic elements for two QMs). Frequently, QMs also include specifications about the level of measurement (e.g., health system or provider) and measurement period, as well as definitions and information about value sets (e.g., ICD-10 codes, Current Procedural Terminology [CPT] codes, Systematized Nomenclature of Medicine [SNOMED] codes) being used. The development of QMs includes multiple phases, including conceptualization of the instrument, its development and specification, and testing. Conceptualization and development of specifications typically involve iterative processes in which available research and information on clinical guidelines and standards are evaluated by technical or domain-level experts. Testing is conducted not only to ensure that the QM is, at a minimum, both reliable and valid but also to examine its feasibility and usability for tools within the context of its intended (quality improvement) purpose. After development, QMs are governed by stewards who continue to assess their quality and frequently track their use within different programs.

TABLE 19–1. Components of quality measures, with examples

	Example 1	Example 2
Measure	Hours of physical restraint use	Depression remission at 6 months
ID	HBIPS-2	MIPS Clinical Quality Measure #411
NQF-ID	N/A	711
Measurement set	HBIPS	CMS MIPS quality measures
Steward	The Joint Commission	Minnesota Community Measurement
Type	Process	Outcome
Measurement description	Total number of hours that all patients admitted to a hospital-based inpatient psychiatric setting were maintained in physical restraint.	Adult patients ≥18 years of age with MDD or dysthymia and an initial PHQ-9 score >9 who demonstrate remission at 6 months, defined as a PHQ-9 score <5. Applies to patients with newly diagnosed or existing depression whose current PHQ-9 score indicates a need for treatment. Also promotes ongoing contact between patient and provider, because patients who do not have a follow-up PHQ-9 score at 6 months (±30 days) are included in the denominator.
Denominator	Number of psychiatric inpatient days. Basis: per 1,000 hours. Included populations: all psychiatric inpatient days.	Adult patients ≥18 years of age with a diagnosis of MDD or dysthymia and an initial (index) PHQ-9 score > 9.
Exclusions	Excluded populations: Total leave days	Patients who die, are permanent residents of a nursing home, or are enrolled in hospice care and patients who have a diagnosis (in any position) of bipolar or personality disorder.
Numerator	Total number of hours that all psychiatric inpatients were maintained in physical restraint. Basis: number of hours of physical restraint; however, algorithm calculates number of minutes to ensure more accurate calculation of the measure. Convert minutes to hours when analyzing and reporting this measure. Included populations: patients for whom at least one physical restraint event is reported during the month.	Adult patients ≥18 years of age with a diagnosis of MDD or dysthymia and an initial PHQ-9 score >9 who achieve remission at 6 months as demonstrated by a 6-month (±30 days) PHQ-9 score < 5.
Risk adjustment	No	Yes

Note. CMS=Centers for Medicare & Medicaid Services; HBIPS=Hospital-Based Inpatient Psychiatric Services; MDD=major depressive disorder; MIPS=Merit-based Incentive Payment System; NQF=National Quality Forum; PHQ=Patient Health Questionnaire.

Health Care Quality in Psychiatry

Problems with the quality of health care are thought to be a major factor contributing to poor outcomes of mental illness and the fact that prevalence rates of psychiatric conditions have not changed over recent decades (Baxter et al. 2014; Global Burden of Disease Study 2013 Collaborators 2015; Jorm et al. 2017). As in other fields of medicine, quality problems in psychiatry include failure to treat or prevent illness, inappropriate care, and unsafe care practices. Currently, several QMs for behavioral health–related conditions are deployed in the most important ongoing quality improvement programs. Many of the organizations that utilize QMs are also involved in their development and governance. In Table 19–2 we introduce some of the most important organizations and programs. Table 19–3 provides information on QMs for behavioral health currently used in these programs.

Failure to Treat or Prevent

When patients who should be treated for a mental illness are not receiving any care at all, it is considered a *failure to treat*. Obstacles to accessing care and insufficient screening and diagnosis are significant contributors to these problems. According to the results of the Substance Abuse and Mental Health Services Administration 2018 National Survey on Drug Use and Health, only 20.6 million of 47.6 million adults (43.3%) with any mental illness and only 7.3 million of 11.4 million adults (64.0%) with severe mental illness received mental health services in 2018 (Substance Abuse and Mental Health Services Administration 2019). The most common reasons reported for not receiving services were inability to afford the cost of care, insufficient time to obtain care, and not knowing where to receive the correct care. Individuals from ethnic minority groups face additional obstacles to receiving needed mental health services (Office of the Surgeon General 2001). In 2018, less than 20% of 20.1 million people in the United States who were thought to need substance use treatment received it. The most common reasons for not receiving substance use treatment included lack of perceived need for treatment (99.4%) and lack of desire to quit substance use, but in one out of three cases in which patients perceived a need for treatment but did not receive it, lack of insurance coverage or inability to afford treatment was cited. Of all QMs currently deployed in federal quality improvement programs, only a few address access and utilization of services; these include three QMs within the National Committee for Quality Assurance's Healthcare Effectiveness Data and Information Set (HEDIS) measurement set. The level of analysis for these measures is health plans, and the data source is claims data. The HEDIS measure "Utilization of Mental Health Services" (NQF None) summarizes the number and percentage of patients receiving mental health services, while "Identification of Alcohol and Other Drug Services" (NQF None) summarizes the number and percentages of patients receiving substance use services. Another HEDIS measure, "Initiation and Engagement of Alcohol and Other Drug Abuse or Dependence Treatment" (NQF 0004), measures the degree to which a health organization initiates and continues treatment for alcohol and substance use disorders once a need has been identified.

In addition to problems with access, missed or significantly delayed diagnoses are common problems for patients with psychiatric conditions. For almost all psychiatric conditions, evidence has shown missed or delayed diagnoses in routine health care, in-

TABLE 19–2. Quality measures (QMs) for behavioral health in federal quality improvement programs

National Quality Forum (NQF), www.qualityforum.org

Not-for-profit membership organization with the goal of promoting and ensuring patient protection and health care quality through measurement and public reporting. Operates as a *consensus-based entity* in the creation of *consensus standards* that are defined by the National Technology Transfer and Advancement Act of 1995. Uses a multistep consensus development process to vet potential QMs and endorses those measures that meet the following criteria:

Importance to measure and report

Scientific acceptability of measure properties

Feasibility

Usability and use

NQF does not organize quality improvement programs itself, but NQF-endorsed measures are preferred by federal programs. A database with detailed information on all QMs and reports with information about their use is freely available on the website. Evaluated QMs receive an identification number (e.g., NQF # 0104). In chapter text, this number is used to reference QMs wherever possible.

National Committee for Quality Assurance (NCQA), www.ncqa.org

Not-for-profit organization established in 1990 with support from the Robert Wood Johnson Foundation. Manages voluntary accreditation programs for individual physicians, health plans, and medical groups and is involved in developing and maintaining QMs. Developed and maintains the Healthcare Effectiveness Data and Information Set (HEDIS), one of the most widely used QM sets in the managed care industry. Information on NCQA's QMs is available on the website. Most of the HEDIS QMs are also endorsed by NQF, and information is available in the NQF database.

The Joint Commission (TJC), www.jointcommission.org

U.S.-based nonprofit organization that accredits more than 21,000 U.S. health care organizations and programs. Developer and steward of the Hospital-Based Inpatient Psychiatric Services QM set as part of its ORYX Quality Initiative, and the National Patient Safety Goals program, which includes specifications for quality standards in the context of suicide risk assessments and suicide prevention. Also recently added requirements to its accreditation process for implementing components of measurement-based care utilizing standardized assessment tools for behavioral health.

Centers for Medicare & Medicaid Services (CMS), www.cms.gov

Organizes the largest ongoing federal-level efforts to improve health care quality in the United States. Program participation is either required as part of accreditation (see NCQA and TJC above) or incentivized through pay-for-performance reimbursement programs. Currently uses QMs for behavioral health in its Inpatient Psychiatric Facility Quality Reporting Program and recently established Quality Payment Programs.

CMS Inpatient Psychiatric Facility Quality Reporting (IPFQR) Program, www.qualitynet.org/ipf/ipfqr/measures

Pay-for-reporting program mandated by the U.S. Congress and implemented in 2012. Intended to equip consumers with quality-of-care information to make more-informed decisions about health care options and to encourage hospitals and clinicians to improve inpatient care quality. Inpatient psychiatric facilities are required to submit a specific set of QMs to CMS to avoid financial penalties to their standard federal rate. Data provided by psychiatric inpatient facilities to CMS are publicly available on the website.

TABLE 19–2. Quality measures (QMs) for behavioral health in federal quality improvement programs *(continued)*

CMS Quality Payment Programs (QPPs), qpp.cms.gov
The Medicare Access and CHIP Reauthorization Act of 2015 provisioned significant changes to physician reimbursement for treating patients enrolled in Medicare. This change was aimed toward transitioning from a fee-for-service system to a pay-for-performance system. Since 2017, CMS has been advancing these efforts through two distinct QPPs, the Merit-based Incentive Payment System (MIPS) and the Advanced Alternative Payment Models. Older CMS pay-for-performance programs that utilized quality metrics included the Physician Quality Reporting System and the "meaningful use" electronic health record incentive payment program, both of which were rolled over into the current QPPs. Information and specifications for QMs used in MIPS are available on the QPP website.

cluding mood and anxiety disorders (Borner et al. 2010; Cheung et al. 2017; Coyle et al. 2003; Ko et al. 2012; Schonfeld et al. 1997; Williams et al. 2002); psychotic disorders (Marshall et al. 2005); PTSD, in particular when comorbid with other mental illness (Zammit et al. 2018); ADHD (Taylor 2017); and personality disorders (Bozzatello et al. 2019). Several widely used QMs target processes for appropriate screening and assessment of psychiatric conditions; however, only a few psychiatric conditions are specifically covered. Most QMs for this purpose measure screening and assessment for depressive disorders and alcohol and substance use disorders. A few QMs in the ongoing federal quality improvement programs measure assessment of behavioral and psychiatric symptoms in patients with dementia or Parkinson's disease.

One of the most apparent problems related to poor quality of screening and assessment is the failure to prevent suicides. Every year, more than 47,000 Americans die by suicide (Centers for Disease Control and Prevention 2019), and there is widespread belief that this number could be reduced if many quality problems were addressed. Most suicides are due to mental illness (Bachmann 2018), and many individuals who die by suicide make contact with primary care providers or mental health services before the suicide. For example, it has been shown that approximately 15% of suicide victims age 35 and younger saw a mental health professional within 1 month of their suicide, and approximately 23% saw a primary care provider (Luoma et al. 2002).

Patients undergoing psychiatric inpatient treatment continue to be at high risk for suicide as well. Estimates of the number of occurrences of hospital inpatient suicides in the United States vary substantially. Some sources estimate the number per year to be around 1,500 (Powell et al. 2000; "Practice Guideline for the Assessment and Treatment of Patients With Suicidal Behaviors" 2003); however, a more recent analysis of data from various hospital reporting databases estimated a much lower number, averaging between 48.5 and 64.9 cases per year, of which approximately 70% occurred during psychiatric treatment (Williams et al. 2018). The fact that many patients die by suicide in the period immediately after a psychiatric hospitalization (Chung et al. 2017) points to quality problems not only in screening but also in discharge planning and transition of care of patients at high risk for suicide. Implementation of suicide risk assessments is currently measured for adults and children with a diagnosis of major depressive disorder (MDD) in the Merit-based Incentive Payment System Quality Payment Program (NQFs 0104 and 1365) and one QM in The Joint Commission's ORYX Quality Improvement Program (NQF 1922).

TABLE 19–3. Quality measures (QMs) in federal programs

	NQF endorsed 2019	TJC ORYX 2019	NCQA HEDIS 2019	CMS IPFQR 2019	CMS MIPS 2019
Total number of QMs	542	4	68	8	268
Number of QMs specific to behavioral health	41	4	18	8	25
Percentage of QMs for behavioral health	8%	100%	26%	100%	9%
Type of QMs (only behavioral health)					
Outcome	5	0	1	0	3
Process	36	4	12	8	22
Structure	0	0	0	0	0
Target population by condition					
Depressive disorders	11	0	4	0	9
Anxiety disorders	0	0	0	0	0
Bipolar and related disorders	1	0	1	0	0
Schizophrenia/Psychotic disorders	5	0	2	0	1
Trauma- and stressor-related disorders (including PTSD)	0	0	0	0	0
ADHD	1	0	1	0	1
Neurocognitive disorders (including dementia)	0	0	0	0	5
Alcohol and substance use disorders	9	0	2	1	4
Unspecified disorder	15	4	3	7	1
Age range					
Adult (or not specified, sometimes includes adolescent or all age groups)	36	4	12	8	16
Child (includes children and adolescents)	5	—	4	—	2
Geriatric	—	—	—	—	5
Quality construct target					
Medication best practices	3	1	4	2	4
Screening or assessment of psychiatric condition or alcohol or substance use (not suicide)	10	1	1	1	10
Screening/monitoring or coordination of care for comorbid medical conditions or medical risk factors	12	0	2	0	1
Follow-up after psychiatric treatment event (e.g., emergency or inpatient)	3	0	3	1	1
Symptom severity or disorder status outcome	5	0	1	0	2
Seclusion/Restraint	0	2	0	2	0
Suicide risk assessment	2	1	0	0	2

Note. CMS=Centers for Medicare & Medicaid Services; HEDIS=Healthcare Effectiveness Data and Information Set; IPFQR=Inpatient Psychiatric Facility Quality Reporting Program; MIPS=Merit-based Incentive Payment System; NCQA=National Committee for Quality Assurance; NQF=National Quality Forum; TJC=The Joint Commission.

Inappropriate Care

In addition to failures to treat that result from lack of access and missed diagnosis, poor outcomes in psychiatry also arise from provision of low-quality treatment during routine practice. Routine mental health care is highly variable across regions and providers. Variations in care are appropriate when clinicians tailor therapeutic regimens to patients' unique clinical conditions or patients' preferences; however, in many cases variations are undesirable and lead to poor treatment outcomes. Overall adherence to specific clinical practice guidelines for treating psychiatric patients is poor (Bauer 2002; Nguyen et al. 2020). For example, in four industrialized countries, no change in the prevalence of common mental disorders was observed, despite evidence for increased provision of treatment (Jorm et al. 2017). This discrepancy is believed to arise from failures to provide care consistent with scientific evidence.

Many QMs are aimed at quantifying the alignment of care processes with empirically based treatments. Regarding medication management, some widely used QMs assess the use of antidepressants, antipsychotics, and ADHD medications. For example, one QM (NQF 105) quantifies how many patients diagnosed with MDD who were prescribed antidepressant medication in the past continue to receive antidepressant medication. Other commonly used QMs assess best practices of antipsychotic prescribing, including adherence to medication among patients with schizophrenia and the extent of concurrent use of multiple antipsychotics (NQFs 1879 and 0560). Several QMs quantify compliance using known guidelines for monitoring common medication-related side effects and recommended assessments for comorbid medical problems in patients with mental illness (e.g., NQFs 1932–1934, 2601–2604). Best practices in care coordination are also commonly assessed, including follow-up after inpatient psychiatric hospitalization or emergency department visits for mental health or substance use disorders (e.g., NQFs 0576, 2605, 3488).

Unsafe Care

Of the many practices considered to be forms of *unsafe care*, the one most debated in psychiatry is the use of seclusion and restraint. Although coercive measures are thought to be unavoidable in some situations to avoid risks for patients and others, seclusion and restraint clearly carry a significant risk for psychological and physical harm. An abundance of evidence shows the effectiveness of care processes to reduce the incidence of coercive measures; however, despite this knowledge, these measures are still frequently being used (Chieze et al. 2019). Currently, two QMs that quantify the total amount of time that psychiatric inpatients spent in seclusion or restraint are being utilized in the ORYX program and the CMS IPFQR program (NQFs 0640 and 0641).

Current State of Quality Measures in Behavioral Health Care

Overall, there is little evidence that the quality of psychiatric health care has significantly improved over the past two decades. Compared with general medicine, the impact of federal programs on quality of behavioral health care seems to be marginal. A recent article examining QM data obtained from insurers for the year 2014 showed that best practices were followed less than half of the time in four areas of behavioral health, whereas six cardiovascular and diabetes measures showed 72% compliance. Although QMs for diabetes and hypertension showed slow incremental improvement over time, behavioral health measures showed an average quality *decline* for two out of three payers (Pincus et al. 2016). Some argue that this is due to a lack of appropriate QMs and underutilization of QMs relevant for routine psychiatric health care in current quality improvement programs. Compared with QMs for other fields of medicine, there is a dearth of QMs designed for behavioral health care that are suitable for "high-stakes" accountability purposes, such as public reporting and value-based purchasing. For example, of more than 500 measures endorsed by NQF, fewer than 30 are specifically designed for behavioral health care. In addition, QMs for behavioral health care are underrepresented in current federal quality improvement programs (see Table 19–3). Of the more than 500 measures for behavioral health care identified in large national databases, only about 5% are utilized in major quality reporting programs (Patel et al. 2015). Underlying factors for these deficits include insufficient efforts to coordinate and provide funding for the development of clinical practice guidelines and associated QMs, as well as insufficient training of the clinical workforce in the use of QMs and clinical practice guidelines (Pincus et al. 2016).

Measurement-Based Care and Patient-Reported Outcomes

Efforts to prioritize the development of QMs that incorporate patient-reported outcome measures (PROMs) and the implementation of MBC in routine clinical practice for behavioral health care have accelerated. *Measurement-based care* has been broadly defined as the practice of basing clinical care on data about the patient. Specifically, in MBC, providers base clinical decision-making on information about a patient's health and well-being that is systematically collected throughout the treatment process. PROMs are standardized psychometric instruments including symptom rating scales and questionnaires that probe patients' level of functioning or quality of life. These instruments are completed by patients or their proxies, such as family members or caregivers.

The primary benefit of MBC is better treatment outcomes. Patients enrolled in treatment programs that incorporate MBC methodologies achieve better outcomes than patients undergoing "usual care." This phenomenon has been demonstrated across many treatment settings and for many conditions, including inpatients with depression (Adli et al. 2002; Bauer et al. 2009), patients with MDD treated in outpatient psychiatric care (Trivedi et al. 2004), patients with late-life depression in primary care settings (Unützer et al. 2002), patients with bipolar disorder treated in community mental health clinics (Simon et al. 2006), and patients with anxiety disorders in primary care clinics (Roy-Byrne et al. 2010). In addition, many empirically supported types of psychotherapy utilize key processes of MBC, namely systematic monitoring of patient progress as part of the treatment process.

There is compelling evidence that adding systematic monitoring and feedback can improve any type of therapy with respect to outcomes, such as degree of psychological disturbance, interpersonal problems, social role functioning, and quality of life (Krägeloh et al. 2015; Lambert 2003). The positive effects of MBC on treatment outcomes are thought to result from a combination of factors. Primarily, the ability to quantify symptoms through PROMs and other standardized measures improves clinicians' understanding and awareness of where patients' symptoms are at baseline and how they fluctuate throughout treatment. Continuous feedback of this type of data can facilitate optimal treatment decisions.

Not surprisingly, in addition to improving outcomes, MBC—when used to facilitate treatment guidelines and algorithms—leads to fewer changes of the treatment plan and lower use of psychotropic medication (Bauer et al. 2009). At the same time, it leads to earlier detection of symptom worsening and better appreciation of residual symptoms (Hatfield et al. 2010; Walfish et al. 2012), and it is thought to facilitate changes in the treatment plan when clinically indicated (Henke et al. 2009; Shimokawa et al. 2010; Zimmerman and McGlinchey 2008a). In addition to the primary benefits for treatment monitoring, PROMs improve screening and diagnosis and care-related communication. They can streamline the assessment process and aid clinicians in making a differential diagnosis (Kroenke et al. 2001), which can help overcome the problems surrounding low diagnostic accuracy observed in routine clinical care (Rettew et al. 2009). PROM utilization also improves patient engagement in the treatment process (Dowrick et al. 2009; Eisen et al. 2000) and can facilitate communication across the care teams (Unützer and Park 2012).

Various secondary benefits of MBC and routine PROM data collection have been proposed for all levels of stakeholders in behavioral health care. Providers can utilize data obtained in the context of MBC to objectively assess the effectiveness of various treatments or treatment components in a range of clinical contexts and use this information to become better clinicians. In addition, aggregated MBC data can be used for quality improvement efforts for clinical programs. At the health care organization level, such data can be utilized to demonstrate efficacy of the services delivered and lead to increased revenue through value-based-care incentive payments.

Despite evidence for the benefits of MBC and PROMs, only 18% of psychiatrists and 11% of psychologists in the United States routinely utilize symptom rating scales in their clinical practice (Hatfield et al. 2010; Zimmerman and McGlinchey 2008b). Different reasons for this low utilization have been identified. For clinicians, these include lack of training (Ionita et al. 2016; Meehan et al. 2006) and problems with access to PROM instruments and with implementing MBC processes into routine clinical work due to resource constraints (Ionita et al. 2016; Kotte et al. 2016). Other concerns reported by clinicians include possible negative impacts to treatment and anxiety about data being used for performance evaluation (Meehan et al. 2006; Ionita et al. 2016).

The Sheppard Pratt Journey to Measurement-Based Care and Patient-Reported Outcome Measures

In 2018, Sheppard Pratt started an initiative with the goal enabling MBC using PROMs at the point of care. PROM data are collected using electronic questionnaires that patients can answer remotely or using tablet computers provided in waiting rooms and on inpatient units. Data are analyzed and reported immediately in real time to the treating clinicians through integration with Sheppard Pratt's electronic medical record system.

As of August 2020, 15 adult and child/adolescent programs have implemented MBC. These include various outpatient clinics, crisis services, inpatient units, partial hospital programs, and intensive outpatient programs and an adolescent residential treatment center. In total, 10,000 unique patients have used the PROM system during their care episode to report about their health and well-being. More than 160,000 PROM instruments have been completed to date (using a specific standardized questionnaire; e.g., Patient Reported Outcomes Measurement Information System [PROMIS]—Depression, Patient Health Questionnaire–9, World Health Organization Disability Assessment Schedule [WHODAS]) within more than 24,000 assessments (battery of instruments collected at the same time).

The American Psychiatric Association National Mental Health Registry

Sheppard Pratt, firmly believing that it is imperative to give people the ability to make informed decisions about their care through meaningful outcomes data, was the first health system to join PsychPRO, the American Psychiatric Association's national patient registry. A core feature to highlight is the registry's ability to support dedicated physicians and care providers to better automate their reporting of quality data and maintain their board certification. In time, the registry will be able to guide future research and to develop new diagnostics, therapeutics, and QMs.

References

Adli M, Berghöfer A, Linden M, et al: Effectiveness and feasibility of a standardized stepwise drug treatment regimen algorithm for inpatients with depressive disorders: results of a 2-year observational algorithm study. J Clin Psychiatry 63(9):782–790, 2002 12363118

Allen-Duck A, Robinson JC, Stewart MW: Healthcare quality: a concept analysis. Nurs Forum 52(4):377–386, 2017 28407249

Bachmann S: Epidemiology of suicide and the psychiatric perspective. Int J Environ Res Public Health 15(7):1425, 2018 29986446

Bauer MS: A review of quantitative studies of adherence to mental health clinical practice guidelines. Harv Rev Psychiatry 10(3):138–153, 2002 12023929

Bauer M, Pfennig A, Linden M, et al: Efficacy of an algorithm-guided treatment compared with treatment as usual: a randomized, controlled study of inpatients with depression. J Clin Psychopharmacol 29(4):327–333, 2009 19593170

Baxter AJ, Scott KM, Ferrari AJ, et al: Challenging the myth of an "epidemic" of common mental disorders: trends in the global prevalence of anxiety and depression between 1990 and 2010. Depress Anxiety 31(6):506–516, 2014 24448889

Borner I, Braunstein JW, St Victor R, Pollack J: Evaluation of a 2-question screening tool for detecting depression in adolescents in primary care. Clin Pediatr (Phila) 49(10):947–953, 2010 20724330

Bozzatello P, Bellino S, Bosia M, Rocca P: Early detection and outcome in borderline personality disorder. Front Psychiatry 10:710, 2019 31649564

Centers for Disease Control and Prevention: Suicide and self-harm injury. 2019. Available at: www.cdc.gov/nchs/fastats/suicide.htm. Accessed December 15, 2021.

Centers for Medicare and Medicaid Services: Hospital Quality Initiative (online). Baltimore, MD, Centers for Medicare and Medicaid Services, 2020. Available at: www.cms.gov/Medicare/Quality-Initiatives-Patient-Assessment-Instruments/HospitalQualityInits. Accessed December 20, 2019.

Cheung R, O'Donnell S, Madi N, Goldner E: Factors associated with delayed diagnosis of mood and/or anxiety disorders. Health Promot Chronic Dis Prev Can 37(5):137–148, 2017 28493658

Chieze M, Hurst S, Kaiser S, Sentissi O: Effects of seclusion and restraint in adult psychiatry: a systematic review. Front Psychiatry 10:491, 2019 31404294

Chung DT, Ryan CJ, Hadzi-Pavlovic D, et al: Suicide rates after discharge from psychiatric facilities: a systematic review and meta-analysis. JAMA Psychiatry 74(7):694–702, 2017 28564699

Coyle JT, Pine DS, Charney DS, et al: Depression and Bipolar Support Alliance consensus statement on the unmet needs in diagnosis and treatment of mood disorders in children and adolescents. J Am Acad Child Adolesc Psychiatry 42(12):1494–1503, 2003 14627885

Dowrick C, Leydon GM, McBride A, et al: Patients' and doctors' views on depression severity questionnaires incentivised in UK quality and outcomes framework: qualitative study. BMJ 338:b663, 2009 19299474

Eisen SV, Dickey B, Sederer LI: A self-report symptom and problem rating scale to increase inpatients' involvement in treatment. Psychiatr Serv 51(3):349–353, 2000 10686242

Global Burden of Disease Study 2013 Collaborators: Global, regional, and national incidence, prevalence, and years lived with disability for 301 acute and chronic diseases and injuries in 188 countries, 1990–2013: a systematic analysis for the Global Burden of Disease Study 2013. Lancet 386(9995):743–800, 2015 26063472

Hatfield D, McCullough L, Frantz SHB, Krieger K: Do we know when our clients get worse? An investigation of therapists' ability to detect negative client change. Clin Psychol Psychother 17(1):25–32, 2010 19916162

Henke RM, Zaslavsky AM, McGuire TG, et al: Clinical inertia in depression treatment. Med Care 47(9):959–967, 2009 19704353

Institute of Medicine Committee on Crossing the Quality Chasm: Adaptation to Mental Health and Addictive Disorders: Improving the Quality of Health Care for Mental and Substance-Use Conditions (Quality Chasm Series). Washington, DC, National Academies Press, 2006

Institute of Medicine Committee on Quality of Health Care in America: To Err Is Human: Building a Safer Health System. Washington, DC, National Academies Press, 2000

Institute of Medicine Committee on Quality of Health Care in America: Crossing the Quality Chasm: A New Health System for the 21st Century. Washington, DC, National Academies Press, 2001

Ionita G, Fitzpatrick M, Tomaro J, et al: Challenges of using progress monitoring measures: Insights from practicing clinicians. J Couns Psychol 63(2):173–182, 2016 26651210

Jorm AF, Patten SB, Brugha TS, Mojtabai R: Has increased provision of treatment reduced the prevalence of common mental disorders? Review of the evidence from four countries. World Psychiatry 16(1):90–99, 2017 28127925

Katsambas A, Marketos SG: Hippocratic messages for modern medicine (the vindication of Hippocrates). J Eur Acad Dermatol Venereol 21(6):859–861, 2007 17567336

Ko JY, Farr SL, Dietz PM, Robbins CL: Depression and treatment among U.S. pregnant and nonpregnant women of reproductive age, 2005–2009. J Womens Health (Larchmt) 21(8):830–836, 2012 22691031

Kotte A, Hill KA, Mah AC, et al: Facilitators and barriers of implementing a measurement feedback system in public youth mental health. Adm Policy Ment Health 43(6):861–878, 2016 27000148

Krägeloh CU, Czuba KJ, Billington DR, et al: Using feedback from patient-reported outcome measures in mental health services: a scoping study and typology. Psychiatr Serv 66(3):224–241, 2015 25727110

Kroenke K, Spitzer RL, Williams JB: The PHQ-9: validity of a brief depression severity measure. J Gen Intern Med 16(9):606–613, 2001 11556941

Lambert MJ: Is it time for clinicians to routinely track patient outcome? A meta-analysis. Clinical Psychology: Science and Practice 10:288–301, 2003

Landrigan CP, Parry GJ, Bones CB, et al: Temporal trends in rates of patient harm resulting from medical care. N Engl J Med 363(22):2124–2134, 2010 21105794

Luoma JB, Martin CE, Pearson JL: Contact with mental health and primary care providers before suicide: a review of the evidence. Am J Psychiatry 159(6):909–916, 2002 12042175

Makary MA, Daniel M: Medical error–the third leading cause of death in the US (comment). BMJ 353:i2139, 2016 27143499

Marshall M, Lewis S, Lockwood A, et al: Association between duration of untreated psychosis and outcome in cohorts of first-episode patients: a systematic review. Arch Gen Psychiatry 62(9):975–983, 2005 16143729

Meehan T, McCombes S, Hatzipetrou L, Catchpoole R: Introduction of routine outcome measures: staff reactions and issues for consideration. J Psychiatr Ment Health Nurs 13(5):581–587, 2006 16965478

Nguyen T, Seiler N, Brown E, O'Donoghue B: The effect of clinical practice guidelines on prescribing practice in mental health: a systematic review. Psychiatry Res 284:112671, 2020 31732189

Office of the Surgeon General: Mental Health: Culture, Race, and Ethnicity: A Supplement to Mental Health: A Report of the Surgeon General. Rockville, MD, Substance Abuse and Mental Health Services Administration, 2001

Patel MM, Brown JD, Croake S, et al: The current state of behavioral health quality measures: where are the gaps? Psychiatr Serv 66(8):865–871, 2015 26073415

Pincus HA, Scholle SH, Spaeth-Rublee B, et al: Quality measures for mental health and substance use: gaps, opportunities, and challenges. Health Aff (Millwood) 35(6):1000–1008, 2016 27269015

Powell J, Geddes J, Deeks J, et al: Suicide in psychiatric hospital in-patients: risk factors and their predictive power. Br J Psychiatry 176:266–272, 2000 10755075

Practice guideline for the assessment and treatment of patients with suicidal behaviors. Am J Psychiatry 160(11 suppl):1–60, 2003 14649920

Rettew DC, Lynch AD, Achenbach TM, et al: Meta-analyses of agreement between diagnoses made from clinical evaluations and standardized diagnostic interviews. Int J Methods Psychiatr Res 18(3):169–184, 2009 19701924

Roy-Byrne P, Craske MG, Sullivan G, et al: Delivery of evidence-based treatment for multiple anxiety disorders in primary care: a randomized controlled trial. JAMA 303(19):1921–1928, 2010 20483968

Schacht LM, Hines H: Recent applications of risk adjustment for performance measures used by state inpatient psychiatric facilities. Harv Rev Psychiatry 11(4):220–224, 2003 12944130

Schonfeld WH, Verboncoeur CJ, Fifer SK, et al: The functioning and well-being of patients with unrecognized anxiety disorders and major depressive disorder. J Affect Disord 43(2):105–119, 1997 9165380

Shimokawa K, Lambert MJ, Smart DW: Enhancing treatment outcome of patients at risk of treatment failure: meta-analytic and mega-analytic review of a psychotherapy quality assurance system. J Consult Clin Psychol 78(3):298–311, 2010 20515206

Simon GE, Ludman EJ, Bauer MS, et al: Long-term effectiveness and cost of a systematic care program for bipolar disorder. Arch Gen Psychiatry 63(5):500–508, 2006 16651507

Substance Abuse and Mental Health Services Administration: Key Substance Use and Mental Health Indicators in the United States: Results From the 2018 National Survey on Drug Use and Health (HHS Publ No PEP19-5068, NSDUH Series H-54). Rockville, MD, Substance Abuse and Mental Health Services Administration, 2019

Taylor E: Attention deficit hyperactivity disorder: overdiagnosed or diagnoses missed? Arch Dis Child 102(4):376–379, 2017 27821518

Trivedi MH, Rush AJ, Crismon ML, et al: Clinical results for patients with major depressive disorder in the Texas Medication Algorithm Project. Arch Gen Psychiatry 61(7):669–680, 2004 15237079

Unützer J, Park M: Strategies to improve the management of depression in primary care. Prim Care 39(2):415–431, 2012 22608874

Unützer J, Katon W, Callahan CM, et al: Collaborative care management of late-life depression in the primary care setting: a randomized controlled trial. JAMA 288(22):2836–2845, 2002 12472325

Walfish S, McAlister B, O'Donnell P, Lambert MJ: An investigation of self-assessment bias in mental health providers. Psychol Rep 110(2):639–644, 2012 22662416

Williams JW Jr, Noël PH, Cordes JA, et al: Is this patient clinically depressed? JAMA 287(9):1160–1170, 2002 11879114

Williams SC, Schmaltz SP, Castro GM, Baker DW: Incidence and method of suicide in hospitals in the United States. Jt Comm J Qual Patient Saf 44(11):643–650, 2018 30190221

Zammit S, Lewis C, Dawson S, et al: Undetected post-traumatic stress disorder in secondary-care mental health services: systematic review. Br J Psychiatry 212(1):11–18, 2018 29433609

Zimmerman M, McGlinchey JB: Depressed patients' acceptability of the use of self-administered scales to measure outcome in clinical practice. Ann Clin Psychiatry 20(3):125–129, 2008a 18633738

Zimmerman M, McGlinchey JB: Why don't psychiatrists use scales to measure outcome when treating depressed patients? J Clin Psychiatry 69(12):1916–1919, 2008b 19192467

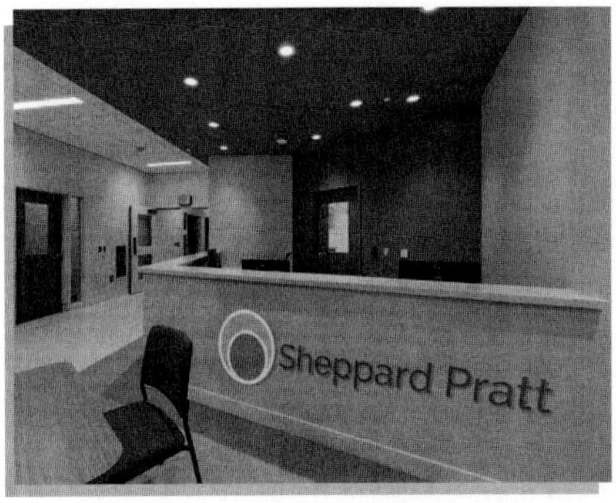

CHAPTER 20

Risk Management

Jerry Halverson, M.D.
Nathaniel Clark, M.D.
Terri Schultz, R.N., M.B.A.
Steven Hertig, B.A., CHPC

Psychiatric hospitals must manage many of the same risks that multispecialty hospitals do, in addition to confronting several challenges unique to the behavioral health specialty practice. To manage these risks, a well thought out and functional risk management system is of primary importance to the hospital and can help to guarantee its ability to serve the community in the face of various threats. A solid risk management system is a cornerstone of good psychiatric practice for all behavioral health providers because it gives the patients and employees the security and stability they need to do the lifesaving work that occurs in a psychiatric hospital. A risk management system comprises the policies, protocols, and procedures that keep patients, employees, and other interests of the hospital safe and whole by identifying and addressing threats. Many of these threats have been discussed extensively elsewhere and have been consistent throughout the years (i.e., patient and staff safety), and some are newer and have evolved with societal or technological changes (i.e., patient health data safety or cybersecurity). In this chapter, we explore the common risks and liabilities that psychiatric hospitals must manage to protect their patients, their staff, and their ability to maintain access to their services.

Patient Rights

Patient rights are the basic rules of conduct between patients and medical caregivers, as well as the institutions and people that support them. A patient is anyone who has requested to be or is being evaluated by any health care professional. Medical caregivers include hospitals and health care personnel, as well as insurance agencies or any payers of medical-related costs. This is a broad definition of patient rights, but there are other, slightly more specific definitions. For example, a legal definition is as follows: *patient rights* is a general statement adopted by most health care professionals that covers such matters as access to care, patient dignity, confidentiality, and consent to treatment. No matter what definition is used, most patients and doctors are finding that many of the details of patient rights have changed and are continuing to change over time.

Often, patients do not realize their specific rights at the time of their care because those rights are not clearly defined or described in the bundle of papers that patients need to sign during the registration or admission process. An example of one of these fundamental rights that is not clear to all is that all patients who seek care at an emergency department (ED) or hospital have the right to a screening examination and that patients who cannot afford to pay are not turned away. These rights are detailed in the Emergency Medical Treatment and Active Labor Act (EMTALA) in the United States. Further, many patients do not understand the nature of their rights, for example, thinking that their rights are only applicable between themselves and their doctor. This is not true. As stated in the first definition, patient rights can be extensive and exist between many people and institutions. Most notably, they can exist between patients, any medical caregiver, hospitals, laboratories, insurers, and even support staff or housekeepers who may have access to patients or their medical records.

It is not possible to list all patients' rights. However, most written rights that doctors and health care personnel have patients read (and sign) are abbreviated statements that summarize all or parts of the American Medical Association's Code of Medical Ethics.

The Affordable Care Act also offers rights and protections. Some rights and protections apply to plans in the Health Insurance Marketplace or other individual insurance, some apply to job-based plans, and some apply to all health coverage. The law provides patients with protections to obtain coverage for those with preexisting conditions. It provides coverage for pregnancy and free preventive care, no lifetime or yearly dollar limits on coverage of essential health benefits, and health plan communications written in language the patient can understand. The law also makes it illegal for health insurance companies to cancel patients' health insurance just because they get sick, protects patients' right to choose their provider of choice, and prevents employer retaliation. Additionally, it provides for free birth control and counseling and coverage for mental health and substance abuse services, and ensures the right to appeal a health plan decision and the right to choose an individual Marketplace plan rather than the one provided by the patient's employer.

In addition to the Affordable Care Act, patient rights have also been written into state law. If a health care organization is found to have violated any of these state or federal statutes, violations may result in fines or even prison time. Each medical caregiver has the responsibility to become familiar with these statutes and understand how they must be applied in medical practice. In addition, all medical caregivers must ensure patients can exercise their rights while in treatment. Each patient or patient representative has the right to file a complaint or grievance with the physician or organization, and organizations must have a detailed policy for dealing with patients' grievances related to patient care, specific client rights issues, allegations of abuse or neglect, issues related to the organization's compliance with regulatory agency requirements, and any billing complaint related to patient rights.

If a patient provides the physician or organization with a rights or care complaint that cannot be resolved at the time of the complaint, is postponed for later resolution, is referred to other staff for later resolution, requires investigation, or requires further actions for resolution, then the complaint should be considered a *grievance*. That complaint can only be considered resolved when the patient is satisfied with the actions taken on their behalf or the organization is unable to validate the claim. All medical caregivers and organizations must ensure that filing of a grievance by the patient will have no adverse effect on that patient's treatment. Each allegation or occurrence must be investigated, and caregivers must remain objective to the presenting concern and ensure all patients are protected from retribution. If a grievance or concern is brought on behalf of a patient by another person who is not the parent (if the patient is a minor) or guardian, your organization's client rights specialist must meet with the patient to determine if they wish to have the complaint investigated. All of this must be understood by an organization's medical caregivers to ensure patients can exercise their rights while in treatment.

Patient and Staff Safety

The inpatient psychiatric hospital faces many challenges to keep their high-risk patients safe. Despite the safeguards put in place to avoid critical incidents, some such incidents may occur. This section addresses critical incidents and what can be done if they occur. Examples of critical incidents may include the following:

- Elopement from a locked unit
- Serious suicide attempt causing injury or necessitating transfer to another level of care
- Reported sexual encounter
- Alleged caregiver misconduct
- Substantiated Health Insurance Portability and Accountability Act (HIPAA) violation/breach
- Potential EMTALA violation
- Patient death

In each of these scenarios, staff must know what immediate actions need to be taken to address the situation and keep patients safe and to reduce risk to the organization. The hospital should develop a critical incident response policy that staff can refer to as soon as a critical incident is identified. A checklist that can be followed is also recommended. These incidents pose considerable challenges to an organization in terms of both the need to respond intelligently to their occurrence and the need to deal with their aftermath. The challenge is to find a way forward that provides the necessary support for the people involved while ensuring that the lessons of the incident are learned by both the individual staff members and the overall organization (Vincent 2003).

Root cause analysis is a widely used process for investigating critical incidents and sentinel events and can be found on the website of The Joint Commission (TJC) (The Joint Commission 2017). By utilizing this tool or a similar tool, investigators are guided through a process that helps with learning from the incident and determining action items that can be implemented to prevent it from occurring in the future. This process also assists the organization in adjusting its processes and procedures to better keep patients safe. Although not all incidents can be prevented, it is important to review each significant incident, perform a full investigation, and make changes based on that investigation to prevent reoccurrence. Some health care organizations have developed their own tools and techniques to address critical incidents. Developing an organization policy will help with standardization and response.

Use of Seclusion and Restraint

Seclusion and restraint should only be used as a last resort intervention when caring for patients. Use of seclusion and restraint poses a high risk of injury to staff and to the patient as well as a potential risk of death for the patient. Other interventions must be taken prior to implementing seclusion and restraint and need to be fully documented. Legally, every person has the right to be free of a restraint; therefore, a physician order is required with documentation that the seclusion and restraint be used to prevent that patient from harming themselves or others. There are many regulations surrounding the use of seclusion and restraint, and because of this complexity and controversy, the topic will be covered in more detail in Chapter 21.

Safety in the Context of Inpatient Suicide

According to the Centers for Disease Control and Prevention, suicide was the tenth leading cause of mortality in the United States in 2019, with 47,511 deaths reported (Kochanek et al. 2019). Suicidal ideation or suicide attempts are among the most common chief complaints leading to inpatient psychiatric hospitalization. Recent evidence has shown that in the 3-month period after discharge from a psychiatric facility, patients' suicide rates remain markedly elevated, significantly above baseline risk for the general population (Chung et al. 2017). Furthermore, suicide risk can often affect hospitalization itself. An analysis of data available through two national databases demonstrated that between 48.5 and 64.9 hospital inpatient suicides occur per year in the United States, with 31.0–51.7 occurring in the inpatient psychiatric setting. This number is less than what was previously widely accepted (Mills et al. 2008), but management of patients at risk for suicide continues to be a challenging and difficult issue given that one of the purposes of inpatient psychiatry is to address suicidality.

Assessment, mitigation of risk, prevention, and continuity treatment following discharge all compose vital components of managing suicide risk in the inpatient setting. The challenges in the hospital are identifying those at risk of suicide, determining whether they are able to verbalize this, and offering a therapeutic environment where suicidality and underlying behavioral health diagnoses, as well as stressors, may be addressed, while at the same time ensuring that there are strong limits on any accessible means for suicide. Balancing a warm environment with the stark need for precautions is by no means an easy task, but it is necessary to fulfill our obligation to our patients to improve health and do no harm.

The Joint Commission and Ligature Risk

TJC classifies an in-hospital suicide as a sentinel event and a "never event." Accrediting agencies have placed a premium on evaluating suicide risk in all health care settings, with the hope of preventing in-hospital suicides. In 2007, TJC established National Patient Safety Goal 15.01.01 on suicide prevention in health care settings, and in 2016, it released Sentinel Event Alert 56 (now retired), which highlighted the importance of detecting and treating suicidal ideation in all medical settings. It recommended that all patients in medical hospitals be screened for suicide risk with a brief, standardized, evidence-based screening tool and that appropriate interventions and follow-up be undertaken for those who screen positive.

In 2018, TJC issued a report on the National Patient Safety Goal for suicide prevention and altered its recommendations with the hope of improving the care of patients in the hospital identified as being at high risk of suicide (The Joint Commission 2018). This included a new requirement, effective July 1, 2019, that all patients being evaluated or treated for behavioral health conditions as their primary reason for treatment be screened using a validated screening tool (The Joint Commission 2019). The verbiage was broad, and no clear definition of behavioral health conditions, clear guidance on which screening tool to use, or instruction for how to implement it effectively was provided. The mandates to attain a "ligature-resistant" environment have been somewhat controversial due to the manner of implementation, the costs associated, and the greater harms of psychiatric units being closed rather than having hospital funds invested in bringing them up to code. According to the National Association for Behavioral Healthcare, the ligature risk regulations impose approximately $880.4 million in compliance costs nationwide per year. For a case example regarding ligature risk, refer to Chapter 23, "Architecture and Thoughtful Design."

Case Vignette

A 25-year-old white male with a prior history of schizophrenia and substance use disorder (cannabis) presented to the ED. He was brought in by police after his parents reported they had found him in his vehicle with the engine running, the windows up, and the exhaust pipe blocked. After evaluation and appropriate diagnostic tests, the ED physician and staff determined that he had no obvious signs of injury or impairment, and he was considered medically appropriate for transfer to inpatient psychiatry. The patient was evaluated by the on-call psychiatrist and confirmed that he had made a suicide attempt and that his goal had been to "go to the afterlife, because there is nothing left for me on earth." The patient had been nonadherent with his outpatient regimen of a long-acting injectable antipsychotic, and the psychiatrist noted the presence of delusions with strong religious and persecutory themes. The patient's affect was noted to be flat, his attitude was guarded, and his eye contact was poor.

After admission to the inpatient ward, the patient's antipsychotic medication was resumed, and he was placed on one-to-one precautions because he continued to report having thoughts of suicide. After 3 days, he reported improvement, and the inpatient team noted his delusions appeared to be less intense. His precaution status was changed to eyesight. Several mental health technicians and nurses' notes indicated that he was not attending groups and was isolative. When asked about thoughts of suicide, he reported that "there's no way for me to commit suicide here" and at times did not respond to the questions. He continued to report believing he "belonged in the afterlife." Given his overall improvement in affect and organization of thoughts, he was switched to 15-minute precautions. That evening, he took his bedtime medications with a bottle of water. During the overnight shift, he was discovered during a 15-minute check to be unconscious in his bed, covered with blood. He had ripped the plastic bottle into shards, which he used to cut his wrists. A rapid response was called, and he was transferred to the ED, where his condition was stabilized.

Background

Determining whether a patient has had recent thoughts, intent, or a plan to commit suicide is a challenge. Although suicide is the tenth leading cause of death in the United States, the overall rate of suicide as of 2017 was 14.0 per 100,000 (Hedegaard et al. 2018). In 2015, it was estimated that 3.9% of the U.S. population reported having suicidal thoughts, and 1.1% had formulated a plan for suicide (Centers for Disease Control and Prevention 2015). The relative rarity of suicidality contributes to the difficulty of identifying and stratifying risk in the general population. However, among a selected population of those admitted to a psychiatric hospital, screening and risk assessment form a foundational skill set and obligation to good patient care. A history of a prior suicide attempt is among the strongest predictors of future suicide attempts (Phillips et al. 2005). Psychiatric diagnosis, including major depressive disorder, bipolar disorder, schizophrenia, addiction disorders, borderline personality disorder, anxiety disorder, and PTSD, increases suicide risk (Angst et al. 1999; Jamison 2000; Nepon et al. 2010; Soloff et al. 1994; Substance Abuse and Mental Health Services Administration 2016). Psychological factors such as hopelessness, despair, isolation, impulsivity, loss, and stress have also been identified as being associated with suicide (Institute of Medicine 2002; Lee and Jung 2006; Osgood 1991). Other, more broadly applicable risk factors include male gender, access to firearms, family history of suicide or violence, exposure to others' suicidal behavior, medical illness, and being younger than 24 or older than 60 years (National Institute of Mental Health 2016).

Although risk factors permit identification of those currently or chronically at risk, at present there is no consistent or reliable method of predicting which individuals will attempt or complete suicide. Within the psychiatric setting, therefore, performing a thorough assessment at admission and interval reassessment during the inpatient stay, treating underlying conditions, addressing psychological factors, reassessing patients before changing their level of treatment, and offering an appropriate level of continuity treatment after discharge are all essential components of the treatment plan. In addition, the treatment facility should assess its treatment program (including policies and procedures around appropriate monitoring of the patient) and physical facilities to ensure that a safe and therapeutic environment is offered to patients.

Assessments

Overview

The initial evaluation for suicidality should be included in the psychiatric history and physical examination. Although many elements of the patient's current history of present illness and psychiatric history will inform the assessment of their suicide risk

(Table 20–1), some elements must be specifically queried (Table 20–2). Furthermore, the initial assessment—which needs to be a thorough inventory—is distinct from reassessments during the hospital course, which must be efficient and track the course of a patient's symptoms related to suicide. In *any* assessment, the most accurate formulations regarding diagnosis, treatment, and risk cannot come solely from a single source; the necessary face-to-face interview with patients may fail to shed light on symptoms that they are unable or unwilling to articulate. Family members, friends, or other supports and patients' outpatient caregivers, including therapists and psychiatric providers, typically provide helpful and important collateral information about the patients' recent presentation, particularly suicidal thoughts, behaviors, or plans.

Assessment Tools

Several structured suicide risk assessment tools have been developed that address the need to complete a comprehensive assessment across a variety of medical providers and treatment settings, including the inpatient psychiatric setting. The Columbia-Suicide Severity Rating Scale (C-SSRS)—Risk Assessment version is a three-page questionnaire that can be administered as part of a comprehensive assessment. It consists of a checklist inventory of risk and protective factors. Although administering the scale produces a total score derived from the ratings in individual categories, the "interpretation will be derived from a thorough clinical assessment, client history, and clinical expertise" (Center for Deployment Psychology 2016). Research on the C-SSRS has yielded "promising data on the convergent and divergent validity, predictive validity, sensitivity, specificity, sensitivity to change, and internal consistency" (Posner et al. 2011, p. 1277), and the scale has been recommended by the National Institutes of Health, the Substance Abuse and Mental Health Services Administration, the National Action Alliance for Suicide Prevention, the U.S. Department of Defense, the Centers for Disease Control and Prevention's National Center for Injury Prevention and Control, and the FDA.

The Scale for Suicide Ideation—Worst (SSI-W; Beck et al. 1997) and the Beck Scale for Suicide Ideation (BSI; Beck et al. 1997) exhibit strong internal reliability as well as discriminant, construct, and convergent validity. The SSI-W is an interviewer-administered scale, whereas the BSI is a self-report instrument. Notably, hopelessness on the BSI predicted eventual suicide over a 10-year prospective study (Beck et al. 1985).

In addition to the use of structured instruments at admission, reassessments for suicide risk should be conducted regularly, particularly for those who have suicidal ideation, those who attempted suicide prior to admission to the hospital, and those who have risk factors for suicide. No expert consensus has been reached on the recommended frequency of reassessments, although it is reasonable and considered best practice for physicians to assess on a daily basis or for nursing staff to reassess once per shift. These assessments should be focused on eliciting the presence or absence of suicidal ideation, along with plan, intent, and access. A screening rating scale may be used as part of the assessment (Intermountain Healthcare 2014), and clinicians should include this conversation as part of the regular daily interview.

Unfortunately, some obstacles intrinsic to inpatient psychiatry may make interviews or assessment tools challenging. The rate of involuntary hospitalization is not well tracked or recorded, and international studies demonstrate a broad range in the proportion of involuntary admissions (Lebenbaum et al. 2018; Sheridan Rains et al. 2019).

TABLE 20–1. Elements of suicide assessment

History of present illness
Suicidal thoughts, suicide plan, suicide means, suicide intent
Comorbid psychiatric conditions
Comorbid substance use disorders
Chronic medical conditions
Past history
Previous history of suicide attempts, including dates, means, and hospitalizations, including medical sequelae and psychiatric inpatient stays
Previous history of suicidal ideation
Previous history of self-harming behaviors
Past history of treatment therapies helpful for suicidality (including lithium and clozapine)
Family history
Family history of suicide attempts, deaths by suicide
Psychosocial history

More research needs to be conducted on the ability to assess the suicide risk of patients admitted involuntarily. In one study, suicidality and hostility were assessed following involuntary treatment (Giacco and Priebe 2016), and significant hostility was present after admission and after 1 month of treatment. These findings underscore the importance of establishing a therapeutic alliance with all patients, regardless of whether their hospitalization is voluntary or involuntary. One meta-analysis demonstrated the positive effect of a strong therapeutic alliance (mainly on outpatients) on suicidal ideation and suicide attempts (Dunster-Page et al. 2017). According to the American Psychiatric Association (2003) *Practice Guideline for the Assessment and Treatment of Patients With Suicidal Behaviors*, "The ability of a psychiatrist to connect with the patient, establish rapport, and demonstrate empathy is an important ingredient of the assessment process." A strong therapeutic alliance provides the environment in which suicidal thoughts and related issues may be explored nonjudgmentally and empathically, with the ultimate goal of reducing the potential for suicide. The Aeschi approach to building alliances with suicidal patients involves reaching a "shared understanding of the patient's suicidality" (Michel et al. 2009). This is in contrast to an expert–patient relationship and instead elevates patients' narratives to the forefront. Hopelessness has been identified as a major risk factor for future suicide attempts; in addition, the period following a suicide attempt or severe ideation is a highly vulnerable time for patients, and finding times when they have the capacity to discuss and process their experiences is crucial for interpreting their suicide risk while in the hospital.

At times when patients are unable to express their level of suicidality, being able to assess their suicide risk independent of their expressed intentions can be helpful. The Sheppard Pratt Suicide Risk Assessment Instrument (SPSRAI; Figure 20–1) was developed as a tool similar to other risk assessments that is meant to supplement clinical judgment and to bring together risk factors on one sheet of paper for a consolidated review. It establishes three categories of risk: 1) expressed intentions, 2) mental status findings, and 3) relevant history. It can be scored at the conclusion of a thorough psychiatric history. This tool is recommended for use at patients' admission and whenever

TABLE 20–2. Suicide assessment interview

Ideation			
Currently suicidal	Are you currently having thoughts of suicide?		Yes/No
Recent attempt	Have you recently made a suicide attempt?		Yes/No
Frequency	How frequently are you having thoughts of suicide? Or, when was the last time you had thoughts of suicide?		***
Intensity	How intense are the thoughts? (1=least, 10=most)		1 2 3 4 5 6 7 8 9 10
Duration	How long has this been going on?		***
Plan			
Plan	Do you have a plan to commit suicide?	Yes/No	
	What is the plan?	***	
	Do you have access to a firearm?	***	
	Where are you now in thinking about suicide?	***	
Timing	When did you plan to commit suicide? What was the situation?	***	
Location	Where were you planning to attempt suicide?	***	
Lethality	What was the means by which you were planning to commit suicide?	***	
Availability	Did you have access to that means?	Yes/No	
Preparatory acts	Did you prepare for the attempt or for events after your death?	Yes/No	
Intent			
Intent	Do you or did you expect to carry out the plan, or do you or did you believe the plan was lethal?	Yes/No	
Attempts			
Previous attempts	Have you previously attempted suicide? (Review history of attempts.)	***	
Treatment history			
Lithium	***		
Clozapine	***		
Antidepressants	***		
Electroconvulsive therapy	***		
Psychotherapy	***		
Inpatient	***		
Self-injurious behavior	***		
Family history of suicide	***		

***Patient response when not a yes/no question.

Sheppard Pratt
HEALTH SYSTEM

ADDRESSOGRAPH

SUICIDE RISK ASSESSMENT

FACTORS THAT MAY INCREASE RISK

	CATEGORY	DESCRIPTION	YES	NO
1.	Recent suicide attempt?	Seriously attempted suicide immediately prior to admission	☐	☐
2.	Imminent suicidal intent?	Currently expressing a desire to kill self in program	☐	☐
3.	Actionable plan?	Has specific plan that can be acted upon in the program	☐	☐

Questions 1 - 3 ask about the patient's intentions, expressed in words or behavior.

If the answer is Yes to items 1, 2, or 3, a high level of observation should be considered. If the answer is Yes to items 2 and 3, "SO arm's length" should be ordered unless an equally intensive but more individualized plan is preferred; if so, the reasons for the choice should be clearly documented.

4.	**Psychological pain or anguish?**	**Shows signs of extreme psychological anguish or distress**	☐	☐
5.	**Self-hatred?**	**Shows signs of extremely poor self-esteem and feelings of worthlessness and guilt**	☐	☐
6.	**Hopelessness?**	**Does not believe that he/she will ever feel better**	☐	☐
7.	**Agitation?**	**Is visibly restless and tense**	☐	☐
8.	**Psychosis?**	**Has delusions, especially delusional guilt, or hallucinations**	☐	☐
9.	**Wish for death?**	**Feels death would bring relief**	☐	☐

Questions 4 - 9 ask about features of the patient's mental status.

If the answer is Yes to one or several of items 4 - 9, a high level of observation should be considered even if the patient denies suicidal thoughts.

10.	Family / Peer suicidal history?	Has a history of suicidal behavior or successful suicide by family members / friends	☐	☐
11.	Substance abuse?	Has recent history of substance abuse or dependence	☐	☐
12.	Recent severe stressor?	Has experienced a devastating loss, disappointment or threat	☐	☐

Questions 10 - 12 ask about aspects of the patient's history.

If the answer is Yes to item 12, a high level of observation may be appropriate even if the patient denies suicidal thoughts, especially if the answer is Yes to any of the items 4 - 9.

FACTORS THAT MAY REDUCE RISK

1.	Presence of dependents?	Is pregnant or has children in home	☐	☐
2.	Responsibility?	Has a strong sense of responsibility to family or pets	☐	☐
3.	Sources of support?	Has the following sources of support:		
		a. friends, relatives, co-workers	☐	☐
		b. belonging to a faith based community	☐	☐
		c. a positive therapeutic relationship with a professional	☐	☐
4.	Hope / Future oriented?	Describes reasons for living	☐	☐
		If yes, specify: ______________________		

Remember to document rationale for all interventions in the patient's medical record.

Print Name ______________________

Signature ______________________ Date ____________

0101040 SPHS (R 8/6/2014) (F3F) CF

FIGURE 20–1. Sheppard Pratt Suicide Risk Assessment Instrument.
Source. Reprinted with permission of Sheppard Pratt Health System, Inc. Copyright © 2006.

a change in observation is considered. The three expressed-intentions questions establish some of the main risk factors for future suicide attempts and concern whether a recent suicide attempt has been made, whether patients are currently experiencing suicidal ideation, and whether patients have an actionable plan in the hospital. Most suicide attempts in the psychiatric hospital are by hanging (75% as reported to TJC; Williams et al. 2018), occurring most often in isolated or unexpected areas, such as bathrooms, bedrooms, and closets (Sakinofsky 2014). Thus, it is imperative to query about plan feasibility. No psychiatric unit is completely safe from suicide attempts, but areas of vulnerability must be monitored or a plan be in place for known areas of risk.

When patients do not express thoughts of suicide, mental status examination findings may be valuable to the assessment. The items scored on the SPSRAI are thought to be helpful in assessing risk, although only hopelessness is felt to be predictive; the other items are commonly cited as risk factors and are psychological pain or anguish, self-hatred (involving poor self-esteem, worthlessness, or guilt), agitation, psychosis (particularly delusional guilt), and a wish for death. The historical elements assessed include family or peer suicidal history, poor social supports (including a support network, employment or school, and spiritual community), substance use disorders, and recent stressors (highlighting devastating losses or threats). These are not alterable elements and do not require reassessment, but they bring to bear the strongest risk factors together with the other categories for the clinician to review. For the first two sections, on expressed intentions and mental status, a single positive response is enough to alert clinicians that a high level of observation should be considered. The final item (recent severe stressor) should be combined with any positive items from the mental status examination to elevate the concern of the scoring clinician.

Physical Environment

In the medical-surgical setting, jumping was the most common method of completed suicide, although hanging, cutting, and poisoning were also significant means (Ballard et al. 2008). The advantages of the psychiatric setting are the expectations of and the regulatory requirements for a safe physical environment. These carry their own burdens of cost and effort to maintain compliance with potentially rapidly changing environmental technology. Hanging is the most frequent cause of suicide in the psychiatric inpatient setting, accounting for more than 70% of suicides (Williams et al. 2018). About 80% of these suicides occurred in the bathroom or bedroom and frequently involved use of a door handle, door hinge, shower bar or pipe, or other fixture. TJC's emphasis on a ligature-resistant environment or the ability to provide continuous one-to-one monitoring arose from this data analysis. Access to items that could be used to injure patients quickly should be removed, including items fashioned from glass (e.g., mirrors or vases), eating utensils that could be used to harm oneself (e.g., metal knives or forks), sharp or tense plastic items, and pens. A ligature-resistant environment lacks any points to which material could be attached to form a loop for use in a suicide attempt. Ligature resistance is most important in areas such as patient rooms, bathrooms, and common patient care areas but not, for example, in the nurses' station or behind a self-locking door only accessible to staff. TJC (The Joint Commission 2020) and the American Hospital Association (Beebe 2018) recommend following the American Society for Health Care Engineering's tools and resources related to ligature risk. These consist of checklists, virtual rounding tools, and decision-support tools for self-assessing physical environment safety. For a case example regarding ligature risk, refer to Chapter 23.

Patient Elopement

Elopement can be a high-risk event in terms of potential harm to patients, issues with regulators, legal implications, and public loss of confidence. Breaches to patient safety due to elopement can result in a Centers for Medicare & Medicaid Services finding of immediate jeopardy. Between 2006 and 2009, the number of cases of elopement increased by 38%. It is vital for staff to understand organizational policies and what they can, as well as cannot, do during an elopement situation. Procedures vary geographically based on expectations of local agencies, including law enforcement.

Elopement prevention procedures should be detailed and be incorporated into general staff trainings. It is helpful to ascertain each patient's elopement risk. For those deemed to be high risk, potential preventive measures can include selection of room location on the unit, wearing distinctive-color gowns, and utilizing technology solutions (i.e., radio-frequency identification or other geolocation tag). A response plan in the event of an elopement can include searching the floor by clinical staff and notifying security if the patient is not found, searching the facility and grounds, calling a mass notification alert similar to "code orange," clearly delineating how far staff can chase patients or use physical means to bring patients back, and parameters for notifying law enforcement and the patient's family. Documentation is critical throughout the elopement period, and all such events should be reviewed utilizing a root cause analysis to learn how to improve organizational processes.

Sexual Harassment and Assault

Sexual harassment and assault on psychiatric units remain ongoing concerns for both adult and pediatric populations. People have a right to feel and be safe while accessing treatment in mental health wards. The hospital has a duty—and must make it a priority—to ensure that people using health care services are kept safe and their privacy and dignity are maintained. This means ensuring patients are protected from sexual safety incidents and supporting those who may behave inappropriately due to their condition.

Code Response

Severe weather events, such as hurricanes, tornadoes, flooding, and storm surges, can cause hospital power and connectivity outages or in other ways disrupt crucial services and processes that are core to delivering care. If the unit is not prepared for such circumstances, they can lead to chaos and an unsafe care environment. A hospital being unable to admit patients for even 1 day can lead to large financial losses and the inability to help meet the community's need for services. Furthermore, it may be necessary to evacuate or to take in patients from another hospital or health care facility that has been evacuated. Day-to-day weather events such as snow and ice events can also put patients in danger while accessing care and staff in danger coming to or heading home from work.

Every hospital must have an emergency operations plan for addressing response to and recovery from all hazards. Essential services are those that are central to an organization's mission and cannot be stopped or delayed without a threat to or negative impact on organization stakeholders. Prioritizing essential services for continuity of operations will depend on multiple factors, but the significance of the impact and the amount of time a facility can safely do without the service are key considerations. A continuity of operations plan can supplement this framework by prioritizing the essential services an organization must perform even in an emergency and identifying the resources required to make certain that these services continue. For hospitals, such a plan helps ensure services for current patients and maintains the ability to respond to a patient surge situation. Important questions to consider include

- What resources are needed to restore critical functions if they go down?
- If critical functions cannot be restored, what resources are needed to replicate these services in a mobile facility, partner location, or alternate care site?
- Are there business-related functions that can also be a part of your essential services, to keep lines of communication open and information available?
- Are alternative facilities available, such as mobile command centers or alternative work-sites where desks, wireless internet, telephones, and computers are immediately accessible?
- Can you readily turn to your data backup facility to access critical patient records? The facility should be beyond the reach of severe weather events that could affect your facility.
- Is there an emergency plan in place? The Centers for Medicare & Medicaid Services requires that emergency plans include policies and procedures to maintain the confidentiality and availability of patient medical information to protect continuity of services even if patients must be transferred to another facility.
- Has an incident command structure been established and the emergency plan been rehearsed regularly?

Electronic Health Record and Cybersecurity

Electronic health records (EHRs) are critical enterprise systems leveraged by health care organizations to improve the facilitation of treatment, clinical decision-making, and monitoring of outcomes and to streamline operations. The EHR is a significant repository of protected health and consumer information, and its security is vital for the operations of health care organizations and their reputations. Protecting high-risk information systems is a significant undertaking with material costs that requires due diligence. Regular formal risk assessments should be done, and broader executive leadership should be included in decisions around security initiatives.

Cybersecurity for EHRs can be broken into two large categories: networking and applications. Role-based security is the most typical approach to securing access to application-based information and requires broader infrastructure to be successful. Each organization should have formalized policies around applications access and processes in place, such as access control lists, to prescribe the procedure for authorizing access. Deviations from documented procedure should be run through appropriate governance committees for approval. Role-based security involves finding the right balance between giving people access to what they need to know and not creating operational barriers to the delivery of optimal patient treatment.

Applications are run from end-user devices and are only as secure as those devices. Ensuring the health of end-user hardware is just as important to protecting sensitive information as protecting the application itself. Regular security updates, patches, antivirus scans, and auto logouts are some traditional methods of protecting devices. Given the success of phishing attacks, health care organizations also need to focus on external threats to devices typically transmitted through email. Advanced threat analytic and protection strategies must be implemented to defend devices against social engineering tactics. At the end of the day, it is not a question of *if* the system will be attacked but *when*, and if the facility is ready.

Phishing remains the most effective social engineering method for bypassing technical defenses. Employee education and awareness represent the final line of defense for any organization. Cybersecurity training must be provided to each new employee and added to regular competency checks for existing employees. Phishing test campaigns are methods by which health care organizations can monitor their susceptibility to phishing attacks, and serve as a platform for further education of those who may fail the exercises.

Remote hosting services are an effective strategy for gaining more network security at a cheaper price than using an in-house approach. Network security is a diverse and complicated field that requires many specialists to operate. The best of the human resource pool tends to prefer working for large technology companies rather than hospitals, so aligning with these companies will likely be a safer decision for most organizations. Perimeter defenses, firewalls, antithreat protection, web filters, and regular updates and patching of hardware are critical for network security. Security is more of a cat-and-mouse game than a one-and-done situation. Hybridizing security engagement is an effective strategy to reduce the most risk at the lowest price. The makeup of any hospital technology department should be more heavily focused on roles that enable better treatment of patients, while outsourcing functions that do not directly deliver that value to internal and external customers.

Coding and Fraudulent Billing

As the employed provider becomes more common, the known liability to providers for coding-related issues spreads somewhat more to the hospitals. Each hospital must have a culture that encourages reporting concerns about fraud. Health care organizations must audit coding practices on a routine basis. Coding and reimbursement systems in psychiatric practice are very complex but clearly important for providers and hospitals as a revenue stream. However, they also carry substantial risk of liability with regard to accusations of health care fraud by payers and patients. Such accusations could lead to substantial fines and put the hospital's mission at risk. Billing and coding fraud is now a primary target for regulators and prosecutors.

Inpatient psychiatry is known as one of the top coding risk areas for hospitals. The Health and Human Services Office of the Inspector General is specifically examining Medicare outlier payments to hospitals for inpatient psychiatric services because total Medicare payments for inpatient psychiatric services have been increasing. Examples of health care fraud include providers billing for services not rendered, using duplicate billing, coding without appropriate medical documentation, using improper diagnosis codes to justify the performance of medically unnecessary services, and billing a procedure code for a more complex, higher-paying service than was performed or was medically necessary. Hospitals should put safeguards in place throughout the coding and bill submission process to mitigate liability. Hospitals must have a current coding compliance policy in which all providers consistently use the same official coding rules, conventions, guidelines, and definitions. Providers must use codes that are clearly and consistently supported by authenticated clinical documentation in accordance with Current Procedural Terminology guidelines. This policy should be evaluated and updated annually.

Providers must understand the codes that they are using and the associated documentation. They must understand the concepts of medical necessity regarding the frequency and intensity of visits and the payer's regulations and the specific contract that the hospital system/provider has with that payer. Mistakes can happen as well, such as transposition of numbers in a code or just plain human error, and systems must be in place that can detect and correct those mistakes. Every hospital must have a compliance program with periodic risk assessments and auditing to ensure compliance. Best practices include auditing a random sample of medical and billing records to monitor compliance. Prospective or real-time review of the records has the benefit of possibly correcting claims before they are submitted and payment is received from the payer. Findings and education should be timely to correct trends at the provider or medical staff level. Periodic external audits can help verify that the current process is valid. Many hospitals have added a "compliance hotline" for employees to report fraud concerns anonymously if desired without fear of retaliation. Any hospital that does not provide such an option may be found negligent for not doing everything possible to encourage reports of fraud.

Vignette

Dr. Thompson is seeing an inpatient in follow-up for a suicide attempt. It is hospital day 8, and the patient is no longer actively suicidal. Medication changes were made earlier in the patient's stay that seem to have helped with sleep and anxiety. The patient continues to feel depressed but is not in need of further medication changes and is expected to be transferred to a residential level of care in the next couple of days. They discuss medication, side effects, groups, progress, and discharge planning. Dr. Thompson delivers a high-intensity visit and codes for a high-intensity visit, a 99233. She also completes an appropriate note because her understanding is that this patient is very ill, ill enough to be on the inpatient unit, and she delivered to what her knowledge is the appropriate level of intensity for an acutely ill patient. This code is transcribed and submitted without any internal audit process that evaluates medical decision-making or medical necessity of the intensity of the visit. This visit may now be at risk of being questioned by regulators and payers as to whether the intensity level of the visit was medically necessary. Was this the right visit at the right time? Even though the patient was on an inpatient unit, was an intensive medical visit the right level of intensity?

Anti-Kickback Statute and Physician Self-Referral Laws (Stark Law)

Anti-kickback laws and Stark Law violations are a continued focus of law enforcement, with agencies evaluating hospital–physician relationships and unlawful payments to and financial relationships with referral sources. Hospitals, employed physicians, and physicians with other financial relationships with hospitals must be aware of these laws. The federal Anti-Kickback Statute is a criminal statute that prohibits the exchanging of or offering to exchange anything of value in an effort to induce or reward the referral of any business reimbursable by federal health care programs. Possible penalties include fines of up to $25,000, up to 5 years in jail, and exclusion from Medicare and Medicaid care program business.

The physician self-referral laws (Stark Law) are U.S. federal civil laws that prohibit physician self-referral—specifically a referral by a physician of a Medicare or Medicaid patient to an entity with whom the physician or a family member has a financial arrangement. This is a noncriminal statute, but it can entail significant financial penalties and exclusion from the Medicare/Medicaid programs.

Conclusion

No chapter can fully cover every risk. Systematically defining and managing risks in your organization or program is an important task. Utilizing structured risk assessments, particularly for suicide risk, is paramount for patient safety. It is imperative for all organizations to provide staff education and training in core skills and keep staff updated periodically. The best risks are those that we can successfully mitigate to prevent harm to our patients or staff.

References

American Psychiatric Association: Practice Guideline for the Assessment and Treatment of Patients With Suicidal Behaviors. Washington, DC, American Psychiatric Association, November 2003

Angst J, Angst F, Stassen HH: Suicide risk in patients with major depressive disorder. J Clin Psychiatry 60 (suppl 2):57–62, discussion 75–76, 113–116, 1999 10073389

Ballard ED, Pao M, Henderson D, et al: Suicide in the medical setting. Jt Comm J Qual Patient Saf 34(8):474–481, 2008 18714750

Beck AT, Steer RA, Kovacs M, Garrison B: Hopelessness and eventual suicide: a 10-year prospective study of patients hospitalized with suicidal ideation. Am J Psychiatry 142(5):559–563, 1985 3985195

Beck AT, Brown GK, Steer RA: Psychometric characteristics of the Scale for Suicide Ideation with psychiatric outpatients. Behav Res Ther 35(11):1039–1046, 1997 9431735

Beebe C: Ligature-risk requirements: separating fact from fiction in suicide prevention. HFM Magazine November–December:30–34, 2018

Center for Deployment Psychology: Columbia Suicide Severity Rating Scale (C-SSRS) Fact Sheet. Bethesda, MD, Uniformed Services University of the Health Sciences, October 2016

Centers for Disease Control and Prevention: Suicide: Facts at a Glance. Atlanta, GA, Centers for Disease Control and Prevention, 2015. Available at: www.cdc.gov/suicide/facts/index.html. Accessed November 26, 2021.

Chung DT, Ryan CJ, Hadzi-Pavlovic D, et al: Suicide rates after discharge from psychiatric facilities: a systematic review and meta-analysis. JAMA Psychiatry 74(7):694–702, 2017 28564699

Dunster-Page C, Haddock G, Wainwright L, Berry K: The relationship between therapeutic alliance and patient's suicidal thoughts, self-harming behaviours and suicide attempts: a systematic review. J Affect Disord 223:165–174, 2017 28755624

Giacco D, Priebe S: Suicidality and hostility following involuntary hospital treatment. PLoS One 11(5):e0154458, 2016 27171229

Hedegaard H, Curtin SC, Warner M: Suicide mortality in the United States, 1999–2017. NCHS Data Brief No 330, November 2018

Institute of Medicine, Committee on Pathophysiology and Prevention of Adolescent and Adult Suicide: Reducing Suicide: A National Imperative. Edited by Goldsmith SK, Pellmar TC, Kleinman AM, et al. Washington, DC, National Academies Press, 2002

Intermountain Healthcare: Suicide prevention: inpatient. Best Practice Flash Card. Salt Lake City, UT, Intermountain Healthcare, 2014

Jamison KR: Suicide and bipolar disorder. J Clin Psychiatry 61 (suppl 9):47–51, 2000 10826661

The Joint Commission: Framework for Root Cause Analysis and Corrective Actions. Oakbrook Terrace, IL, The Joint Commission, October 2017. Available at: www.jointcommission.org/-/media/tjc/documents/resources/patient-safety-topics/sentinel-event/rca_framework_101017.pdf?db=web&hash=B2B439317A20C3D1982F9FBB94E1724B&hash=B2B439317A20C3D1982F9FBB94E1724B. Accessed November 30, 2021.

The Joint Commission: Revisions to National Patient Safety Goal Regarding Suicide Prevention. The Joint Commission Perspectives, December 2018. Available at: www.jointcommission.org/resources/patient-safety-topics/suicide-prevention. Accessed October 25, 2021.

The Joint Commission: National Patient Safety Goal 15.01.01. 2019. Available at: www.jointcommission.org/-/media/tjc/documents/standards/r3-reports/r3_18_suicide_prevention_hap_bhc_cah_11_4_19. Accessed November 30, 2021.

The Joint Commission: Suicide Prevention Resources to Support Joint Commission Accredited Organizations Implementation of NPSG 15.01.01. Revised July 2020. Available at: www.jointcommission.org/-/media/tjc/documents/resources/patient-safety-topics/suicide-prevention/suicide_prevention_compendium_5_11_20_updated-july2020.pdf.

Kochanek KD, Xu J, Arias E: Mortality in the United States, 2019. NCHS Data Brief No. 395. Data table for Figure 4. Atlanta, GA, Centers for Disease Control and Prevention, 2019. Available at: www.cdc.gov/nchs/data/databriefs/db395-tables-508.pdf#page=2. Accessed October 4, 2021.

Lebenbaum M, Chiu M, Vigod S, Kurdyak P: Prevalence and predictors of involuntary psychiatric hospital admissions in Ontario, Canada: a population-based linked administrative database study. BJPsych Open 4(2):31–38, 2018 29467057

Lee SI, Jung H-Y: Psychosocial risk factors for suicide. Psychiatry Investig 3(2):15–22, 2006

Michel K, Jobes D, Leenaars AA, et al: Meeting the Suicidal Person: The Guidelines for Clinicians. Aeschi, Switzerland, Aeschi Working Group, 2009

Mills PD, DeRosier JM, Ballot BA, et al: Inpatient suicide and suicide attempts in Veterans Affairs hospitals. Jt Comm J Qual Patient Saf 34(8):482–488, 2008 18714751

National Institute of Mental Health: Suicide in America: Frequently Asked Questions (DHHS Publ No TR 18-6389). Bethesda, MD, National Institute of Mental Health, 2016

Nepon J, Belik SL, Bolton J, Sareen J: The relationship between anxiety disorders and suicide attempts: findings from the National Epidemiologic Survey on Alcohol and Related Conditions. Depress Anxiety 27(9):791–798, 2010 20217852

Osgood NJ: Psychological factors in late-life suicide. Crisis 12(2):18–24, 1991 1935192

Phillips KA, Coles ME, Menard W, et al: Suicidal ideation and suicide attempts in body dysmorphic disorder. J Clin Psychiatry 66(6):717–725, 2005 15960564

Posner K, Brown GK, Stanley B, et al: The Columbia-Suicide Severity Rating Scale: initial validity and internal consistency findings from three multisite studies with adolescents and adults. Am J Psychiatry 168(12):1266–1277, 2011 22193671

Sakinofsky I: Preventing suicide among inpatients. Can J Psychiatry 59(3):131–140, 2014 24881161

Sheridan Rains L, Zenina T, Dias MC, et al: Variations in patterns of involuntary hospitalisation and in legal frameworks: an international comparative study. Lancet Psychiatry 6(5):403–417, 2019 30954479

Soloff PH, Lis JA, Kelly T, et al: Risk factors for suicidal behavior in borderline personality disorder. Am J Psychiatry 151(9):1316–1323, 1994 8067487

Substance Abuse and Mental Health Services Administration: Substance use and suicide: a nexus requiring a public health approach. In Brief, 2016. Available at: https://sprc.org/sites/default/files/resource-program/SAMHSA_SbstncUsSuicdNxsPblcHlthAprch2016.pdf. Accessed November 30, 2021.

Vincent C: Understanding and responding to adverse events. N Engl J Med 348(11):1051–1056, 2003 12637617

Williams SC, Schmaltz SP, Castro GM, Baker DW: Incidence and method of suicide in hospitals in the United States. Jt Comm J Qual Patient Saf 44(11):643–650, 2018 30190221

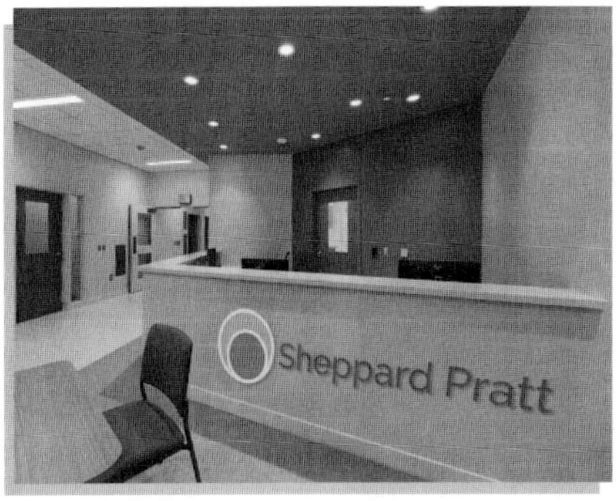

CHAPTER 21

Preventing Conflict, Violence, and Use of Seclusion and Restraint

Kevin Ann Huckshorn, Ph.D., M.S.N., R.N., ICADC
Janice L. LeBel, Ph.D., ABPP

Violence in Mental Health Settings: Issues and Costs

Violence in mental health settings has a significant impact on quality of care, the safety of service users and staff, staff morale, and staff retention (Joint Commission 2005). Research supports the growing acknowledgment that violent incidents are often preceded by behavioral signs but that these signs are often difficult for untrained staff to note. Duxbury (2002) identified the need to combine evidence on patient propensity (individual characteristics) for violence with environmental triggers in order to prevent conflict and aggression in inpatient settings, with a focus on improving safety for all.

Seclusion and Restraint

Seclusion is defined as "the involuntary confinement of a person in a room where they are physically prevented from leaving or think they are" (Huckshorn et al. 2021). *Restraint* is defined as a "manual method or mechanical device, material, or equipment attached or adjacent to the patient's body that he or she cannot easily remove that restricts the patient's freedom or normal access to one's body" (Huckshorn et al. 2021). Seclusion and restraint are used in mental health settings to "manage" aggressive behaviors and have been the object of increased interest, oversight, and regulatory attention by legislators and policy makers since 1998 (Substance Abuse and Mental Health Services Administration 2004; U.S. General Accounting Office 1999). This interest appears to be due to increasing awareness of the short- and long-term physical and emotional consequences of these procedures for both patients and staff (LeBel et al. 2014).

The *Hartford Courant* Series

In 1998, the *Hartford Courant*, a newspaper in Connecticut, released a series of reports titled "Deadly Restraint: A Nationwide Pattern of Death" (Weiss et al. 1998). Driven by the tragic death of an 11-year-old boy, this investigative series cataloged the largely unregulated and unreported deleterious effects of seclusion and restraint on children and adults (Busch and Shore 2000). These publications sent tremendous reverberations throughout the mental health system in the United States (National Association of State Mental Health Program Directors 1999a, 1999b, 2001; U.S. General Accounting Office 1999). The investigative team (Weiss et al. 1998) interviewed health care officials, federal and state regulatory agencies, consumers, family members, advocacy organizations, and other stakeholders to piece together a picture of violence and the use of seclusion and restraint in mental health and intellectual disability care settings. The reporters canvassed all 50 states and the District of Columbia regarding the propensity for violence and the use of seclusion and restraint. From 1988 to 1998, 142 deaths were attributed to restraint or seclusion. Harvard University's Center for Risk Analysis reviewed these findings and estimated that 50–150 deaths occur annually as a result of these practices.

The *Courant* noted that seclusion and restraint–related deaths were occurring in a variety of venues, including hospitals, residential facilities, group homes, and other types of inpatient settings. These reports revealed the disproportionate number of deaths of children for merely refusing to obey staff directives, such as to move to another seat or to give up a contraband family photograph (Weiss et al. 1998). Finally, this series detailed the deaths of a medically ill woman after 558 hours of restraint, a 15-year-old girl who used a pencil to threaten staff, and 33 others who died by asphyxiation after being restrained facedown (U.S. General Accounting Office 1999). Most troubling were the lack of formalized reporting of seclusion and restraint use, the lack of standardized federal regulations guiding practice, the lack of a national database recording serious injuries and deaths, and the lack of accountability for use, injuries, or deaths in health provider organizations (Lieberman et al. 1999). The *Hartford Courant*'s findings were subsequently substantiated and expanded in a Congress-commissioned study on seclusion and restraint use by the U.S. General Accounting Office (1999).

Consequences of Seclusion and Restraint Use

When conflict leads to violence and seclusion or restraint, the result can be physical and emotional injury to all parties (Robins et al. 2005; U.S. General Accounting Office 1999).

Restraint interventions alone were estimated to cause up to 1,240 deaths or serious injuries among service users each year in the United States, according to The Joint Commission in 2005 (Joint Commission 2005). The incidence of staff injury has been less studied, but one survey, conducted in three states, reported 26 injuries for every 100 mental health technicians (Love and Hunter 1996). This reported injury rate surpassed those found in the lumber, construction, and mining industries and highlighted the safety problems in inpatient mental health environments (Love and Hunter 1996). The legal consequences of inappropriate physical containment have led to increasingly frequent court findings of civil damages, administrative sanctions, and criminal prosecution (Haimowitz et al. 2006). Seclusion and restraint procedures are believed to be high risk and potentially dangerous for both clients and staff and have resulted in federal, state, and legal mandates to significantly reduce or eliminate use (Centers for Medicare and Medicaid Services 2006; Health Care Finance Administration 1999, 2001; Substance Abuse and Mental Health Services Administration 2004).

Factors in Conflict and Violence Causality

National and international literature reviews have identified the inconsistent and often idiosyncratic decisions that are frequently present when seclusion and restraint are used (Busch and Shore 2000; Hinsby and Baker 2004; Smith et al. 2005). These research studies suggest that cultural and facility-specific biases affect the decision to use seclusion and restraint. Patient characteristics such as sex and gender, race, and age; staff perceptions; and administrative attitudes inform these practice choices and are often valued as more important variables than other factors, such as understanding actual antecedents to conflict (Busch and Shore 2000; Legris et al. 1999). Current research demonstrates that conflict and violence causality goes beyond the traditional focus on patient characteristics and that conflict and violence frequently emerge as a result of environmental factors, such as staff attitudes and facility cultures (Duxbury 2002; Hinsby and Baker 2004).

Medical leaders should understand the internal and external factors that may contribute to conflict and violence. These include patient factors, such as having a history of violence or of being in seclusion or restraints, and environmental and agency norms (Okin 1985; Ray and Rappaport 1995). It is telling that several studies have found very dissimilar practices in very similar settings (LeBel et al. 2004; Steinert and Needham 2007). Similarly, it is imperative that leadership appreciate the tangible impact of violence in health care settings. The use of seclusion and restraint derails treatment and day-to-day unit operations. These violent episodes translate into significant disruptions, staff time away from service users, longer lengths of stay, higher staffing costs, and greater staff turnover and absenteeism (LeBel and Goldstein 2005). On-unit violence has a direct impact on clinical care, service quality, and the fiscal "bottom line" (LeBel and Goldstein 2005).

Mental health care clinicians, especially physicians, must become better educated about their roles in improving workplace safety and use that knowledge to practice in a manner that prevents normal conflict from escalating to violence (Joint Commission 2002). This is key to workforce retention. According to study by Duncan and colleagues (2000), 46% of nurses reported workplace violence during their five most recent shifts, and one-third of these nurses experienced physical assault on the job. Safety has been cited as a key factor in staff retention; without efforts to improve the safety of the work environment, staff will leave direct care settings, and safety will further deteriorate (Joint Commission 2005).

The Call to Transform Mental Health Care

Long before the *Hartford Courant* series on seclusion and restraint was published, some organizations had started to reduce the use of seclusion and restraint in their respective facilities. A few of these programs and facilities were highlighted in the report by the U.S. General Accounting Office in 1999 and are examples of what could happen given leadership, creativity, and the will to change practice patterns. These include model programs in Pennsylvania, Massachusetts, and New York. Many of these projects were co-led by physicians.

Following the *Courant* series, federal regulators promulgated policy and regulatory revisions in an attempt to ensure the safer use of seclusion and restraint practices (Centers for Medicare and Medicaid Services 2006; Health Care Finance Administration 1999, 2001). However, these regulations did not specifically address the prevention of conflict or violence and are considered minimum standards, not best practices (L. Norwalk, Director, Centers for Medicare & Medicaid Services Behavioral Health Standards, personal communication, January 18, 2007). In 1999, the National Association of State Mental Health Program Directors (NASMHPD) unanimously approved a policy statement committing to the reduction and eventual elimination of seclusion and restraint, and its Medical Directors Council authored a series of technical reports on seclusion and restraint use and recommendations for change (National Association of State Mental Health Program Directors 1999a, 1999b, 2001). The President's New Freedom Commission Report on Mental Health was published in 2003, and the Institute of Medicine published a report in 2006 titled *Adaptation to Mental Health and Addictive Disorders: Improving the Quality of Health Care for Mental and Substance-Use Conditions* (Institute of Medicine Committee on Crossing the Quality Chasm 2006). These works provided strong support for transformative change in the delivery of mental health care that included significant attention to the reduction of conflict, violence, and coercive measures.

The United States is not alone in the growing concern about use of coercive interventions. International standard-bearing organizations have explicitly articulated the essential rights of people who receive mental health care and experience seclusion and restraint. The United Nations adopted a resolution titled *Principles for the Protection of Persons With Mental Illness and for the Improvement of Mental Health Care* in 1991 and outlined inviolable basic rights recognized by the international community, including 1) the right to be protected from harm or abuse and 2) the right to be free from restraint or seclusion unless it is used as the "only means available to prevent immediate or imminent harm to the patient or others" (United Nations 1991). Despite these and other fundamental protective covenants adopted by the European Union and other countries, harm to individuals in psychiatric settings persists nationally and internationally (Declaration of Dresden Against Coerced Psychiatric Treatment 2007; Mental Disability Advocacy Center 2003).

Mental health consumers and advocates have been concerned about the use of coercive interventions in mental health settings for years (Bluebird 2004). In recent decades, the mental health advocacy movement has grown beyond its modest beginnings, and groups of ex-patients have become more organized, holding conferences, publishing newsletters, and lobbying legislators for recognition of their issues (Bluebird 2004). The mental health consumer movement is now well established in the national arena; it is recognized as a significant, viable, and effective stakeholder group. Many states have added consumer affairs staff to their state mental health agencies, and most states now host peer-run drop-in centers. Peer specialists are now in most states, and 39 state Medicaid programs now recognize and reimburse peer support services, which is a rapid increase from 2008, when only 8 states reimbursed peer support services (Open Minds 2018). Mental health providers are recognizing peer support, peer-provided services, paid peer staff, and self-help as critical in recovery-oriented systems of care (Huckshorn et al. 2021).

The involvement of service users as full partners is still limited in the private and public sectors due to a combination of fear, distrust, and discomfort (Ashcraft et al. 2012). However, as noted in the President's New Freedom Commission on Mental Health (2003) report and the Institute of Medicine Committee on Crossing the Quality Chasm (2006) report, the sincere and meaningful inclusion of consumers and advocates in every component of the service system not only is absolutely critical but also is a mandatory best practice that distinguishes the new mental health system from the old.

Consumer and Staff Experiences

It has become clear to clinical and policy experts that it is incumbent upon the mental health system to listen and give value to self-reports by people who have personally experienced violence in health settings and staff who are expected to use these procedures (Huckshorn et al. 2021). Personal vignettes provide a picture of individual experiences that should not and cannot be minimized or ignored, even though they may not reach the level of empirical research. The following experiences were recorded from patients and staff who were involved in violent events in mental health settings (Huckshorn et al. 2021):

> I would just like to say that I only jumped in the restraint because, in my eyes, staff were hurting a patient, and it brought back memories for when I was being hurt by people and no one was there to help me....I figured that patient might have thought no one was there to help her, but I was. (Female patient, age 16 years)

> One of the things that doesn't get talked about very much is the trauma of the staff. We talk about the trauma paradigm for our clients or people in recovery. But not very often in my 20 years of work in the field of mental health have I heard much about what happens to us, the workers, and I think that's an area where we need to do some work. I've seen some pretty traumatic things from when I first started 20 years ago. Some of those things still haunt me. (Female direct care staff member)

> It became a "war of words" all about who had the power. I was restrained and forcibly injected. I did not speak to anyone for the next 2 days, and developing any sort of trusting relationship was seriously delayed. (Male patient, age 32 years)

> I got put in the quiet room for pulling the alarm. I pulled the alarm because my grandma did not visit with me, so I felt really bad and did not know what to do. (Male patient, age 16 years)

> I had never seen such a thing…a blue mattress with restraints. They strapped me in face-down. I have a memory that they also gave me an injection, but that might have been from another time. I remember whispering to the nurse, "What happens now?" I was petrified because all their behavior and equipment seemed so weird. She said, "Just try to sleep." (Adult female patient)

> The first time that I helped with a restraint, a four-point restraint, I walked out of the room in tears because it was one of the most horrible things I had ever seen. (Female direct care staff member)

> I've been injured from time to time. Nothing severe. I have bruises, yeah, sometimes I get headaches. I get shaky. (Male direct care staff member)

Some unexpected vignettes also identified practices that appeared to help individuals cope with being put in restraints or seclusion, in the aftermath of the event.

> She asked if I would be safe if she took off the restraints, and I said yes. She said, "Well, that is a good safe." When she took the restraints off of my wrists and legs, I was unable to move my right hand and shoulder. It was very swollen. She couldn't believe how swollen I was and immediately called for medical attention. It was her passion and conviction about the fact that I had not received any medical attention. She was screaming to whoever it was. Then she got me up and helped me take a shower and got me food. In her face I could see that she cared for me, and also in her voice. (Adult female patient)

> It was a Palm Sunday and I wanted to go to Mass. It was a Catholic hospital. The nurse let me go though she knew that I was expressing suicidal thoughts. When I came back one and a half hours later, I was put in seclusion. The nurse did not talk to me. Nobody talked to me. I was on a little mat in the room. When my doctor [psychiatrist] came back 2 days later, after being gone on a long weekend, he was furious. He talked to the nurse and told her, "You had no right doing that." He got me out of seclusion. He then spent time with me. (Adult female patient)

Principles Underlying Trauma-Informed Systems of Care

A core construct believed to be critical in reducing the use of seclusion and restraint is the emerging science of trauma-informed care. The implementation of the principles of trauma-informed care is a "universal precaution" when attempting to prevent conflict or violence (Huckshorn et al. 2021). These principles have been developed and studied by clinicians and researchers for two decades but have only now begun to receive significant attention (Moses et al. 2003; National Association of State Mental Health Program Directors 2005).

Mental health literature reports are now replete with studies on the high prevalence of traumatic life experiences in the general public and in the lives of adults and children in the public mental health system (Cusack et al. 2004; Mueser et al. 1998; Saxe et al. 2003). *Traumatic life events* are defined as those that involve a direct threat of death, severe bodily harm, or psychological injury that the person, at the time, finds intensely distressing (Rosenberg et al. 2001). *Trauma* and *traumatic events* are defined as "the personal experience of interpersonal violence including sexual abuse, physical abuse, severe neglect, loss and/or the witnessing of violence" (Huckshorn et al. 2021). Epidemiological studies estimate that between 36% and 81% of the general population has experienced some kind of significant traumatic event, and the rates are even higher for people who seek clinical services from public mental health and substance abuse treatment providers (Cusack et al. 2004; Mueser et al. 1998).

Kessler et al. (1995) conducted a nationally representative study of the general population in the United States, and in face-to-face interviews with 5,877 people ages 15–54 years, 60% of men and 51% of women reported at least one traumatic event at some time in their lives. In a widely cited groundbreaking report titled "Origins of Addictive Behavior: Evidence From a Study of Stressful Childhood Experiences," Felitti (2003) noted that the "compulsive use of nicotine, alcohol and injected street drugs increase[d] proportionally in a strong, graded, dose-response manner that closely parallel[ed] the intensity of adverse childhood experiences" (p. 3) in a population-based study of more than 17,000 middle-class American adults. The impact of traumatic life events, characterized by subjectively perceived threats of harm, has also been clearly defined and linked positively to PTSD, acute stress disorder, poor treatment outcomes, and personal distress (Jennings 2004).

Individuals who experience trauma sometimes develop PTSD, a clinical disorder characterized by stress and anxiety-related acute and chronic signs and symptoms (Frueh et al. 2000). PTSD is considered to be chronic and debilitating and to have serious adverse effects on social, familial, and occupational functioning. Studies demonstrate a high prevalence rate of PTSD in people with mental illness (≤43%) and even higher rates of traumatic exposure in the same population (51%–98%) (Cusack et al. 2003; Kessler et al. 1995; Mueser et al. 1998). Other studies have found trauma prevalence rates of 52%–90% in persons with schizophrenia, schizoaffective disorders, major depression, and co-occurring disorders (Cusack et al. 2004; Frueh et al. 2002; Green et al. 2000; Mueser et al. 1998). Leading researchers have concluded that the syndrome of PTSD is associated with significant psychiatric and medical comorbidity, social maladjustment, and poor quality of life (Frueh et al. 2006). Research on the neurobiology of PTSD indicates that although it is strikingly similar to major depression, it has several distinctive features, including hyperactivity of the hypothalamic-pituitary-adrenal system and hypersecretion of corticotropin-releasing factor in the presence of normal to low cortisol levels (Newport and Nemeroff 2003). Considerable evidence also shows that early traumatization is associated with adoption of high-risk behaviors, substance abuse, revictimization, reduced treatment adherence, poor quality of life among HIV-infected individuals, and increased morbidity (Whetten et al. 2006).

On balance, the literature regarding PTSD is compelling. This complex psychiatric disorder not only results in emotional distress but also has far-reaching effects, including impaired social and work functioning, negative life-course consequences, and increased likelihood of repeat traumatic experiences, and often lasts for many years (Kessler 2000). The significance of trauma in the lives of people with mental conditions cannot be ignored in mental health environments. The following principles of trauma-informed systems have been identified as critical in preventing adverse events and in reducing the use of seclusion and restraint (Fallot and Harris 2002; Huckshorn et al. 2021):

1. An understanding of the neurological, biological, psychological, and social effects of trauma and violence in human experience.
2. An appreciation of the high prevalence of traumatic experience in the lives of the people who receive mental health services.
3. The use of a standardized, early, and thoughtful trauma assessment on admission to any mental health service or setting, with positive results informing treatment.
4. A recognition and sincere attempt to minimize the fact that mental health treatment environments are often traumatizing, both overtly and covertly.
5. Valuing the consumer in all aspects of care, including highly individualized treatment planning and shared decision-making.
6. The use of neutral, objective, supportive, person-first language in policies, procedures, and daily usage.
7. Workforce development activities that seek to increase staff awareness and understanding of trauma in the lives of people served and to instill humility related to the power these staff have over persons in care. This principle also includes ongoing reviews of organizational rules, practices, and policies that are possibly homogenizing, demeaning, disrespectful, confusing, or worse.
8. Organization-wide practices that seek to minimize the use of coercive practices such as seclusion, restraint, punishment, consequences, and forced medication.

In some settings, the implementation of these principles alone has completely transformed the culture of care and reduced or eliminated the use of seclusion and restraint (Azeem et al. 2017; Huckshorn et al. 2021). These principles are believed to be not only a universal precaution against conflict and violence in our treatment settings but also a core component in creating a recovery-based service system, as articulated by the President's New Freedom Commission on Mental Health (2003) and the Institute of Medicine Committee on Crossing the Quality Chasm (2006).

More recently, neuroscience has begun to shape the design of policies, programs, and practices for people who have experienced traumatic events (Dannlowski et al. 2012; De Bellis et al. 2011; Weems et al. 2021). Some trauma experts cite neuroimaging research, which illustrates what happens in the brain under situations of threat and fear and underscores the importance of building relationships that create a sense of safety and trust. This information supports the contention that being "trauma informed" is not enough and results in a distorted focus on trauma without a corresponding focus on strengths. These experts believe that active efforts must be made to solicit strengths, resources, and protective factors from clients to foster hope, recovery, and skill development. This shift in focus to strengths promotes "resilience-informed care," which "moves trauma information to neuroscience-based action with practical skills to build greater capacity for self-regulation and self-care in both providers and clients" (Leitch 2017, p. 1).

Last, another closely related phenomenon, rarely discussed or studied, is related to conflicts and violence. Staff behaviors toward patients may include subtle—but sometimes overt—discrimination and disrespect that can result in escalating behaviors. Such behaviors reflect an abuse of staff's power over persons who are being served in that setting (Huckshorn 2013; Papadopoulos et al. 2012). Although relatively rare, this phenomenon is significant in more than a few settings.

To date, three violence models have been portrayed in the literature. The first is the "blame the patient" model that is predicated on beliefs that if the person in care stopped being aggressive, the violence levels would decrease. In this model, violence is attributed to symptoms of mental illness or substance use and to volitional behaviors related to antisocial and other character disorders (Huckshorn et al. 2021). The model is best illustrated by statements from staff such as "These patients are much more violent these days"; "He knew what he was doing and needs consequences"; or "I would not let my kids get away with that behavior."

The second model is the "environmental factors model" (Huckshorn et al. 2021), which holds that the persons receiving care in psychiatric inpatient and residential settings become violent as a result of "triggers" in the care environment itself. These triggers include crowded settings, lack of privacy, poorly managed environmental temperatures, and poor quality or quantities of food, all of which lead to general physical discomfort and feelings of distress. Additional triggers may include institutional rules that make little sense to the person in care and feel dehumanizing, such as being expected to line up for services, having enforced wake-up and sleep times, being forced to receive unwanted medications, and having nothing productive to do while in the facility (Huckshorn et al. 2021).

The third model, which currently appears to be most useful to those working in the field, is informally known as the "situational model" (Huckshorn et al. 2021; Wikstrom and Treiber 2009). This model combines the learnings that have emerged from the first two models, resulting in an understanding that violence in inpatient and residential settings is a complex phenomenon and is difficult to study. This model posits that patient, staff, and environmental factors are often interrelated and must be taken into account when one is trying to determine the root causes of adverse events (Huckshorn 2013; Wikstrom and Treiber 2009).

During literature reviews conducted to develop the curriculum training manual *Six Core Strategies to Prevent Conflict and Trauma in Behavioral Health Settings* (Huckshorn et al. 2021), we found several studies and articles that discussed additional, although not often mentioned, causes of conflict and violence specifically related to the outcomes when human beings are placed in restricted settings. Several of these studies described typical mental health locked-service settings, whereas others portrayed prison settings. More recently, the literature on violence has expanded, and more insights have emerged about humans in locked settings, particularly related to the power differential between facility staff and patients (Duxbury et al. 2019a; Gaynes et al. 2017; Guzman-Parra et al. 2021; Riahi et al. 2016). Although we cannot review all of these articles in this chapter, we summarize a few here.

In 1973, David Rosenhan conducted a study designed to examine the impact of environment via how being involuntarily admitted and confined to a psychiatric facility might, in and of itself, change the way an individual patient would be perceived and valued (Rosenhan 1973). (The article reporting the study results was titled "On Being Sane in Insane Places.") Eight people, hereafter known as "pseudopatients," volunteered to act as though they were mentally ill to gain admission to an inpatient facility. These pseudopatients, three women and five men, were a graduate student, three psychologists, a pediatrician, a psychiatrist, a homemaker, and a painter.

Over the length of the study, these research subjects were admitted to care in 12 hospitals in 5 states by alleging psychotic symptoms. Other than their alleged symptoms and false names and vocations, they portrayed the truth about themselves and their life histories. Once admitted, the pseudopatients immediately reverted to their usually normal behaviors and reported that their symptoms had remitted. Other than being anxious, checking the medications prescribed to them, being bored, and worrying about being exposed, they behaved as they had prior to their admission. They cooperated with staff directions, noted they were "fine" when asked, interacted with other patients, and devoted their time to taking copious notes on their experiences. Even so, these eight pseudopatients were never discovered, and all were eventually discharged with a diagnosis of schizophrenia, in remission (Rosenhan 1973).

One finding was particularly significant. In the notes that the pseudopatients kept were many recorded events in which actual patients' distress had been misinterpreted by staff. Often, a patient was observed to become extremely agitated because of staff mistreatment. Staff rarely asked the patient the cause of the agitation but, rather, would assume the distress was due solely to the patient's pathology. Never did the staff consider that either the structure of the hospital environment or a staff member's behaviors had anything to do with the behavior.

Rosenhan followed his initial study with another that used a slightly reversed methodology. In this study, staff at one psychiatric hospital were informed of a high probability that some "fake" patients would be admitted over the next 3 months. When asked to identify which patients, of the 193 patients admitted to their hospital during that period, were the fake patients, at least one staff member identified 41 patients, one psychiatrist suspected 23 patients, and a psychiatrist and another staff person identified 19 patients (Rosenhan 1973). In reality, no fake patients had been admitted to the hospital.

Rosenhan suggested that when a person is given a psychiatric label, that label assumes a life of its own and exerts a strong influence regardless of any actual behaviors that person may exhibit. Once such a diagnosis has been bestowed, earned or not, the person is always viewed through that lens and consequently expected to behave in predetermined ways that are consistent with the diagnosis. Perfectly normal behaviors become distorted and pathologized through this diagnostic lens. Rosenhan believed that eventually and inevitably, the diagnosis becomes a self-fulfilling prophecy. His second study also addressed the phenomenon of depersonalization. Rosenhan wrote of this experience through the notes taken by his research team that documented the extreme frequency with which psychiatric patients were observed to be shamed, humiliated, ignored, verbally taunted, and physically abused for not following rules that the staff had set. The pseudopatients wrote about the "overwhelming sense of powerlessness" they felt when assuming the role of patient (Rosenhan 1973, p. 183) and described the deprivation of basic rights, loss of credibility regarding complaints and concerns, loss of freedom, and lack of privacy. At times, the pseudopatients reported feeling invisible and being treated as such (Rosenhan 1973).

Many studies, including international data reviews, have demonstrated that hospitals and hospital systems' use of seclusion and restraint varies significantly and the differences are not fully attributable to patient behavior or demographics (Huckshorn et al. 2021; Raboch et al. 2007; Schneeberger et al. 2017; Steinert et al. 2010). What has repeatedly emerged is institutional bias regarding the use of these procedures (Huckshorn et al. 2021) Several studies of restraint and seclusion use identify racial bias as well (Price et al. 2004; Schnitzer et al. 2020; Wong et al. 2021).

In 1989, Eileen Frances Morrison, a nurse researcher, conducted a multimonth ethnographic study on three inpatient units. She titled this study "The Tradition of Toughness: A Study of Nonprofessional Nursing Care in Psychiatric Settings." Morrison defined *violence* as "any verbal, nonverbal or physical behavior that is threatening (to self, others or property), or physical behavior that actually did harm" (Morrison 1990, p. 32). She found that the care environment was characterized by a "tradition of toughness" and organizational values that emphasized control and safety. Her research documented that both staff and the organization believed that patients "are sick and must be treated as such" (p. 34) and that acting-out behaviors were symptoms of mental illness, whereas the patients described their behaviors as tools "to get these people off my back" (p. 34). Although licensed nurses were available, they had rigidly defined roles, which resulted in nonlicensed staff interacting with patients most of the time.

Morrison (1990) found that the hospital's policies and its enforcement of rules derived from those policies "inevitably [lead] to violence through the process of confrontation and escalation of the violent situation" (p. 35). The defined role of the nonprofessional staff members (mental health assistants) was called "enforcing." The enforcers used thematic strategies they called "policing," "supermanning," and "putting on a show" to enforce rules designed to control patient behaviors, sanction the physical behaviors of like-minded staff, protect the remaining staff, and receive positive reinforcement from other staff members, and they were highly skilled in hiding these strategies from facility administrators (p. 35).

In summary, these types of studies are rarely developed or done but should not be ignored.

Effective Strategies to Prevent Violence and Improve Safety

Facilitating recovery, independence, and illness self-management is the goal of a transformed mental health service system (Institute of Medicine Committee on Crossing the Quality Chasm 2006; President's New Freedom Commission on Mental Health 2003). Implicit in the recovery model are principles and values that require a reduction in coercive, violent, and involuntary procedures done to persons with mental illness as part of a major shift in practice. The National Consensus Statement on Mental Health Recovery was developed by the Center for Mental Health Services (2004) and describes the recovery process and key principles. Simply stated, transformed systems of care that are recovery focused and trauma informed are not characterized by rigid rules, coercive practices, or "one size fits all" treatment. As such, these principles are important in understanding the rationale for preventing violence and improving safety.

Preventing Violence Through a Formal Plan

For a mental health facility to begin a conflict and violence prevention effort, including a reduction in its use of seclusion and restraint, a facility-specific strategic action plan should be developed and structured that includes identification of the responsible parties, due dates, and expected outcomes. A facility-specific action plan should work to incorporate the six core strategies as the framework, as this model continues to integrate effective practices from across the country that have been proven successful

(Huckshorn et al. 2021). These strategies form the training curriculum that has been developed to assist psychiatric facilities in preventing both violence and the use of seclusion and restraint. Although designed for use with mental health populations, the strategies have been successfully adapted and applied to other populations and care settings as well. They are not meant to replace evidence-based and other clinical approaches, meaningful treatment activities, or effective pharmacological management but, rather, are designed to be used in conjunction with these methods. The six core strategies to improve workplace safety are summarized below.

Leadership Toward Organizational Change

This strategy outlines the role of the executive director or facility administrator and other executive staff. Reduction in the use of seclusion and restraint must start with clear, focused leadership. Leaders must define and articulate a mission and philosophy for reducing seclusion and restraint and outline the roles and responsibilities of all facility staff (Huckshorn 2006). Development and implementation of a prevention plan is a leadership responsibility that requires full and consistent participation by a facility administrator or chief executive officer who is firmly committed to this effort. The plan should be presented in a continuous quality improvement framework that understands that culture change takes time and that "we learn as we go."

A core element of this strategy is elevating the oversight of every seclusion and restraint event by executive management. This requires paying a very different level of attention to these events than has historically been practiced (Riahi et al. 2016). It ensures a timely (minimum weekly) senior administrative review of all incidents that captures detailed information needed for determining necessary prevention activities. It takes advantage of facility leaders' organizational position, power, and influence to ensure policy changes are implemented quickly. Leadership strategies include developing a facility-wide policy statement outlining the seclusion and restraint prevention/reduction approach for all staff, determining data-driven goals to reduce use, announcing "kickoff" events and routinely celebrating successes, identifying seclusion and restraint reduction champions at all levels of the organization, and assigning these staff to specific prevention roles. Another effective action step is voluntarily raising the minimum standards of practice, such as by reducing the maximum seclusion or restraint orders from 4 hours to 2 hours.

Leadership strategy should include supporting staff practice change through frequent communication from and hospital rounds done by executives. It should ensure the inclusion of consumers, family members, and advocates in all aspects of the effort and create mechanisms so that this involvement will occur, be understood by staff, and be viewed in a positive manner (Bluebird 2004). The key issue here, based on real reduction experiences, is that leadership is essential. If leaders are committed to the effort, significant organization-wide culture change will occur. If they are not, it will fail. In summary, the critical function of organizational leadership is to take an active, visible role, prioritize the initiative, "preach and teach," and hold people accountable for all aspects of the plan.

Use of Data to Inform Practice

Reducing seclusion and restraint through the thoughtful use of data includes tracking core measures, such as seclusion and restraint episodes and hours, and supplemental measures, such as the use of emergency involuntary (usually intramuscular) medication administration, the incidence of consumer and staff injuries, and qualitative reporting of consumer and staff satisfaction (Bluebird 2004). The facility should highlight seclusion and restraint use by graphing and posting these data on all units so that they are clearly visible for staff and consumers. The facility's baseline use of seclusion and restraint should be identified and recorded at the start to set performance improvement goals, monitor use over time, and track progress (or lack thereof) (Hardenstine 2001). Data-driven goals should be set and communicated to staff.

Using data in this way includes analysis of facility seclusion and restraint use by unit, shift, day, and staff member involved, although this last-mentioned strategy should be recorded confidentially for identifying individual staff training and supervisory needs and not for disciplinary actions in general (Huckshorn 2006). These data should be used in a nonpunitive manner to generate healthy competition among facility units or wards and to elevate the general oversight and knowledge of seclusion and restraint use in real time for everyone involved (Hardenstine 2001; Huckshorn 2006). This helps the facility's administration identify successful staff and specific units so that effective seclusion and restraint prevention practices can be shared.

Workforce Development

The strategy focuses on creating a treatment environment in which policies, procedures, and practices are based on the knowledge and principles of recovery and the characteristics of trauma-informed systems of care (Huckshorn 2006). This strategy is implemented primarily through staff training, education, and human resources development activities and provides guidelines for choosing seclusion and restraint application training vendors, particularly vendors who have data demonstrating success in seclusion and restraint reduction with their particular model. This strategy ensures that staff are given the opportunity to develop and practice individualized treatment planning and practice skills that integrate seclusion and restraint prevention strategies for persons served. Included are activities that ensure adequate staff education about the experiences of consumers and staff with seclusion and restraint, address the common myths associated with use, introduce the rationale and characteristics of trauma-informed care, explain the neurobiological and psychological effects of trauma and the power differential between patients and staff, and embody a prevention-based approach to reduction.

Also included is facility leadership's understanding that many seclusion and restraint events occur because of win/lose conflicts set up by facility rules and the staff's roles in enforcing these rules. Because of this institutionally driven risk issue, leadership must understand the value of allowing staff to "suspend" institutional rules and procedures when necessary to avoid or resolve conflicts when addressing individual needs (Huckshorn 2006). Examples of this important construct are rigid policies regarding attendance at activities, wake and sleep times, curfews, smoke breaks, and mealtimes, and other rules designed to keep order that do not consider individual needs or the signs and symptoms of mental illness. Other important activities include discussing the facility's seclusion and restraint reduction plan in new-hire interviews and incorporating expectations in job descriptions, performance evaluations, and new-staff orientation activities (Huckshorn 2006). Senior management must ensure that the seclusion and restraint prevention plan is communicated early and is consistently reinforced, that staff clearly understand their important role in the plan, and that adequate supervision of staff is provided throughout the process so that learning can occur.

Use of Seclusion and Restraint Prevention Tools

This strategy reduces the use of seclusion and restraint through a variety of preventive tools and risk assessments that are integrated into hospital policy and procedure and each individual consumer's treatment plan. This intervention includes using tools for identifying risk for violence (including previous seclusion and restraint history), persons with medical risk factors for death and injury, and persons with psychological risk factors that would be informed by a trauma assessment; for developing and using de-escalation or safety plans (including psychiatric advance directives); for creating sensory-based interventions to teach self-calming and soothing; for making changes to the physical environment (including the development of comfort or sensory rooms); and for implementing daily meaningful treatment activities.

Each of these tools has a specific purpose and associated goals, such as identifying people at higher risk for seclusion and restraint use based on past incidents or those at higher risk for injury or death due to health conditions such as obesity, respiratory disease, or cardiac anomalies; medication side effects; recent ingestion of food; prone positioning; or past trauma histories. De-escalation or safety plans help the service recipient learn illness self-management by identifying emotional triggers and developing awareness of interpersonal or environmental stressors that could lead to conflict or emotional dyscontrol. Proactive strategies can be practiced in advance of a crisis. A behavior scale can offer a set of guidelines to staff to ensure that their response is appropriate to the behavior demonstrated by the service recipient. This helps to ensure that behavior truly meets the criterion of imminent dangerousness before seclusion and restraint are implemented. Many seclusion and restraint incidents are initiated prematurely, before the level of "imminent danger" occurs, often because staff do not know any other approach to use.

One of the most promising practices to aid in reduction efforts and the creation of alternatives is the use of sensory interventions. Sensory interventions can be applied across the range of milieu-based services. This approach requires knowledge of occupational therapy, an assessment of each service user's "sensory diet" (Ayers 1979), an understanding of specific sensory needs (sensory seeking or avoiding), and creation of person-centered care plans based on that knowledge. Applying these concepts to clinical service leads to meaningful, creative therapeutic activities, sensory education and intervention practice, greater instruction in self-calming and soothing techniques, and consideration of unit environments. Implementing sensory interventions at the environmental level shifts the focus from "unit space" to "unit place." The former indicates physical location and boundaries, whereas the latter connotes therapeutic meaning and purpose within the environment (Hasselkus 2002). This can be readily achieved with thoughtful attention to the full range of sensory experience throughout the unit, by attending to color, sound, aroma, lighting, furniture placement, plants, murals—the "softscape"; by creating specific rooms to enhance calm, such as comfort rooms or sensory rooms; or simply by creating quiet areas or smaller seating arrangements that offer greater privacy, sanctuary, and an opportunity to restore (Oostermeijer et al. 2021). The use of sensory rooms and interventions has been attributed to decreased perceived distress, reduced maladaptive behaviors, and enhanced participation and task performance among consumers in treatment settings (Ashby et al. 1995; Champagne 2006; Champagne and Sayer 2003; Hutchinson and Haggar 1991). Moreover, sensory room/comfort room development has been identified as an integral component to many successful restraint-reduction efforts in psychiatric facilities throughout the country (Champagne and Stromberg 2004; Huckshorn et al. 2021; LeBel and Goldstein 2005). Some hospitals have reported significant reductions (54%–91%) in restraint and seclusion use once this preventive alternative was implemented (Champagne and Stromberg 2004; LeBel and Goldstein 2005).

Full Inclusion of Consumers and Advocates

The full and formal inclusion of consumers or "persons in recovery," as well as family members and external advocates, in various roles in the organization assists in the reduction of seclusion and restraint (Bluebird 2004). These roles can be developed by converting vacant positions and hiring consumers into full- or part-time jobs, such as director of advocacy services, peer specialist, drop-in center director, and consumer advocate. These roles are immeasurably valuable if the facility and staff understand and are open to the depth and breadth of knowledge that consumers bring to an organization. The roles and their importance should be defined for staff, and consumer staff should report to managers who understand and support these roles. The new role of a consumer in an inpatient facility can be daunting, intimidating, and difficult; all staff should clearly understand these new roles and attention should be given to orienting and training those who undertake them. It is equally important that inclusion be real and that consumers be empowered to do their jobs, including making mistakes or receiving additional training (Bluebird 2004). Similarly, the inclusion of family members and external advocates can be extremely valuable and is necessary in children's units where service recipients are too young to participate in these kinds of roles. Inviting the local protection and advocacy organization to be involved can be helpful in preventing problems and developing a transparent organization committed to quality improvement.

Rigorous Debriefing Activities

The final strategy uses event debriefing procedures (defined as rigorous analysis) to examine the knowledge gained from a careful review of seclusion and restraint events in order to reduce their occurrence. This knowledge is used to inform policies, procedures, and practices to avoid repeated incidents in the future (Huckshorn 2006). A secondary goal of this strategy is to mitigate harm and the potentially traumatizing effects of a seclusion and restraint event for staff, consumers, and all witnesses to the event.

Debriefing activities are separated into two distinct but equally important activities. The first is an immediate postevent discussion led by a nursing supervisor or a senior staff person who was not involved in the event. The purpose is to ensure the safety of all involved parties, review the documentation, interview staff and others who were present, and attempt to return the unit to the precrisis milieu. The use of an interview guideline and the documentation of activities immediately following the event are highly recommended. The second activity is a more formal meeting that occurs 24–48 hours later. It includes the treatment team, the attending psychiatrist, and a representative from management and uses rigorous problem-solving methods, such as root cause analysis, to review and analyze the event. The goal is to identify what happened and what can be changed to avoid an event in the future and to ensure that, as much as possible, traumatic sequelae are mitigated for everyone involved. Establishing and maintaining a nonpunitive environment is essential to creating a safe space for staff to share their thoughts and feelings.

Inclusion of the consumer's perspective is also critical. A recently secluded or restrained individual may be too intimidated to attend a large meeting, however, and alternatives are recommended. For example, the patient's perspective can be included and represented by a staff advocate if the recipient is able and willing both to agree and to communicate their perspective. This alternative is not meant to patronize or otherwise assume inability of the service recipient to participate; it is intended only to make facility staff aware that patients may have covert feelings of coercion or helplessness in the face of a group of professionals.

In summary, the six core strategies (Huckshorn et al. 2021) are part of a comprehensive performance improvement plan for reducing both conflict and the use of seclusion and restraint (Huckshorn 2006). They are focused on prevention and incorporate the most current and effective approaches known. These strategies have been substantiated in the literature and appear to be a common thread in successful projects (Azeem et al. 2011; Barton et al. 2009; Huckshorn 2014; Lewis et al. 2009; Riahi et al. 2016; Wale et al. 2011).

A Prevention Framework

The avoidance of conflict and violence starts with the use of prevention tools that train staff in best practices (Huckshorn 2006). An obvious place to start this effort is by focusing on the reduction of seclusion and restraint procedures. This is an attainable goal that has been achieved by many facilities throughout the United States and is well within the reach of every committed organization. Changing these practices is much more than rethinking the use of coercive procedures. The essence of this effort is about transforming practice, changing treatment cultures, and reflecting on how we *think* about the people we serve and how to educate the staff who serve them. At its core, this work is about improving safety and using every preventive technique that is known and effective.

Traditional mental health practices have most often placed the reasons for conflict and the use of seclusion and restraint on the shoulders of the consumer—attributing acts of aggression in isolation from the environment and devoid of environmental triggers. A prevention approach is one way for physicians to take a lead role in reorganizing agency operations and can change the way that violence in mental health settings is currently viewed.

In physical health, the public health prevention model is a model of disease prevention and health promotion and a logical fit with a practice issue such as seclusion and restraint (National Association of State Mental Health Program Directors 1999a). This approach directs efforts to anticipate conflicts, immediately resolve situations when they arise, and learn new prevention strategies from an analysis process when these events do occur. This model is best understood through the constructs of primary prevention, secondary prevention, and tertiary prevention to guide the development of reduction activities (Huckshorn et al. 2021).

Primary prevention interventions speak to the development of treatment environments that anticipate the potential for conflict to occur. Strategies include the implementation of trauma-informed visions, values, and principles of care; thorough analysis of organizational values to ensure they are reflected in current practices; ongoing revision of policies and procedures; and early individualized assessments of risk factors for violence, injury, or death. *Secondary prevention* activities speak to the immediate and effective use of early interventions to mitigate conflict or aggression when they occur. These interventions include staff training focused on attitudes and behaviors when faced with a conflict situation, competency-based negotiation and de-escalation skills, and the use of individually developed crisis plans that assist in teaching emotional self-management (Huckshorn et al. 2021). *Tertiary prevention* interventions address the most effective ways to minimize the damage done to consumers, staff, and others witnessing a seclusion and restraint event once it occurs. These strategies include rigorous problem-solving activities in event analyses and include the mandatory involvement of the involved service recipient. These types of interventions are also focused on identifying people who may require specific treatment for trauma.

Conclusion

Were seclusion and restraint regulated substances, the FDA would probably have banned their use, given the number of people who have died and continue to die from these procedures. Consumers are not the only victims; staff have also died or been seriously injured while implementing these practices (Huckshorn et al. 2021). The advantage of publicized reports of seclusion and restraint deaths is that these often spur calls for practice reforms, and such reforms are now occurring domestically and internationally (Department of Health 2005; Mental Disability Advocacy Center 2003; Huckshorn et al. 2021). Despite well-codified local and worldwide human rights and patient protections, the harm to consumers and the staff who serve them persists (Declaration of Dresden Against Coerced Psychiatric Treatment 2007; Mental Disability Advocacy Center 2003).

The good news is that the knowledge about how to do this work is readily available and in the public domain. Many "success story" facilities provide contemporary testaments to transformed mental health services and lived recovery experiences (Duxbury et al. 2019b). None of these stories could be told without courageous leaders who were willing to take an unpopular stand, manage staff anxieties, weather perpetual challenges, and seriously commit to this initiative. Mental health facilities are encouraged to develop their own individualized safety plan that includes violence prevention objectives. Adopting prevention-oriented and trauma-informed principles by implementing the six core strategies will help facilitate an organizational culture change process if committed medical and administrative leaders are willing to chart and stay the course and commit time and personal capital to the mission.

References

Ashby M, Lindsay W, Pitcaithly D, et al: Snoezelen: its effects on concentration and responsiveness in people with profound multiple handicaps. Br J Occup Ther 58:303–307, 1995

Ashcraft L, Bloss M, Anthony WA: Best practices: the development and implementation of "no force first" as a best practice. Psychiatr Serv 63(5):415–417, 2012 22549524

Ayers JA: Sensory Integration and the Child. Los Angeles, CA, Western Psychological Services, 1979

Azeem MW, Aujla A, Rammerth M, et al: Effectiveness of six core strategies based on trauma informed care in reducing seclusions and restraints at a child and adolescent psychiatric hospital. J Child Adolesc Psychiatr Nurs 24(1):11–15, 2011 21272110

Azeem M, Aujla A, Rammerth M, et al: Effectiveness of six core strategies based on trauma informed care in reducing seclusions and restraints at a child and adolescent psychiatric hospital. J Child Adolesc Psychiatr Nurs 30(4):170–174, 2017 30129244

Barton SA, Johnson MR, Price LV: Achieving restraint-free on an inpatient behavioral health unit. J Psychosoc Nurs Ment Health Serv 47(1):34–40, 2009 19227108

Bluebird G: Redefining consumer roles: changing culture and practice in mental health care settings. J Psychosoc Nurs Ment Health Serv 42(9):46–53, 2004 15493495

Busch AB, Shore MF: Seclusion and restraint: a review of recent literature. Harv Rev Psychiatry 8(5):261–270, 2000 11118235

Center for Mental Health Services: National Consensus Statement on Mental Health Recovery. Washington, DC, U.S. Department of Health and Human Services, Substance Abuse and Mental Health Services Administration, 2004. Available at: http://mentalhealth.samhsa.gov/publications/allpubs/sma05-4129. Accessed April 9, 2008.

Centers for Medicare and Medicaid Services: Final Rule, Medicare and Medicaid Programs. Hospital Conditions of Participation: Patients' Rights (42 CFR Part 482, Section 13). Baltimore, MD, U.S. Department of Health and Human Services, 2006

Champagne T: Creating sensory rooms: environmental enhancements for acute inpatient mental health settings. American Occupational Therapy Association. Mental Health Spec Interest Sect Q 29:1–4, 2006

Champagne T, Sayer E: The effects of the use of the sensory room in psychiatry (online). OT-Innovations.com, 2003. Available at: www.ot-innovations.com/wp-content/uploads/2014/09/qi_study_sensory_room.pdf. Accessed September 18, 2007.

Champagne T, Stromberg N: Sensory approaches in inpatient psychiatric settings: innovative alternatives to seclusion and restraint. J Psychosoc Nurs Ment Health Serv 42:35–44, 2004

Cusack KJ, Frueh BC, Hiers TG, et al: The Impact of Trauma and Posttraumatic Stress Disorder Upon American Society: Report to the President's Commission on Mental Health. Unpublished paper, 2003

Cusack KJ, Frueh BC, Brady KT: Trauma history screening in a community mental health center. Psychiatr Serv 55(2):157–162, 2004 14762240

Dannlowski U, Stuhrmann A, Beutelmann V, et al: Limbic scars: long-term consequences of childhood maltreatment revealed by functional and structural magnetic resonance imaging. Biol Psychiatry 71(4):286–293, 2012 22112927

De Bellis MD, Spratt EG, Hooper SR: Neurodevelopmental biology associated with childhood sexual abuse. J Child Sex Abus 20(5):548–587, 2011 21970646

Declaration of Dresden Against Coerced Psychiatric Treatment: The Declaration of Dresden Against Coerced Psychiatric Treatment: consensus statement of the World Network of Users and Survivors of Psychiatry, European Network of Ex-Users and Survivors of Psychiatry, Bundesverband Psychiatrie-Erfahrener, and Mind-Freedom International. Presented at the World Psychiatric Association thematic conference Coercive Treatment in Psychiatry: A Comprehensive Review, Dresden, Germany, June 2007

Department of Health: Delivering Race Equality in Mental Health Care: An Action Plan for Reform Inside and Outside Services and the Government's Response to the Independent Inquiry Into the Death of David Bennett. London, Crown, 2005. Available at: www.dh.gov.uk/en/Publicationsandstatistics/Publications/PublicationsPolicyAndGuidance/DH_4100773. Accessed January 10, 2007.

Duncan S, Estabrooks CA, Reimer M: Violence against nurses. Alta RN 56:13–14, 2000

Duxbury J: An evaluation of staff and patient views of and strategies employed to manage inpatient aggression and violence on one mental health unit: a pluralistic design. J Psychiatr Ment Health Nurs 9(3):325–337, 2002 12060377

Duxbury J, Baker J, Downe S, et al: Minimising the use of physical restraint in acute mental health services: the outcome of a restraint reduction programme ("REsTRAIN YOURSELF"). Int J Nurs Stud 95:40–48, 2019 31009823

Duxbury J, Thomson G, Scholes A, et al: Staff experiences and understandings of the REsTRAIN Yourself initiative to minimize the use of physical restraint on mental health wards. Int J Ment Health Nurs 28(4):845–856, 2019b 30887624

Fallot RD, Harris M: The Trauma Recovery and Empowerment Model (TREM): conceptual and practical issues in a group intervention for women. Community Ment Health J 38(6):475–485, 2002 12474935

Felitti VJ: Origins of addictive behavior: evidence from a study of stressful childhood experiences [in German]. Prax Kinderpsychol Kinderpsychiatr 52:547–559, 2003

Frueh BC, Dalton ME, Johnson MR, et al: Trauma within the psychiatric setting: conceptual framework, research directions, and policy implications. Adm Policy Ment Health 28(2):147–154, 2000 11194123

Frueh BC, Cousins VC, Hiers TG, et al: The need for trauma assessment and related clinical services in a state-funded mental health system. Community Ment Health J 38(4):351–356, 2002 12166921

Frueh BC, Cusack KJ, Grubaugh AL, et al: Clinicians' perspectives on cognitive-behavioral treatment for PTSD among persons with severe mental illness. Psychiatr Serv 57(7):1027–1031, 2006 16816289

Gaynes BN, Brown CL, Lux LJ, et al: Preventing and de-escalating aggressive behavior among adult psychiatric patients: a systematic review of the evidence. Psychiatr Serv 68(8):819–831, 2017 28412887

Green BL, Goodman LA, Krupnick JL, et al: Outcomes of single versus multiple trauma exposure in a screening sample. J Trauma Stress 13(2):271–286, 2000 10838675

Guzman-Parra J, Aguilera-Serrano C, Huizing E, et al: A regional multicomponent intervention for mechanical restraint reduction in acute psychiatric wards. J Psychiatr Ment Health Nurs 28(2):197–207, 2021 32667113

Haimowitz S, Urff J, Huckshorn KA: Restraint and Seclusion: A Risk Management Guide. Alexandria, VA, National Association of State Mental Health Program Directors, 2006

Hardenstine B: Leading the Way Toward a Seclusion and Restraint–Free Environment: Pennsylvania's Success Story. Harrisburg, Office of Mental Health and Substance Abuse Services, Pennsylvania Department of Public Welfare, 2001

Hasselkus B: The Meaning of Everyday Occupation. Thorofare, NJ, Slack, 2002

Health Care Finance Administration: Interim Final Rule, Medicare and Medicaid Programs. Hospital Conditions of Participation: Patient's Rights (42 CFR Part 482, Section 13). Baltimore, MD, U.S. Department of Health and Human Services, 1999

Health Care Finance Administration: Interim Final Rule, Medicaid Program. Use of Restraint and Seclusion in Psychiatric Residential Treatment Facilities Providing Psychiatric Services to Individuals Under Age 21 (42 CFR Parts 441 and 483). Baltimore, MD, U.S. Department of Health and Human Services, 2001

Hinsby K, Baker M: Patient and nurse accounts of violent incidents in a medium secure unit. J Psychiatr Ment Health Nurs 11(3):341–347, 2004 15149383

Huckshorn KA: Re-designing state mental health policy to prevent the use of seclusion and restraint. Adm Policy Ment Health 33(4):482–491, 2006 16244812

Huckshorn KA: Reducing seclusion and restraint use in mental health settings: a phenomenological study of hospital leader and staff experiences. Dissertation Research; UMI Number 3553916. Ann Arbor, MI, ProQuest LLC, 2013

Huckshorn KA: Reducing seclusion and restraint use in inpatient settings: a phenomenological study of state psychiatric hospital leader and staff experiences. J Psychosoc Nurs Ment Health Serv 52(11):40–47, 2014 25310675

Huckshorn KA, LeBel J, Caldwell B (eds): Six Core Strategies to Prevent Conflict and Trauma in Behavioral Health Settings: An Evidence-based Practice Curriculum Training Manual. Originally developed with the National Association of State Mental Health Program Directors (2002–2009): Alexandria, VA, National Association of State Mental Health Program Directors, 2021
Hutchinson R, Haggar L: The Whitinghall Snoezelen Project. Chesterfield, Derbyshire, England, North Derbyshire Health Authority, 1991
Institute of Medicine, Committee on Crossing the Quality Chasm: Adaptation to Mental Health and Addictive Disorders: Improving the Quality of Health Care for Mental and Substance-Use Conditions. Quality Chasm Series. Washington, DC, National Academies Press, 2006
Jennings A: The Damaging Consequences of Violence and Trauma: Facts, Discussion Points, and Recommendations for the Behavioral Health System. Alexandria, VA, National Association of State Mental Health Program Directors, National Technical Assistance Center, 2004
Joint Commission: Health Care at the Crossroads: Strategies for Addressing the Evolving Nursing Crisis. A JCAHO Public Policy Initiative. Oakbrook Terrace, IL, The Joint Commission, 2002. Available at: www.jointcommission.org/-/media/deprecated-unorganized/imported-assets/tjc/system-folders/topics-library/health_care_at_the_crossroadspdf.pdf. Accessed July 14, 2007.
Joint Commission: The Joint Commission's sentinel event policy: ten years of improving the quality and safety of health care. Jt Comm Perspect 25(5):1, 3–5, 2005 15969297
Kessler RC, Sonnega A, Bromet E, et al: Posttraumatic stress disorder in the National Comorbidity Survey. Arch Gen Psychiatry 52(12):1048–1060, 1995 7492257
Kessler RC: Posttraumatic stress disorder: the burden to the individual and to society. J Clin Psychiatry 61 (suppl 5):4–12, discussion 13–14, 2000 10761674
LeBel J, Goldstein R: The economic cost of using restraint and the value added by restraint reduction or elimination. Psychiatr Serv 56(9):1109–1114, 2005 16148326
LeBel J, Stromberg N, Duckworth K, et al: Child and adolescent inpatient restraint reduction: a state initiative to promote strength-based care. J Am Acad Child Adolesc Psychiatry 43(1):37–45, 2004 14691359
LeBel JL, Duxbury JA, Putkonen A, et al: Multinational experiences in reducing and preventing the use of restraint and seclusion. J Psychosoc Nurs Ment Health Serv 52(11):22–29, 2014 25310674
Legris J, Walters M, Browne G: The impact of seclusion on the treatment outcomes of psychotic in-patients. J Adv Nurs 30(2):448–459, 1999 10457248
Leitch L: Action steps using ACEs and trauma-informed care: a resilience model. Health Justice 5(1):5, 2017 28455574
Lewis M, Taylor K, Parks J: Crisis prevention management: a program to reduce the use of seclusion and restraint in an inpatient mental health setting. Issues in Mental Health Nursing 30:159–164, 2009
Lieberman J, Dodd C, DeLauro R: Testimony to the Senate Committee on Finance. Washington, DC, U.S. Senate Proceedings, March 1999
Love CC, Hunter ME: Violence in public sector psychiatric hospitals: benchmarking nursing staff injury rates. J Psychosoc Nurs Ment Health Serv 34(5):30–34, 1996 8732980
Mental Disability Advocacy Center: Cage Beds: Inhuman and Degrading Treatment in Four EU Accession Countries. Budapest, Hungary, Mental Disability Advocacy Center, 2003
Morrison EF: The tradition of toughness: a study of nonprofessional nursing care in psychiatric settings. Image J Nurs Sch 22(1):32–38, 1990 2400419
Moses DJ, Reed BG, Mazelis R, et al: Creating Trauma Services for Women With Co-occurring Disorders: Experiences From the SAMHSA Women With Alcohol, Drug Abuse and Mental Health Disorders Who Have Histories of Violence Study. Rockville, MD, Substance Abuse and Mental Health Services Administration, 2003
Mueser KT, Goodman LB, Trumbetta SL, et al: Trauma and posttraumatic stress disorder in severe mental illness. J Consult Clin Psychol 66(3):493–499, 1998 9642887

National Association of State Mental Health Program Directors: Medical Directors Council Technical Report. Reducing the Use of Seclusion and Restraint: Findings, Strategies, and Recommendations. Alexandria, VA, National Association of State Mental Health Program Directors, 1999a

National Association of State Mental Health Program Directors: NASMHPD Position Statement on Seclusion and Restraint. Alexandria, VA, National Association of State Mental Health Program Directors, 1999b

National Association of State Mental Health Program Directors: Medical Directors Council Technical Report. Reducing the Use of Seclusion and Restraint: Findings, Principles, and Recommendations for Special Needs Populations, Part Two. Alexandria, VA, National Association of State Mental Health Program Directors, 2001

National Association of State Mental Health Program Directors: Position Statement on Services and Supports to Trauma Survivors. Alexandria, VA, National Association of State Mental Health Program Directors, 2005. Available at: www.nasmhpd.org/general_files/position_ statement/NASMHPD%20TRAUMA%20Positon%20 statementFinal.pdf. Accessed July 14, 2007.

Newport DJ, Nemeroff CB: Neurobiology of posttraumatic stress disorder. Focus 1(3):313–321, 2003

Okin RL: Variation among state hospitals in use of seclusion and restraint. Hosp Community Psychiatry 36(6):648–652, 1985 4007818

Oostermeijer S, Brasier C, Harvey C, et al: Design features that reduce the use of seclusion and restraint in mental health facilities: a rapid systematic review. BMJ Open 11(7):e046647, 2021 34233981

Open Minds: 39 state cover peer support services for behavioral health—Open Minds releases reference guide on Medicaid reimbursement for peer support services. April 26, 2018. Available at: www.globenewswire.com/news-release/2018/04/27/1488741/0/en/39-States-Cover-Peer-Support-Services-For-Behavioral-Health-OPEN-MINDS-Releases-Reference-Guide-On-Medicaid-Reimbursement-For-Peer-Support-Services.html. Accessed November 7, 2021.

Papadopoulos C, Ross J, Stewart D, et al: The antecedents of violence and aggression within psychiatric in-patient settings. Acta Psychiatr Scand 125(6):425–439, 2012 22268678

President's New Freedom Commission on Mental Health: Achieving the Promise: Transforming Mental Health Care in America. Final Report (DHHS Publ No SMA 03-3832). Rockville, MD, U.S. Department of Health and Human Services, 2003

Price TB, David B, Otis D: The use of restraint and seclusion in different racial groups in an inpatient forensic setting. J Am Acad Psychiatry Law 32(2):163–168, 2004 15281418

Raboch J, Kališová L, Kallert T; EUNOMIA Study Group: Comparison of the clinical use of individual coercive measures during hospitalization across the EUNOMIA study sites. BMC Psychiatry 7 (suppl 1):S31, 2007

Ray NK, Rappaport ME: Use of restraint and seclusion in psychiatric settings in New York State. Psychiatr Serv 46(10):1032–1037, 1995 8829784

Riahi S, Dawe IC, Stuckey MI, Klassen PE: Implementation of the six core strategies for restraint minimization in a specialized mental health organization. J Psychosoc Nurs Ment Health Serv 54(10):32–39, 2016 27699424

Robins CS, Sauvageot JA, Cusack KJ, et al: Consumers' perceptions of negative experiences and "sanctuary harm" in psychiatric settings. Psychiatr Serv 56(9):1134–1138, 2005 16148329

Rosenberg SD, Mueser KT, Friedman MJ, et al: Developing effective treatments for posttraumatic disorders among people with severe mental illness. Psychiatr Serv 52(11):1453–1461, 2001 11684740

Rosenhan DL: On being sane in insane places. Science 179(4070):250–258, 1973 4683124

Saxe G, Vanderbilt D, Zuckerman B: Traumatic stress in injured and ill children. PTSD Research Quarterly 14:1–7, 2003

Schneeberger AR, Kowalinski E, Fröhlich D, et al: Aggression and violence in psychiatric hospitals with and without open door policies: a 15-year naturalistic observational study. J Psychiatr Res 95:189–195, 2017 28866330

Schnitzer K, Merideth F, Macias-Konstantopoulos W, et al: Disparities in care: the role of race on the utilization of physical restraints in the emergency setting. Acad Emerg Med 27(10):943–950, 2020 32691509
Smith GM, Davis RH, Bixler EO, et al: Pennsylvania State Hospital system's seclusion and restraint reduction program. Psychiatr Serv 56(9):1115–1122, 2005 16148327
Steinert T, Needham I: Seclusion and restraint in different European countries: incidence and interventions. Symposium presentation at the World Psychiatric Association thematic conference Coercive Treatment in Psychiatry: A Comprehensive Review, Dresden, Germany, June 2007
Steinert T, Lepping P, Bernhardsgrütter R, et al: Incidence of seclusion and restraint in psychiatric hospitals: a literature review and survey of international trends. Soc Psychiatry Psychiatr Epidemiol 45(9):889–897, 2010 19727530
Substance Abuse and Mental Health Services Administration: Matrix SAMHSA: The Matrix Priority Programs: Addressing Unmet and Emerging Needs. Rockville, MD, Substance Abuse and Mental Health Services Administration, 2004
United Nations: Principles for the Protection of Persons With Mental Illness and for the Improvement of Mental Health Care (Resolution 46/119). New York, United Nations General Assembly, 1991
U.S. General Accounting Office: Mental Health: Improper Restraint or Seclusion Use Places People at Risk (GAO/HES-99-176). Washington, DC, U.S. General Accounting Office, 1999
Wale JB, Belkin GS, Moon R: Reducing the use of seclusion and restraint in psychiatric emergency and adult inpatient services—improving patient-centered care. Perm J 15(2):57–62, 2011 21841927
Weems CF, Russell JD, Herringa RJ, Carrion VG: Translating the neuroscience of adverse childhood experiences to inform policy and foster population-level resilience. Am Psychol 76(2):188–202, 2021 33734788
Weiss EM, Altimari D, Blint DF, et al: Deadly restraint: a nationwide pattern of death. The Hartford Courant, October 11–15, 1998
Whetten K, Leserman J, Lowe K, et al: Prevalence of childhood sexual abuse and physical trauma in an HIV-positive sample from the Deep South. Am J Public Health 96(6):1028–1030, 2006 16670226
Wikstrom P-OH, Treiber KH: Violence as situational action. Int J Conf Violence 3(1):75–96, 2009
Wong AH, Whitfill T, Ohuabunwa EC, et al: Association of race/ethnicity and other demographic characteristics with use of physical restraints in the emergency department. JAMA Netw Open 4(1):e2035241, 2021 33492372

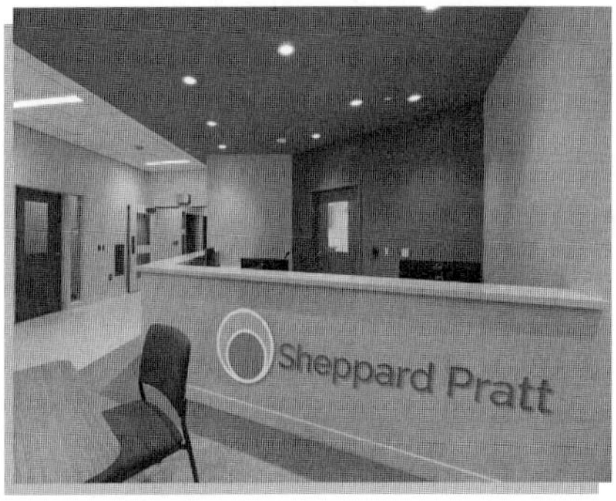

CHAPTER 22

Lean and Operational Excellence

Sunil Khushalani, M.D., DFAPA, FASAM

The core values of Sheppard Pratt are to meet a need, to care, to respect, and to lead the way. Like every health care organization, Sheppard Pratt also has the difficult task of providing psychiatric services in a world in which there are significant and perpetual challenges to resources. The difficulty of this task is compounded by the fact that care is delivered in an incredibly complex and fragmented health care environment. To deliver high-quality care with high reliability requires paying attention to operational indicators of safety, quality, and care delivery while also taking care of our employees. This may seem formidable, and it is in this context that health care organizations have looked to other industries to learn about how to optimize their own systems. The net effect has been the adoption of performance improvement methodologies, with Lean and Six Sigma being two such examples.

The field of medicine was drawn to operational excellence methodologies to reduce errors, reduce wasted resources, improve value, reduce variation, standardize processes, and deliver data-driven care more efficiently and in a cost-conscious way. Lean is a quality improvement methodology based on the Toyota Production System, an approach that Toyota Motor Corporation has used for decades and that has made inroads into many hospitals over the past two to three decades with good results (Kenney 2012; Merlino et al. 2014; Toussaint and Gerard 2010). These hospitals have found it to be an effective way to deal with the challenges of under-resourced systems with ever-growing expectations and complexities.

Sheppard Pratt adopted Lean as a continuous performance improvement methodology because it aligned well with our organizational mission and core values. Lean is not meant to be a list of quality improvement tools. Instead, it is a way of being, leading, and guiding others to work harmoniously with the goal of best utilizing existing resources to achieve ever-increasing heights of improved quality and safety. Which industry or business can say that this is not applicable to its environment and setting?

Why Lean?

There are ever-growing calls for improvement in quality and safety of care. Ever since publication of *To Err Is Human* (Institute of Medicine 2000) and *Crossing the Quality Chasm* (Institute of Medicine Committee on Quality Health Care in America 2001), reports by the Institute of Medicine, much greater attention has been paid to quality and safety of care in hospitals. Concepts such as waste, value, and being patient centered have appeared with greater frequency in medical journals and at presentations during medical conferences. Payers, regulators, patients, and family members are also more sensitized to these issues and consequently have greater expectations in this regard.

Psychiatric hospitals or psychiatric units in general hospitals all over the world are in limited supply. The number of psychiatric beds in the United States is much lower than the demand for them, and the number and availability of such beds have fallen over the years for a multiplicity of reasons (Torrey et al. 2012). As a resource, psychiatric facilities are faced with multiple challenges. The demand for mental health services continues to increase as the stigma of mental health illnesses decreases and the awareness of the importance of mental health keeps growing. This has led to a huge mismatch between supply and demand of psychiatric beds and many unintended consequences, such as boarding patients in emergency departments. In addition, length of stay in these beds has dramatically decreased. It is not uncommon to see patients with serious mental illnesses discharged from psychiatric units into the community less than a week from the time they were admitted (Glick et al. 2011). Because of the number of medications and therapies available for many psychiatric conditions, these conditions are being treated by general practitioners before hospitalization is even considered. The numerous barriers to psychiatric hospitalizations limit their use only for very complex or severe cases, and typically for a short span of time. This has made the work of caring for psychiatric inpatients quite challenging.

The workforce in psychiatric hospitals faces significant challenges due to multiple pressures. A large proportion of the psychiatric workforce is aging (Satiani et al. 2018), and the pipeline of new psychiatrists is not robust enough to keep up. In addition to the increasing complexity of the people being treated, there are exhaustive requirements for documenting information about the care rendered. The amount of time spent documenting care is disproportionate to the total time at work.

The introduction of electronic medical records (EMRs) has further complicated the delivery of psychiatric care. Rather than speeding up documentation, EMRs have inadvertently added to the time spent on documentation, and there is a pervasive sentiment that the quality of face-to-face encounters has diminished. In addition, the practice of medical and psychiatric care has become harder because of an increase in administrative and regulatory burdens. It should not come as a surprise that this especially affects psychiatric care. The ability to pay attention to what is conveyed through affect, expressions, and body language can be lost if a provider's gaze is fixed to a computer screen. The provider is being guided by busy computerized templates with various prespecified fields that need to be completed in a certain order. The progression of questions in these templates (at times required for billing) sometimes artificially leads the conversation along a defined path that is unnatural and not in keeping with how the conversation naturally unfolds or in-sync with the moment-to-moment needs of the patient. This can also lead to newer kinds of errors, such as orders being entered for the wrong patient or things getting missed because of too many notifications, and these errors can affect patients much more rapidly.

Vignette 1

A psychiatrist laments how a new evaluation that used to take 45 minutes and approximately 15 minutes to write up now takes at least 90 minutes. Every day, she takes work home and spends 1–2 hours completing her notes. Her kids have never seen her at home without her computer. Sometimes she sits down to write her notes at bedtime after a busy day at work and home. She has caught herself dozing off while writing her notes. She feels that the joy of practicing medicine has been lost somewhere and wonders if she is burnt out.

A group of experts at the Institute for Healthcare Improvement has articulated the "triple aim" (Berwick et al. 2008) of improving patient experience and improving population health while reducing costs. In 2014, Bodenheimer and colleagues elaborated on this concept, coining the term *quadruple aim* (Bodenheimer and Sinsky 2014), which refers to an additional goal of improving the work life of health care providers, including clinicians and other employees. This quadruple aim has become the guiding light for many organizations.

Medical education and research focus on improving the understanding of the etiology, diagnosis, and treatment of medical conditions. Hardly emphasized, however, is how to uniformly implement these findings in various practice settings or to recognize factors within various contexts that hinder the uniform implementation of this evidence. For instance, if research says that a long-acting antipsychotic injectable should be given to patients with greater risk of nonadherence to antipsychotics, the implementation of such a recommendation depends on the conditions within each practice setting and whether this method of administration is even available to patients in that setting.

Such variations in health care are ubiquitous. A greater degree of variability leads to organizations having more quality and safety issues. Unless health care professionals are taught to be proactive problem solvers, to remove barriers in order to diminish variability and create higher reliability, both health care systems and the workforce over time will become less effective and less capable in maintaining and improving quality. This proactive approach will require leaders, managers, and providers to pay more attention not only to the content (what) delivered but also to the structures (where), processes (how), and capabilities of individuals (who) delivering the care interventions.

Vignette 2

A physician notices that a few patients were sent to the emergency department for severe constipation. Looking at these cases more closely, he realizes that these patients have all been prescribed either Suboxone or methadone. He also sees that they have not been reliably ordered any medications to prevent constipation, which can be expected in patients who use opioids. He decides to work with other physicians to improve the opioid order set and ensure that agents that prevent constipation are included.

What Is Lean?

Lean matured at Toyota after decades of knowledge from early quality improvement pioneers in the United States. Following World War II, the automobile industry in Japan had challenges, similar to those of modern health care systems, that forced it to accelerate the improvement of the quality of products and efficiency of processes to compete in the world market despite limited resources. Hence, the pioneers at Toyota sought to deeply understand waste, with the assumption that underneath every wasted step was a quality problem to be improved.

In Lean as applied to health care, *waste* is defined as any activity that does not help patients or does not move them toward being discharged or cured (Graban 2016). A common example of waste in health care is "waiting"—waiting for an order, a supply of medication, or discharge. Taiichi Ohno, one of the pioneers of Lean, is known to have classified waste into seven different types (Ohno and Kimoto 1987). Later, an eighth type was added.

1. Defects (e.g., medication errors)
2. Overproduction (e.g., inpatient units receiving food trays after patients have been discharged)
3. Waiting (e.g., in the emergency department for an inpatient bed)
4. Nonutilized talent (e.g., a large portion of the day going to copious documentation)
5. Transportation (e.g., sending a patient from an inpatient unit for a venous Doppler to rule out thromboembolism)
6. Inventory (e.g., overstocking supplies and medications)
7. Motion (e.g., looking in multiple rooms for a chart or looking all over the intranet for a policy)
8. Extra processing (e.g., staff from multiple disciplines asking the same questions to the patient on the day of admission)

One of the fundamental principles of Lean is that *problems are not hidden but surfaced*. Many Lean tools serve the purpose of bringing waste into focus. Waste is any action or step in a process that does not add value to the customer or patient. Knowing all types helps teams identify and call out these types of wastes (or problems) in the process.

A complementary principle is the concept of *value*. Value has been articulated as health outcomes based on the resources spent on them over time. In simpler and client-centric terms for any service industry, value is defined as benefits received for burdens endured (Berry 1999). The two pillars of this improvement methodology as defined by Toyota are "continuous improvement" and "respect for people." One important component of "respect for people" is that employees should perform at the height of their potential. Lean says all employees should be taught the improvement methodology so that as part of their daily work, they can contribute to improving their workplace and work processes. When implemented, this creates an "army of problem solvers" who iteratively keep improving the company. As is said of Lean, "With Lean, you will keep changing your definition of what 'good' is" (Toussaint and Berry 2013, p. 74).

How Was Lean Implemented?

A little more than a decade ago, when Sheppard Pratt leadership sought a consistent performance improvement process from all the available improvement methodologies, Lean was chosen as the preferred methodology. This was partly inspired by an article that described the application of Lean methodology as adapted by hospitals (Spear 2005). Spear and colleagues wrote about how two dozen hospitals in Pittsburgh had succeeded in solving vexing problems such as decreasing central-line infections by 50%–90% and improving ventilator-associated pneumonias, postsurgical infections, primary care, and nursing care, among many other clinical and nonclinical processes (Spear 2005). The article asserted that it was "possible to manage the contributions of dozens, hundreds, and even thousands of specialists in such a way that their collective effort not only is capable and reliable in the short term but also improves steadily in the longer term" (Spear 2005, p. 81).

The conclusion we drew from this was that if these methods could be applied to general medical and surgical settings, mental health care settings could also benefit from such thinking and methods. Ultimately, any work can be broken down into processes that can be improved. The activities, connections, and pathways in each setting might be different, but they can all be amenable to improvement (Spear 2004). It introduced our organization to Lean methodology and how it is employed by companies as varied as Toyota, Alcoa, Vanguard, and Southwest Airlines. This inspired our health system to learn these methods and apply them in the context of a mental health setting.

Lean built upon the "plan-do-check-act" (PDCA) method that was already being used by the quality team. *The goal was to move such thinking and application beyond the scope of the quality department to involve as many professional and nonprofessional employees in quality improvement efforts as possible and bring about a cultural change in the health system.* To define the goals and driving principles of the new quality improvement efforts, the leadership came up with a vision statement: To create a health system in which problems are embraced as opportunities for improvement and everyone is motivated, trained, and empowered to spot and solve problems, all with the goal of making Sheppard Pratt a constantly improving place to receive care and in which to work. The idea was to encourage all staff to think of this approach as a "collaborative, innovative approach to improve the quality of care for everyone we serve." Our continuous improvement philosophy would be "person-centered, outcomes-oriented, data-driven, and value-centric."

Lean was found to be intuitive and easy to learn, understand, and teach, regardless of the learner's background or level of experience. Enough basic principles and tools could be taught to get individuals started on their own improvement journeys. Lean was deployed in several ways, at first with the help of consultants and then by hiring our own set of experts. Our health system began with a three-pronged approach:

1. Rapid process improvement (RPI) events
2. Lean Problem-Solving Course
3. Lean daily management or "daily huddles"

Rapid Process Improvement Events

RPI events are highly focused events that can last anywhere from 1 to 5 days. A multidisciplinary team comes together to solve a particular challenge within the health system. These are generally problems encountered in the course of daily work and may be recurring, chronic, or pervasive problems. Sometimes they are complex and involve processes that traverse multiple interconnected departments. For example, one of the first challenges we tackled was improving our discharge planning process on one inpatient unit.

In an RPI event, the team works together to articulate the "business case" and figure out why the improvement is needed by the organization at that time. The questions to be answered here are

1. Why is the improvement necessary?
2. Why is it needed now?
3. How can the organization benefit from this improvement?
4. What is the downside of doing nothing?

Determining why is a good motivator to inspire action by all the team members or stakeholders. An important concept is to develop "process literacy" (Ogrinc et al. 2012). First, the team observes the process they are trying to improve, in person, from start to finish. It is important that the observation occur from the patient's perspective *at the location* where the work occurs. This is not to be drawn from someone's mind in some remote meeting room. In-person observation captures the process not as one imagines or desires it to be but as it actually takes place. Any variations, wasteful steps, and detours are thus brought to the surface and illustrated on a process map like that shown in Figure 22–1. The key steps of the process are listed first. Then, after team discussion, the observed problems, gaps, or defects in the process that may negatively affect or get in the way of desired outcomes are highlighted. These are depicted as "storm clouds." The team can also highlight the things that work well and should be preserved or enhanced. As they brainstorm ways to remove all kinds of waste, they gradually enhance the proportion of value within that process, thereby improving quality and safety with every bit of waste that is reduced or eliminated.

The idea of an RPI event is to become aware of improvement opportunities in order to devise countermeasures and solutions—to "try-storm" (as opposed to just brainstorming)—within the time frame of the event and do planned pilot experiments. It is helpful to create and perform small pilot projects that may then be cascaded and inform other areas of the system. One improvement effort often reveals four or five other improvement opportunities.

In the example of improving discharge planning on an inpatient unit, one of the first small pilot projects was to organize a closet of patient belongings. It was observed that disorganized belongings led to extra effort (waste of motion [Figure 22–2], extra processing, and waiting) when gathering patient belongings from various locations (storage, security, and pharmacy). Items forgotten or lost had to be mailed or replaced (waste of defects) at the time of discharge, which led to not only increased delays in discharges but also increased expenses, decreased satisfaction, and increased complaints. This gave rise to the idea of a checklist for organizing belongings at the time of discharge. This

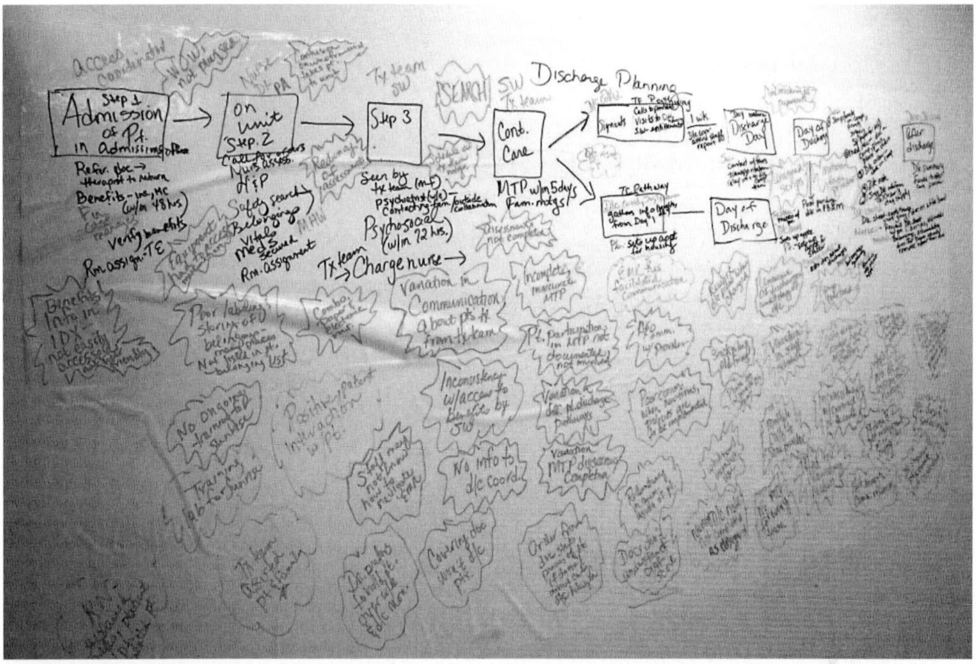

FIGURE 22–1. Process map of the journey of a patient from admission to discharge.
To view this figure in color, see Plate 3 in Color Gallery.

checklist project then demonstrated another type of waste: the lack of clarity of various individual roles with respect to discharge, as seen in Figure 22–3. Some tasks were being handled by multiple individuals whereas other tasks were being forgotten.

When new workflows or process improvements are derived from successful experiments, the team can then create a new "standard work" document. This document includes process steps, key points of each step, and reasons why each step is carried out. Standard work documents allow for communication of the proposed process to everyone, including people from every shift, so that all can provide suggestions for improvement or express concerns. Involving everyone affected by changing the process is important to achieve buy-in and ensure sustainment of the change. In addition, ideas conceived by one set of individuals may not anticipate all the unintended consequences of an improvement effort that occurs downstream. A standard work document becomes a template for all to follow and provides a baseline for the next improvement cycle.

It is also important to articulate how the team measures improvement. Donabedian (1966) spoke about structural, process, and outcome measures as one "family" of measures. Alternatively, one could measure input, process, and output measures. It is important that the improvement process be data driven, which is best communicated to the stakeholders and leadership graphically.

Vignette 3

Checking patient responses to as-needed medications after they are administered is a regulatory requirement. The quality officer heard about the number of times these checks were missed on different inpatient units but stated in absolute numbers. The quality of-

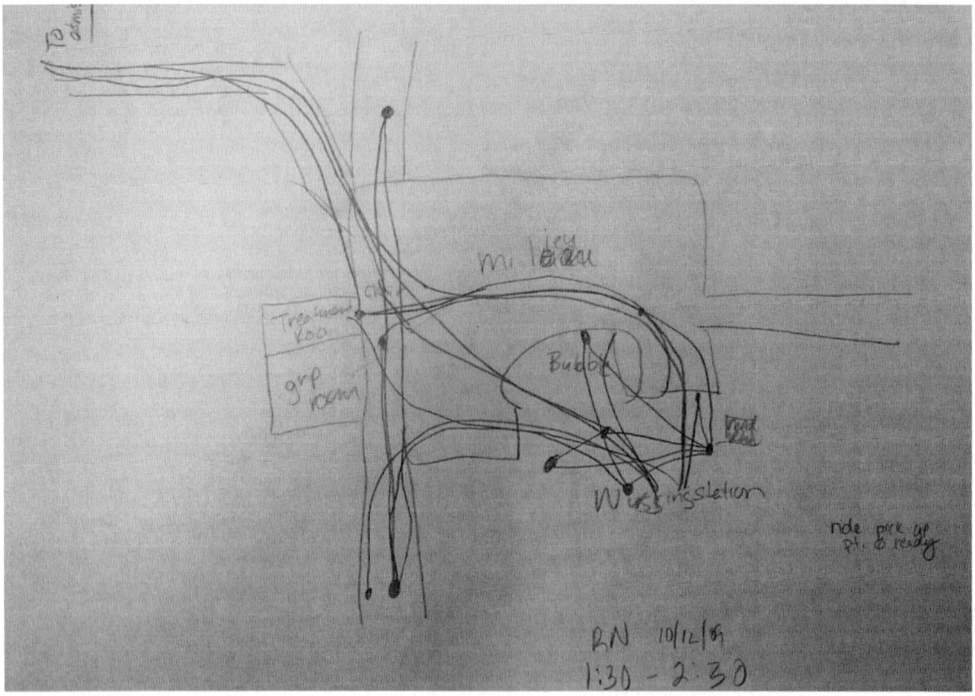

FIGURE 22–2. A "spaghetti diagram" tracks a nurse's movements as she prepared a patient for discharge (waste of motion visualized).

ficer suggested that these missed checks be reported as a percentage of total number of medications administered (which would then be reported as a rate and allow for inter-unit comparison) and graphically reported as a run chart with a reference target. This allowed everyone else to see each unit's relative performance over time. If a unit improved, they could share their success story with others. If a unit did not improve, that could easily be seen by the local managers, who could then investigate further.

Lean Problem-Solving Course

To engage more individuals outside the quality department in the improvement process, a continuing education course titled Lean Problem-Solving Course was conceptualized. The idea was to incorporate Lean thinking into more areas and layers of the organization. The course was aimed at familiarizing participants with the organization's vision and strategic objectives, Lean principles and methodology (waste and value), and basic tools of improvement. In addition to didactic presentations and discussions, teaching methods included simulations, hand-on exercises, and reflections.

The biggest, most significant element of the course was an experiential component to ensure a deeper learning of the material. Each participant was asked to pick a current, relevant problem to solve, and supervisor approval and participation were required. As long as the problem affected any of the important strategic objectives at that time (safety, quality, service delivery, employee engagement, or customer satisfaction), it was deemed a suitable project. The participant was to choose a scope for the project that would allow it to be completed before the end of the 4-month course. Each class of about 10–12 participants would work with a team from their department, and they would re-

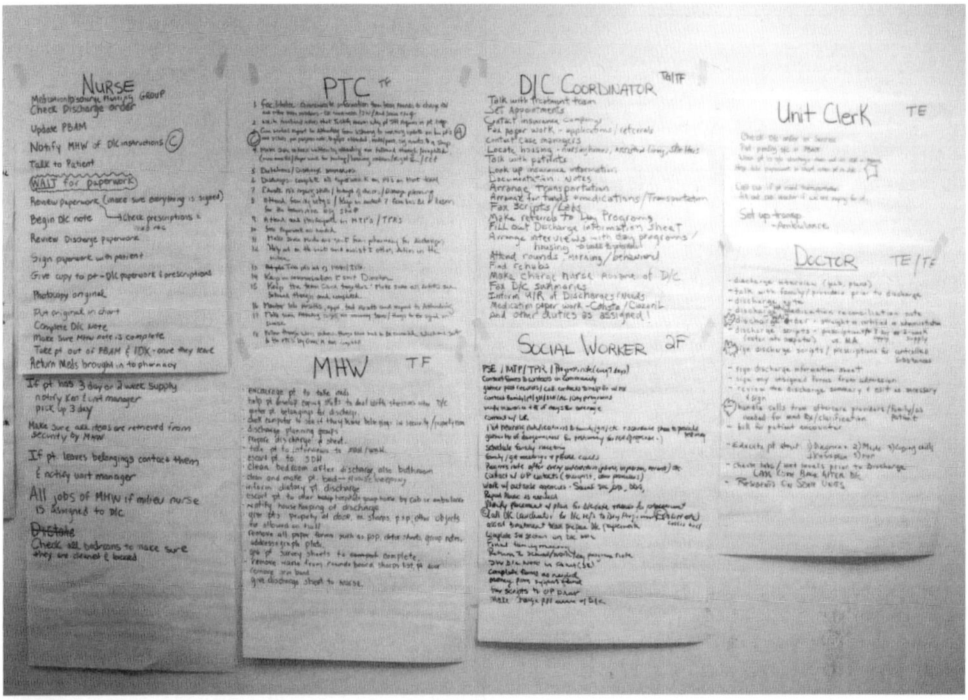

FIGURE 22–3. Role clarification of various disciplines in order to reduce ambiguity and increase role clarity.

To view this figure in color, see Plate 4 in Color Gallery.

ceive feedback from other class participants, the class instructors, and their supervisors. Individual coaching was provided as needed. At the end of the course, all participants presented their completed project to the organization.

The framework that each participant followed was a structured A3 template (A3 refers to the size of the paper: 11″×17″) (Shook 2010). The idea was to fit the entire project summary on a single page (Figure 22–4). Historically, a paper of this size was chosen because that was the largest page that could be faxed to leadership at Toyota. Because it was just one page, ideas had to be conveyed succinctly and preferably visually (with data and charts). The various steps of this structured template provided the necessary structure and progression. It allowed others to see and learn from an individual's project. This template incorporated the "plan" (entire left side of the page, which included the business case, understanding customers and stakeholders, process map and baseline data, goal, and root cause analysis) as well as "do" (listing solutions and experiments), "check" (improvement confirmation and lessons learned), and "act" (follow-up action plan) sections.

Lean Daily Management or "Daily Huddles"

The Lean Problem-Solving Course taught quality improvement principles, which raised awareness of these ideas in the organization. However, many more of the organization's employees were exposed to Lean through the creation of brief daily huddles. If any organization is to achieve the quadruple aim—simultaneously improving the

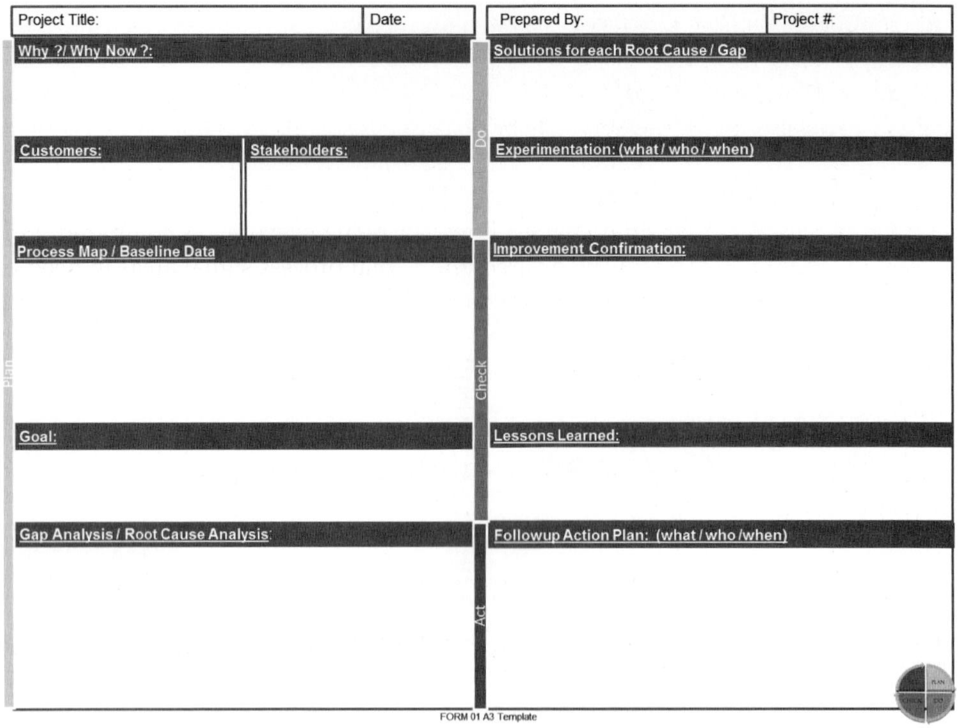

FIGURE 22–4. The standardized A3 template.
To view this figure in color, see Plate 5 in Color Gallery.

health of the population, enhancing the experience and outcomes of the patient, and reducing per capita cost of care while improving joy at work—it will have to improve across all domains of safety, quality, and care delivery and act as a good steward of all available resources. Leadership cannot accomplish all this by itself or even in conjunction with small quality departments. Facilitating audits to keep up with ever-increasing regulatory pressures will not engage everyone; it is neither inspiring nor enough to keep up with all the demands of performance improvement. Leaders can achieve this monumental task by creating an infrastructure and culture that will allow all employees not only to do their jobs well but also to be fully engaged in improving the system as they work.

Based on this time-tested Lean philosophy, the Lean daily management system (also described as daily huddles) is one tool to achieve performance improvement for any selected strategic initiative. It engages both the frontline providers of care and the organization's management in a disciplined, daily problem-solving exercise that focuses attention on improving processes within the organization to meet strategic goals. John Toussaint, in his book *Management on the Mend: The Healthcare Executive Guide to System Transformation*, described the Lean daily management system as "a constructive pipeline for intelligence from the front line that flows up through the organization and an equally robust line of communication and strategy from the top back to the front line" (Toussaint and Adams 2015, p. 87). If implementation of the system is effectively orchestrated, not only do problems get solved and participants get more engaged but the organization can also get optimally aligned to tackle complex systemic challenges. Providers can surface problems, do a quick root cause analysis, and shed light on systemic barriers to performance improvement and value creation.

These huddles at Sheppard Pratt, which took place in many different departments, helped groups of individuals practice brief "improvement drills" or "improvement kata" (Rother 2009). Even the daily huddle discussions follow the PDCA logic. To begin, a process is selected for improvement, and the scope and metrics are agreed upon. Then the process is tracked daily to see how it is being executed as compared with a desired standard. Gaps between desired and actual process signal areas in need of improvement. The expertise, resourcefulness, and creativity of the frontline team are used to solve complex issues impacting the process. A monthly run chart shows the performance trend over time, and an action plan keeps the entire team aligned and on target.

Huddles last around 5–10 minutes each day. The framework used is as follows: Employees gather around a presentation board. (We tried using a whiteboard and placing hand-drawn charts physically on the wall and finally decided on making these presentations virtually via a large screen mounted on the wall in the nurses' station. The latter came in handy during COVID-19 because team members could participate virtually from their offices and maintain physical distancing.) Figure 22–5 shows an example of the digital board, called a "four-block." The top left box is the monthly run chart of the process being monitored. At the top of this block is an agreed-upon target goal and the previous month's observed data. The top right box is the daily check, which tracks daily progress; colors are used as a visual to indicate if performance is as desired (*green*) or not (*red*). This leads the discussion to the lower left corner, which either notes the frequency of the problem or creates a Pareto chart to assess factors contributing to the problem. The team could also draw on this section to do a root cause analysis of the problem using a five-why process or a fishbone diagram, which are tools for this purpose. Last, the lower right section is the current action plan, which is derived after discussion with the team and outlining actions or strategies for preventing a similar problem in the future. Each action is assigned to a particular team member and includes a due date for future discussion. This system provides a continuous daily improvement drill.

Once performance is consistently above the target, a standard work document is created to capture the improved process. At this point, the local departmental team is joined by a leadership team, which performs a complementary "coaching drill" or "coaching kata" by asking Socratic questions to strengthen the improvement mindset and skills of the departmental team members. The leadership team also helps the local department resolve any systemic barriers that come up. Finally, the leadership team shares the best practices and innovative strategies developed by the local team throughout the organization to cascade their use.

These three methods were used at Sheppard Pratt to inculcate Lean thinking in various individuals within our organization. Ongoing learning and improvement cycles can ultimately lead to a gradual cultural transformation. These methods require active leadership involvement to transform a system's culture. Delegating this function to local departments leads to uneven change and does not lead to the desired organization-wide alignment or results. Recently, the Lean Department at Sheppard Pratt

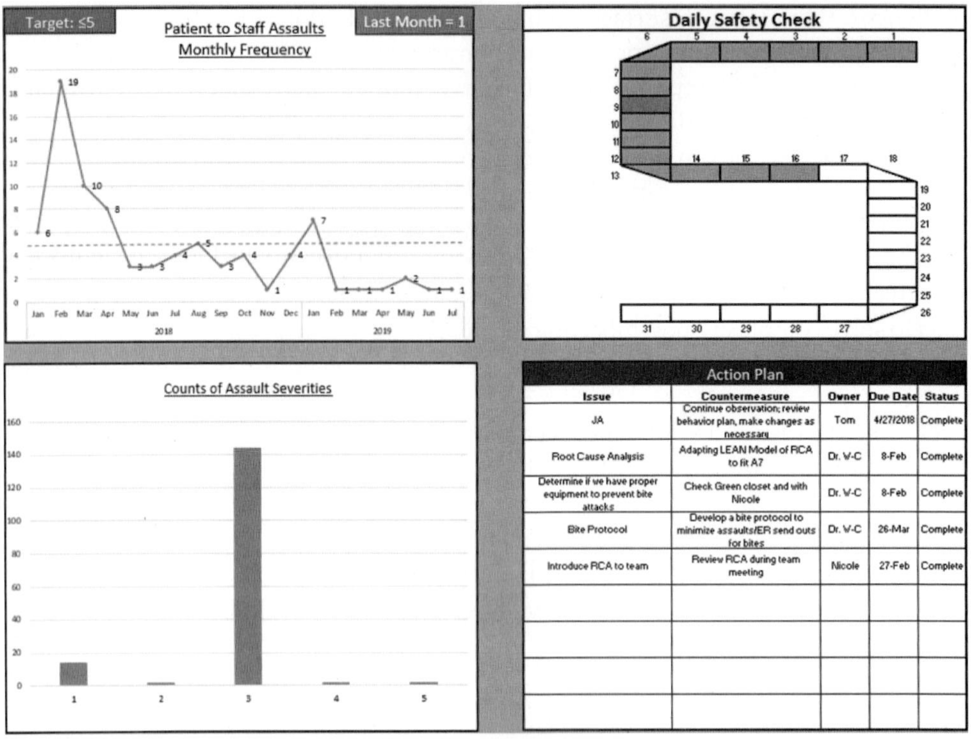

FIGURE 22–5. The four-block daily huddle board.
To view this figure in color, see Plate 6 in Color Gallery.

was renamed Operational Excellence out of a desire to utilize tools from other methodologies, such as Six Sigma, depending on the need of the situation. Just as Lean has been highly effective in reducing waste, Six Sigma approaches have been useful in reducing variation. Six Sigma is a process improvement methodology that was developed at Motorola in the late 1980s. It is a highly disciplined, meticulous, and statistically driven approach to quality improvement. The primary objective of this methodology is to reduce variations in product, process, or service opportunities. Defect levels are measured in terms of parts per million or defects per million opportunities. Six sigma denotes an approach to reduce variation to an extent that the level of defects is reduced to less than 3.4 per million process, product, or service opportunities (Urdhwareshe 2011). Six Sigma is often combined with Lean, in practice, and called "Lean Sigma" or "Lean Six Sigma." This is made possible since both approaches value data and are systematic improvement methods (KaiNexus 2021).

We have industrial engineers working side by side with mental health professionals utilizing these various performance improvement tools to repair wasteful processes, redesign inefficient or ineffective workflows, and plan new ventures and developments. Mental health professionals are becoming more comfortable with an entirely new language and set of tools, and industrial engineers are becoming sensitized to the vocabulary of psychiatry and the formidable challenge of measuring, standardizing processes, and reducing variability in mental health care. The overarching idea is to optimize the functioning of the behavioral health system given its existing resources at any given moment in time. We aim to continuously improve our health system so that it can demonstrate all of our core values and become a highly desirable place to work.

Conclusion

The field of medicine can consistently apply performance improvement (or operational excellence) methodologies to reduce errors, reduce waste, improve value, reduce variation, standardize processes, and deliver data-driven care more efficiently and in a cost-conscious way. Many other industries have done so successfully. Problems should be embraced as opportunities for improvement. Employee motivation, training, and empowerment to spot and solve problems are all important for continuously improving the health care infrastructure and environment and becoming truly value driven and patient centered.

Continuous improvement is one of the best ways to sustain improvement. This monumental task is made easier once we demonstrate respect for everyone: all of those whom we serve and all of our employees. Adoption of performance improvement methodologies will be necessary for survival of health care organizations, and further advancements will come from learning and adopting methodologies from other, nonmedical disciplines. As the complexity of health care rises, so will the need to train everyone to become not only competent health care professionals but also adept problem solvers. Each health care worker will have to learn to repair, redesign, and devise innovative ways to provide care. Robust performance improvement methodologies such as Lean and Six Sigma will need to be utilized in order to meet the ambitious quadruple aim of enhancing patient experience, improving population health, reducing costs, and improving the work life of employees universally.

References

Berry LL: Discovering the Soul of Service. New York, Free Press, 1999, pp 12–13

Berwick DM, Nolan TW, Whittington J: The triple aim: care, health, and cost. Health Aff (Millwood) 27(3):759–769, 2008 18474969

Bodenheimer T, Sinsky C: From triple to quadruple aim: care of the patient requires care of the provider. Ann Fam Med 12(6):573–576, 2014 25384822

Donabedian A: Evaluating the quality of medical care. Milbank Mem Fund Q 44(3, suppl):166–206, 1966 5338568

Glick ID, Sharfstein SS, Schwartz HI: Inpatient psychiatric care in the 21st century: the need for reform. Psychiatr Serv 62(2):206–209, 2011 21285100

Graban M: Lean Hospitals: Improving Quality, Patient Safety, and Employee Engagement. Boca Raton, FL, CRC Press, 2016

Institute of Medicine: To Err Is Human: Building a Safer Health System. Washington, DC, National Academies Press, 2000

Institute of Medicine Committee on Quality Health Care in America: Crossing the Quality Chasm: A New Health System for the 21st Century. Washington, DC, National Academies Press, 2001

Kainexus: What is six sigma? Process improvement methodology. 2021. Available at: www.kainexus.com/improvement-disciplines/six-sigma. Accessed November 7, 2021.

Kenney C: Transforming Health Care: Virginia Mason Medical Center's Pursuit of the Perfect Patient Experience. Boca Raton, FL, CRC Press, 2012

Merlino JP, Omi J, Bowen J (eds): Lean Behavioral Health: The Kings County Hospital Story. New York, Oxford University Press, 2014

Ogrinc G, Headrick L, Moore S, et al: Fundamentals of Health Care Improvement: A Guide to Improving Your Patient's Care. Oak Brook Terrace, IL, The Joint Commission, 2012

Ohno T, Kimoto LM: The Toyota Production System. Monterey, CA, Monterey Institute of International Studies, 1987

Rother M: Toyota Kata: Managing People for Improvement, Adaptiveness, and Superior Results. New York, McGraw-Hill Education, 2009

Satiani A, Niedermier J, Satiani B, Svendsen DP: Projected workforce of psychiatrists in the United States: a population analysis. Psychiatr Serv 69(6):710–713, 2018 29540118

Shook J: Managing to Learn: Using the A3 Management Process to Solve Problems, Gain Agreement, Mentor and Lead. Cambridge, MA, Lean Enterprise Institute, 2010

Spear SJ: Learning to lead at Toyota. Harv Bus Rev 82(5):78–86, 151, 2004 15146738

Spear SJ: Fixing health care from the inside, today. Harv Bus Rev 83(9):78–91, 158, 2005 16171213

Torrey EF, Fuller DA, Geller J, et al: No Room at the Inn: Trends and Consequences of Closing Public Psychiatric Hospitals, 2005–2010. Research From the Treatment Advocacy Center. Arlington, VA, 2012. Available at: www.treatmentadvocacycenter.org/storage/documents/no_room_at_the_inn-2012.pdf. Accessed July 21, 2020.

Toussaint J, Adams E: Management on the Mend: The Healthcare Executive Guide to System Transformation. Appleton, WI, ThedaCare Center for Healthcare Value, 2015

Toussaint JS, Berry LL: The promise of Lean in health care. Mayo Clin Proc 88(1):74–82, 2013 23274021

Toussaint J, Gerard R: On the Mend: Revolutionizing Healthcare to Save Lives and Transform the Industry. Cambridge, MA, Lean Enterprise Institute, 2010

Urdhwareshe H: Six Sigma for Business Excellence: Approach, Tools and Applications. Pearson Education India, May 2011

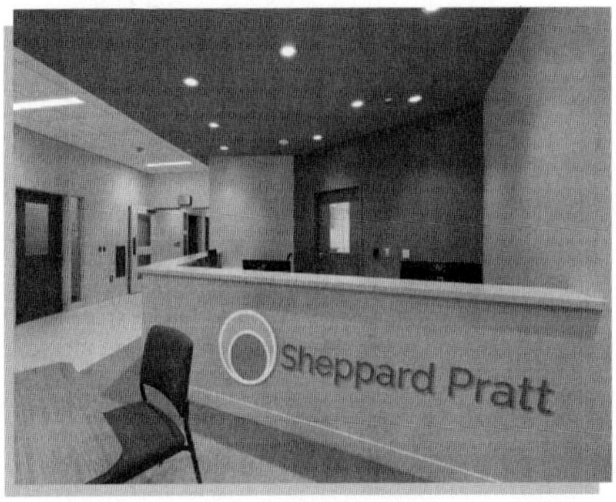

CHAPTER 23

Architecture and Thoughtful Design

Harsh K. Trivedi, M.D., M.B.A
Michelle S. Hooper, M.S.H., AIA
Antonio DePaolo, Ph.D.
Thomas D. Hess, M.B.A.
Roger Daub

At Sheppard Pratt, the importance of architecture and thoughtful design has guided the creation of transformational therapeutic spaces from our inception in 1853 to the building of our newest hospital, which opened in June 2021 (Figure 23–1). Moses Sheppard's initial bequest specified architectural and design directives as well as his intentions of how the space should be utilized. A few excerpts are given below, as presented by Forbush (1971, p. 18), to illustrate the vision:

> Courteous treatment and comfort of all patients be given first consideration in the plans for the grounds, buildings, and medical care.
>
> All patient rooms shall be above ground and all should have privacy with ample sunlight and fresh air.
>
> Combine every feature that science and experience might indicate as requisite or desirable to minister to the greatest possible advantage of the patients.

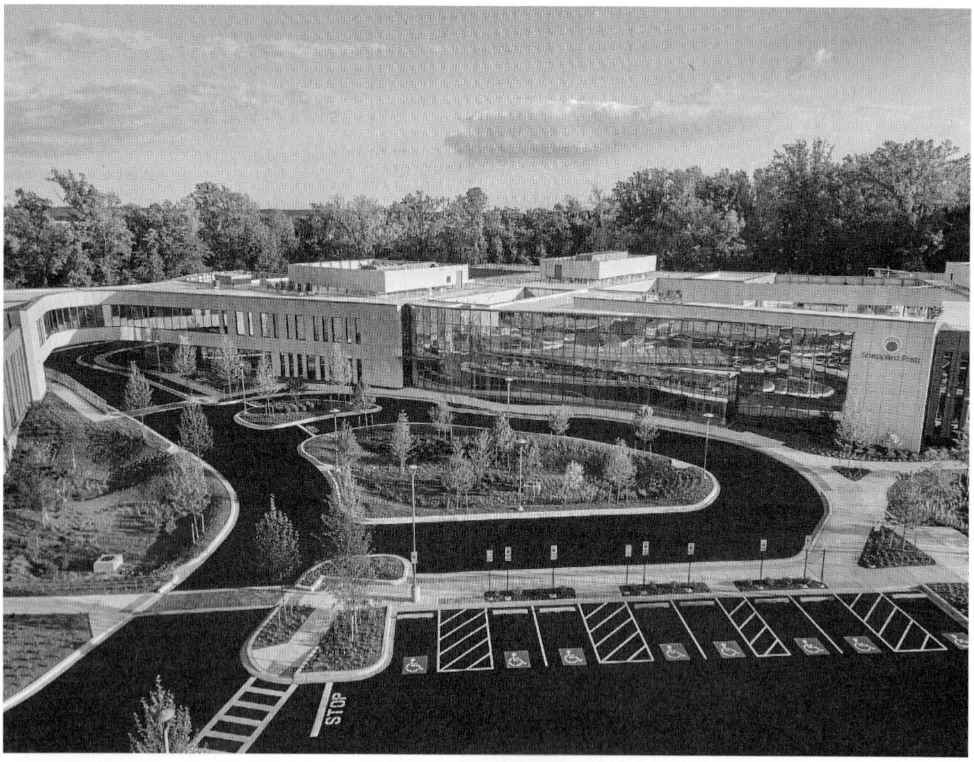

FIGURE 23–1. Sheppard Pratt Baltimore/Washington campus.
To view this figure in color, see Plate 7 in Color Gallery.
New state-of-the-art behavioral health facilities incorporate thoughtful design and set the standard for psychiatric and behavioral health care.

Anything suggestive of a prison-like appearance is to be avoided.

Buildings are to be fireproof as far as possible, and to feature many windows.

Although attitudes toward the stigma of mental illness, the nature of psychiatric treatment in each era, and the balance between therapeutic benefit and engineering safety have intertwined and changed over time, we have been fortunate that Moses Sheppard's directives have guided the architecture and thoughtful design of Sheppard Pratt such that there is a fundamental belief in the dignity of every life and an unyielding focus on the patient experience.

The Moral Treatment Movement

The early care of persons with mental illness in America occurred primarily among family members and within informal structures. As time passed, it "became common for towns to provide subsidies to families dealing with an insane family member.…If families were unable to care for their insane or did not have the financial means, many ended up in jails or public poorhouses" (Osborn 2009). The initial psychiatric asylums were public, created by state governments to treat the insane (see Chapter 1).

The Eastern Lunatic Asylum of Virginia, opened in 1773, was the first such hospital in the United States (Grob 1994). By the mid-1800s, there were still few hospitals for the mentally ill. Not unlike today, the mentally ill were all too often poor and confined to prisons (Jones et al. 1856).

Design of Care Environments

The built environment plays an important role not only in our physical health but also in our mental health. The architectural design of care environments has the ability to either impair or promote psychological well-being. Behavioral health facilities span a wide range of care environments, including psychiatric hospitals, psychiatric units of general hospitals, addiction treatment facilities, mental health clinics, day hospitals, and outpatient treatment centers. These facilities provide treatment and recovery for patients with behavioral and mental health conditions who require temporary or long-term inpatient care. A quality environment for behavioral health patients is directly tied to the architectural design. Design guidelines for behavioral health facilities are limited because of the variety of settings and diagnoses. Designers have access to several guides, standards, and research by experts, but evidence-based design is limited to postdischarge patient surveys and interviews with staff. There is no direct correlation linking one design element to a particular patient outcome.

In addition to research by experts in the field, the following resources are available to designers:

- "Guidelines for Design and Construction of Hospitals" (Facility Guidelines Institute 2018), developed by the Facility Guidelines Institute, provides minimum design standards for general hospitals, freestanding emergency facilities, critical access hospitals, psychiatric hospitals, rehabilitation hospitals, children's hospitals, and mobile/transportable medical units.
- *The Behavioral Health Design Guide* (Hunt et al. 2019), published by Behavioral Health Facility Consulting LLC, addresses leading practice design challenges of the built environment for adult inpatient behavioral health care units.
- *Mental Health Facilities Design Guide* (U.S. Department of Veterans Affairs 2017), published by the U.S. Department of Veterans Affairs Office of Construction and Facilities Management, is a planning tool intended to provide design strategies and technical specifications for new construction and renovations of psychiatric inpatient, outpatient, and residential settings.
- *Patient Safety Standards, Materials and Systems Guidelines* (New York State Office of Mental Health 2021), published by the New York State Office of Mental Health in association with architecture+, offers guidance for patient safety features in the inpatient psychiatric environment, and applies to new construction and major renovations.

In psychiatry, building or renovating a unit is a capital project that does not happen often. The design process is an opportunity for the clinical staff to change the culture of their institution through the reinvention of their clinical processes. Planning and designing a new facility not only changes the physical environment but also transforms patients' experience of care (Pitts 2018). Most design guides and research recommend "therapeutic" design, which is the result of the deinstitutionalization trend, starting in the mid-twentieth century, of closing publicly funded behavioral health institutions. Patient recovery is promoted not only through therapeutic programs but also through therapeutic facility design. A therapeutic design provides an environment that prevents harm and promotes healing.

There is no one-size-fits-all solution for designing a therapeutic environment. Medical comorbidities complicate patient care. Providing treatment and promoting recovery for psychiatric patients have traditionally focused on safety and mitigating the risk of self-harm and harm to others. A therapeutic environment helps patients be more receptive to the provided treatment by creating a nonthreatening atmosphere where patients feel comfortable and relaxed. Patients can exhibit symptoms such as suicidal ideation or suicide attempts, aggression, self-harm, psychosis, or difficulty with executive function as they receive care for their anxiety, depression, schizophrenia, dementia, substance addiction, or eating disorders. Environments that aggravate these symptoms can make patients feel watched, judged, or isolated. Especially after a crisis event, the stress of being admitted to inpatient care can be exacerbated by design elements that trigger feelings of hopelessness, being trapped, isolation, guilt, shame, sensory overload, boredom, or being watched. Recovery is aided by design elements that instill a sense of self-control, environmental control, individuality, freedom, creativity, and a connection to nature. Although there is little evidence focused on designing for medical patients with behavioral health comorbidities, research suggests that certain design features are important for behavioral health treatment facilities or units (Karlin and Zeiss 2006; Shepley and Pasha 2013; Shepley et al. 2016). The range of diagnosis means that while some design features are likely to help everyone, other design features are more applicable to certain patient populations.

Design elements that promote psychological well-being in hospitals include the following (Center for Health Design 2017) (Figure 23–2):

- A deinstitutionalized, well-organized setting
- Access to daylight, views of nature, and the outdoors
- A sense of safety, security, and privacy
- Acoustic control
- Patient control over their own environment
- Places for social interaction
- Positive distraction

Some of these design elements are more important to specific populations. When designing for a specialized program, stakeholders need to carefully balance therapeutic design with appropriate safety. Design elements selected and implemented should minimize harm and maximize benefits. Risk factors can include both individual and external conditions, including the built environment. Methods of self-harm typically include hanging, jumping, cutting, intentional drug overdose, and strangulation (Hunt et al. 2019). Mitigating risk includes designing ligature-resistant environments in addition to considering latent conditions that contribute to elopement and/or harm to others (Taylor and Zborowsky 2019), including the following:

- Access to high-risk areas such as windows, porch, balcony, and roof
- Uncontrolled egress

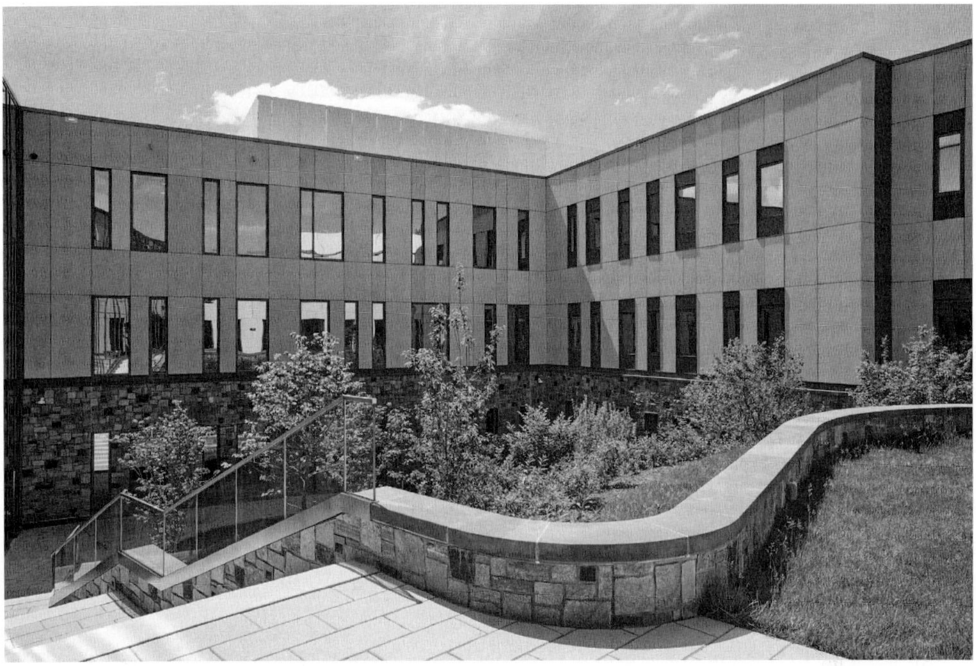

FIGURE 23–2. Interior courtyard.
To view this figure in color, see Plate 8 in Color Gallery.
Patient rooms and units that face wooded areas or interior courtyards offer well-lit spaces and capitalize on the healing effects of nature.

- Poor visibility/accessibility to patient-occupied areas (both interior and exterior)
- Unauthorized access to staff areas and high-risk areas, such as team stations and environmental services
- A lack of secure holding (unit seclusion, emergency departments)
- Unsafe finishes or design elements (toxic or flammable elements)
- Furniture that can be used for projectiles, barricades, entrapment, or suicide
- Access to ligature points on plumbing fixtures, mechanical (HVAC) systems, electrical fixtures/outlets, and doors
- Other issues that may contribute to patient negative perceptions (e.g., lighting, colors, signage)

Latent conditions can be partially mitigated through planning the building design categories using a security risk assessment. Guidelines by Hunt et al. (2019) and the New York State Office of Mental Health (2021) organize the risk levels of concern as high, medium, and low on the basis of a functional statement of intended use. The highest-risk areas are those where the patient is alone or unsupervised, such as bedrooms and bathrooms. Areas where the patient is in a highly agitated condition, such as admission areas, exam rooms, and seclusion rooms, also have high risk potential. Typical medium-risk areas include living rooms, dining rooms, group rooms, and corridors, where patient access is controlled and use is supervised. The lowest-risk areas are those that are under constant supervision or are not in use by patients, such as medication rooms, offices, and utility rooms.

Patient behavior is not always predictable, and this makes planning and designing for these conditions complex. Using a layered approach that considers patients, staff, organizational culture and procedures, and challenges of the existing built environment will help designers to strike a balance between safety and recovery. A design process that keeps the needs of the patient at the forefront can also mean designing an environment that does not further isolate the patient. Clinical staff can better focus resources on patient recovery in a facility that is designed to promote healing and manage risk. We cannot underscore enough the importance of maintaining therapeutic spaces. Often, we see projects proudly displaying the installation of forensic hardware in nonforensic settings based on recommendations of consultants. If you, or your mom or your child, needed to access psychiatric care, would you want to be in a bathroom with a cold metal toilet used at jails and prisons across our nation? Would you allow yourself or your loved one to use a bathroom or shower stall with no door and no ability to prevent anyone else from just walking in?

Symptom control is most challenging with respect to elopement, suicide, self-harm, and violence. Most psychiatric patients are not allowed to choose when to leave; therefore, facilities must accommodate secure doors, windows, staff areas, maintenance, outdoor structures, and fences. However, it is important to give patients the environment in which to succeed without making them feel like they are caged in or have had to give up their dignity to access lifesaving care.

All design elements must be evaluated and selected for ligature resistance, impact resistance, and vandal or tamper resistance. Ligature resistance prevents a point of attachment that may result in self-harm. Impact resistance is a measurement of force that an object can sustain without breaking. Vandal or tamper resistance is the ability of an object to withstand abuse so that its broken pieces cannot be used inappropriately. Product designers must balance aesthetics and physics by incorporating features that can withstand a high level of abuse without looking institutional or correctional.

Effectively planning an environment of care involves bringing together an interdisciplinary, experienced team of stakeholders, including clinicians, facilities managers, designers, and contractors. This integrated team should work collaboratively to envision, plan, and design an environment to support a new model of care for the particular population being served. The design process should include a safety/risk assessment, design charettes, a mock-up of a patient room with actual finishes and furniture, simulation/role-playing, and postoccupancy evaluations. It is helpful to tour other treatment facilities and learn from the experience of others as well. At each step of decision-making, the question should be asked: *"If my loved one needed care, is this the care experience I would want for them?"*

The design elements can be organized from broad to specific, addressing the following topics, and should be appropriate to the type of care setting and needs of the patients served.

Exterior/Site

Secure the outdoor perimeter in accordance with the needs of the population being served. Fences or walls to mitigate elopement are appropriate for managing involuntary or forensic patients, and in situations where there is concern about patient elopement. Preventing elopement through access to roofs, porches, and balconies needs to be considered. Where patients have access to outdoor areas, select landscaping that does not impede visibility or have branches that can be used to climb over barriers or as weapons. Provide patients with visual and physical access to nature as appropriate for the population.

Building Envelope/Structure

Specify security glazing as appropriate for the risks associated with the use of the room. If operable windows are required, limit the opening size to mitigate the jumping risk. Coordinate specifications of the exterior wall with the exterior windows with respect to force protection. Provide floor-to-floor heights that allow for ceiling heights that mitigate the risk of access to ceiling fixtures.

Common Areas and Staff Support

Provide patients with a choice of spaces for social interaction or reflection (Figure 23–3). Design the lighting, finishes, and furniture of the common spaces to be welcoming. Patients tend to congregate near the nurse station, so there should be ample space and seating around this area. Open nurse stations encourage interaction between staff and patients and reduce the institutional perception. Maximize visibility and accessibility to all patient-occupied areas, and eliminate blind spots. Separate the circulation paths of staff from patients. Provide a safe place for staff respite. Provide secure rooms for at-risk patients, as warranted, with visual access for staff.

Patient Rooms and Bathrooms

Single-occupant patient rooms with private bathrooms (Figure 23–4) are the single most important feature in reducing aggression and stress in patients (Sheehan et al. 2013). Ensure bathroom doors, if included, are designed to reduce ligature points. Make sure doors swing out to prevent barricading from the inside. If bathroom doors lock, provide locks designed for emergency access. Patient rooms and bathrooms present higher risk because they are more private, and should be designed accordingly. Providing some level of environmental control within the patient room will support stress coping. Examples of such features include partly operable windows, controllable lighting, and artwork.

Placemaking/Configuration

Central to promoting a sense of calm in patients are design features that enhance their connection to their surroundings, or "place attachment." Consider providing smaller groups of patient rooms, or "neighborhoods," to make it easier for patients to navigate relationships and to address crowding stress that can lead to aggressive behavior. Using the "treatment mall" care model increases responsibility, provides choices, and promotes independence. Designing for flexibility in configuration is helpful in that it allows for patient rooms between two units to be assigned to one or the other unit when a change in census occurs.

Interior Design

Strike a balance between ensuring safety and promoting healing when planning the interior design, as well as the architectural design. Safety considerations include pro-

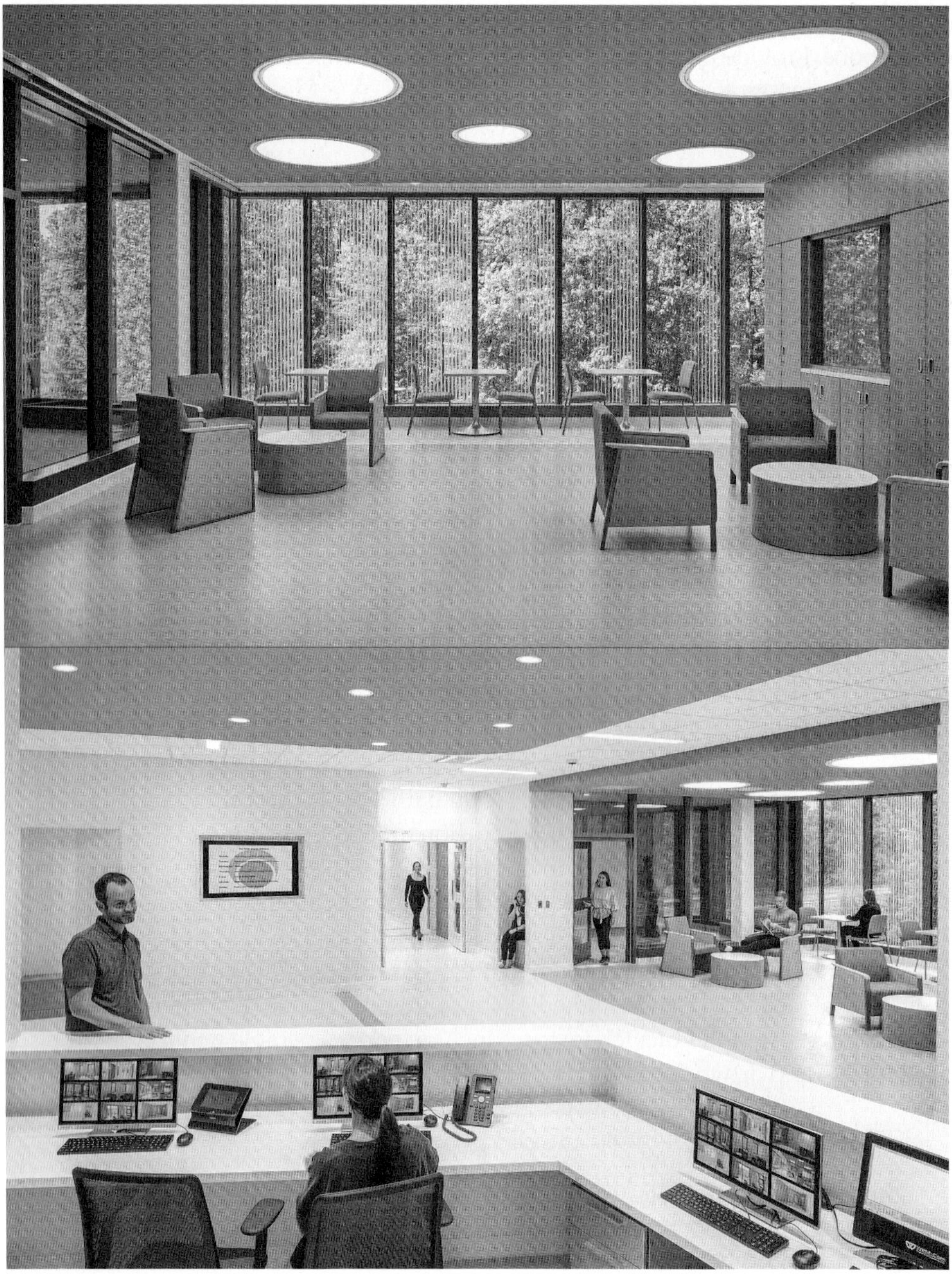

FIGURE 23–3. Patient care area.

To view this figure in color, see Plate 9 in Color Gallery.

Patient care areas offer contemplative and restorative spaces where patients can learn skills to help them succeed in the long term.

viding hard ceilings in patient rooms; using nonpick finishes, anti-ligature hardware, and nonbreakable materials and nonsharp edges; and eliminating spaces where contraband can be hidden. Acoustic and noise control are important in creating a calming atmosphere.

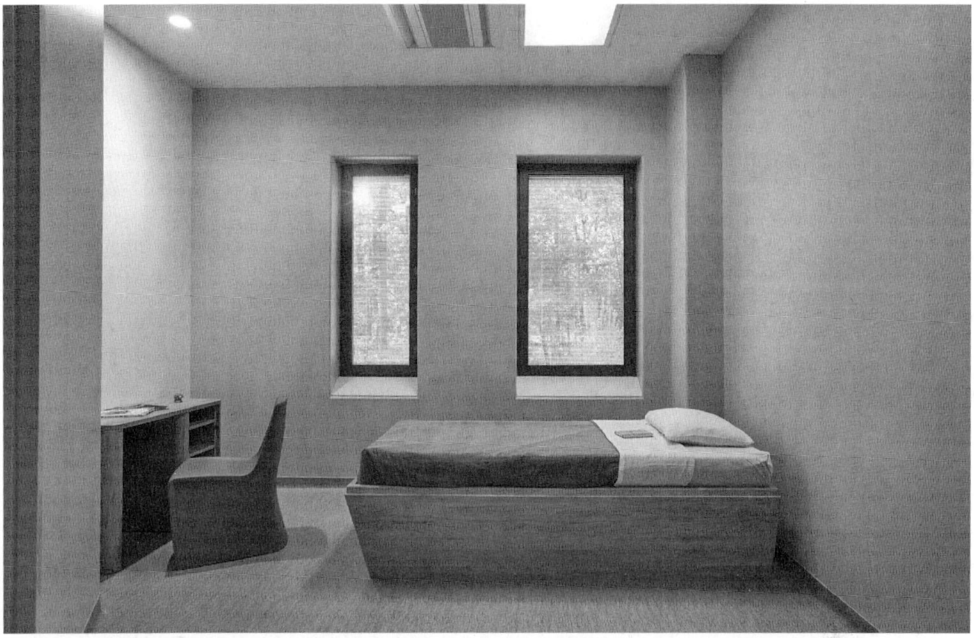

FIGURE 23–4. Patient bedroom.
To view this figure in color, see Plate 10 in Color Gallery.
Single-occupant patient rooms with private bathrooms are the single most important feature in reducing aggression and stress in patients.

Biophilic design incorporates natural materials, natural light, and the spatial qualities of nature to create a sense of calm, safety, and well-being for patients by appealing to the basic human inclination to connect with nature (Stance Healthcare Inc. 2017). Lighting strategies can be used to support natural sleep-wake cycles, impacting healing and well-being. Lighting color and intensity influence physiology and can reinforce patient and staff circadian patterns. Research indicates that blue light has an alerting effect, while warm light has a calming effect (Clark and Brennan 2017). Night lighting is an important feature in both patient bedrooms and bathrooms and can help patients maintain circadian rhythms.

Patterns can agitate patients with sensory issues or visual hallucinations. Avoid patterns that randomly appear to move or change shape or color. Studies show that art depicting scenes of nature is less taxing and physiologically stressful to the visual system and brain (Ulrich et al. 2018) and more effective in reducing aggressive behavior than abstract art.

Furniture needs to respond to the risk level in each application. In high-risk settings, it may be physically attached. In medium- or low-risk settings, weight needs to be considered to prevent self-harm or harm to others, as patients may use lighter furniture as a barricade, projectile, or for entrapment.

Mechanical, Electrical, and Plumbing

Select all anti-ligature HVAC and electrical components to mitigate patient tampering and self-harm or harm to others. Eliminate or control electrical outlets. Design service access for mechanical, electrical, and plumbing to be from outside the patient room.

Renovations to Existing Spaces

Architects and engineers are well versed in the Facility Guidelines Institute guidelines (Facility Guidelines Institute 2018). The challenge is applying the guidelines to conditions of existing spaces, facilities, and properties. Because the environments of care for child, adolescent, and adult patients are very different, converting existing space and designing around a greenfield site's various constraints requires a unique approach to design and a crucial collaborative engagement by a qualified contractor. Contractors now understand that although mental health is health care, constructing health care is not building mental health care.

Modifying existing and constructing new behavioral and mental health facilities have introduced a whole new set of challenges for owners, designers, and contractors. The Joint Commission (TJC), an independent, not-for-profit organization, recognizes the 2018 Facility Guidelines Institute guidelines on design and construction of behavioral and mental health facilities, both for renovation and for new construction, as the standards for design and construction (Facility Guidelines Institute 2018). These stringent guidelines are enforced through periodic inspections, known as "surveys," conducted over several days on-site within the facility. Survey results can have a significant bearing on a facility's accreditation and ability to operate. We offer our own case example below to show what is possible.

Sheppard Pratt's Lean Journey at the Intersection of Ligature Risk

Introduction to The Joint Commission Survey and Emphasis on Ligature Risk

On August 8, 2017, TJC conducted a routine triennial assessment and accreditation for deemed status by the Centers for Medicare & Medicaid Services (CMS). This survey in 2017 cited Sheppard Pratt Health System (SPHS) for ligature risks in patient bedrooms and bathrooms (Joint Commission 2018). We had had numerous positive surveys in previous years and had led the country in engineering patient safety into the design and operation, as evidenced by our participation in creating Facility Guidelines Institute standards when a new hospital was constructed in 2010. This year's survey, conducted in the same locations as previous surveys, found deficiencies in faucets, toilet pipes, door handles, door hinges, showerheads, and bed rails across multiple locations. An immediate review of all ligature risk exposure was ordered, with a focus on ensuring a safe environment and remedying all citations—within the prescribed time period (without requesting time extensions) and without decreasing access to care. Given that Sheppard Pratt is the largest provider of acute psychiatric services in Maryland and a referral site for patients from more than 40 states and 20 foreign countries annually, any decrease in bed capacity would lead to substantial emergency room boarding locally and impact access to lifesaving psychiatric care far beyond.

Baseline of Sheppard Pratt Health System Ligature Risk

Once TJC provided ligature risk citations to SPHS, the plant operations team went into action and spent 3 days conducting a full survey and inventory of every patient bedroom, bathroom, and seclusion room across two inpatient campuses. They also ordered hardware samples in order to begin the process of gaining organizational approval, to determine installation time, to determine ongoing maintenance for each product, and to determine logistics/sourcing time.

The survey identified replacement hardware that was needed:

- 550 door hinges
- 625 door locks
- 295 sink faucets
- 40 shower faucets and heads
- 250 toilet enclosures—custom-made
- 3,000-linear-foot handrail upgrade

Timeline to Fix the Problem (45 Days)

By postsurvey day 3, a full baseline was reported to the leadership team in terms of approximate time and cost to complete the project. Emergency disbursement of capital was secured with board approval for an initial estimated cost of $1.5 million. Once the demonstrations were completed and reviewed by both clinical and plant operations staff, the hardware was chosen based on both the need to be "ligature risk free" and the need to adhere to the principles of Sheppard Pratt's founder, Moses Sheppard. Sheppard stated, "To meet a need that would otherwise not be met…everything must be done for the comfort of the patient." This founding principle led the SPHS team to make choices based on maintaining the look of a therapeutic environment without using fixtures that resembled those used in an institutional or correctional facility. By postsurvey day 8, the work on correcting the physical environment had already commenced.[1]

The plant operations team developed plans that reflected the need to reduce risk within the first 45 days and concentrated efforts on bedrooms, bathrooms, and seclusion rooms. However, SPHS also had a goal of keeping units open and accepting patients while completing the necessary work. Maryland and the greater geographical region rely on SPHS to maintain patient access to care. Thus, to complete each phase, the facilities team staggered the work to ensure that it did not significantly impact any particular milieu or unit. This required joint planning with physicians, nurses, plant operations, environmental services, and support services personnel. For example, while one unit was getting new door hardware, another unit was getting new faucets. Instead of batching the processes, which would close down entire units, the facilities team developed a staging and planning process to help maintain forward momentum one piece of hardware at a time until all rooms were in compliance with the new standard, without impacting patient care.

The full launch of a three-phase plan was put into place on postsurvey day 10. To help effectively manage and report daily project progress, the facilities team developed and implemented a dashboard with color coding. It allowed a visual monitoring

---

[1]Note that we know that there is no truly "ligature-free" hardware in the hands of someone who wishes to inflict self-harm, but the terminology used here reflects the terminology used at the period of time.

of the progress of each room. The dashboard was updated in real time, and unit staff were updated on the mitigation plan for their area for that day on their particular shift. An example of the visual dashboard for Phase I is shown in Figure 23–5.

Expert installation teams were created for each type of repair to improve time of completion. As opposed to one plant operations team doing all repairs for a given room, a specific team became the faucet installation specialists and refined their execution over successive installations. As the work progressed, teams were decreasing their installation time, and additional work could be pulled ahead into the work schedule. Installation teams worked 7 days a week and across multiple shifts a day to complete the task in a timely manner. An example of the visual dashboard for Phase II by fixture type is shown in Figure 23–6.

Thinking Outside the Box

When the necessary hardware was not available from distributors because every hospital was finding itself in the same quandary, the SPHS team worked directly with the manufacturers to procure the parts in time for installation. In one case, SPHS inserted itself into the supply chain of a hardware vendor. To speed up the process, our staff worked with a tier-three supplier in Puerto Rico that manufactured the core products needed for a final assembly shop in New York. SPHS chartered a flight to move the parts to New York in between two major hurricane storms in order to ensure timely manufacturing, shipping, assembly, and arrival of hardware.

Imposed Constraints Lead to Creativity

TJC gave SPHS 45 days to implement major changes, and such time constraints have their challenges. To achieve such a monumental feat, SPHS was also required to employ creativity within the process. During the review of products, we found that "ligature risk free" patient beds and toilet pipe covers were not available from manufacturers or that the existing products did not meet our internal environmental standard of comfort and therapeutic effectiveness.

Patient bed requirement. SPHS has two types of beds for psychiatric patients. The first type is a platform bed with restraint rails on the side to allow for restraint straps when needed. Whereas many psychiatric units use restraint chairs or a specific room to conduct restraints, SPHS works to limit the discomfort and trauma of restraints by ensuring that restraint can be carried out within the privacy of the patient's own bedroom and in the comfort of their own bed. This also allows the maximum use of milieu space for all patient needs. However, this practice was not acceptable to TJC because there were ligature points in the design of the bed. To remove this risk, the plant operations team removed the restraint rails from each bed and plugged all remaining fastener holes. However, the hospital still had an issue with how to care for those who were compelled to harm themselves. To account for this need, the plant operations team designed a custom "restraint board." After three variations, the final design was tested by staff, put into trial use, and disseminated to all patient units.

The second type of bed is the medical bed. Within every medical bed, there are several ligature points. However, when there is a need to care for the elderly or other medically compromised patients at SPHS, the clinical team has no alternative but to use a medical bed. After reviewing other medical beds on the market, SPHS deter-

LIGATURE RISK PHASE I COMPLETION DASHBAORD

AREA	RM #	STATUS	AREA	RM #	STATUS	AREA	RM #	STATUS	AREA	RM #	STATUS
	1	100%		1	91%		1	100%		1	82%
	2	91%		2	82%		2	91%		2	91%
	3	100%		3	91%		3	91%		3	73%
	4	100%		4	100%		4	100%		4	82%
A	5	91%	E	5	82%	I	5	91%	M	5	73%
	6	100%		6	100%		6	100%		6	91%
	7	100%		7	91%		7	91%		7	73%
	8	100%		8	100%		8	100%		8	91%
	9	91%		9	91%		9	91%		9	91%
	1	91%		1	100%		1	100%		1	91%
	2	91%		2	91%		2	82%		2	100%
	3	91%		3	91%		3	100%		3	91%
	4	100%		4	91%		4	100%		4	100%
B	5	91%	F	5	91%	J	5	100%	N	5	73%
	6	100%		6	100%		6	91%		6	100%
	7	91%		7	91%		7	100%		7	100%
	8	91%		8	100%		8	91%		8	73%
	9	100%		9	82%		9	100%		9	91%
	1	100%		1	100%		1	91%		1	91%
	2	100%		2	82%		2	91%		2	64%
	3	91%		3	100%		3	91%		3	
	4	100%		4	91%		4	91%		4	
C	5	100%	G	5	73%	K	5	100%	O	5	100%
	6	100%		6	91%		6	100%		6	91%
	7	100%		7	100%		7	100%		7	100%
	8	100%		8	82%		8	100%		8	82%
	9	100%		9	100%		9	100%		9	82%
	1	100%		1	82%		1	100%		1	91%
	2	100%		2	100%		2	100%		2	82%
	3	100%		3	91%		3	100%		3	91%
	4	100%		4	91%		4	100%		4	82%
D	5	100%	H	5	91%	L	5	100%	P	5	100%
	6	100%		6	100%		6	100%		6	100%
	7	91%		7	91%		7	100%		7	82%
	8	100%		8	100%		8	100%		8	91%
	9	91%		9	91%		9	91%		9	100%
STATUS BY TYPE	Door Handle	Roton Hinge	Sink Pipe Cover	Toilet Pipe Cover	Faucet	Bed	Shower Head	Dresser/ Wardrobe	Tub	PTAC Bar	
% Complete	73%	93%	90%	76%	99%	100%	99%	100%	100%	100%	

FIGURE 23–5. Visual dashboard for completion of Phase I of Sheppard Pratt Health System project to reduce ligature risk.
To view this figure in color, see Plate 11 in Color Gallery.

mined that there was no existing alternative design that was acceptable. Thus, there was no practical way to remove this risk entirely. SPHS focused on limiting the exposure by procuring and installing inserts to cover holes in the medical beds where they could; and removing the medical beds from the milieu unless there was a specific medical need. If a patient was both medically compromised and exhibiting suicidal ideation, then a nurse or mental health worker would observe the patient at all times. This mitigation strategy was acceptable to TJC.

Toilet pipe covers. The other ligature risk SPHS needed to address was covers for the toilet pipes. Since there was no cover on the market that would fit the toilets, we had to either procure new toilets or design and implement a custom cover. The decision was made to design and implement a cover for each toilet pipe exposure. After trial, review, and approval, we worked with a local metal fabricator to procure the required number of pieces and install them within the first 45 days after the TJC survey.

Costs

The final costs incurred by the health system amounted to $1.3 million in materials and approximately $500,000 in labor expense, for a total approximate cost of $1.8 million. This was a significant financial and organizational undertaking. It is unclear whether many other psychiatric hospitals or units could bear this unexpected expense. Likewise, the added complexity of product manufacturers also being caught

LIGATURE RISK PHASE II COMPLETION DASHBAORD

STATUS BY TYPE / Area	Door Handle	Roton Hinge	Sink Pipe Cover	Toilet Pipe Cover	Faucet	Shower Head	Shower Diverter	Tub Diverter	Other
A	100%	100%	97%	50%	97%	100%	100%	100%	100%
B	100%	100%	100%	55%	100%	100%	100%	100%	100%
C	100%	100%	94%	50%	94%	100%	100%	100%	100%
D	100%	100%	100%	55%	100%	100%	100%	100%	100%
E	100%	100%	100%	50%	100%	100%	100%	100%	100%
F	100%	100%	100%	50%	100%	100%	100%	100%	100%
G	100%	100%	95%	50%	95%	100%	100%	100%	100%
H	80%	80%	65%	25%	65%	100%	100%	100%	100%
I	50%	0%	50%	50%	50%	100%	100%	100%	100%
J	53%	50%	53%	53%	53%	100%	100%	100%	100%
K	50%	0%	100%	50%	100%	100%	100%	100%	100%
L	0%	0%	33%	33%	100%	100%	100%	100%	100%
M	0%	0%	93%	100%	93%	80%	100%	100%	100%
N	0%	0%	100%	78%	100%	100%	100%	100%	67%
O	0%	10%	57%	100%	52%	57%	100%	100%	100%
P	0%	0%	43%	64%	43%	57%	100%	100%	100%
TOTALS									

PHASE II PERCENT COMPLETE	79%

FIGURE 23–6. **Visual dashboard for completion of Phase II of Sheppard Pratt Health System project to reduce ligature risk.**
To view this figure in color, see Plate 12 in Color Gallery.

off guard with changing requirements for ligature risk led to logistical issues in procuring new hardware in a timely manner. Indeed, certain hospitals decided to close psychiatric beds or succumb to regulatory pressure in a manner that decreased the therapeutic effectiveness of their care environment. In addition, despite our heroic efforts, there was continued uncertainty within the TJC engineering team as to which solutions would be deemed acceptable or where indeed CMS would land on the final regulation interpretation.

Next Steps

With the end of the audit period and full accreditation, SPHS did not stop working to reduce ligature risk. Phase III reflected the ongoing need to continue to address items not currently seen as ligature risks. The leadership team felt it was imperative to continue working proactively on removing ligature risk and improving clinical processes. That work has since been concluded and allows us to lead the way in providing the care that you would expect for your own loved one.

Results

Today, because of the hard work by many people across SPHS, the organization is safer in regard to ligature risk. The entire task was completed within the 45 days allotted and was effectively implemented because of a well-nurtured culture of safety and development of a robust Lean program across the health system (see Chapter 22). When a TJC surveyor returned on the 45th day, the results showed that SPHS had adequately addressed the ligature risk citation and the organization achieved accreditation. Active advocacy with TJC has also led to further guidance from TJC regarding ligature risk.

Conclusion

For decades, society has been challenged to make changes to deinstitutionalize psychiatric patient care and meet the growing mental health crisis. Deinstitutionalization has elevated the level of care offered and improved the quality of care and of treatment patients receive within various care environments and facilities. Health systems are including mental and behavioral health practices and centers within their existing facilities and taking them into account in the planning and design of new facilities. Dedicated and stand-alone facilities are now being placed adjacent to acute care facilities, and enhanced partnerships have broadened patients' access to psychiatric care.

The future of behavioral health design will need to address the millennial generation (now larger than the generation of baby boomers), who represent a large percentage of potential behavioral health patients (Figure 23–7). Engaging millennials in the health care system is difficult, and marketing messages need to appeal to this digitally connected population (Miller 2017). Mobile devices such as smartphones and tablets provide new ways to access help, monitor progress, and increase understanding of mental well-being. Mental health technology may lag behind physical health technology in terms of advancements, but it is gaining ground. Designated spaces for telemedicine can be created, essentially the size of an office, with lighting, technology, and acoustical privacy.

Dedicated behavioral health crisis centers stabilize and assess people in crisis in an environment designed specifically to serve their needs. The need for these centers is on the rise because too many people are arriving in hospital emergency departments and are not being well served in that setting. Quick assessment and treatment response yields better patient outcomes. These behavioral health crisis environments often are associated with extended observation units that provide treatment in a less restrictive setting than a hospital.

The shortage of mental health beds can be alleviated by strengthening community and outpatient services. Community mental health services include day hospitals and substance abuse treatment clinics and are part of a pattern of services to help patients recover in the least restrictive setting. Additionally, the model of integrated care in which mental and physical health care are integrated in one setting is being used to treat a patient's behavioral and medical needs, with shared medical records access. This growing model of care treats the whole person and has the potential for more positive health outcomes and cost-effective care. Additional consultation rooms within clinics provide work space for these clinicians, because a typical exam room is not the appropriate setting for these conversations.

Specialty programs are on the rise, addressing the needs of specific populations, including older patients, children and adolescents, patients with eating disorders, and patients with trauma disorders, as well as LGBTQ+ patients and forensic patients. Commonalities exist in designing for these populations, such as natural light, security, and safety, but there are also specific design solutions that can support the different treatment approaches required.

The design trends noted above all contribute to reducing the stigma of behavioral health care. Technology will increase access, community programs will increase awareness, and the treatment environments will be more therapeutic. Destigmatizing mental

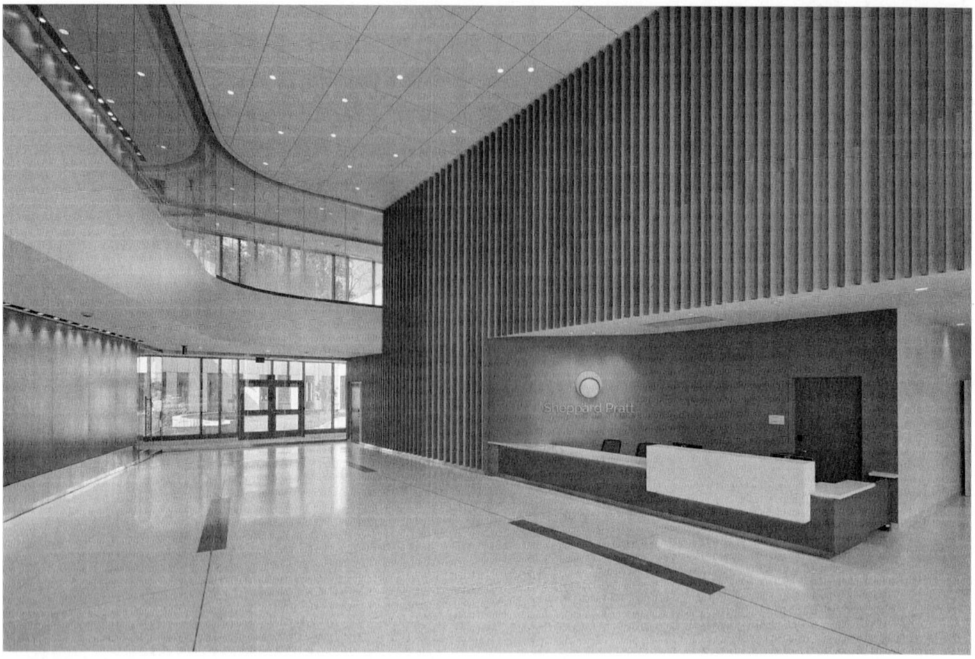

FIGURE 23–7. Lobby.
To view this figure in color, see Plate 13 in Color Gallery.
The need for mental health treatment spaces is rising, and modern, well-designed spaces can contribute to the healing and therapeutic benefit of the patient.

illness will assist in early diagnosis, crisis prevention, and the provision of appropriate services for those who need them.

References

Center for Health Design: Understanding the Unique Needs of Behavioral Health Facilities, an Interview With James Hunt, AIA, NCARB. Concord, CA, The Center for Health Design, 2017

Clark E, Brennan M: Natural remedy: biophilic design supports behavioral health. Healthcare Design Magazine, 2017

Facility Guidelines Institute: Guidelines for Design and Construction of Hospitals. New York, Facility Guidelines Institute, 2018

Forbush B: The Sheppard & Enoch Pratt Hospital, 1853–1970: A History. Philadelphia, PA, JB Lippincott, 1971

Grob GN: The Mad Among Us: A History of the Care of America's Mentally Ill. New York, Free Press, 1994

Hunt JM, Sine DM, Murray KN: The Behavioral Health Design Guide. Behavioral Health Facility Consulting, 2019

Joint Commission: Revisions to the National Patient Safety Goal on Reducing the Risk for Suicide. November 26, 2018. Available at: www.jointcommission.org/-/media/tjc/documents/newsletters/bhc_suicide_npsg_prepub_emb.pdf?db=web&hash=5C7704E3B251F735CA1EA6CB44DAC00B. Accessed February 27, 2021.

Jones CF, Chubbuck J, Germain G, et al: Report and Memorial of the County Superintendents of the Poor of This State on Lunacy and Its Relation to Pauperism, and for Relief of Insane Poor. New York, 1856

Karlin BE, Zeiss RA: Best practices: environmental and therapeutic issues in psychiatric hospital design: toward best practices. Psychiatr Serv 57(10):1376–1378, 2006 17035554

Miller J: Eight Behavioral Health Trends for 2018. Psychiatry and Behavioral Health Learning Network, 2017

New York State Office of Mental Health, in association with architecture+: Patient Safety Standards, Materials and Systems Guidelines, 25th Edition. Albany, New York State Office of Mental Health, January 31, 2021

Osborn LA: From beauty to despair: the rise and fall of the American state mental hospital. Psychiatr Q 80(4):219–231, 2009 19633958

Pitts FM: Using the Design Process to Create Safe and Comfortable Behavioral Health Environments. Concord, CA, The Center for Health Design, 2018

Sheehan B, Burton E, Wood S, et al: Evaluating the Built Environment in Inpatient Psychiatric Wards. Washington, DC, American Psychiatric Association, 2013

Shepley MM, Pasha S: Design Research and Behavioral Health Facilities. Concord, CA, The Center for Health Design, 2013

Shepley MM, Watson A, Pitts F, et al: Mental and behavioral health environments: critical considerations for facility design. Gen Hosp Psychiatry 42:15–21, 2016 27638966

Stance Healthcare: Biophilic Design in Behavioral Healthcare. Kitchener, ON, Canada, Stance Healthcare, 2017

Taylor E, Zborowsky T: Reducing Injury and Harm: Safety for Behavioral and Mental Health (2016, Revised). Concord, CA, The Center for Health Design, February 2019

Ulrich RS, Bogren L, Gardiner SK, Lundin S: Psychiatric ward design can reduce aggressive behavior. J Environ Psychol 57:53–66, 2018

U.S. Department of Veterans Affairs, Office of Construction and Facilities Management: Mental Health Facilities Design Guide (2010, Revised). Washington, DC, U.S. Department of Veterans Affairs, 2017

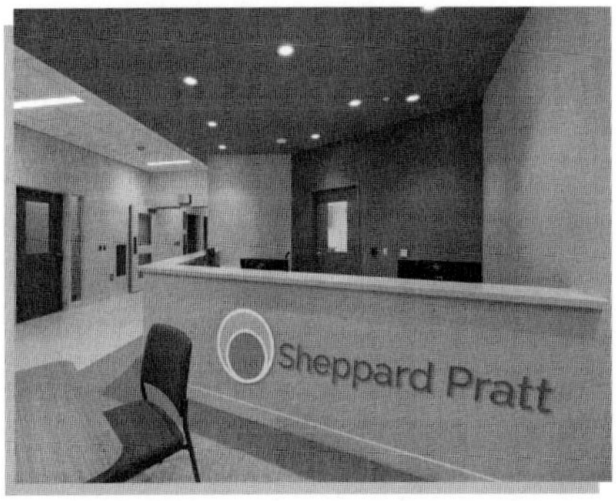

PART 4

Workforce and Special Issues

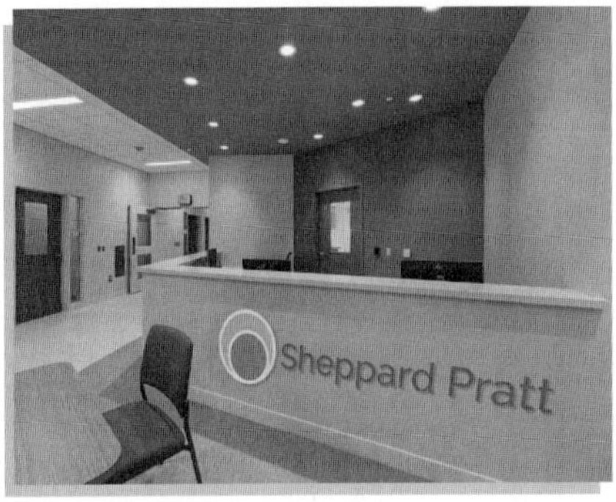

CHAPTER 24

Psychiatrists, Psychiatric Nurse Practitioners, and Psychologists

Todd Peters, M.D.
Kathleen Hilzendeger

In this chapter, we discuss the roles of psychiatrists, psychiatric nurse practitioners, and psychologists in treating patients in the hospital setting. We also review methods for compensating clinicians and how practices are evolving to meet the needs of patients and our community.

Psychiatry Work Settings and Roles

Roles of the Psychiatrist in the Hospital Setting

Hospitals use various employment and staffing models to ensure their services are staffed appropriately and that patients are receiving quality mental health care. Although there is a desire to reduce hospitalization because it is expensive, inpatient care will continue to be necessary because it provides a safe environment for treating acute mental illness. Hospital-based services may include inpatient care, partial hospital care, or intensive outpatient treatment, as well as emergency, evaluation, or consultation-liaison (C-L) services. Supplemental treatments such as electroconvulsive therapy or transcranial magnetic stimulation are also generally part of the service portfolio.

Team Lead

A large portion of the psychiatrist role in hospital-based care environments is being the team lead for the treatment team, which often includes psychologists, nurses, social workers, and other specialty team members such as nutritionists, art therapists, and occupational therapists. The psychiatrist is responsible for the overall care of the patient in the medical setting and is responsible for creating and implementing a customized master treatment plan, which is a map that guides the therapeutic efforts of every member of the team. Psychiatrists often meet with their patients each day to determine if they are progressing toward achieving the goals of the treatment.

Another major role for the psychiatrist in hospital services is psychopharmacological management, with less emphasis on providing therapy. The psychiatrist assumes responsibility for taking a psychiatric history of the patient, performing a mental status examination, performing a general physical and neurological examination, and reviewing the results of diagnostic tests. The admitting psychiatrist also consults with family and referring psychiatrists to get collateral information. In some programs, physician participation in individual and family therapy is part of the treatment model. Examples would be programs with complex patient populations, such as individuals with a history of trauma. When programs are not funded by insurance and are self-paid, there is flexibility for providing more extensive treatment programming, such as access to more physician-led therapy and supplemental programming.

Most inpatient care facilities have seasoned psychiatrists providing medical director or unit director leadership. These roles include not only managing other psychiatrists and medical issues that arise but also developing programmatic details and protocols for the delivery of psychiatric services. In addition, directors work with hospital leadership to develop or modify services and may serve on committees, such as the medical credentialing committee or medical executive committee, that are responsible for the overall quality of medical care at the hospital.

Consultation-Liaison

C-L psychiatry is a standard practice of hospital-based psychiatric care. C-L is the discipline of providing psychiatric care to hospital patients who are admitted for somatic reasons but have comorbid psychiatric symptoms that emerge during their hospital stay. One study found that more than 27% of acutely medically ill patients had mental illness with a DSM-IV (American Psychiatric Association 1994) diagnosis, including depression, anxiety disorders, and dependence disorders (Silverstone 1996). Therefore, the value of providing access to psychiatry specialists during hospital stays is high.

There are several models for providing C-L services. In the most common model, a psychiatrist provides a psychiatric consultation when requested by the primary hospital care team. The psychiatrist provides recommendations or advice regarding treatments and risk management. In other, more proactive models, multidisciplinary mental health teams are embedded in assigned units, working as team members with the medical care team. Cases that require psychiatric consultation may be identified as part of screening medical records or nursing reports at the request of the primary medical provider. The psychiatric care is more collaborative in nature, with follow-up care provided by the psychiatric team during the hospital stay. Research indicates that a proactive model is more effective, provides better outcomes, and creates a more unified team between the medical and psychiatric care providers (Munjal 2018).

Collaborative/Integrated Care

A more recent evolution for the delivery of mental health care is a collaborative-care or integrated-care services model, which is an extension of C-L services. This model brings psychiatry and mental health expertise into general medicine outpatient practices, making it easier and more convenient for patients to access needed care. Often, social workers or therapists are implanted within the practice to provide patients with counseling when they attend primary care appointments. Primary care providers may provide patients with a brief mental health questionnaire at the onset of their appointment and, if any questions related to depression, anxiety, or substance abuse are answered with a positive response, refer the patient to the on-site therapist. Therapists may also offer groups that focus on decreasing frequent medical conditions such as obesity, smoking, or diabetes. Many of these conditions are treatable, but patients who struggle with mental illness may be unable to sustain the behavior modifications required to correct them.

Psychiatrists can also come to the practice or be available by telemedicine for primary care physician consultation. This is generally a consultation model in which the psychiatrist does not add the patient to their outpatient practice. This approach allows the primary care physician to provide mental health services and prescribe psychopharmacological medications while being able to consult with a psychiatry expert. The objective is to better utilize primary care practitioners for improved access to mental health care but to do so in a way in which they can access specialty knowledge to provide the best outcome for their patients. Providing this service not only improves care but may also offer the general medicine practice the opportunity to apply for financial incentives or higher billing rates. This is a growing field in psychiatry; many novel models have been implemented and improved over time. The goals are to ensure a seamless flow of patients between primary care providers and mental health experts, to help patients feel more comfortable accessing mental health care, and to create sustainable financial models of care.

Telepsychiatry

Besides hospital-based psychiatry, there are many other settings for the delivery of care. These include residential treatment programs, schools, outpatient practices, and correctional facilities. One recent trend that aims to improve access to care is the delivery of telepsychiatry services or telemedicine. This is a growing trend in psychiatry because of the many underserved areas with limited or no access to a general or specialized psychiatrist. Different models of care for telepsychiatry services are being provided; most are outpatient focused, but telemedicine has also been used on inpatient units that have staffing issues. Telepsychiatry is an excellent mechanism for delivering required medical services where there are staffing shortages so that institutions do not need to close inpatient beds.

Specific guidelines for telepsychiatry must be adhered to when providing services. In 2016, the American Medical Association adopted a new policy outlining ethical rules for telemedicine. Some guidelines require physicians to inform patients about limitations of the relationship and services provided and to recognize the limitations of the technology and take steps to overcome them (e.g., have another health care provider at the patient's location) (Farouk 2016). Other organizations have reviewed the use of telemedicine and provided standards for its use as well. The Telepsychiatry Committee of the American Academy of Child and Adolescent Psychiatry (2014) outlined specifications for the successful use of this technology, including patient appropriateness, physical location attributes, therapeutic space attributes, and factors to improve the clinical experience. For example, they described the importance of making eye contact with young patients and their parents and the need for greater animation to build an effective rapport with patients. State and accreditation organizations also have standards related to telemedicine that require research and adherence.

Care Models That Include Psychiatric Nurse Practitioners

Because of the large national shortage of psychiatrists, many organizations have added advanced practice nurses, such as clinical nurse specialists or psychiatric nurse practitioners, to their treatment teams. According to the Substance Abuse and Mental Health Services Administration (Center for Behavioral Health Statistics and Quality 2016), nearly one in five Americans has a mental health condition. There are 111 million people living in mental health care shortage areas—half of the counties in the United States—where there are no psychiatrists providing services. Two out of three primary care physicians experience difficulty referring patients for mental health services. More than 60% of practicing psychiatrists are older than 55 years, one of the highest proportions among specialties, which projects a significant loss in psychiatrists due to retirement in the upcoming years (Weiner 2018). According to the National Council for Behavioral Health reports, the number of patients going to the emergency department for mental health services has increased 42%. The shortage of psychiatrists combined with the increasing need for mental health services will create a situation in which advanced practice nurses will have to bridge the widening gap (Theccant 2015).

Regulations dictating the scope of practice for use of advanced practice nurses vary among states. For example, some states allow clinical nurse specialists to independently prescribe medications, whereas other states prohibit this practice. Some require nurse practitioners to have designated mentors or collaborators, whereas others allow fully independent practice. Some state regulations affect a psychiatric nurse practitioner's ability to provide hospital-based services, with some requiring that psychiatrists certify patients, administer emergency intramuscular injections for severe agitation, and appear at court hearings. Because there is such a shortage of providers, there is a trend toward decreasing these regulations to allow expanded use of midlevel providers. More states are allowing nurse practitioners full practice authority and allowing them to prescribe buprenorphine (Albright 2017). Finally, psychiatric nurse practitioners have a specific scope of practice that may prohibit them from managing other underlying medical conditions. This is not the case with psychiatrists, who have extensive medical training and are often required to treat medical conditions during inpatient psychiatric hospitalizations.

There are varying models of care for the integration of psychiatric nurse practitioners into teams providing hospital-based care. Some organizations allow psychiatric nurse practitioners to take a full attending role in which they serve as the primary psychiatric medical provider, similar to the role of a psychiatrist. Some hospitals utilize hybrid models in which psychiatric nurse practitioners share patients with psychiatrists. In these models, psychiatric nurse practitioners serve as physician extenders, allowing the physician to carry a larger patient volume because the partnering nurse practitioner can also see patients throughout their inpatient stay. Some other models rotate which provider sees patients on a given day. For example, the psychiatrist may be responsible for admitting patients, seeing them every other or every few days, and discharge. On the days that the psychiatrist does not see patients, the psychiatric nurse practitioner provides follow-up care. These models rely on good communication and teamwork to ensure quality care is being provided.

Many psychiatric nurse practitioner training programs are available. Like those for any specialty, these programs are of varying quality. Most full-time nurse practitioner training is 16–24 months in duration and includes approximately 500 supervised clinical hours, which is considerably shorter than the total training required for a psychiatrist (Theccant 2015). Employers have utilized varying approaches to ensure the quality of the services provided. Many participate in nurse practitioner training by offering practicums, which allow employers to test skills prior to offering positions. This also allows nurse practitioners to receive training that aligns with an organization's treatment style and medical protocols, thereby allowing for an easier transition to an attending role. Other organizations provide mentoring and may reduce targeted patient volumes until newer nurse practitioners complete more clinical hours and show a competence in psychopharmacology.

Many psychiatric nurse practitioners are very experienced and can immediately offer services at a caliber similar to that of a psychiatrist, but, just as with any other type of clinician, individual skills must be assessed by the medical leadership team to ensure there is no reduction in the quality of care provided. Some studies suggest that patients relate more easily to an advanced practice nurse. In addition, skilled advanced practice nurses can reduce lengths of stay and decrease costs for hospitalized patients (Theccant 2015).

It is important to note that in some areas, physician assistants can specialize in psychiatric/mental health practice and provide mental health services under the supervision of a physician. Nationally, only about 1% of physician assistants practice in this specialty, equaling about 1,200 providers total (National Commission On Certification of Physician Assistants 2017).

Roles of the Psychologist in the Hospital Setting

Psychologists who have hospital privileges are a critical part of inpatient treatment teams. In some facilities, they may serve as the attending clinician, but this is not the norm. They most often provide evidence-based psychotherapy, such as cognitive-behavioral therapy and dialectical behavior therapy, in a group or individual setting. Psychologists can also contribute significantly to diagnostic formulation development of admitted patients. One significant way they contribute is through performing psychological or neuropsychological testing, providing assessments that the multidisciplinary team can use to address specific clinical questions. Psychologists can also contribute to safety initiatives within hospital settings, such as suicide assessment strategies, and smoking cessation interventions. Psychologists may participate in hospital-based research initiatives, which are well suited for large psychiatric institutions that have a large amount of patient data and numerous patients for therapy and behavior modification studies. The psychologist is a critical part of the treatment team, along with other professionals such as nurses, social workers, and mental health technicians.

Compensation Models

There are different types of compensation models for psychiatrists, psychiatric nurse practitioners, and psychologists. The market for mental health clinicians is highly competitive, and a wide range of compensation and associated work volumes are available. Academic settings generally have lower compensation but may offer other, nonmonetary incentives that are attractive to candidates, including prestige, being part of a world-class practice group or health system, research grant funding, academic appointments, and the ability to teach trainees.

The two basic types of compensation are guaranteed salaries and productivity-based compensation systems. Salaries are generally geared toward administrative positions and positions for which there are no direct billable services through Current Procedural Terminology (CPT) codes, such as work within multidisciplinary environments in schools and residential treatment centers. Clinicians often feel most comfortable with guaranteed incomes and without the pressure of volume targets. In addition, salary contracts are more easily understandable and less complex, reducing the need for clinicians to do research during employment negotiation. This is a comfortable employment arrangement that is typically the easiest to negotiate in a difficult employment market. However, that comfort may be its greatest shortfall. Because there are no volume targets, misalignment may arise between compensation expense and revenue generated that compromises the financial position of the clinical program or hospital. In addition, clinicians have no incentive to provide extra work, which is often needed when staffing shortages occur or extra weekend coverage is required.

Most hospital-based services provide compensation based on productivity or on volume expectations. Some models use revenue as the key metric: a targeted amount of revenue must be achieved, or payment is a percentage of the revenue received for services. One benefit of this type of compensation is clinicians have incentive to ensure that all requirements for the services are billed and collections are completed. Other organizations use clinician-generated service volumes or CPT codes. This may be measured in work relative value units, which are effort units assigned by the Centers for Medicare & Medicaid Services. These units are associated with CPT codes and are equal across all medical specialty areas. Productivity-based compensation systems require back-end processes or systems so that actual work is measured/reported by clinicians, used to pay bonus incentives, and managed by the practice administrator(s) and medical leadership team. Systems can get very complex, but they incentivize extra work because they offer an avenue for achieving bonuses that is easily within the control of the clinician.

Such productivity-based systems are often best combined with a short-term guaranteed salary. These provide clinicians with a guaranteed salary for some duration (e.g., 1 year), and the compensation can be adjusted in the subsequent employment term if targets are exceeded or missed. Clinicians have the comfort of knowing their fixed salary amount while also benefiting from the opportunity to complete and be compensated for extra work. Employers can set volume targets required to meet profitability goals that better ensure financial viability of the program or unit. Productivity systems are easy to benchmark within the industry where data are available that show total collected compensation, total revenue, and even work relative value units in different geographical regions and psychiatry specialty and subspecialty areas.

Compensation includes much more than base salary and productivity bonuses. Because there is a large amount of competition between employers, offers are generally packaged with other incentives. One hiring incentive that may be quite lucrative to potential employees is a loan repayment benefit. Some organizations offer loan repayment with very high values to attract talent, especially in hard-to-staff remote locations or underserved areas. This benefit is generally attached to a several-year commitment to the organization. In addition to employer-based loan repayment, employers can assist clinicians in applying for available government-sponsored loan repayment programs. For example, programs may offer incentives for clinicians who work at not-for-profit organizations, allowing clinicians to pay a fixed monthly loan repayment and, after a certain period of service is completed (potentially 10 years), eliminating the balance of the loan. In addition to loan repayment, signing bonuses are often offered. Other incentives include immigration support, continuing education stipends, payment of licensure fees or association dues, and protected time for research.

Given the shortage of psychiatrists, nurse practitioners, and psychologists, making an investment in staff is necessary to hire new talent and retain current staff. The competitive market adds pressure on hospitals and other employers to ensure mental health clinicians have positive experiences in the workplace. Recruiters are actively calling psychiatrists each day, making it evident that psychiatrists have many employment options available to them. Given the wide range in compensation available to psychiatrists and other mental health providers, hospitals must ensure they continue to offer competitive pay and other nonmonetary incentives.

Decreasing turnover is essential to maintaining a healthy and financially viable practice group. Clearly, from a patient care perspective, maintaining doctor-patient relationships over time builds trust, and may lead to better outcomes. Clinician turnover results in a significant loss of knowledge to the hospital care team. Time to fill positions can be long, ranging from months to even years due to the national shortage of providers and the timelines necessary to complete state licensing and credentialing requirements. Being short-staffed often impacts revenue streams, especially if hospital beds are blocked for admission. In addition, the remaining psychiatry team members may be asked to increase their patient volumes to maintain the hospital census, which may lead to lower morale over time. Hiring temporary or *locum tenens* staff during periods of staffing shortages is an expensive option. Recruitment costs to locate and hire new staff can also be very high, including advertising, interview expenses, signing bonuses, and recruitment fees, which are typically $35,000 or more per psychiatrist hired. Therefore, having a strong psychiatric medical leadership team supplemented by an experienced practice group administrative team is necessary to hire and maintain the needed psychiatry talent to staff hospital units.

Conclusion

The modern psychiatric hospital must continuously review service models and provide new service offerings to stay responsive to patients, families, and referrers. It is the full expectation that hospital-based psychiatric services will continue, but a wide range of mental health services will be necessary to provide patients with different levels of care and reduce hospitalization. This includes providing improved access to care through collaborative care and telepsychiatry.

In addition, models for how to best utilize clinicians will also continue to evolve. The use of advanced practice nurses will expand to help to bridge some of the supply shortage of psychiatrists. State regulations may change over time to help reduce strains on the supply, requiring hospital administrators to assess and reassess practitioner care models to ensure advanced practice nurses are providing services up to their full scope of practice. These models will need to balance the high need to provide services with preserving the quality of care provided in psychiatric hospitals.

As the supply shortage continues or worsens, there will be added pressure to offer mental health care providers with competitive compensation packages. These packages include not only competitive pay but also other incentives, such on sign-on bonuses, loan repayment, and protected time. Creating a workplace where clinicians want to work will decrease turnover rates and create considerable savings from recruitment costs, reduction in services due to long recruitment timelines, and loss of intellectual capital.

References

Albright B: Midlevel practitioners help workforce shortage. Behavioral Healthcare Executive, July 19, 2017. Available at: www.psychcongress.com/article/midlevel-practitioners-help-workforce-shortage-psychiatry. Accessed November 14, 2019.

American Academy of Child and Adolescent Psychiatry, Telepsychiatry Committee: Key Considerations in the Practice of Child and Adolescent Telepsychiatry. Washington, DC, American Academy of Child and Adolescent Psychiatry, May 2014. Available at: www.aacap.org/App_Themes/AACAP/docs/clinical_practice_center/business_of_practice/Telepsych/TPC%20Key%20Considerations_091814.pdf. Accessed November 10, 2019.

American Psychiatric Association: Diagnostic and Statistical Manual of Mental Disorders, 4th Edition, Washington, DC, American Psychiatric Association, 1994

Center for Behavioral Health Statistics and Quality: Key Substance Use and Mental Health Indicators in the United States: Results From the 2015 National Survey on Drug Use and Health (DHHS Publ No SMA 16-4984, NSDUH Series H-51). Rockville, MD, Substance Abuse and Mental Health Services Administration, 2016. Available at: www.samhsa.gov/data/sites/default/files/NSDUH-FFR1-2015/NSDUH-FFR1-2015/NSDUH-FFR1-2015.pdf. Accessed November 24, 2021.

Farouk A: Telemedicine prompts new ethical ground rules for physicians (online). Chicago, IL, American Medical Association, June 13, 2016. Available at: www.ama-assn.org/practice-management/digital/telemedicine-prompts-new-ethical-ground-rules-physicians. Accessed November 15, 2019.

Munjal S: Proactive consultation: a new model of care in consultation-liaison psychiatry. Curr Psychiatr 17(10):e3–e5, 2018. Available at: www.mdedge.com/psychiatry/article/175926/practice-management/proactive-consultation-new-model-care-consultation. Accessed November 15, 2019.

National Commission on Certification of Physician Assistants: 2016 Statistical Profile of Certified Physician Assistants: An Annual Report of the National Commission on Certification of Physician Assistants. Johns Creek, GA, National Commission on Certification Of Physician Assistants, 2017. Available at: https://prodcmsstoragesa.blob.core.windows.net/uploads/files/2016StatisticalProfileofCertifiedPhysicianAssistants.pdf. Accessed February 21, 2021.

Silverstone PH: Prevalence of psychiatric disorders in medical inpatients. J Nerv Ment Dis 184(1):43–51, 1996 8551289

Theccant SM: Integrating psychiatric nurse practitioners into psychiatric practice settings. Psychiatr Serv 66(9):913–915, 2015. Available at: https://ps.psychiatryonline.org/doi/10.1176/appi.ps.201500040. Accessed November 13, 2019.

Weiner S: Addressing the escalating psychiatrist shortage (online). Washington, DC, Association of American Medical Colleges, February 12, 2018. Available at: www.aamc.org/news-insights/addressing-escalating-psychiatrist-shortage. Accessed November 15, 2019.

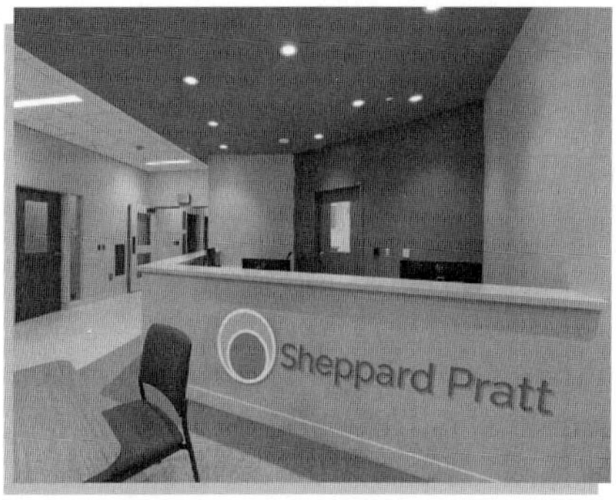

CHAPTER 25

Psychiatric Mental Health Nursing

Laura Lawson Webb, M.S.N., R.N., PMHN-BC

Inpatient psychiatric care environments are managed by nurses and behavioral health staff. The therapeutic environment is a 24-hour operation where structure and intentional activities guide interactions between patients and staff (Czekanski 2016). Standards and competencies for psychiatric nurses guiding unit practice are set by the American Psychiatric Nurses Association and the International Society of Psychiatric Nurses (Czekanski 2016). The care team managing the milieu has input in developing the plan of care and providing the observation of each patient that is required for safety. Developing relationships, continual assessment, astute observation of social interactions, medical and physical care provision, and empowerment of patients and families embody the role of psychiatric nurse.

There is a recognized shortage of mental health professionals, including nurses and physicians. Psychiatric mental health nurse practitioners have the education and licensure to fill in the provider gap and increase access to services (Delaney 2017). The care environment and organization must be clear on the practice parameters to have nurse practitioners work to the very top of their license. Expressing this adequately on the unit creates a positive environment with clarity for the entire team. The nurse practitioner brings a patient-centered, holistic approach to the team while also understanding managed care (Delaney 2017). Education and growth of unit-based teams are essential because the unit will rely on these providers in the future to guarantee access to care, even when shortages occur.

Changing the Culture of Psychiatric Inpatient Care

Throughout history, psychiatric inpatient care has been shrouded in mystery, stigma, and risk. Shifting the culture to a patient-centered model with shared decision-making and planning can remove a culture of nursing that maintains safety and reduces risk through containment, authority, and medication (Slemon et al. 2017). The paternalistic approach of the past is being replaced by recovery-focused care (RFC), an approach that partners with patients to achieve positive outcomes without assuming they will become aggressive or threatening (Lim et al. 2019). Strategies to keep patients safe may be rationalized as necessary to keep them alive or keep others from harm. Practices such as removal of patients' personal clothes and belongings, control of their free movement around the unit, and enforcement of arbitrary rules create a restrictive environment in the name of safety that reflects the institutional practices of long ago. RFC transforms the culture by emphasizing individualized knowledge of each patient's lived experience (Lim et al. 2019). It deeply intertwines trauma-informed care (TIC) practices with a therapeutic relationship that promotes trust and patient partnership toward safe behaviors.

Courageous Conversations

Having started work on a psychiatric unit more than 30 years ago, I remember the awkward observations and silences. Recognizing patterns of negative culture is easier for a new eye to do. Seeing and hearing staff members get into control battles and struggle to answer "why" when asked about rules. It is healthy conversations that sift out safety from convenience and interventions from punishments. More experienced or senior staff members may be resistant to questions or concerns, but creating a safe space for conversations among staff, physicians, social workers, and leadership fosters a positive culture. Brené Brown (2018) described 10 behaviors and cultural barriers that can also be aptly applied to inpatient units:

- Avoiding tough conversations, which leads to lack of clarity, loss of trust, and possible passive-aggressive behaviors
- Managing problem behaviors instead of addressing fears and feelings
- Losing trust through lack of connection and empathy
- Maintaining status quo by not sharing bold ideas or radical thinking out of fear of ridicule
- Focusing on setbacks instead of building and healing
- Shaming and blaming instead of being accountable and learning
- Moving away from lasting change and trust by avoiding uncomfortable conversations around diversity and inclusivity
- Demoralizing teams by focusing on ineffective solutions
- Presenting organizational values as aspirations rather than as behaviors that can be measured and evaluated
- Demanding perfection, which stops people from the messiness of learning

Keeping these things in mind, it is essential to embrace questions, ideas, and observations. Vulnerability is not a weakness but the very foundation of courage and growth. Be kind, compassionate, and open to the conversation, no matter how awkward or difficult.

Person-First Language

The culture of recovery orientation can be heard in the linguistics used on the unit or in the program. Person-first language focuses on the person rather than the diagnosis (Jensen et al. 2013). An example of this would be "a person with schizophrenia" rather than "a schizophrenic." The culture is reflected in language of respect, compassion, and dignity. One common label is "borderline," which refers to a patient who either is diagnosed with or exemplifies traits of borderline personality disorder. Calling that patient "needy" or "manipulative" lends itself to negativity toward the patient. Directing energy toward compassion and understanding and trying to get the person's needs met in that moment or situation is a more positive approach.

Safety and Staffing

The Centers for Medicare & Medicaid Services began including inpatient psychiatric facilities in quality measurement reporting on October 1, 2012 (National Association for Behavioral Healthcare 2019). There are six core measures for these facilities, and nursing has an important role in driving these outcomes. Documentation around safety policy, interventions, behaviors requiring seclusion or restraint, changes in treatment plans related to these issues, and direct work with quality is the current landscape of care due to reimbursement requirements. The Centers for Medicare & Medicaid Services and Joint Commission standards are the same. Integrating this knowledge into the daily work of psychiatric nursing and using standard language to measure quality outcomes are essential (Frauenfelder et al. 2013). This inherently expands nurse–patient advocacy and collaborative work to achieve positive outcomes.

The environment of care can be assessed for risk by noting the observation level status; the patient's risk of harm to self and others, sexual inappropriateness, impulsivity, falling, and elopement are some of the considerations. The reasons for inpatient admission place the patient in a high-risk category to be further explored. Does the patient have the means, opportunity, and continued desire to harm? Based on observations and knowledge obtained, nursing staff, in collaboration with the patient, physician, social worker, and other therapy disciplines, establish a risk level for that patient. Unit mental health staff provide rounds, environmental rounds, and preventive tactics to mitigate risk, including the risk of suicide.[1] The Joint Commission has established a National Patient Safety Goal to reduce the risk of suicide, with specific elements of

[1]*Rounds* are the routine roundings based on the observation status of the patient. This is policy driven by the organization, but it is most important to see the patient head-to toe, assess respirations if the patient is asleep, and note location of patient. The check assures the patient was seen and free from harm. *Environmental rounds*, which are also driven by the policy of the organization, are regular checks of all patient areas, including bedroom and bathrooms, for risk or items that could cause harm. This is also documented in the interval determined.

performance; nursing and physician staff use an evidence-based process and tools to assess a patient's risk, and then implement mitigation strategies (National Association for Behavioral Healthcare 2019).

Staffing numbers can play a role in positive and negative outcomes. It is important to have nursing staff who thrive in the activity of the milieu (Deacon et al. 2006). One nurse may change a dressing, feed a patient, administer medications, break up a fight, and calm a confused family member, all in the regular course of a day. Mental health nurses must find this meaningful and validating, because they may find it difficult to put into words what they do all day (Deacon et al. 2006). It is important to carefully evaluate the influx of new patients and risks with the numbers of staff providing care. This can vary depending on the shift, activities, and ancillary therapeutic staff available during those times. Factors such as admissions, discharges, experience, mix of staff, medical comorbidity, and technology issues influence staffing needs (American Psychiatric Nurses Association 2012).

Raising observational status to 1:1 and adding a staff member to the milieu to provide care are required for safety in some cases. Using this practice in the place of a much more successful practice of collaborative conversations about when to use one-to-one as opposed to another level of observation is necessary because the choice may depend on the behavior and situation. For example, a highly sexualized patient may need time alone in their room, whereas another patient may require more monitoring when outside the room. Nurses may always raise a patient's level of precaution as necessary. Each unit should reflect on quality of care outcomes in relation to staffing nuances and decision-making to inform the staffing matrix practice (i.e., to identify the ratio of staff to patients that is needed based on observation levels and identified risks requiring intervention and monitoring) (American Psychiatric Nurses Association 2012).

Changes in Acuity

Someone once told me that "the acuity goes up when they are here" (D. Greene, personal interview, March 1991), referring to the acuity on a unit and its response to a particular staff member ("they"). Being new, I needed clarification. He explained that this staff member walked in anxious and afraid. Admissions, discharges, and other seemingly normal unit events caused her to become upset and say the unit was short-staffed. However, it was really the experience, mindset, and confidence of the team that were short. Learning to brave these topics as a unit allowed for difficult conversations and vulnerability.

Medication Management

The psychiatric nurse is responsible for the safe reconciliation, monitoring, documenting, and administration of medication. The Joint Commission made improving the safety of medication administration a National Patient Safety Goal for 2020, including the reconciliation of medications at admission (National Association for Behavioral Healthcare 2019). Nursing staff educate the patient regarding new medications, new doses, and the importance of adherence. Hospital-based inpatient psychiatric services measure the prescribing of polypharmacy at discharge and document the reasoning behind it. Nurses are excellent advocates to observe the effectiveness and streamline the use of medications, including as-needed drugs. The therapeutic relationship between the nurse and the patient may provide information important to the administration of medications.

The nursing framework of long ago in psychiatric units made use of a charge nurse and a medication nurse. A more personalized approach offers a greater engagement opportunity to meet patients where they are on the unit and administer medications instead of patients having to line up at a medication room door. Medication errors have been linked to groups of patients causing chaos outside the door to the medication room (Keers et al. 2018). It is important to have an efficient process, from ordering to administration, that includes technology to catch errors in a fast-paced acute environment (Steele et al. 2018).

As part of the TIC approach, nurses who used a calm tone of voice when explaining changes in medications were met with fewer outbursts and problems than those who employed an abrasive manner and tone (Delaney et al. 2017). Smiling and engaging in friendly conversation during the medication interaction have also been noted to increase compliance and positivity (Delaney et al. 2017). Nurses can feel pressed for time, and increased acuity is often used as the reason for errors. Nurses who intentionally engage with each patient on their assignment may ultimately save time by improving the culture and tone in the milieu. Allowing and encouraging patients to partially own the medication administration process is another important control shift that supports patient empowerment (Chandler 2008).

Trauma-Informed Care

TIC strategies acknowledge the presence of trauma in individuals and align with mental health recovery principles (Isobel and Edwards 2017). The approaches used are based on recovery and establishing a patient's autonomy. Patients may experience retraumatization during seclusions, restraints, searches, forced administration of medications, and observations (Niimura et al. 2019). Autonomy may reduce negative attempts at coping, such as self-harm and drug use (Sweeney et al. 2018). Adopting these interventions and practices requires the entire multidisciplinary team to be adept in recovery language and attention to self-behaviors and tone, and to view coercion as a last resort only (Niimura et al. 2019).

Caregivers also must be emotionally connected to their own reactions and trauma that may pop up during engagement. This is where clinical processing in a debriefing group or supervision can allow staff members to reflect and learn. For example, while interacting with a young adult male patient, a young nurse feels overly friendly and warm in the connection. This is vital to recognize and discuss in a safe space in order to plan for the next interaction. Having experienced psychiatric nurse leaders available to manage these opportunities helps promote the TIC culture.

Team Collaboration

The necessary transition from a rigid, control-centered model to one that creates a sense of safety calls for a power transition from staff to patient (Chandler 2008). Decreasing use of seclusion and restraints is a clear example of this transition. Maintaining collaboration with patients, families, physicians, and others increases a sense of support and accomplishment (McTiernan and McDonald 2015). Nurses who report feeling supported by the organization and having a strong team collaboration experience less burnout (McTiernan and McDonald 2015). Staff must feel assured of their safety and the opportunity to revisit situations to guide practice changes and growth. Nurses in high-acuity areas are under great stress when balancing demands. Without the opportunity to engage and collaborate with the patient in a meaningful way, they are at risk of resorting to superficial therapeutic interventions and rigid milieu management.

Case Vignette

Nine-year-old Lucas came onto a child inpatient general psychiatric unit overnight without his parents or belongings. As I walked toward his room to make my first morning round on shift, I noticed two staff members standing at his doorway firmly stating, "Get down right now!" They continued to direct him from a distance; his room was dark as he stood on the window ledge approximately 3 feet from the ground. He had climbed up and was simply standing there, refusing to get down. I approached his room and set out to do a few things:

- Determine what was going on in the moment (what did he need)
- Address his newness and fear
- Ask to partner with him to have a better morning together
- Orient him to the day
- Orient him to the people and place

I asked him if I could turn the light on, and he said no. I respected that and asked if I could come talk with him. He gave permission, and we had a conversation. We discussed his standing on the ledge, his admission the night before, and his feeling scared and not liking the hospital scrubs. I offered to find him some clothes, and he said, "Please don't give me used clothes; the kids will laugh at me." I found some new sweats, and he happily put them on to come out and eat breakfast. He said he had not slept much the night before out of fear. I introduced him to the staff and to some of the patients while he ate. He needed information and needed to express his feelings. It is important to take the mystery out of the environment—to explain what is going on and to allow the patient to talk and be heard.

Nurse-Patient Therapeutic Relationship

Hildegard Peplau established the nurse-patient therapeutic relationship as fundamental for mental health care in 1951. A modern aim of safety without this focus may undermine the art and skill in this relationship. Recent studies report that many nurses perceive seclusion as an essential aspect of patient care (Slemon et al. 2017). Enclosed nursing stations may be used instead of proactively managing risks and decreasing disempowering situations (Slemon et al. 2017). Harmonious team discussions and planning support and direct care staff in handling emotional reactions to patient behaviors. Anticipation of patient needs through relationships can prevent many instances of anger and hostility that may arise in a restrictive, oppressive environment. Promoting a person-first approach and language within the multidisciplinary team fosters a positive culture and makes the shift needed for compassion and boundaries without rigidity and stigma. Every small check in place within the care team promotes a positive culture and expresses it to every patient.

Seclusion and Restraint

Seclusion and restraint are physical ways to manage behaviors emergently. More than one-quarter of child or adolescent patients treated in a psychiatric facility have at least one episode of seclusion or restraint while hospitalized (Valenkamp et al. 2014). These measures are associated with negative outcomes for staff and patients both emotionally and physically. The Joint Commission has established clear guidelines for documenting and reporting these events. Culturally, forcing patients to behave or progress in a way that is against their own wishes can be seen and felt as coercive (Paterson et al. 2013). The culture and milieu of a unit may embrace the threat of seclusion, restraint, and medication and lose sight of patient empowerment, compassion, and TIC.

Nurse education and leadership in the milieu can inform practice and improve outcomes. Nurse leadership can be a strong advocate for TIC interventions and a multistrategy approach with the multidisciplinary team. Six core strategies based in TIC have been developed by the National Association of State Mental Health Program Directors (Azeem et al. 2017, as summarized by Valenkamp et al. 2014):

- Leadership commitment to organizational change
- Use of data and consistent methods to inform decision-making
- Workforce development
- Use of tools such as sensory rooms and behavioral intervention strategies, and involving the patient and possibly the family in these tools and strategies
- Consumer roles
- Debriefing, assessing, and analyzing the patient's perspective to identify a need for change

Effective milieu management that includes a schedule of activities with little transition time and ambiguity, staff identification boards with pictures, moving staff out of the nursing station to engage with patients, and clearly written patient rights and expectations reflects a healthier environment and less use of seclusion and restraint as a first line of action (Espinosa et al. 2015).

Communication

Changes in communication styles and intervention choices are education intensive. A supportive tone should be used (e.g., "I am so happy you made it to group today" instead of "You are 5 minutes late to group and may not come in"). Constant positive language and neutrality require that nursing staff feel comfortable with the multidisciplinary plan and process. Listening to patients' complaints of boredom and strife and redeveloping the schedule accordingly empowers patients and sets up an opportunity for a therapeutic exchange. For example, if a patient says it is boring waiting in line to have vital signs taken, the nurse might attempt to avoid boredom and conflict by going to the patient when it is their turn rather than forming a line. This is an insightful and creative means of problem solving in a patient-focused, personalized manner. The paradigm shift is from one of control to one of collaboration, in which the patient learns coping skills with less restrictive measures (Chandler 2008).

Tolerating Behavior

Allowing behaviors that may seem disruptive or harmful does not mean avoiding conflict. It simply allows the reaction or action a patient is exhibiting in the moment while maintaining a calm presence. It can be common to see a restraint for "posturing, scratching, cursing, threatening, and/or banging." Most of these behaviors are benign and, with the proper support, will extinguish. Clinical decision-making in that moment must be free of control battles. Reacting in an immediate way can make a stressful situation worse. If you deeply understand the nature of trauma and neurological development, you know that behaviors do not change rapidly or because you set firm limits. It is a better approach to foster resiliency and acceptance. Creating a calm environment and nurturing positive coping strategies happen outside those stressful behaviors, not during. It is vital that unit staff and nursing not demand that a patient "talk about his feelings" when in a disrupted, dysregulated state. The dysregulation in those moments can make it difficult to put words to feelings, leading to deep shame and anxiety (van der Kolk 1996).

Motivational Interviewing and Communication

Motivational interviewing does not aim at controlling the patient; rather, it aims at increasing the desire for changing unwanted behaviors (Bullington et al. 2019). The psychiatric nurse uses compassionate listening and targeted comments to point out patient strengths and resources. The graceful use of empathy in a phenomenological approach helps the nurse put aside their own feelings to validate the patient's experience. For example, when a patient discusses disliking themself or their appearance, the nurse does not aim to teach skills to change or improve but listens and explores opportunities for support that the patient may recognize. Ultimately, listening and reflecting back the feelings communicated by the patient is effective communication that takes training to fully embrace and foster (Bullington et al. 2019). Communication competency is important to instill in the milieu.

Accurate handoff communication between nurses, shifts, and transfers is essential for good outcomes. This includes sharing information from the family with the care team. Using elements in the electronic medical record, nursing staff may collate the information into a concise handoff tool that includes the essentials of the patient's history, diagnosis, medications, and precaution level. Nurses should also prioritize reporting critical laboratory values, changes in suicidality, and incidents immediately to the physician.

Communication in daily activities and transition on the unit is vital. Removing a patient from their room to meet with the team without communicating this to the nursing staff may cause panic! Staff are constantly rounding, counting, and communicating the whereabouts of patients, from the restroom to the therapy rooms. The multidisciplinary team falls into this cadence in the milieu. Nursing staff may experience anxiety because the burden of safety often rests on them (Slemon et al. 2017). Adopting a shared responsibility model with patients and the entire care team recenters risk management.

Conclusion

The more a nurse is engaged with a patient on an acute unit, the more positive outcomes, patient satisfaction, and staff satisfaction will be (McAllister et al. 2019). Creating a compassionate and collaborative care environment using trauma-informed principles supports safety for all by reducing use of seclusion and restraint, power struggles, and staff burnout. Individual nurse choices for education may cause variations in skills and performance; thus, to add reliability to the inpatient unit, it is important to provide professional education across team members (McAllister et al. 2019). Balancing unit tasks with initiatives informed by a specific theoretical approach to engagement and milieu management can be challenging and lead to conflicting priorities.

Working collaboratively with physicians, social workers, mental health workers, and other team members, the nurse can receive support and gain knowledge from within the team. Physician explanation of the medication approach to a patient's diagnosis within the treatment team may lead to an enlightened, less tense conversation between that patient and the nurse when the medication is administered. Social workers provide essential information for understanding the patient's current situation, family, and opportunity. Developing a treatment collaboratively interconnects the team and provides a safe feeling for every patient. Recognizing the traumatic experiences of every patient, even if they are not reflected in the presenting reasons for admission, is part of offering person-centered care (Truesdale et al. 2019). Education and awareness are essential to caring for the increasing population of patients needing mental health care (Truesdale et al. 2019). Care providers in the milieu cannot engage with patients or deliver trauma-informed care without learning how, and communication cannot become lateral without staff across the unit learning how.

References

American Psychiatric Nurses Association: APNA position statement: staffing inpatient psychiatric units. J Am Psychiatr Nurses Assoc 18(1):16–22, 2012 22344589

Azeem M, Aujla A, Rammerth M, et al: Effectiveness of six core strategies based on trauma informed care in reducing seclusions and restraints at a child and adolescent psychiatric hospital. J Child Adolesc Psychiatr Nurs 30(4):170–174, 2017 30129244

Brown B: Dare to Lead: Brave Work, Tough Conversations, Whole Hearts. New York, Random House, 2018

Bullington J, Söderlund M, Bos Sparén E, et al: Communication skills in nursing: a phenomenologically based communication training approach. Nurse Educ Pract 39:136–141, 2019 31487674

Chandler G: From traditional inpatient to trauma-informed treatment: transferring control from staff to patient. J Am Psychiatr Nurses Assoc 14(5):363–371, 2008 21665779

Czekanski E: Empowering staff nurses with essential skills: training strategies for success. Nurs Adm Q 40(3):237–243, 2016 27259127

Deacon M, Warne T, McAndrew S: Closeness, chaos and crisis: the attractions of working in acute mental health care. J Psychiatr Ment Health Nurs 13(6):750–757, 2006 17087679

Delaney KR: Psychiatric mental health nursing advanced practice workforce: capacity to address shortages of mental health professionals. Psychiatr Serv 68(9):952–954, 2017 28502249

Delaney KR, Shattell M, Johnson ME: Capturing the interpersonal process of psychiatric nurses: a model for engagement. Arch Psychiatr Nurs 31(6):634–640, 2017 29179832

Espinosa L, Harris B, Frank J, et al: Milieu improvement in psychiatry using evidence-based practices: the long and winding road of culture change. Arch Psychiatr Nurs 29(4):202–207, 2015 26165973

Frauenfelder F, Müller-Staub M, Needham I, van Achterberg T: Nursing interventions in inpatient psychiatry. J Psychiatr Ment Health Nurs 20(10):921–931, 2013

Isobel S, Edwards C: Using trauma informed care as a nursing model of care in an acute inpatient mental health unit: a practice development process. Int J Ment Health Nurs 26(1):88–94, 2017 27291292

Jensen ME, Pease EA, Lambert K, et al: Championing person-first language: a call to psychiatric mental health nurses. J Am Psychiatr Nurses Assoc 19(3):146–151, 2013 23698977

Keers R, Placido M, Clayton K, et al: What causes medication administration errors in a mental health hospital? A qualitative study with nursing staff. PLoS One 13(10):e0206233, 2018 30365509

McAllister S, Robert G, Tsianakas V, McCrae N: Conceptualising nurse-patient therapeutic engagement on acute mental health wards: an integrative review. Int J Nurs Stud 93:106–118, 2019 30908958

McTiernan K, McDonald N: Occupational stressors, burnout and coping strategies between hospital and community psychiatric nurses in a Dublin region. J Psychiatr Ment Health Nurs 22(3):208–218, 2015 25490860

National Association for Behavioral Healthcare: Hospital-Based Inpatient Psychiatric Services Core Measure Set. 2019. Available at: www.nabh.org/policy-issues/quality/hbips-core-measures. Accessed December 15, 2021.

Niimura J, Nakanishi M, Okumura Y, et al: Effectiveness of 1-day trauma-informed care training programme on attitudes in psychiatric hospitals: a pre-post study. Int J Ment Health Nurs 28(4):980–988, 2019 31081263

Paterson B, McIntosh I, Wilkinson D, et al: Corrupted cultures in mental health inpatient settings: is restraint reduction the answer? J Psychiatr Ment Health Nurs 20(3):228–235, 2013 22632655

Slemon A, Jenkins E, Bungay V: Safety in psychiatric inpatient care: the impact of risk management culture on mental health nursing practice. Nurs Inq 24(4):1–10, 2017 28421661

Steele ML, Talley B, Frith KH: Application of the SEIPS model to analyze medication safety in a crisis residential center. Arch Psychiatr Nurs 32(1):7–11, 2018 29413076

Sweeney A, Filson B, Kennedy A, et al: A paradigm shift: relationships in trauma-informed mental health services. BJPsych Adv 24(5):319–333, 2018 30174829

Truesdale M, Brown M, Taggart L, et al: Trauma-informed care: a qualitative study exploring the views and experiences of professionals in specialist health services for adults with intellectual disabilities. J Appl Res Intellect Disabil 32(6):1437–1445, 2019 31169970

Valenkamp M, Delaney K, Verheij F: Reducing seclusion and restraint during child and adolescent inpatient treatment: still an underdeveloped area of research. J Child Adolesc Psychiatr Nurs 27(4):169–174, 2014 25100241

van der Kolk BA: The complexity of adaptation to trauma: self-regulation, stimulus discrimination, and characterological development, in Traumatic Stress: The Effects of Overwhelming Experience on Mnd, Body, and Society. New York, Guilford, 1996

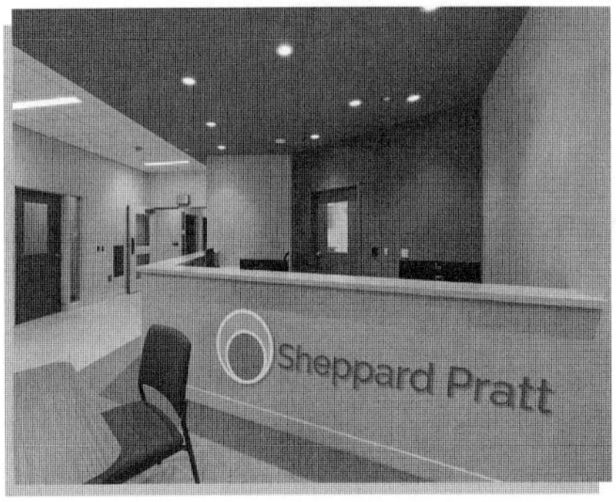

CHAPTER 26

Social Work and Rehabilitation Therapies

Carrie Etheridge, LCSW-C
Vaune Kopeck, OTR/L
April Sobiech, LCSW-C

Social Work

Social workers have an integral role in the evolving landscape of inpatient psychiatric care. They are the face of the organization as liaisons to families and agencies, gatekeepers to community resources, and providers of clinical treatment. The role and specific responsibilities of a social worker can vary widely according to the patient population and specialized treatment needs. In an inpatient psychiatric setting, social workers function as part of a collaborative and dynamic interdisciplinary team that often consists of psychiatrists, nurses, occupational therapists, rehabilitation therapists, and mental health workers. Social workers and other treatment team members meet regularly with the patient to assess clinical status, identify progress toward treatment goals, engage in meaningful family therapy, and plan next interventions.

Infrastructure of Social Work

Inpatient social workers may be working on units that serve either a general or a more specialized psychiatric population. These inpatient units are often organized as part of a larger hospital service line. Social workers report to a social work supervisor who is responsible for coordination of staffing, administrative supervision, clinical supervision of social workers who are working toward advanced licensure, clinical consultation for complex case dynamics, and process improvement of social work practice. Social work supervisors of various hospital service lines report to a director of social work who provides the vision and direction for social work practice and policies.

Establishing a clinical ladder on which social workers can develop new skills and attain advanced levels of competence and responsibility is vital for building the social work discipline. Responsibilities within the clinical ladder can include lead social worker on a unit or service line, chairperson of social work committees, clinical supervisor, and acting as a social work supervisor. Social workers apply for different levels of the ladder that are commensurate with their level of competency and professional experience. The application and interview process can involve a peer committee and social work leadership.

To promote standardization and advancement of their practice, social workers participate in regular meetings with social work colleagues and leadership. These meetings are focused on both clinical and administrative matters. Expectations for documentation standards and processing barriers regarding workflow are identified and addressed. A more clinical focus is optimizing care for hospitalized patients by identifying opportunities to mobilize patient strengths, engaging family supports to facilitate family dynamics, identifying new community resources for patients and families, and providing consultation for difficult cases. The overarching goal of these roles is to advance social work practice through excellence in patient care and service delivery within the hospital.

Continuing education opportunities are critical to providing social workers with current information about advancements in psychiatry and best practices in social work. These educational seminars and lectures help promote the knowledge and competence of social workers regarding specialized patient populations, treatment modalities, and available community supports and services. Social workers are often able to earn credits toward renewal of their professional license by participating in these educational venues. Scholarly work by social workers includes studying the efficacy of treatment modalities, evaluating the effectiveness of clinical programs, and investigating the impact of public policies and administrative practices.

Social Work Interventions With Patients

Adult Populations

In working to identify needs and establish goals with adult patients, a social worker must be attuned to patients' right to self-determination. "Self-determination, the concept that individuals are qualified to make their own decisions about their lives, is a central concept in the social work profession" (Akbar 1980, p. 9). Social workers have to balance their approach and recommendations with patients' self-identified needs and goals. This can be a clinical pitfall for social workers when they believe patients are not making decisions within their own best interests.

There are five primary social work interventions with patients in an inpatient psychiatric setting: assessment, supportive counseling, psychoeducational groups, case management, and aftercare planning. Psychosocial assessments (Table 26–1) are an assessment tool used by social workers to identify the complex influences and factors that impact a patient's current clinical presentation. Social work assessments focus on individuals in the "context" of their home environment, family dynamics, and "wider social circumstance" (Hamilton et al. 2004, p. 684). Information for the psychosocial assessment is often gathered from multiple sources, including the patient, family members, and other hospital or emergency department records available. These evaluations can be valuable in providing a holistic picture of the treatment needs.

Because of the brief length of stay and focus on stabilization, individual therapy is not traditionally provided in an inpatient psychiatric setting. Supportive counseling is provided by social workers to help optimize patients' treatment progress. Social workers meet individually with patients to provide psychoeducation and identify incremental steps in working toward short- and long-term goals. They process concerns about returning to the community while reinforcing coping strategies and develop a safety plan in preparation for discharge.

Psychoeducational groups, often facilitated by social workers, are a core component of inpatient psychiatric treatment. Based on the treatment needs of a specific patient population, the structure, time frame, and content of groups can look quite different. Group treatment has significant value in decreasing feelings of isolation among group members while working to increase knowledge, skills, and functioning. As described by Schaub et al. (2016),

> Illness management programs include psychoeducation but also teach cognitive-behavioral strategies aimed at improving treatment adherence, coping with symptoms and stressors, developing a relapse prevention plan, and modifying dysfunctional beliefs about the illness and oneself. The primary goal of these programs is to enhance the patients' ability to manage their illness in collaboration with others. (p. S82)

Cognitive-behavioral therapy (CBT) and dialectical behavior therapy (DBT) are treatment modalities that have evidence-based effectiveness with several patient populations. According to Chapman (2006), "The patient populations for which DBT has the most empirical support include parasuicidal women with borderline personality disorder (BPD), but there have also been promising findings for patients with BPD and substance use disorders (SUDs), those with symptoms meeting criteria for binge-eating disorder, and elderly patients with depression" (p. 62). When groups are being planned, the cognitive and developmental level of the patient population should be considered. For example, for group work with patient populations with intellectual and developmental disabilities, the content, language, and group materials must be adapted accordingly.

Case management is a core responsibility of social workers in an inpatient psychiatric setting. It involves assisting patients with social, financial, legal, and psychiatric barriers to obtain needed supports and services. "Case management has a long tradition in social work, where the social worker intervened at the environmental level on behalf of the client to mobilize resources for the client" (Aviram 2002, p. 626). In looking at social determinants of mental health, we know that certain patient populations are more likely to have mental health issues related to their demographics, social environment, and personal life experiences. In a review of studies, by Silva et al. (2016), higher rates of mental disorders were associated with social disadvantage, including low income, limited education, lower occupational status, and financial strain. They also identified a lack of social support, high-demand work, low control over work, crit-

TABLE 26–1. Elements of a psychosocial assessment

These assessments involve obtaining comprehensive information pertaining to the following domains of a patient's personal and psychiatric history:
Demographics
Outpatient providers
Employment history
Educational level
Leisure interests and hobbies
Income and insurance
Presenting concerns leading to inpatient hospitalization
Stressors
Detailed history of psychiatric illness and previous treatment encounters
History of suicide attempts, aggression, and other risk behaviors
Family of origin and current family dynamics
Traumatic life experiences

ical life events, unemployment, adverse neighborhood characteristics, and income inequality as psychosocial risk factors that may negatively affect mental health. These risk factors are often identified in the psychosocial assessment and help provide social workers with a plan for needed interventions. For example, if a patient has no health insurance, this will be a significant barrier to accessing needed services and medications and maintaining psychiatric stability after discharge. A social worker may help the patient apply for health insurance or explore pro bono or sliding-scale treatment options in the community and find pharmacies that offer low-cost copays for generic formulations of psychiatric medications.

It is common for inpatient social workers to make referrals for aftercare programs, housing, and other patient supports, such as transportation. They may provide documentation to a patient's employer to substantiate an absence or help the patient apply for Family and Medical Leave Act leave or short-term disability assistance through their employer. Social workers also provide education about applying for various entitlements through a local department of social services office. Patients with pending legal issues may need documentation for their probation officer or the court system. An important aspect of case management is coordinating patients' care with involved community providers and providing a handoff of care to subsequent providers prior to discharge. Ensuring a quality handoff of care between treating providers helps promote continuity of treatment, support, and monitoring of a patient's needs in the community setting.

Aftercare planning is a continuous process throughout hospitalization. During the psychosocial assessment process, social workers obtain information regarding the status of patients' housing, insurance coverage, and outpatient providers. Patients' tentative plans regarding housing, outpatient treatment, and daily structure are discussed. Depending on patients' mental status at admission, aftercare planning is sometimes unable to occur until they achieve some stability. This is particularly the case when working with patients who are experiencing an acute psychotic or manic episode or a severe withdrawal from substances or who present with catatonia. In work with a vulnerable adult who has a legal guardian of person, aftercare planning is a collaborative process between the social worker and guardian. Aftercare planning is a fluid process because many factors and circumstances can change during hospital treatment. Patients may be ambivalent about housing or treatment services options due to concerns about loss of independence and quality of care. Lack of available treatment or housing may lead to limited viable options. Effective aftercare planning involves continuous and coordinated efforts among the patient, family, treatment team, and involved outpatient providers.

Patients' readiness for discharge is determined by a number of factors: their clinical presentation in treatment team rounds with the psychiatrist and other clinicians, their behavioral presentation on the unit, feedback from family regarding their baseline functioning, and their own perception of readiness. The treatment team must determine what level of care can adequately meet a patient's psychological, developmental, and medical needs postdischarge. The focus is on identifying a level of care in treatment services that will promote the patient's stability and decrease the risk of illness relapse. According to Smith et al. (2017),

> For individuals with more severe illnesses, comorbid conditions, housing instability, or multiple care coordination needs, routine discharge planning practices may have little impact on transition to outpatient care. These individuals likely require intensive care transition interventions that have been shown to improve linkages to outpatient services for…psychiatric patients at high risk of readmission. (p. 94)

Step-down levels of care from an inpatient psychiatric setting can include a residential treatment center, substance abuse rehabilitation program, nursing home placement, partial hospitalization program, intensive outpatient program, and outpatient mental health services. Outpatient mental health care includes a broad spectrum of services, such as individual therapy, medication management, group therapy, case management, assertive community treatment, psychiatric rehabilitation programs, supported employment programs, and supported living arrangements. Formalized discharge plans are often a blend of the treatment team's recommendations, the patient's preferences and choices, and input from the patient's family. Because supportive housing and outpatient programs in the community are generally voluntary, patients must give informed consent and be willing to commit to engagement in these services.

Child and Adolescent Patients

Psychiatric social workers on child and adolescent inpatient units provide mental health services to children and adolescents in an acute stabilization setting, with an average length of stay of 5 days to 2 weeks. Nationally, there is a lack of sufficient access to appropriate step-down services or community placements, which adds to hospital length of stays. Social workers are responsible for completing a psychosocial assessment, facilitating family meetings, and creating the aftercare and discharge plan. These tasks are often being changed, updated, and adjusted depending on the patient's functioning, the desires of both the family and the treatment team, and the constraints of program availability and insurance barriers. In a study by Moore et al. (2017) related to social work in emergency departments, the role was broken down into categories that define the complexity of the role: a social investigator, gatekeeper, resource broker, care coordinator, problem solver, crisis manager, advocate, and discharge planner. Inpatient stays may also be the beginning of a transition for children and adolescents who need a higher level of care, such as a residential treatment center or a diagnostic center for more intensive stabilization.

The role of inpatient psychiatric social workers usually begins with the process of obtaining collateral information for the psychosocial evaluation. They identify the presenting issues that have led to the patient's hospitalization and obtain critical information from the child, family, and other involved outside parties, such as the school, outpatient treatment teams, and social service workers. This information is critical to identifying the patient's needs, influencing the course of treatment, and contributing to a multifaceted approach. Regardless of the child or adolescent patient's age, it is important to include them in this interview process. The social worker interviewing a patient for the first time can use this opportunity not only to gain the child's perspective on their crisis or family dynamics but also to screen properly for neglect and abuse. For some children and adolescents, this is an opportunity to tell "their side of things" and express themselves in a safe environment. This is often the first step in forming a therapeutic alliance with the patient, which will promote a better outcome for family meetings.

The intimate nature of the psychosocial interview gives the social worker an opportunity to normalize the thoughts and feelings expressed by the patient and explore risk factors that may be minimized by the patient and family. Risk factors highlighted in the psychosocial evaluation impact the treatment plan and establish the groundwork for safety planning prior to discharge. A study conducted on a child and adolescent unit in Turkey (Demirgoren et al. 2017) identified the following individual risk categories at admission: history of violent behavior, use of sharp objects or weapons, threatening behaviors, destroying or harming property, hurting animals, illegal behaviors or punishments, self-harm, recent suicidal thoughts or attempts, alcohol/substance use, abuse (emotional, physical, sexual), inappropriate sexual behaviors, and the presence of any physical disability. Family risk factors measured included insufficient supervision at home, conflicts in the family, a lack of cooperation with school, a history of psychiatric disorder, self-harm or suicide in the family, a lack of social support, and unemployment/poverty in the family environment (Demirgoren et al. 2017).

Severe episodes of aggression, suicide attempts, self-harm, and impulsivity are the predominant risk behaviors that precipitate an inpatient psychiatric admission. Counseling on safety planning for the patient is paramount. On the basis of risks assessed at admission, along with information gathered from the psychiatric evaluation, a unit-based safety plan is developed to decrease the frequency and intensity of unsafe behaviors. Another safety plan is completed prior to discharge, with input from the patient and family, that focuses on the skills, supports, and environmental factors needed to promote safe behavior in the community.

Social workers are also responsible for psychoeducation and skill building with the child or adolescent patient. In either an individual or group setting, they meet with patients to identify needed skills and increase patients' capacity to utilize those skills. Social workers also prepare patients for family meetings by identifying the goals for the meeting, eliciting feedback from the patient about needs and concerns, and explaining the role of the social worker as a mediator.

Children and adolescents often have multiple agency involvement at the time of inpatient hospitalization, including the local school system, the department of social services, foster care agencies, and the outpatient treatment team. Social workers are responsible for ensuring that proper communication is carried out with and information is gathered from these various entities, some of which require parental permission for release of information. Obtaining feedback from the school counselor, with consent from the parents, can be helpful for gathering data about the child's functioning, interpersonal dynamics, possible impact of behaviors on academic functioning, and behaviors that present exclusively in the school setting. Children's expression of emotions and behavioral presentations can vary depending on the structure and their expectations in different environments.

Discharge planning begins at admission. Throughout the hospitalization, it is important to keep involved agencies aware of a child's discharge plan to make the transition as smooth as possible for both the patient and the family. Although a discharge date is not set at assessment, planning must begin to address complicated aftercare needs, such as identifying outpatient psychiatric providers, in-home therapeutic support services, and possible referrals for a diagnostic treatment center or a residential treatment center. The goal is for the child to have the needed resources to function optimally within the community, school, and family settings ready upon discharge. At times, it may be determined that it is not safe for the child to return home with the parents or guardians, and alternative placement must be sought. This could include another family member, foster home, group home, or diagnostic center or residential treatment center. Fontanella (2008) studied the impact of various influences on readmission rates of adolescents in psychiatric institutions. It was discovered that one important factor was ensuring that discharge planning considered the stability of the patient's discharge placement, because such intervention reduces readmissions, specifically among adolescents in foster care, who are the most vulnerable to readmission.

Length of hospital stay is often affected by time and the efforts needed to initiate referrals to a higher level of care, such as a diagnostic treatment center or residential treatment center. Depending on the need, social workers gather documents and letters of recommendation from physicians and educate families and guardians throughout the process. The family and the treatment team are often unfamiliar with the intricacies of the process, timelines, and financial and educational roadblocks. Often, patients may need another level of care in the community to meet their clinical needs and maintain their safety. Although ultimately the recommendation for this level of care, such as a residential treatment facility or a group home, must be made by the attending physician, the request is often initiated by patients' families or guardians in the community, such as a state agency (e.g., department of social services, department of juvenile services). Each state has guidelines that govern admission criteria for residential treatment.

Inpatient psychiatric stays are the most restrictive options for children and adolescents who are in crisis. The psychiatric social worker should specialize in the clinical field or be in training and supervised by a clinical social worker to meet the needs of the patients and their caregivers and family. While children with various diagnoses and needs come into care in the inpatient setting, common themes include behavioral issues in the school, home, or community involving aggression toward others, self-harm, suicidal thoughts/attempts, and substance abuse. Because of the short length of stay and the need for stabilization of complicated issues, the role of the social worker focuses on what may be called "social work triage," or assessing the needs of patients, including community resources for the family, such as health insurance, food stamps, and educational assessments. A plan must be compiled relatively quickly that will best address the needs of the presenting situation, as well as address longer-term issues by ensuring referrals to follow-up care, potential educational assessments, and patients' safety when they return home.

Case Vignette

Christopher, a 14-year-old biracial male, presented to the hospital from the emergency department because of aggression at home, use of drugs and alcohol, and threats to his siblings and parents. His outpatient psychiatrist had diagnosed him in the past with oppositional defiant disorder, SUD, and ADHD. Christopher's parents were divorced, and although his mother was less involved than his father, whom he primarily lived with, they both retained joint custody and guardianship. Christopher's mother and father disagreed significantly about what they thought their son needed in regard to treatment. Christopher's father signed him in to the hospital when his crisis occurred. At that time, the social worker asked for copies of the custody agreement to show current status. The father had tried multiple times to get his son to see a therapist, but Christopher periodically refused to attend sessions, leading to inconsistent medications and therapeutic interventions over the past year. Christopher's father made it clear that he and his ex-wife did not get along and that Christopher "gets away with murder" when he is with his mother. His father reported that he would like his ex-wife to have minimal involvement in his treatment; he was not telling her about the admission right now and did not include her on the visitors list or phone list for his son.

A few days into Christopher's stay, his mother attempted to call the unit. She was panicked and seeking information, which she was unable to receive initially because she was not on the approved list. When the custody paperwork was reviewed, however, it showed that both parents had legal custody with no parameters, meaning Christopher's mother could visit him and be involved in his treatment. As his inpatient stay progressed, the physician recommended that Christopher be referred to a residential treatment center for multiple reasons, including his severe and worsening aggression at home and at school, his refusal to get treatment in the community, and his multiple hospitalizations in the past year, which had increased in frequency and intensity. He had also made minimal progress in the inpatient setting, where he continued to have behavioral outbursts that were too dangerous for placement in a temporary foster care home. Christopher's mother did not agree with the idea of placement, but his father agreed with the team.

The goal is always for a patient to be in the least restrictive setting. This is especially important with children and adolescents because this experience can be traumatic in and of itself and should be reserved for patients who need 24-hour treatment for an extended period in order to stabilize. Although discharge directly to a residential treatment center is preferred, the likelihood of that transition occurring is low because it typically takes a weeks- to months-long process due to minimal bed availability, and parents must endure the bureaucratic process involved in filing a voluntary placement agreement through the department of social services. Although the decision occurs on an individual basis, it usually preferred that the child or adolescent return home prior to going to the residential treatment center because remaining on the locked inpatient unit is more restrictive and often contributes to patients' decline in functioning over an extended period of time.

Several family meetings occurred with both parents present, and it was agreed that all calls would occur at set times with both parents on the phone to minimize miscommunication and offer the opportunity for the parents to share their thoughts and opinions about the treatment options. Once Christopher had stabilized on his medication regimen and demonstrated an ability to control his more impulsive and aggressive behaviors, the physician and team determined it was time for him to discharge to a less restrictive setting while he waited for placement at the in-state residential center, which would not have a bed available for 2 months. Christopher's father felt strongly that he needed to go straight to the residential center from the hospital, fearing that once Christopher left the structure, accountability, and locked doors of the inpatient unit he would refuse his medications, leave home, and revert to his aggressive and violent behavior toward him and other children. The father did not feel comfortable having Christopher in his home. However, Christopher's mother was willing to have him in her home, with some supportive services through the department of social services, until a bed became available.

The social worker discussed the importance of having Christopher in the least restrictive environment and pressured the department of social services to hold a family intervention meeting at the hospital with the local agency to determine the best plan. Such pressure was necessary because local agencies often do not feel a sense of urgency to move forward if they believe the patient is in a safe place, and disregard the importance of keeping a child in the least restrictive environment. During this meeting, led by the social worker, although Christopher's father did not want his son discharged home before residential placement and did not think his ex-wife could handle Christopher in her home, the social services representative decided that the agency would provide supports to Christopher's mother to help her during the 2 months he lived with her while waiting for placement. Christopher was discharged to his mother's home after being in the hospital for more than a month, with supportive services in place that included in-home supports, an assertive community team, and a social services caseworker.

Social Work Interventions With Families

Adult Patients and Their Families

Social workers are the primary liaison between the treatment team and the patient's family members. This relationship is critically important for patients and their families. Families themselves are often in crisis and experiencing a grief process regarding their loved one's illness. The line of communication between the social worker and the family can significantly ease anxiety, promote an improved understanding of the treatment process, and assist the treatment team in identifying when a patient is reaching baseline functioning in treatment.

For adult patients, written consent is often required under law to release treatment information to family members, except in situations in which patients are admitted on a certified status. When a patient is admitted under a certified status, social workers can gather collateral information regarding imminent dangerousness in preparation for the certification hearing without the patient's consent. Social workers obtain information from family regarding a patient's safety toward self and others prior to hospital admission and assess for any safety concerns in the home, such as possession of firearms or other weapons.

Facilitating meetings with family members or others in a patient's support system is a best practice of inpatient psychiatric treatment. In a review of literature, Lopez (2003) found that family psychoeducation can be effective in reducing relapse of illness when the following elements are incorporated: "provision of emotional support, education, resources during periods of crisis and problem solving skills" (p. 1). The aims of a family meeting can be multifold: psychoeducation, discussing ways to improve communication, highlighting and promoting insight into family dynamics, safety planning, and identifying concrete ways that the family can support the patient's stability after discharge from hospitalization. For specialized patient populations, such as individuals with schizophrenia, providing family psychoeducation can be critical because "clinical intervention for schizophrenia is now considered a solid evidence-based effective practice for reducing relapse and hospitalizations, and for several functional outcomes, especially in conjunction with effective psychiatric medication" (Lucksted et al. 2012, p. 103). Because of their clinical training, social workers are skilled in identifying family dynamics that may be impeding a patient's psychiatric stability, such as high expressed emotion in the family. As Heru (2006, p. 964) notes, "High expressed emotion is a 'significant and robust' predictor of relapse in many illnesses, such as schizophrenia, depressive disorders, acute mania, and alcoholism. Criticalness is one of the essential components of expressed emotion and is associated with the poorest patient outcomes." The goal is to bring these dynamics into the patient's and family's awareness while providing concrete interventions, such as education regarding boundary and limit setting; identifying reasonable expectations for their relationship in the context of the patient's illness; and helping the family practice ways to effectively communicate emotional needs. Because the inpatient psychiatric setting is brief and focused on stabilization, social workers are often beginning family work that will need to continue on a long-term basis in the community setting.

Safety plans are a tool for decreasing suicide risk following discharge from hospitalization. A safety plan "incorporates evidence-based suicide risk reduction strategies such as lethal means reduction, brief problem solving and coping skills, increasing social support and identifying emergency contacts to use during a suicide crisis" (Brodsky et al. 2018, p. 33). The development of a safety plan is guided by a clinical professional, with high engagement from the patient. Ideally, this plan is developed in the context of a family meeting in which the patient's support system can provide feedback and have a concrete understanding of the plan. The first step is to identify the warning signs: internal and external cues that a patient is deteriorating. This leads to the next step, which involves identifying specific coping and distraction strategies that can be utilized to decrease emotional distress. The next two steps involve identifying layers of the personal and professional support system the patient can access if the patient continues to deteriorate and escalates into a crisis. The last step is to identify ways the patient can alter aspects of the environment to promote safety and decease access to means for attempting suicide.

Case Vignette

Sara was a 33-year-old white, married female who was employed as a schoolteacher. She and her husband had two young children, ages 4 and 6 years. She was admitted for inpatient psychiatric hospitalization because of worsening depressive symptoms and suicidal ideation with a plan to overdose. This was her first inpatient psychiatric hospitalization. Sara had been receiving treatment in an outpatient setting with a psychiatrist for medication management and a licensed clinical social worker for therapy for the past 2 years. Sara had had multiple antidepressant medication trials that were ineffective in improving her symptoms. In the context of job stressors, Sara's condition had rapidly deteriorated over the 2 months prior to hospitalization.

During the inpatient hospitalization, a social worker met with Sara to complete a psychosocial evaluation, which highlighted the following: job stressors, a strong support system (husband, sister, and best friend), a history of childhood sexual abuse, two suicide attempts during adolescence, and current self-injurious behaviors (mild skin picking). Sara identified her goals for treatment as being better able to manage stressors and experiencing an improved mood. When the social worker explored her stressors, it was identified that Sara had been recently assigned a new classroom and new student population. Her supervisor had been giving her frequent negative feedback about her job performance, and Sara acknowledged that she struggled with asserting herself and asking for the supports she needed to be more successful.

Sara requested assistance in providing documentation to her employer to cover her absence. She also inquired about the process for applying for Family and Medical Leave Act leave, as Sara noted she was unsure she would be able to immediately return to work following discharge from hospitalization. She provided consent to involve her husband in her treatment. The social worker contacted Sara's husband to obtain collateral information at admission. He noted that Sara often did not communicate her distress to him and that he would not be aware that she was struggling until things had reached a "crisis point." Over the 2 months prior to hospitalization, he noted that Sara had been staying in bed for most of the day on weekends, only getting up to feed the children and complete necessary tasks. He wanted to be more supportive to Sara but was not sure how to do so. The social worker maintained ongoing communication with Sara's husband throughout the hospitalization to provide clinical updates, discuss planned treatment interventions, and obtain feedback about whether he believed Sara was approaching her baseline functioning.

In the social worker's consultation with Sara's outpatient therapist, they discussed that Sara had inconsistent compliance with prescribed antidepressant medication. The therapist noted that Sara really struggled with emotional dysregulation and that the focus of their sessions had been on increasing her distress tolerance skills using a DBT framework while also challenging some of her thought processes using a CBT framework. In the supportive counseling meetings with Sara, the social worker provided psychoeducation regarding depression and the importance of medication compliance in promoting stability. Factors surrounding her inconsistent medication compliance were explored and identified. Sara and the social worker worked collaboratively on identifying ways to increase the consistency of her medication compliance. The social worker reinforced the distress tolerance skills Sara had been working on with her outpatient therapist and identified some ways that Sara could effectively assert her needs with her supervisor at work. To increase her comfort level, the social worker role-played some scenarios with Sara to help her practice assertive communication. Outside of these meetings, the social worker provided Sara with worksheets to help her identify thought distortions and practice cognitive restructuring.

Prior to discharge, the social worker facilitated a family meeting with Sara and her husband. The social worker had worked with them on developing goals for the meeting, including providing psychoeducation about depression, identifying barriers in communication, assisting Sara with being able to ask her husband for specific support, and developing a safety plan. Symptoms, contributing factors, and treatment modalities for depression were discussed. Sara talked about the impact of her traumatic childhood experiences on her ability to openly and effectively communicate her emotional needs to her husband. Sara's husband expressed frustration, helplessness, and confusion regarding Sara's seeming unwillingness to confide in him. The social worker provided some psychoeducation about the impact childhood trauma can have on a person's ability to experience emotional intimacy in their adult relationships.

With guidance and support from the social worker, Sara was able to develop a safety plan. Sara identified signs that indicated she was deteriorating, skills she could use during periods of intense emotional distress, supports she could access (husband, sister, best friend, outpatient therapist and psychiatrist, local and national crisis services), and ways she could reduce or eliminate her access to any lethal means for suicide. Throughout the safety planning process, her husband also provided feedback regarding the feasibility of the plan. The social worker recommended couples therapy for Sara and her husband to continue working on improving their communication, and they were agreeable to doing so. The social worker made a referral to an outpatient couples therapist.

Sara met with the attending psychiatrist, social worker, and a nurse daily for treatment team meetings. The focus of these meetings was to assess Sara's mental status, obtain her feedback about treatment and response to medication changes, and discuss recommendations for next interventions in her treatment. Her readiness for discharge and aftercare planning were regularly discussed. Within 5 days of her admission, Sara began to identify some improvements in mood and a renewed hopefulness about her life. She denied having any suicidal ideation. She reported having a good response to a trial of bupropion 150 mg, with no adverse side effects noted. Following a family meeting with her husband on day 6 of her hospitalization, Sara was discharged on day 7. The social worker communicated aftercare plans with the discharge coordinator throughout Sara's treatment. At discharge, the aftercare plan included a referral to a couples therapist, and Sara returned to her outpatient mental health providers. The social worker and attending psychiatrist provided a verbal handoff to her outpatient providers, and the discharge coordinator faxed them a copy of the discharge summary.

Child and Adolescent Patients and Their Families

Gathering collateral information from the family and outpatient therapist is a critical step in formulating an accurate snapshot of the patient's psychosocial history. Significant factors to inquire about include trauma history, environmental factors contributing to crisis, and functioning of the family or guardian. This is usually the family's first contact with the social worker and establishes the rapport that is critical throughout the hospitalization. It can be challenging for social workers to establish communication channels that satisfy complex families; however, it is important in minimizing conflict and setting structure for families. Divorced parents, parents who disagree with treatment approaches or the need for hospitalization, and parents who have different parenting styles all challenge the social worker's role in an acute hospitalization stay. It is helpful to have established strategies and protocols for these family dynamics, such as having set times for joint phone calls or deciding on one contact person for information, who must then communicate it to the other parent.

The social worker plays an important role in listening to the parents' or guardian's concerns and educating them on various aspects of the patient's diagnosis and behaviors. Psychoeducation about behaviors such as cutting, verbal and physical aggression, and other behavioral and safety concerns is important for helping the family and the social worker prepare for safety planning and for addressing these behaviors in a family meeting. The social worker listens to the patient's perspective and the parents' and often serves as a mediator in making the best plan moving forward. Social workers face a plethora of differing family dynamics for each patient and, while functioning under the same expectation of stabilizing, safety planning, and discharge planning to the community, they employ a skill set specific to social work that relies on addressing family dynamics and setting boundaries and expectations for both the patient and the family.

Although the goal of the family meeting is to focus on acute, short-term solutions to presenting treatment issues, these meetings often veer into other territories that cannot be avoided, given the complexity of patients and families in a mental health crisis. Issues with substance abuse, food scarcity, and financial constraints often weave into family meetings, giving the social worker another opportunity to utilize case management skills to help the family get what they need to support their child. This is particularly challenging at times because of the, in many cases, infrequent number of family meetings that occur during an inpatient stay. Parental psychopathology and high stress levels in the family are associated with poor outcomes. Our results and compatible data from the literature emphasize the importance of working with the family in child and adolescent inpatient units and outpatient follow-ups (Demirgoren et al. 2017).

Future Directions in Social Work

More emphasis is needed on identifying, developing, and standardizing the best practices of social work interventions with inpatient psychiatric populations. Minimal research efforts have been dedicated to this specialized field of social work. A research focus on the impact of social work interventions on patient and family outcomes after discharge from inpatient hospitalization would provide valuable data and insights.

Rehabilitation Services

Rehabilitation services, such as expressive therapies (i.e., art, music, dance and movement, drama), recreational therapy, and occupational therapy, have been utilized as a treatment modality since the arrival of psychiatry during the late 1800s and early 1900s. These rehabilitation therapies help individuals restore and improve the skills and abilities that have been lost or compromised as a result of a physical or mental disease or injury. Educational requirements, credentialing, and licensure vary among each discipline and across states. For example, art therapists enter the field with a master's degree involving coursework in group therapy, research methods, and art therapy assessment. They must complete at least 100 hours of supervised practicum and 600 hours of clinical internship as defined by the American Art Therapy Association (https://arttherapy.org). Occupational therapists need a master's degree for an entry-level position and can also complete their education with a doctoral degree. They are required to complete supervised clinical fieldwork rotations and successfully pass a national certification examination through the National Board for Certification in Occupational Therapy (https://nbcot.org) to practice. Professionals in rehabilitation services are skilled members of the treatment team who augment the ability to connect with patients to better understand their journey and to restore and improve functioning to aid in successful discharge.

Expressive Therapies

Expressive therapies offer individuals forms of expression to grow, heal, and communicate nonverbally through the use of arts, music, dance/movement, and drama. They are very useful with patients who find meaningful verbal communication difficult and, in the instance of a withdrawn or isolative patient, can offer insight into underlying issues contributing to the individual's decreased functioning levels and promote resolution of these challenges (Odell-Miller et al. 2006). Florence Cain, an art therapy pioneer, believed that "human beings perceive the world and process information from it through three main functions: movement, emotion, and thought" and that integrating all of these life functions is an important life goal for improving emotional, academic, and behavioral control (Hinz 2019, p. 17). Through the use of art, dance/movement, and music, one can gain a deeper understanding of a person's most essential feelings and thoughts, which are often buried in the unconscious (Hinz 2019). Art therapy has also been a treatment modality for people who have experienced trauma. The areas of the brain that manage speech and cognition may shut down during a traumatic event, making it difficult for the individual to process the event verbally. Art therapists use the process of creating art to express the event externally (Loumeau-May 2019). This allows the person to express visual and sensory experiences in a concrete manner to promote resolution and improve functioning.

Occupational Therapy

Occupational therapy, as a profession, has been evolving over the past 100 years with a focus on promoting health and well-being so that individuals can participate in "quality, everyday living" (American Occupational Therapy Association 2016). To explain the role of occupational therapy, it is important to answer these three questions:

1. How did occupational therapy evolve?
2. What does "occupation" mean in occupational therapy?
3. What role do occupational therapists play in mental health treatment?

William Rush Dunton Jr., a psychiatrist and educator at Sheppard Pratt, published the first account of occupational therapy as a profession in 1917 and is acknowledged as the "father of occupational therapy." Throughout history, there have been significant changes in the approach to treating individuals with mental illness. Dating back to the third century, people with mental illness were forced to "live a life of confinement" or to live on the streets and were seen as dangerous or as a disgrace to "family honor." During the fifteenth century, these same individuals were placed in asylums and workhouses. The emergence of the humanitarian movement and moral treatment during the mid- to late 1800s was the impetus for many reforms in the treatment of the mentally ill, including the hospital movement by Dorothea Dix (Hardy 2015), which validated the building of 32 state psychiatric hospitals "to protect society and the insane from harm, to cure those amenable to treatment, to improve the lives of the curable, and to fulfill the humanitarian duty of caring for the insane" (Dain 1980, p. 11).

These institutions offered a refreshing emphasis on moral treatment and recognized the need for physical activity and engagement in work tasks. Engaging patients in normal daily routines, work tasks, and play "created a total daily program of organized occupations that minimized the disorganized behavior of the mentally ill. Occupation therapy was created—the forerunner of occupational therapy" (McKay et al. 2008, p. 5). In 1917, during World War I, the U.S. army recruited civilian women to serve as reconstruction aides to care for the wounded and "shell shocked" soldiers on the European front. These aides worked alongside nurses teaching handicrafts and vocational skills to distract the injured soldiers, increase physical activity, and improve morale. Both of these historical events are examples of how "occupation" or meaningful activity can be used to ethically treat individuals through emotions, social interactions, and engagement in purposeful work tasks, as opposed to use of isolation and confinement (American Occupational Therapy Association 2017). George Edward Barton, cofounder of the American Occupational Therapy Association, stated, "Occupational therapy! If there is an occupational disease, why not an occupational therapy?" (American Occupational Therapy Association 2017). Performing occupations at a level that fulfills one's intrinsic needs to maintain a healthy lifestyle is essential to quality everyday life.

Occupational therapists working in behavioral health provide services in various settings across the life span, including state hospitals, acute inpatient hospitals, partial hospitalization programs, community-based settings, forensic settings, and schools. The role of occupational therapy varies across the continuum of care and is largely due to reduced length of stay and payment structures in most settings. Occupational therapists during the early years of the profession were very much a part of the interdisciplinary team treating individuals in state hospital settings. During this time, the length of stay was extensive, and occupational therapists worked to develop patients' skills in the areas of functional living, leisure exploration, work, and social participation. With more recent reduced lengths of stay, occupational therapists now play a large role in helping patients establish consistent daily routines to aid in safe, successful discharge back into the community.

Occupational therapists provide programming focused on helping people find ways to engage in and participate in occupations while in the hospital and in the community after discharge. Acute inpatient psychiatric settings, with very short lengths of stay, limit their role to mainly assessment. Occupational therapists utilize formal assessments, groups, and individual sessions to gather information about patients' level of functioning in the areas of motor and processing skills, personal care and care of others, cognitive processing (as it relates to performance), and sensory processing. They then make recommendations for helping patients manage current challenges with sustaining their performance in occupational roles. Occupational therapy's inclusion of interventional physical activity not only is appreciated by patients but also enhances the intervention's effectiveness (Odes et al. 2011). Within the realm of inpatient services, continued advocacy is needed for the role of occupational therapy in forensic settings, where occupational therapists can provide life skills training and opportunities to explore meaningful interests that are essential for successful reintegration back into the community.

Significant evidence supports the effectiveness of occupational therapy in social skills training interventions that focus on recovery in the areas of establishing life roles and community reintegration for individuals with serious psychiatric disabilities. In community-based and partial hospitalization settings, with longer lengths of stay, occupational therapists can work with patients on developing skills to address specific occupational performance challenges. They can also work with individuals within the context of their own "real life" environments (e.g., work, home, community, school). The context and environment play a large part in influencing a person's access to meaningful work and the quality of and satisfaction with their occupational performance. The context in which a person performs occupations successfully is unique and specific to that person. Changing the context can be crucial to individuals' functioning level in their identified occupation. Occupational therapists recognize that for people to fully participate with meaning and purpose, they must engage comfortably within their environment and context (Amini et al. 2014). Community-based settings provide excellent opportunities for occupational therapists to teach skills within the "real life" context. In both of these settings, inpatient and community based, the role of occupational therapy in building functional skills and recognizing the value of the context/environment is unique within the interdisciplinary team.

Evidence-Based Person-Environment-Occupation Model

An individual's ability to participate in daily occupations depends on the relationship between the person, the occupation, and the environment in which we live, work, and play (Law et al. 1997). The person-environment-occupation (PEO) model is a conceptual framework developed by six Canadian occupational therapists to analyze occupational performance issues within the context of occupational therapy practice (Strong and Rebeiro-Gruhl 2019). In this model, *person* is described as a unique composite of mind, body, and spirit incorporating performance components (i.e., affective, cognitive, and physical) and social and cultural life experiences that impact occupational performance (Law et al. 1997). *Environment* is defined as the context in which an individual performs daily occupations. This includes the physical environment and social (interpersonal relationships), cultural (customs, beliefs), and institutional (state and national institutions [i.e., health care and educational systems]) settings. It is important to understand the context in which occupational performance challenges take place. In this context, *occupation* is defined as the functional tasks and activities in which a person engages while performing various roles throughout the life span (Law et al. 1997). These tasks are defined by the American Occupational Therapy Association as activities of daily living, instrumental activities of daily living, education, work, play, leisure, and social activities in which individuals engage for self-maintenance, expression, and intrinsic gratification (Amini et al. 2014).

The application of the PEO model is a collaborative process between patient and therapist. First, they assess the patient's strengths and barriers in specific occupations. The goal is to determine how the components of person and environment both positively and negatively impact occupational performance. Second, they create an intervention plan that increases support for the patient and removes the barriers that interfere with occupational performance, thus creating an improved balance of person, environment, and occupation. This plan is evaluated throughout the treatment process to determine the right balance between all elements and optimize occupational performance.

Case Vignette

Susan is a 16-year-old female attending a public high school. She is the oldest of three siblings living in a single-family home with a dog in the suburbs of a large city. Her parents both work full time, which requires Susan to come home from school to look after her younger siblings and complete homework and household chores. One of the chores that she enjoys is walking the dog in the neighborhood. Susan is always a bit shy but enjoys school and does very well academically. She has one identified friend in school and is not a big socializer. She does not participate in any extracurricular activities at school. Her goal is to become a veterinarian.

About 6 months ago, Susan began to feel increased anxiety when she was asked to present academic work in front of her peers at school and when attending small gatherings (more than three or four people) outside school with her friend. She noticed that when she was around people and environments that were unfamiliar to her, she thought that people were talking about her. She began isolating in her room after school, and her grades began to drop. She was not answering phone calls from her friend, began avoiding family functions, and started to feel urges to harm herself. Susan was admitted to an inpatient acute care psychiatric unit to address suicidal ideation. While on the unit, Susan was referred to an occupational therapist to help her reengage in occupations that were meaningful to her and to increase social participation.

Assessment

The therapist gathers information about the patient (person), her home and school activities and tasks (occupations), and her home and school (environment) from Susan herself, her family, her treatment team and her teachers and through the use of both formal and informal assessments. The information gathered will include specific information about her strengths and needs in the areas of motor skills, sensory processing skills, and cognitive abilities (person); physical space and cultural and interpersonal skills (environment); and performance in areas of activities of daily living and instrumental activities of daily living, including interests (occupations). The therapist also looks at the PEO component interactions to identify supports and barriers and create the optimal fit for occupational role performance to increase social participation.

There is a poor P-O (person-occupation) fit regarding Susan's ability to believe she has adequate skills to perform occupations at a level that is acceptable to perceived peer expectations, as well as her own, when participating in school and community activities of interest to her (e.g., walking her dog, participating in a social event outside her home). There is also a poor P-E (person-environment) and O-E (occupation-environment) fit, mostly due to her difficulty with managing sensory input in unfamiliar or larger groups of people (see Figure 26–1).

Intervention

The targeted outcome for Susan is to identify an activity in which she will be able to participate with a small group of people upon discharge to increase her opportunities for social participation. When applying the PEO model, the patient, therapist, and family collaborate to create a plan that includes supports and the removal of barriers to increase Susan's social participation. The therapist works to include a client-centered approach that will integrate the patient's identified interests—in this case, Susan's love of animals and her dog. Depending on specific information gathered through assessments (i.e., sensory processing) and the community resources readily available to Susan, the following recommendations could be made:

- Increase her responsibility in the home to include walking her dog daily, with the idea that the route could be modified to include unfamiliar destinations.
- Encourage her to volunteer at an animal shelter walking dogs and to increase her interactions with coworkers as her comfort level increases.
- Encourage her to walk the family dog and ask a peer from school or her neighborhood to join her.

Evaluation/Follow-Up

At discharge, the occupational therapist encourages Susan to verbalize any concerns about these intervention plans as they relate to PEO, utilize her supportive family members, and communicate with the therapist to provide accommodations as needed. After discharge, community-based occupational therapy services can continue to support Susan with identifying her barriers and recognizing her strengths while building additional social participation opportunities and thus increasing her occupational performance.

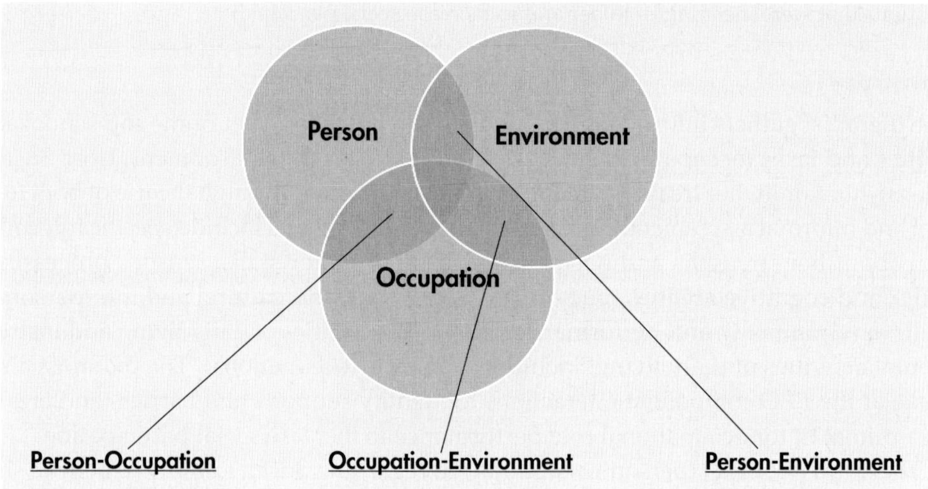

Person-Occupation

Low perception of self-efficacy

Task requirements: Match person's abilities

Comfortable with animals

Motor skills adequate for performing tasks

Occupation-Environment

Participation in academic tasks in large classroom

Feeling people are talking about her when performing tasks

Not engaging in social activities within home or school environments

Person-Environment

High expectations to perform task in large crowd

Availability of family to provide supports to adapt to environmental stressors

Experiences anxiety in large or unfamiliar crowds

FIGURE 26–1. **Analysis of person-environment-occupation transactions (Susan).**
Source. Adapted from Strong et al. 1999.

Rehabilitation Therapy

Rehabilitation therapists measure individuals' functioning through performance-based, experiential modalities. This perspective, combined with traditional forms of psychotherapy, offers valuable information in informing the treatment team, caretakers, and community members when considering discharge recommendations.

Conclusion

The practice of psychiatric care has evolved and become more sophisticated over the past few decades, with patients' needs and the complex systems in which they need to function changing as well. The utilization of social work and rehabilitation services to supplement traditional nursing- and physician-driven models has enhanced the patient's treatment experience. This multidisciplinary intervention approach is essential in promoting recovery and community reintegration and to improve quality of life for individuals diagnosed with a mental health condition that impairs their ability to participate successfully in meaningful life activities. It is imperative that a multitude of clinical professions, including but not limited to social workers, counselors, occupational therapists, rehabilitation therapists, and psychologists, play a role in providing integrated care to patients whose complex needs require their expertise.

References

Akbar GL: Thinking critically about self-determination: a literature review. J Soc Work Values Ethics 16(2):9–17, 1980

American Occupational Therapy Association: AOTA unveils Vision 2025 (online). Bethesda, MD, American Occupational Therapy Association, 2016. Available at: www.aota.org/aboutaota/vision-2025.aspx. Accessed August 4, 2020.

American Occupational Therapy Association: Celebrating AOTA's Centennial: A Historical Look at 100 Years of Occupational Therapy (video). Bethesda, MD, American Occupational Therapy Association, 2017. Available at: www.otcentennial.org/video/history-of-occupational-therapy. Accessed February 27, 2020.

Amini DA, Kannenberg K, Bodison S, et al: Occupational therapy practice framework: domain and process, 3rd edition. Am J Occup Ther 68:S1–S48, 2014

Aviram U: The changing role of the social worker in the mental health system. Soc Work Health Care 35(1–2):615–632, 2002 12365762

Brodsky BS, Spruch-Feiner A, Stanley B: The Zero Suicide model: applying evidence-based suicide prevention practices to clinical care. Front Psychiatry 9:33, 2018 29527178

Chapman AL: Dialectical behavior therapy: current indications and unique elements. Psychiatry (Edgmont) 3(9):62–68, 2006 20975829

Dain N: The chronic mental patient in 19th-century America. Psychiatr Ann 10(9):11–22, 1980

Demirgoren BS, Ozbek A, Gencer O: Factors affecting improvement of children and adolescents who were treated in the child and adolescent psychiatry inpatient unit. J Int Med Res 45(4):1318–1323, 2017 28606027

Fontanella C: The influence of clinical, treatment, and healthcare system characteristics on psychiatric readmission of adolescents. Am J Orthopsychiatry 78(2):187–198, 2008 18954182

Hamilton B, Manias E, Maude P, et al: Perspectives of a nurse, a social worker and a psychiatrist regarding patient assessment in acute inpatient psychiatry settings: a case study approach. J Psychiatr Ment Health Nurs 11(6):683–689, 2004 15544666

Hardy J: A beautiful mind: the history of the treatment of mental illness. History Cooperative, March 14, 2015. Available at: https://historycooperative.org/a-beautiful-mind-the-history-of-the-treatment-of-mental-illness/#more-92. Accessed August 4, 2020.

Heru AM: Family psychiatry: from research to practice. Am J Psychiatry 163(6):962–968, 2006 16741194

Hinz LD: Expressive Therapies Continuum: A Framework for Using Art in Therapy. London, Routledge, 2019

Law M, Stanton S, Polatajko H, et al: Enabling Occupation: An Occupational Therapy Perspective. Ottawa, ON, Canadian Association of Occupational Therapists, 1997

Lopez S: Family interventions for serious mental illness: translating research to practice. World Psychiatry 2(1):34–35, 2003 16946886

Loumeau-May LV: Art therapy with traumatically bereaved youth, in Trauma: Contemporary Directions in Trauma Theory, Research, and Practice. Edited by Ringel S, Brandell JR. New York, Columbia University Press, 2019, pp 206–255

Lucksted A, McFarlane W, Downing D, et al: Recent developments in family psychoeducation as an evidence-based practice. J Marital Fam Ther 38(1):101–121, 2012 22283383

McKay EA, Craik C, Lim KH, Richards G (eds): Advancing Occupational Therapy in Mental Health Practice. Oxford, UK, Blackwell, 2008

Moore M, Cristofalo M, Dotolo D, et al: When high pressure, system constraints, and a social justice mission collide: a socio-structural analysis of emergency department social work services. Soc Sci Med 178:104–114, 2017 28214722

Odell-Miller H, Hughes P, Westacott M: An investigation into the effectiveness of the arts therapies for adults with continuing mental health problems. Psychother Res 16(1):122–139, 2006

Odes H, Katz N, Noter E, et al: Level of function at discharge as a predictor of readmission among inpatients with schizophrenia. Am J Occup Ther 65(3):314–319, 2011 21675337

Schaub A, Hippius H, Möller HJ, Falkai P: Psychoeducational and cognitive behavioral treatment programs: implementation and evaluation from 1995 to 2015 in Kraepelin's former hospital. Schizophr Bull 42 (suppl 1):S81–S89, 2016 27460621

Silva M, Loureiro A, Cardoso G: Social determinants of mental health: a review of the evidence. Eur J Psychiatry 30(4):259–292, 2016

Smith TE, Abraham M, Bolotnikova NV, et al: Psychiatric inpatient discharge planning practices and attendance at aftercare appointments. Psychiatr Serv 68(1):92–95, 2017 27582241

Strong S, Rebeiro-Gruhl K: Person-environment-occupation model, in Occupational Therapy in Mental Health: A Vision for Participation. Edited by Brown C, Stoffel VC, Munoz J. Philadelphia, PA, FA Davis, 2019

Strong S, Rigby P, Stewart D, et al: Application of the person-environment-occupation model: a practical tool. Can J Occup Ther 66(3):122–133, 1999 10462885

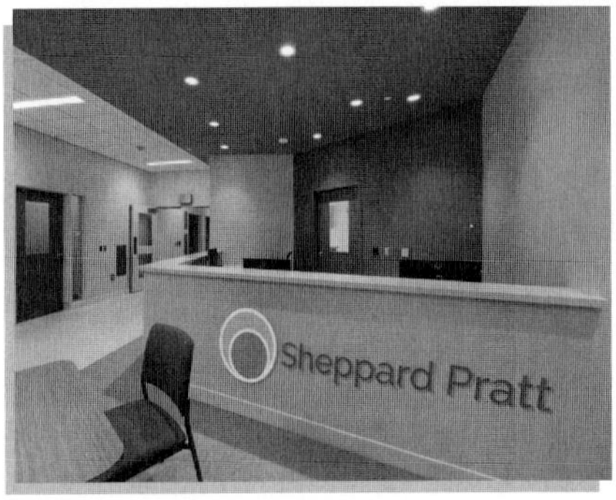

CHAPTER 27

Working With Families

Lisa B. Dixon, M.D., M.P.H.
Thomas Jewell, Ph.D.
Sarah Piscitelli, M.A.

Family members play an integral role in the lives of most persons with serious mental illness (SMI), and the importance of family involvement in the treatment of these persons is widely recognized. Increasingly, international efforts have been made by governments and service providers to invest in family-centered and collaborative treatment models (Nicholson et al. 2015). Moreover, in a large number of randomized trials, family psychoeducation programs have demonstrated robust effects in reducing patients' rates of relapse (Murray-Swank and Dixon 2004). Best-practice treatment guidelines of the American Psychiatric Association (2009) and other professional organizations strongly recommend family involvement in treatment as a critical element of quality care for persons with SMI.

The inpatient phase of care may be an especially critical time to involve family members in the treatment process. During acute periods of illness and crisis, family members often "ramp up" the level of involvement they have with the patient. During these times, family members may provide emotional support and practical assistance (e.g., housing, transportation) and often drive help-seeking, including arranging for the patient to go to the hospital. During the hospitalization, family members may frequently visit the patient and may be an integral part of the patient's support system for discharge planning and successfully connecting with referrals.

In this chapter, we first focus on common themes and issues for clinicians to appreciate in partnering with families in the inpatient setting. Next, we discuss a number of potentially disruptive issues and challenges that clinicians may encounter in their efforts to involve patients' families in the treatment process. Notably, the term *family* is used in a broad and ethical sense to include those whom the patient considers family and does not address the criteria for being a legal patient representative. This chapter focuses on families of adults who are hospitalized. Critical issues in working with family members of child patients, geriatric patients who have substituted consent, people hospitalized in forensic settings, and other patient groups may differ. We also emphasize that in addition to our professional roles as mental health clinicians and researchers focused on the delivery of services for patients with SMIs and their families, we are family members of people living with mental illness. We offer our perspectives grounded in our experience as spouses, siblings, parents, and children of people with mental illness. By considering this topic from these dual vantage points, we hope to provide a useful road map for clinicians to navigate their work with families.

Working With Families in Inpatient Settings: Common Themes and Issues

The experience of having a family member with mental illness varies substantially depending on one's relationship to the patient (e.g., parent, spouse, sibling), the patient's diagnosis and phase of illness, and the family's cultural context. In this section, we discuss four common themes that are critical to appreciate for clinicians who work with families in the inpatient setting.

Range of Emotional Responses

As family members, we have experienced the roller coaster of emotional responses that accompany an acute phase of illness requiring inpatient treatment. This is likely to be a time of instability and chaos in the life of the family. The impact on family members visiting a loved one on an inpatient psychiatric unit can be particularly traumatic, confusing, and fearful. One of us recalled first seeing our loved one hospitalized: "I burst into tears....It was worse than I could have imagined." It can be particularly jarring for family members who have been involved in the involuntary commitment of their loved one. Confronted with the realities of a locked inpatient unit, the family member can be filled with guilt and second thoughts: "Did I do the right thing?" or "Did I do something wrong to cause this to happen?" A reassuring comment at the right moment can be greatly comforting, by showing understanding of the family's concerns (e.g., "Naturally it can be disturbing to see [patient name] in the hospital"), reassuring them that hospitalization was the right course (e.g., "I just want to emphasize that you really did the right thing bringing [patient name] into the hospital, even though he didn't want to come in. I think you might have saved his life. It took real courage and love to do what you did"), and emphasizing that their loved one will receive adequate care and attention (e.g., "We are going to do everything we can to help him get better").

When interviewing family members, clinicians should be attuned to their emotional state and make active efforts to acknowledge and normalize what they might be feeling. Techniques such as reflection (e.g., "It sounds like you are feeling frustrated") and summarizing statements can help family members feel heard and understood. Another way for a clinician to communicate this message could be to say things such as, "I realize that you have really been through a lot during this time. You may be feeling anxious, worried, overwhelmed, angry, or maybe a combination of many different feelings—this is certainly understandable, normal, and to be expected as you are dealing with everything going on with [patient name]."

We also have found it useful to have an awareness of the setting's unique impact on all family members as they become familiar with the unit. It can be helpful to learn what their experience has been like in the past and to provide a sense of how they may be experiencing the current inpatient setting. For example, the clinician might say, "I'm also wondering if you have had any particularly good or particularly bad experiences with inpatient programs before." This can also be a point at which the clinician can orient the family to the unit and the hospital.

Intense Unmet Needs for Information

Research has consistently documented that family members of people with SMI report strong, often unmet, needs for information and support related to their loved one's psychiatric disorder (Tessler and Gamache 2000). In our experience as family members, we have felt the desperation of not knowing where to turn in coping with the mental illness of our loved ones. A lack of knowledge, combined with societal stigma regarding psychiatric disorders, often leaves family members feeling profoundly isolated.

It is important to avoid making assumptions about family knowledge (or to assume a lack of knowledge) because family members may have varying levels of knowledge and views on mental illness. In building an alliance with families, we have found it helpful to meet the family where they are by asking some introductory questions to assess their understanding of their relative's problems. For example, one could begin by saying, "Thanks for meeting with me today about [patient name]'s treatment. To begin, it would be helpful to get your thoughts about what [patient name] is seeking treatment for. If it is okay with you, I would like to ask you some questions to get your input and learn about your understanding of things. Can you tell me a little bit about what you think about [patient name]'s problems?" Follow-up inquiries can include more focused questions such as "What do you think has caused [patient name] to have these problems?"; "Has anybody ever given you a diagnosis for [patient name's] problems?" (if they have been given a diagnosis, it is useful to follow up with "What is your understanding of what that diagnosis means?"); "Are there things that make things better for [patient name]?"; and "Are there things that make things worse?"

Utilizing a culturally humble approach is essential when exploring the family's perspective and can inform how to work with families effectively. Our interpretations of life events not only are personal but also develop out of our participation in diverse social groups that establish traditions of meaning about our worlds. Culture affects how individuals and families understand experiences with illness (e.g., as a biological disorder, spiritual affliction, or lack of motivation), seek help (e.g., from a primary care doctor, faith leader, or police), conceptualize and participate in treatment (e.g., trust of mental health professionals, beliefs about medications, and views on the patient's and family's role in treatment) and develop expectations about recovery. In addition to responding to the world, the world responds to families; families from minority backgrounds, particularly people of color, are often subjected to discrimination on interpersonal, institutional, and structural levels, leading to health disparities such as higher rates of forced hospitalization among people of color and distrust of inpatient staff, administration, and services. Additionally, culture shapes how clinicians interpret the perspectives of patients and families, the patients' and families' capability to accept explanations that are radically different from the Western medical model, and their ability to communicate effectively with patients and families. Clinicians should consider the multiple aspects of family backgrounds that provide a basis for their cultural identity, including age, race/ethnicity, gender, class, faith, sexual orientation, occupation, and, for some, language, immigration, and acculturation. Like fish in water, family members might have difficulty describing their culture. To assist with exploring the impact of culture, inpatient clinicians should consider using the Cultural Formulation Interview, a practical 16-item questionnaire available in DSM-5 (American Psychiatric Association 2013a, 2013b). This tool is designed to improve clinical understanding of the influence of culture on individuals and families, enhance communication, and improve outcomes through the use of questions such as "Sometimes doctors and patients misunderstand each other because they come from different backgrounds or have different expectations. Have you been concerned about this, and is there anything we can do to provide you with the care you need?"

These explorations can help the clinician learn about family members' views of their relative's psychiatric problems and can inform the patient's treatment. For example, family members often have valuable observations about prodromal symptoms that signal risk for relapse or indicate protective factors. Note that these inquiries avoid using terms such as *illness* or *disorder* or other psychiatric terminology. It is best to avoid using this language and to hold off on offering educational information until the interviewer has a good understanding of the family members' views of the patient's problems.

Varying (and Sometimes Misplaced) Expectations

Families may have a wide variety of expectations of hospitalization and treatment. Particularly in the initial years of illness, family members may have misplaced expectations that hospitalization will "fix" the problem and return their loved one "back to normal" on discharge. It is often frustrating for clinicians to encounter such beliefs, and we have certainly felt these frustrations when working with families in our professional roles. It is critical to realize that families' expectations are typically not rooted in a willful denial of their loved one's illness. Instead, their beliefs often reflect a lack of information coupled with an emotional coping process of trying to come to terms with the painful reality of their relative's illness and the uncertainty of the recovery trajectory.

In addressing families' expectations, it can be helpful to provide an orientation to the context of inpatient care. For example:

> It is important for you to know what we do here on the inpatient unit, and the role that we play in [patient name]'s treatment. Typically, the purpose of hospitalization is to help get people through a crisis when their symptoms get worse, to provide an environ-

> ment to ensure their safety, and to make sure they are linked up with appropriate outpatient care as they are discharged. Nowadays, the emphasis of hospitalization is typically focused on helping people get back to the community when they are safe and able to return to their living environment. I know this can be difficult for family members, who sometimes experience a sense of relief when their loved ones are hospitalized. It can be frustrating for all of us to deal with the limits of what we can accomplish while [patient name] is in treatment here. However, we do hope that we can work with you as we help [patient name] start feeling better. We also hope to address your needs for information about [patient name]'s illness and treatment and her plan for care while she is hospitalized here and to work together on a discharge plan that will support her ongoing recovery.

This orientation may also serve as a point of entry to discuss professional and community-based sources of support for family members. For example, some inpatient units have educational family programs that provide a forum for family members to learn about their loved one's illness. Community resources, such as family education programs offered by the National Alliance on Mental Illness, can be recommended for ongoing education and support. We have found it helpful for staff who work with families to have a current, well-organized repository of information about mental illness and referral resources so that information can be provided rapidly and smoothly to families.

Differing Family Organization and Member Roles

Collaboration with families can be strengthened by understanding how the families are organized and the roles that different family members may play. One common theme is that one family member may be the designated spokesperson for the family when the patient is hospitalized. This spokesperson role might be symbolic or literal—for example, non–English speaking families often rely on one or two family members (e.g., siblings of the patient) who speak English. It is critical to take the time to make a positive bond with these spokespersons, because their translations of your message may be the only information from which the family makes its impression of the care. Also, it is important to appreciate that the patient's illness and the forced separation of inpatient stays often prompt a reshuffling of roles in the family.

Moreover, as time passes, there may be generational transitions, such that siblings or other family members may assume a more active role as the patient's parents age. The key point for clinicians is to assess and be sensitive to who in the family are the central figures in the life of the patient. For example, interviewers may inquire, "Who is usually involved in helping [patient name] when he has difficulties?" It is also important to acknowledge and address potentially disruptive issues and barriers to working with families in the inpatient setting.

Potential Barriers and Challenges for Clinicians Working With Families in the Inpatient Setting

In this section, we describe common barriers and obstacles that clinicians encounter while working with families and offer strategies to overcome these challenges and establish an effective working alliance. These challenges can be broken down into clinician-level barriers (e.g., lack of time, confidentiality issues), patients' concerns about involving their family in their treatment, and family-level barriers (e.g., difficulty engaging families and navigating differences of opinions).

Clinician-Level Barriers: Time Limitations and Confidentiality

Contact between clinicians and families may occur in multiple ways. Family meetings may be planned or may occur through more informal avenues, such as during family visits to the patient, family phone calls to the unit, and phone calls from the treatment team to the family. Here we examine two areas that sometimes can create stress between staff and family: time and confidentiality.

For clinicians, the first difficulty is time—not enough of it. Family members may visit and request an unplanned meeting with their loved one's physician or other staff. However, staff are frequently unable to drop everything for such a meeting. Yet we believe that in building an alliance with families, it is critical to communicate the message that family input and involvement in treatment are valued by the clinical team. As family members, we have found it frustrating to be "brushed off" by clinical staff who are completing paperwork or attending to other duties on the unit. Thus, we believe it is important for staff to be attentive to families within the context of their own limited time and other demands. For example, a busy psychiatrist with only 10 minutes to meet with a visiting family could explain: "I only have 10 minutes right now, so let's set priorities in how we might use our time. Perhaps you could tell me about your main questions and concerns, and we can come up with a plan to make sure you are included in the treatment process while [patient name] is being treated here."

Issues of confidentiality can also pose particular challenges. Professional ethics and organizational policies appropriately require clinicians to obtain the consent of patients before releasing specific information about their treatment to family members (although there can be specific exceptions when safety issues, such as suicide and homicide, are active). This consent is typically documented in a written "release of information" form. Perhaps one of the most difficult and common scenarios is when a family member requests information about the patient's treatment but the patient has not provided permission to release information to family. In such situations, clinicians should first reinforce the family member's interest in the patient's treatment and recognize their effort to make contact. For example, "I am so glad that you called, and that you are interested in learning more about [patient name]'s treatment."

Next, the clinician should provide a straightforward explanation to the family member regarding the relevant confidentiality issues. For example, "As you probably know, medical information is private and protected. Therefore, I can't share specific information about [patient name]'s treatment without her permission. I know it's a frustrating situation; it's difficult for us, too, because we really value the opportunity to include patients' families as part of the treatment whenever we can. What I can do is talk with [patient name] the next chance I get, and try to get her permission to talk with you more about her treatment."

It can then be helpful to ask the family member about their needs and offer information that can be shared, such as answering general questions about psychiatric illness, treatment programs, and resources for family members. For example, "Although I can't share specific information about [patient name]'s treatment, I would be happy to answer general questions you might have at this time. Do you have any general questions about our unit or about psychiatric illness?" Families may appreciate a description of the inpatient unit, other treatment resources in the community, programs to support family members of people with mental illness, and general information about psychiatric illness and treatment. Written materials can also be sent to family members (e.g., brochures about mental illness, internet-based information).

Patients' Concerns About Involving Family Members in Their Treatment

For contact with families to be initiated, it is necessary to ask the patient to identify family members and to obtain the patient's permission to speak with them. Although the primary focus of this chapter is on working with families, such work will be brief or nonexistent unless the clinician has done a good job of talking with the patient about involving family members in the treatment process. Furthermore, the involvement of family in treatment should be guided by the patient's preferences and views about the family and the potential role they may play in the treatment process.

Patients may have a wide range of family experiences and preferences regarding family involvement in their mental health care. As a starting point, assess who the patients consider to be their family support system and what role these individuals may play in helping them. For example, "I would like to ask you some questions to better understand your family relationships and support system. Do you have people you would consider to be your family or like family to you?" Significant "family" and potential allies in treatment may include members of the support network who are not relatives (e.g., friend, pastor, 12-step group sponsor). After identifying the key members of the support network, it is helpful to learn about the patient's level of contact with these individuals. Does the patient live with a family member? If not, how close do family members live? How often does the patient talk, text, email, or get together with family members?

Next, it is important to understand the role these individuals play in supporting the patient, including any involvement in the patient's mental health treatment and the patient's preferences regarding involving specific family members at this time. Interviewers should use techniques such as summaries and reflections to gain an understanding of the patient's experiences and preferences. Some examples:

> "So, you have said that you are closest to your two brothers, whom you get together with every couple of weeks. I'm wondering if your brothers have been supportive as you have been dealing with your mental illness?"
>
> "Have they ever attended any kind of educational programs or groups?"
>
> "Would you like to have your brothers involved in your mental health treatment?"
>
> "What might be the possible benefits?"
>
> "What, if any, are your concerns about having them involved?"

Overall, the goals of this discussion are to help patients identify family members who could be allies in their treatment, help patients consider the potential advantages of family involvement in treatment, and identify concerns patients might have about family participation.

In some instances, patients may be ambivalent about involving the family. This is understandable given the complexity of family relationships and the possible presence of abusive family members, as well as the personal nature of mental health treatment. When patients experience mixed feelings about involving family in their mental health care, the primary task of the clinician is to help them explore the potential value of family involvement and to make informed choices, considering the potential advantages and disadvantages of family involvement in care. At times, patients may refuse family involvement, even when the clinical team feels that such involvement would be in their best interest. In these situations, the clinician should revisit the issue during the course of treatment, especially if the patient was acutely ill or in a state of crisis when first asked about involving the family. It may be especially important to consider revisiting family involvement as discharge approaches, with the hope of involving someone who will support the patient upon release from the hospital.

It is always a good practice to talk with patients and obtain their consent before speaking with their family. However, in special situations, safety or other imminent concerns may create the need to speak with family members without the patient's consent. Clinicians should know and follow their relevant local rules and policies in such cases, adhere to principles of good clinical practice, and always try to work as collaboratively with the patient as possible in such circumstances. At times, patients' unwillingness to involve family in treatment may be due to acute symptoms they are experiencing, such as active psychotic symptoms, withdrawal, or disorganization. We have found that the family may be a particularly valuable source of information in these cases and can often provide useful guidance to the clinical team about how to effectively interact with the patient. Thus, special effort is often warranted to get the family involved when encountering this type of reluctance. It is often helpful to remember that involving the family is rarely an "all or none" proposition; it can be useful to present patients with a range of options and to encourage choices regarding how their family can be involved. It is also important to carefully consider all potential family members in the patient's support system. Many patients may be hesitant to involve certain family members in their treatment but willing to allow others to be involved.

In the next section, we focus on two common challenges even when patients are interested in family involvement: difficulties initiating work with family members and addressing situations in which the family has differences of opinion with the clinical team. For a more detailed discussion of clinical intervention with families of persons with SMI (e.g., family psychoeducation), see manuals by McFarlane (2002), Miklowitz (2008), and Mueser and Glynn (1999). These treatment manuals provide a detailed description of strategies to initiate work with patients' families and evidence-based models to provide ongoing therapeutic intervention.

Family-Level Barriers: Difficulties With Engagement and Differences of Opinion

Family members, primarily parents and siblings, are key drivers of help-seeking and integral in supporting treatment engagement. However, family members may have reservations about meeting with their loved one's mental health clinicians or participating in family services. For example, they may be concerned about intruding on their relative's privacy or worried that such participation will add additional caregiving demands. Practical and structural barriers, such as limited time, competing workplace demands, child-care needs, and lack of access to transportation, may also prevent family members from participating in services. Unfortunately, some family members may have past negative experiences with seeking help from the mental health system or participating in family therapy, given prior outdated theories that emphasized the family environment as a causative influence on mental disorders (e.g., the "schizophrenogenic mother"). In this regard, clinicians should appropriately communicate that the illness is *not* the family's fault and provide educational information about what is known about the etiology of psychiatric disorders. For example, when given the opportunity, a clinician can explain thus:

> Relatives often have questions about why their loved one developed schizophrenia. Although the causes are not completely understood, we know that genetics plays a role in determining who is most likely to develop schizophrenia. Also, we know that stressful life events play a role in triggering episodes of the illness. Research has shown that schizophrenia is an illness of the brain. In other words, the symptoms of the illness are caused when certain areas of the brain are not functioning properly and the chemicals that the brain uses to communicate are out of balance. I want to emphasize that schizophrenia is not caused by parenting or family behaviors. In fact, some of the most loving parents I have ever met have had children who go on to develop schizophrenia. On the other hand, we do know that families can play an important role in helping their loved ones manage, cope with, and recover from this difficult illness.

To engage families, clinicians must communicate the value of family involvement to both patients and their relatives. Shea (1998) described several interviewing techniques that can help address the underlying fears family members may bring to the initial meeting. In one technique, the clinician openly acknowledges the immense value of the family member's firsthand longitudinal knowledge of the patient and the patient's care to date. For example, "One of the things I want to emphasize early on is how important your input and background information are in our helping [patient name]. No one in the world knows them better than you. We depend on your input. I also really want to know what you think has worked and what you think hasn't worked." In their discussion of how to best engage families, Mueser and Glynn (1999) offered three useful strategies that clinicians can use to enhance engagement:

1. Letting family know they are not alone
2. Providing support and allowing relatives to vent
3. Instilling hope for change

Persistence and flexibility are also important ingredients in the effort to engage family members as allies in treatment.

Perhaps one of the most challenging scenarios for clinicians is when the family has views that directly contrast with the current biopsychosocial understanding of psychiatric disorders. For example, family members may believe the patient just needs to "pull himself up by the bootstraps" in dealing with his problems and that psychiatric medications are not needed. In these situations, clinicians should attentively listen and understand the family members' perspectives. To the extent possible, they should first validate the family member's concerns or points of view and follow with respectful and culturally appropriate educational information. If the family member opposes medication and believes that the patient just needs to try harder, the clinician can acknowledge this perspective:

> I agree that it's almost always true that people do better if they try harder and believe they can be successful. So, it would be really great if [patient name] could try harder at cleaning up around the house. But one of the things we are learning about the illness of schizophrenia is that chemical changes in the brain change a person's ability to plan and be organized. It can also reduce a person's ability to feel satisfied and proud of completing a task. All of these problems limit someone's ability to pull themselves up.

Regarding medication, an example dialogue may go as follows:

CLINICIAN: I completely understand your hesitation about medication. Can you help me further understand what your concerns are about [patient name] taking the medicine?

FAMILY MEMBER: Well, every time he comes in, it seems like they add more medicines for him to take! And the more medicines you take, the more problems you get—and I don't see any of them helping.

CLINICIAN: I'm glad you raise these concerns. Let me also say that I know it's frustrating to see such limited progress. I wish we had more effective ways to help people get better quicker. Let's talk more about the role that medications might play in helping [patient name]. The overall goal of the medications is to help reduce the symptoms that are part of schizophrenia—things like developing unusual beliefs, not making sense, hearing voices. When he gets sick, these are the kind of symptoms that get worse for him.

FAMILY MEMBER: Yeah, he acts pretty crazy sometimes.

CLINICIAN: For most people, the medicines can help control these kinds of symptoms. Although they won't make everything better, controlling these kinds of symptoms is an important first step. You also raised a concern about the number of medicines he is on and the possible side effects they might have. Let me tell you a little bit about each of his medications and the possible side effects to watch out for. [Clinician provides appropriate information about specific medications.] I'm so glad you raised these questions; things usually work best when we can all work together—[patient name], you, and I—to find the medicines that work best for him and have the fewest negative side effects.

Meaningful Ways to Involve Families in Discharge Planning and Care Transitions

Family caregivers typically have a strong desire to be involved and assist the patient, and they are often directly affected by discharge planning decisions (Cohen et al. 2013). Haselden et al. (2019) found that inpatient staff contact with the patient's family during treatment and throughout discharge planning has an impact on whether a patient connects with an outpatient service provider after leaving the hospital. Thus, one important time to engage families as allies in the treatment process is during discharge planning.

When facing discharge, families are often frightened, unsettled, and anxious about what will happen when the patient is released from the hospital. Questions arise such as Will she go to treatment on her own? Should I try to do anything differently than before she went into the hospital? What if she's not really ready to come home? Even if family members have not yet been involved in the patient's care to this point, this is a good time to consider inviting them to become involved in planning for what happens after the hospitalization ends. This should include conversations about what they can do to help, what to avoid, and the extent to which they have the time and emotional energy to play meaningful roles in supporting the patient's treatment after discharge. In some cases, a patient may be returning home with a family member such as a parent, sibling, or spouse. It can be helpful for staff to assist the patient and family in codeveloping a clear set of shared expectations and agreements about living together and the next steps needed for treatment, which can reduce stress and act as a guide for "hitting the reset button."

If there are safety concerns, families can be meaningfully involved in the patient's discharge plan, including such things as relapse prevention strategies, monitoring for early warning signs of increased symptoms or risk, or involvement in safety planning and supporting the patient if the patient experiences any future high-risk or suicidal thoughts, urges, or behaviors. Patients and families should be provided accurate information about suicide risk and warning signs, as well as how to access community resources if needed. Additionally, they should be encouraged to discuss how the family might be helpful after the discharge in specific ways that are acceptable to both the family members and the patient. For example, family members might become involved in means reduction, such as removing firearms from the home or holding on to medications by keeping them in a locked cabinet and ensuring the person has only a daily supply. Shared decision-making to help families think through choices about how they might be involved after discharge—with the patient's buy-in and consent—is critically important (Substance Abuse and Mental Health Services Administration 2010).

Family members can help ensure a successful transition to referrals by understanding how the follow-up referral can help, where the referred resources are located, when the next appointment is, and the potential repercussions of missing the appointment. Additionally, clinicians might help patients and families identify ways the family might support the transition process both practically (e.g., providing transportation, giving appointment reminders, accompanying patients to appointments) and emotionally (e.g., conveying hope of recovery, using strengths-based language).

Importance of Conveying Messages of Hope and Recovery

As family members, we have all experienced times when we felt hopeless. When connecting with family members on the inpatient unit, it is important to share what is known about recovery and to provide hopeful messages for people. Research has clearly demonstrated that psychiatric illnesses typically are not the "lifelong sentences" that our field once believed. Instead, many people can and do experience improved symptoms, attainment of life goals, and recovery as defined in several different ways—especially as defined by each person for themselves. It is important to convey these messages, such as by saying:

> I know things are difficult now and that [patient name] has experienced a real setback in how he is doing. That can be so hard to witness, and I know it may be hard to remain

> hopeful for his future. Please know that I've seen many people over the years who have had similar setbacks and who go on to experience what I would call "recovery." In my field, we used to think of psychiatric conditions such as schizophrenia as a "life sentence," where people would always have symptoms and would go in and out of the hospital for the rest of their lives. Newer research has shown that this is *not* the case for everyone.

In some cases, it is helpful to direct family members to websites that show videos about recovery and of people telling their personal stories of recovery. One example is Dr. Patricia Deegan's online Recovery Library (https://recoverylibrary.com), which contains many videos, articles, personal narratives, tools, and worksheets for people and families whose lives are touched by mental illness. Resources such as these can be useful in instilling hope for families.

Conclusion and Future Directions

Future, practical challenges for families warrant attention—how to help families set appropriate limits with their relatives, especially upon discharge to a family home or nearby residence. Families could benefit from support and guidance about ways to convey love and support for their relative while also setting limits and communicating appropriate expectations. Future consideration should also be given to exploring the potential role of family advocates in collaborating with hospital staff and meeting the needs of families. More training for staff in how to effectively engage with individuals and families around family involvement is needed. Given the ever-growing diversity in the United States, ways to effectively train staff regarding racial and cultural issues as they relate to family inclusion will be particularly important for the field.

In summary, effectively working with families requires a cross between the clinical skills needed for working with patients and the communication skills needed for interacting effectively with colleagues. In many ways, clinicians are best viewed as consultants to family members, who are often faced with multiple stresses and challenges and can benefit tremendously from practical information, guidance, and support. By establishing an effective working alliance with patients' family members during inpatient hospitalization, clinicians can substantially improve the quality of care, enhance treatment outcomes following hospital discharge, and improve quality of life for both patients and their family members.

References

American Psychiatric Association: Guideline Watch (September 2009): Practice Guideline for the Treatment of Patients With Schizophrenia. Washington, DC, American Psychiatric Publishing, 2009

American Psychiatric Association: Diagnostic and Statistical Manual of Mental Disorders, 5th Edition. Arlington, VA, American Psychiatric Association, 2013a

American Psychiatric Association: Online Assessment Measures (Early Development and Home Background) (online). Arlington, VA, American Psychiatric Association, 2013b. Available at: www.psychiatry.org/psychiatrists/practice/dsm/dsm-5/online-assessment-measures.

Cohen AN, Drapalski AL, Glynn SM, et al: Preferences for family involvement in care among consumers with serious mental illness. Psychiatr Serv 64(3):257–263, 2013 23242515

Haselden M, Corbeil T, Tang F, et al: Family involvement in psychiatric hospitalizations: associations with discharge planning and prompt follow-up care. Psychiatr Serv 70(10):860–866, 2019

McFarlane WR: Multifamily Groups in the Treatment of Severe Psychiatric Disorders. New York, Guilford, 2002

Miklowitz DJ: Bipolar Disorder: A Family Focused Treatment Approach, 2nd Edition. New York, Guilford, 2008

Mueser KT, Glynn SM: Behavioral Family Therapy for Psychiatric Disorders, 2nd Edition. Oakland, CA, New Harbinger, 1999

Murray-Swank AB, Dixon L: Family psychoeducation as an evidence-based practice. CNS Spectr 9(12):905–912, 2004 15616476

Nicholson J, Reupert A, Grant A, et al: The policy context and change for families living with parental mental illness, in Parental Psychiatric Disorder: Distressed Parents and Their Families. Edited by Reupert A, Maybery D, Nicholson J, et al. London, Cambridge University Press, 2015, pp 354–364

Shea SC: Psychiatric Interviewing: The Art of Understanding, 2nd Edition. Philadelphia, PA, WB Saunders, 1998

Substance Abuse and Mental Health Services Administration: Shared Decision-Making in Mental Health Care: Practice, Research and Future Directions (HHS Publ No SMA 09-4371). Rockville, MD, Substance Abuse and Mental Health Services Administration, 2010

Tessler R, Gamache G: Family Experiences With Mental Illness. Westport, CT, Auburn House, 2000

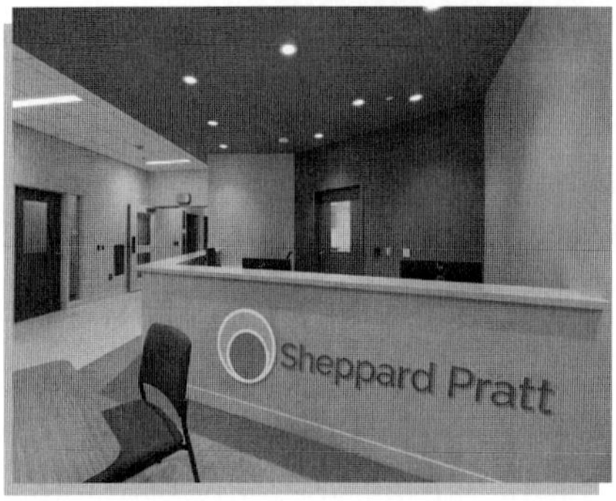

CHAPTER 28

From Within

A Consumer Perspective on Psychiatric Hospitals

Howard D. Trachtman, B.S., CPS, CPRP, COAPS
Kenneth S. Duckworth, M.D.
Reverend Dr. Norma J. Heath
Ziona Rivera

Hospitals that rely solely on the medical model tend to focus primarily on pathology and disease (Mead et al. 2001) and to define *recovery* as a set of predetermined outcomes that emphasize symptom elimination and a return to premorbid functioning. This model of illness can be defeatist because it undermines hope, which has been described by advocates and consumer leaders as "one of the cornerstones of recovery" (Deegan et al. 1988). Consumers of mental health services face many challenges in terms of social attitudes, low social status, and prejudice, yet attitudes are improving and so is knowledge that anyone can have a psychiatric illness at any time in their lives. The challenge for us all is to integrate the best of the consumer movement into the medical service model. The resulting synthesis can continue to improve the quality and experience of care at psychiatric hospitals.

My Experience With Psychiatric Hospitals: Howard D. Trachtman

Prior to my multiple admissions to psychiatric hospitals, I knew very little about mental health, psychiatric treatment, and what happens in a hospital. My "knowledge" was based on what I had seen on television and in movies such as *One Flew Over the Cuckoo's Nest*. As a young person, I was told that a friend of mine had jumped into Niagara Falls, ending his life, an event triggered by a breakup with his girlfriend. At the time, I could not understand why a person would want to end their life. Now I know.

I have been interested in the use of computers for the greater good my entire life and knew that Massachusetts Institute of Technology (MIT) was the best place for me to study artificial intelligence and build robots. I became a freshman at MIT right after my sixteenth birthday in 1981. One of my professors told me about visiting an MIT student who was catatonic in a psychiatric unit. At the time, I did not think I would ever become a psychiatric patient myself. One day, during my freshman year, a friend left a 20-page suicide note that got mixed in with my printouts. Bewildered, I was advised to see a psychiatrist to get this person help. The psychiatrist thought that I also needed treatment, but I do not recall receiving a diagnosis or medication being suggested. I do remember being told that if matters got worse to go to a (specific) hospital.

Just before my eighteenth birthday, I was up all night at the MIT Artificial Intelligence Laboratory. I became convinced that artificially intelligent computers were taking over the world and that I needed to flee. While waiting to change planes, I started thinking that some planes were going to heaven and others were going to hell. I decided that I needed to read the Bible. Because I was acting strangely, the police brought me to a crisis center. When the doctor asked if I heard voices, I answered "Yes" because I thought I was being asked if I could hear people talking, not if I was having auditory hallucinations (I was not). As a result, I was placed in four-point leather restraints and injected with Haldol.

My parents flew up in the morning, and I was discharged to their custody. We flew home, but I was still in crisis and immediately walked out of the house, barefoot, looking for a Bible. My parents initially had difficulty having me admitted to a private hospital, but once they mentioned I thought I was Jesus Christ, I was admitted to a short-term unit. That was enough to be admitted then; I am not sure that would be enough now, in the world of managed care. Although I spent several weeks on the unit and recall being prescribed Thorazine, I was told little about my condition. I was not given a diagnosis, nor did I receive much therapy or education about the importance of remaining on medication. I spent most of my time there reading and watching television and very little time speaking with mental health workers, nurses, or doctors. If I had been told the benefits of speaking with professionals, I would have done so.

I returned to Boston, and soon I was up all night. I was now aware that this was a warning sign that I was not doing well and might be at risk for hospitalization, so I called 911. The police brought me to an emergency department, and I was placed in four-point restraints and told I was being sent to the private hospital recommended by MIT. I felt relieved. However, I felt betrayed when the ambulance brought me to a state hospital instead. I was assigned a psychiatrist who wore black boots, and coupled with her power over me at the hospital, at times I was convinced she was a Nazi.

I spent 9 months on the admissions unit, a coed floor with three large dormitory-style rooms where we slept. Every so often, as the male/female balance changed, we would be moved from one room to another. The staff must have liked me because after a few months I was given my own therapist for an extra hour a week, which I found very helpful. Otherwise, most of my time was wasted: playing games and watching television. I hated not having constructive activities or learning skills to help me live independently after discharge. One lesson I learned at the state hospital was what I now know is called "learned helplessness." When I realized I needed dental care, I went to the hospital dental office, made an appointment, and kept it. When I returned to my unit following the appointment, the staff were angry I had done this on my own.

There were only two groups held per week: privilege group and group therapy. Initially, patients were restricted to the unit; once a week in privilege group you could ask for the next level of freedom, but I was restricted to the unit for several months, possibly because I had refused to sign a voluntary form when admitted. It took me quite a while to move up the privilege ladder because I was never told how a person graduated to the next level. Eventually, I got a staff pass that allowed me to walk around the grounds accompanied by a staff member. The next level, a mutual pass, allowed patients to walk on the grounds accompanied by another patient with a mutual or higher level of privilege, but when I finally reached that level, the other person took off on me. When I returned to the unit alone, I lost all my privileges and had to start over. In time, I reached a level that allowed me to go out on the grounds independently and even to leave the campus. One day, my parents were to take me out on a pass, but I became very anxious and acted out. I thought that I would lose my opportunity to be with them, but the doctor gave me some Ativan and allowed me to go. Her understanding made me very happy and enhanced my respect for her.

Life on the unit was traumatic. One patient kept trying to persuade me to have sexual relations with him; one night, the staff announced that he had hanged himself on the grounds. Another time, a patient assaulted me while I was in bed. There was a hallway of quiet/seclusion rooms where difficult patients would be placed; some spent most of their time in those rooms. The original idea was that people would not be exposed to too much stimulation while in these rooms, but to me they seemed like punishment. When I was sequestered, I would frequently push the door open to get fresh air only to have it pushed back and locked. Once a week I would be asked to sign the required paperwork for being secluded. It was never explained that if I had not opened the door, they would not have locked it, and I would have been let out much sooner. Now, some state hospitals have peers (people with lived experience of mental health treatment) whose job it is to debrief all instances of restraint and seclusion and work to prevent future episodes. I wish that had existed back then. I also wonder why, when I was at my sickest during those 9 months in the state hospital, restraints were never used, but later, in several private hospitals, I was frequently put into restraints. Restraints felt like torture. Several of my friends have stated that they received better care in state hospitals than in some private facilities.

A few months into my state hospitalization, I was told I was being considered for discharge and would move into an adolescent group home. However, a fellow patient convinced me that my medications were bad for me, and I experimented with tonguing (pretending to take them and then throwing them out) which set my treatment back several months. I remember the day of my discharge. I was taken to the Social

Security office to apply for disability benefits; soon after, I was required to apply for welfare and Medicaid. The message I received was that I was profoundly disabled and would never be able to work. I also met my new therapist, whom I saw continuously for over 18 years. I developed a solid rapport with him and can only say good things about not having to continually look for a new therapist.

Even as I became medication compliant, I continued to require hospitalization, but in private facilities. I was able to maintain a romantic relationship for several years, but my housing situation changed a few times, and I felt like ending my life. I went to be evaluated and told the doctor I wanted to kill myself. She noted I had no previous suicide attempts and sent me home. I took a major overdose later that night. Eventually I was prescribed clozapine and required no further hospitalizations for 5 years. I also discovered the peer empowerment movement, which became essential in my recovery. I learned much from my peers; I was mentored by many people and eventually discovered that I had something to offer by helping other people, both individually and systemically. Doing advocacy work was a tremendous boost.

After those quality years on clozapine, I experimented with functioning without medication, but it did not work out well, and I ended up having multiple hospitalizations. I restarted the clozapine, and the hospital added two new medications. However, my outpatient psychiatrist tapered me off the additional medications after my discharge, and I went 6 more years without a hospitalization. I was mentored to do direct action/advocacy-run business meetings and service on nonprofit boards. In 2004, I cofounded the National Alliance on Mental Illness (NAMI) Greater Boston Peer Support and Advocacy Network, and in 2005, I cofounded the Boston Resource Center, a peer-run recovery center at Boston Medical Center. In 2018, the Boston Resource Center became the flagship of the Metro Boston Recovery Learning Community, which today has four recovery centers and a peer support line.

My take-home message is that even though people in the hospital may be acutely ill, there is hope for a recovery in which one's life can become meaningful again. I became a certified peer specialist in 2006 and later became both a certified psychiatric rehabilitation practitioner and a certified older adult peer specialist.

I Am Involved With Inpatient Staff but Not Insurance Companies: Norma J. Heath

I am a 53-year-old Afro Latina woman. I was diagnosed with mental illness in my 20s. My most recent diagnoses are PTSD and bipolar disorder. I also have severe anxiety and depression and have been in and out of psychiatric hospitals for many years. Two things I like most about the inpatient units today are that peers work on the care team and that patients are involved in their own treatment plan. What I dislike is that hospitals are at the beck and call of the insurance companies.

During my inpatient hospitalizations, I realized that the insurance companies have the final say in a patient's care and treatment. I believe this is unethical because the doctors often had to discharge me regardless of whether I was well enough to go home because my insurance would only cover a certain number of days. This caused increased stress. There was once a time when doctors had more control over their patients' care than the insurance companies. If the insurance had not run out and I had not been released prematurely from the hospitals, I likely would not have been in and out of the hospitals so many times.

Peer support made a huge difference in my recovery. My most recent inpatient stay was just a year ago. It was a more pleasant experience because I knew exactly what was going on with my treatment, and the team welcomed my input about what was best for me. The team consisted of a doctor, nurse, social worker, and peer specialist. The peer specialist made a huge difference in the way I felt about my care; I felt that someone who understood me was cheering for me. In the past, the medical team made the decisions about me and told me what was right for me. These days, I can voice my opinion and let them know which medications I do not want to try and how I want to be treated in a crisis.

When it comes to psychiatric care on inpatient units, some things have gotten better while others have gotten worse. Peer specialists should continue to grow in inpatient hospital settings, and the power of the insurance companies should decrease. Programs such as Wellness Recovery Action Plan and Whole Health Action Management are used by peer specialists and have made a positive impact on my recovery. Hospitals need to understand that patients want to be involved in their recovery and do not need the insurance dictating whether we are well.

Generational Psychosis: Ziona Rivera

I believe that psychiatric care is extremely important and should be given to those who need it. Some of my experiences with psychiatric care were nurturing, whereas others were torture, like being in a scary movie. I am now in recovery from institutions and am part of the peer recovery movement for survivors of trauma. We come together with institutions in many ways to inspire hope, courage, and support. My mother participates in this movement as well.

I was born into a dysfunctional family. Everyone in my immediate family is diagnosed with and mostly untreated for substance use disorders and mental illness. My biological father has been diagnosed with paranoid schizophrenic disorder, and my mother was diagnosed with paranoid anxiety, PTSD, depression, and substance use disorder. My older sister has been diagnosed with PTSD, paranoid schizoaffective disorder, adult ADHD, and anxiety and abuses multiple substances. She and I are 9 years apart in age. She was first diagnosed at age 11, and I too received my first mental health diagnosis—delayed sleep phase disorder and depression—at age 11. I believe our diagnoses are related to severe generational abuse and neglect as well as my mother's drug use during pregnancy and other defects that are not her fault.

My mother was undiagnosed for many years and self-medicated with miscellaneous drugs and alcohol. She was good at hiding things and running away from her problems. She would dump my brothers, sisters, and me at anyone's house and run away. This would happen every 2 years for months at a time, like a vicious circle. Sometimes her absence was due to her visits to detox, but her clean time never stuck.

I began to be abused during these stays with the babysitter. My first hospitalization was on an adolescent unit for suicidal ideation shortly after my fourteenth birthday. I had attempted suicide multiple times in the past but had never mentioned it to anyone until this attempt. Sharing my actions provided me with relief, because I no longer carried my burden of darkness alone. When I first arrived on the unit, I was evaluated and asked questions pertaining to my suicidal thoughts and my past attempts. They asked me things I had never been asked before, and I was open to talking about it finally. After 2 hours of questions and paperwork, I was told that I would be taken into a bathroom by two staff members to perform a routine search for dangerous paraphernalia and any self-harm injuries. I did not object because I had nothing to hide, and a part of me was desensitized to being naked around others because of my sexual abuse trauma. Some of the newly admitted patients gave the staff a hard time, arguing that the staff were not medical professionals and the patients were adolescents who should not be naked in a room with an adult. They were right.

Unfortunately, while I was hospitalized, my mother signed over her guardianship of me to the state. I was devastated, and I coped by participating on the unit. During one of my many stays at an adult psychiatric facility, I was using the phone (which is one of my human rights), and no one told me to get off the phone or that it was bedtime, but during my conversation, three staff suddenly physically and chemically restrained me on the floor. The person to whom I was talking became upset because he could not understand what the staff were doing to me and why I had started screaming. My friend felt very helpless and wanted to intervene, but there was nothing he could do.

Although I learned a great deal about mental health terminology and culture, I was shocked to learn I was not permitted to talk about my experiences with any of my adolescent peers on the unit. This was allowed only in clinical group settings, where we were censored and were often interrupted if we raised a passionate subject. It was during one of my involuntary hospital stays that I was invited by a certified peer specialist (a person with lived experience) working on the inpatient unit to take a collaborative problem-solving training. She shared her recovery story with me, and I was amazed to learn so much about her after knowing her off and on for a few years. I also learned that there was a profession for people like me to help others through our story. I ended up participating in the next training cycle that same year.

Psychiatric hospitalizations and rehabilitation have been a vicious circle in my immediate family. Family therapy, individual therapy, medication, and self-care have been the most helpful. Being forced to take medication that did not work and being unjustly restrained were the least helpful. It always made me feel better when everyone had to participate in family therapy and work on our issues together. I learned much about my sister's pain and how I could support her, and it brought us closer. I remember fighting with my mom every week when I was younger; now, I make sure to hug her every day. Self-care is important and looks different for all of us. I enjoy reading and watching movies. Sometimes my self-care is as simple as drinking a cup of juice. Medication does not help everyone living with a mental health diagnosis, but finding the right medication played a huge role in my self-care regimen. Today, I am grateful for peer-run organizations such as NAMI, Recovery Learning Centers and Communities, and others because through them I learned how to heal and to help others who have had similar trauma. I am also grateful for my support system and my family.

Nothing About Us Without Us

The principle "nothing about us without us" illustrates the consumer/peer recovery movement in its essence. Hospitals help vulnerable people obtain a safe course of care to prepare them to move to the next step in their recovery. Although psychiatric hospitals serve a crucial role in the lives of individuals with psychiatric crises, until recently, these specialized hospitals historically rarely involved their patients' experience and feedback in conceptualizing, designing, or improving care. The peer recovery movement has long been about people's choices and being involved in all levels of care. As the culture of welcoming consumer input, evaluation, and design of services continues to develop, material progress can be made toward person-centered care.

What's in a Name?

Psychiatric hospitals have unique power dynamics. The power differential between the people who hold the keys, issue orders, and make decisions about passes and privileges and the people in a locked ward who may be there against their will is a structural fact of inpatient psychiatric care. Language needs to reflect this differential. Words such as *patient* or *chronic,* which may seem benign to doctors, may be quite charged for people receiving psychiatric services who connect being a "chronic" mental "patient" with having very low status or minimal prospects for improvement. Indeed, a significant percentage of inpatients deny having the mental illness with which they are diagnosed by hospital staff.

How we speak about people reflects the beliefs we have about them on many levels. Referring to people with disabilities by the name of the disability—for example, "a schizophrenic," "a paraplegic"—implies that the disability is their defining characteristic. One remedy for defining people by their illness is the use of "person-first" language—for example, "a person with schizophrenia" or "someone with paraplegia." Accepting that people may call themselves *consumers* or *peers* (our terms for this chapter), *residents* (of a living situation), *members* (of a clubhouse), *survivors* (of perceived abuse in the system), or even *prosumers* (consumers who work professionally in the system) gives a glimpse into the varying ways people think about their relationship to the work of recovery and to the care system. Hope and dignity are key elements of recovery, and language should reflect that spirit.

Until more recently, when the philosophy and ideology of recovery began to weave its way throughout the mental health paradigm, consumers were left to foster ideas of hope, well-being, and recovery in a mental health system that "viewed serious psychiatric disorders as harbingers of doom" (Corrigan and Ralph 2005). Pessimistic views about the course of psychiatric conditions, coupled with societal prejudice and language, have historically added to the burden of having a major mental illness. Language is fully under the control of those who use it.

Human rights is an all-encompassing category that incorporates basic human rights within the hospital and efforts to minimize use of restraint and seclusion, provide inpatients access to the outdoors, and make the psychiatric hospital more consumer friendly and treatment focused. Consumers in psychiatric hospital environments are at a vulnerable point in their lives, and service design and delivery need to be mindful of this. Although clinical and human needs are usually met in a healthy and dignified environment and lives are saved, the civil rights division of the U.S. Department of Justice, pursuant to the Civil Rights of Institutionalized Persons Act of 1980, has recounted horrors of care discovered in its state psychiatric hospital investigations in multiple states. Breakdowns of safety systems, excessive use of restraint and seclusion (e.g., as punishment), abuse, inadequate medical care, and poor environmental conditions are among the most common concerns mentioned in its annual reports. Failures of leadership and lack of funding, variables that are out of the control of consumers, are key elements in the difference between respectful, compassionate care and grossly deficient care. Consumers understandably feel safer with guarantees of basic rights and the processes to ensure them.

In 1997, Massachusetts' consumer advocates celebrated the Five Fundamental Rights Act (Commonwealth of Massachusetts 1997) for all persons receiving services from programs or facilities operated by, licensed by, or contracted with the Massachusetts Department of Mental Health. It is still shocking that legislation was needed to guarantee these basic rights, which include the right to "reasonable access" to a telephone for making and receiving confidential calls; the right to send and receive "sealed, unopened, uncensored mail"; the right to receive visitors of one's "own choosing daily and in private, at reasonable times"; the right to a humane environment, including living space that ensures "privacy and security in resting, sleeping, dressing, bathing and personal hygiene, reading and writing and in toileting"; and the right to access legal representation (Commonwealth of Massachusetts 1997). However, penalties for violating this law were not specified, and consumers continue to report violations of these basic rights (Rice 2007).

Access to outdoor space, a right taken for granted in most correctional settings, is a recent addition to basic human rights for inpatients of psychiatric hospitals. Consumers who are denied access to the outdoors report feeling demoralized and contained, which can result in an increase in symptoms and lead, in turn, to an increased length of stay. Because some hospitals have allowed only smokers the "privilege" of going outside, some individuals have tragically started smoking while inpatients because doing so is their only means of outdoor access (Melo 2007). Consumers believe that fresh air is good for the body and soul, decreasing depression, stifling aggressiveness, and ultimately leading to better therapeutic results. In Massachusetts, legislation was enacted that added enforcement provisions to the Five Fundamental Rights Act and established a sixth right, the right to fresh air and the outdoors.

Reducing Restraint and Seclusion as a Human Rights Issue

After a 1998 *Hartford Courant* investigative series (Weiss 1998) exposed the large number of deaths nationwide resulting from the use of restraint and seclusion, consumer advocates and policy makers combined their efforts to reduce and work toward elimination of the use of these procedures. Although people vary in their descriptions of their experiences, a range of difficult experiences, including "torture," are described in a NAMI report entitled *Cries of Anguish* (National Alliance on Mental Illness 2000). Even patients and staff who witness restraint and seclusion can be traumatized, especially those who already have a trauma history. The state medical directors put together a game-changing restraint and seclusion reduction analysis that defined *restraint* as seclusion—not as treatment, but as treatment *failure*. This public health framework of prevention helped move the culture toward working with inpatients and not simply stopping their behavior.

Peers are at the forefront of working to reduce and eliminate restraint and seclusion. NAMI's Consumer Council created a Restraint and Seclusion Committee, which is now the NAMI Peer Leadership Council's Advocacy Committee, and peers are also active with Protection and Advocacy for Individuals with Mental Illness (PAIMI) advisory councils. PAIMI programs are mandated by federal statute to address abuse and neglect as a top priority. Gayle Bluebird, a peer who is also a registered nurse, has championed the conversion of seclusion rooms into comfort or quiet rooms that function as sanctuaries where patients may choose to go to take a break from unit activities (Bluebird 2005). With extensive occupational therapy input, hospitals in many states have designed similar consumer-friendly spaces to help people calm themselves (Champagne 2006).

In 2014, the Substance Abuse and Mental Health Services Administration developed the six principles of trauma-informed care to help guide leaders and practitioners in creating safe and therapeutic settings: safety, trustworthiness and transparency, peer support, collaboration, empowerment voice and choice, and attention to historical gender and culture issues. These principles are not designed only for inpatient care, but they apply very well in that setting. A trauma-informed inpatient care model creates positive and collaborative ways to help inpatients recognize distress and find ways to help defuse it without unnecessary use of restraint or seclusion.

More importantly, because hospital care is treatment focused, involving patients in their own treatment planning is essential. Forming a treatment alliance that includes shared decision-making, while treating patients with respect and courtesy, helps demonstrate that the patients have value. Such valuation should continue through supportive outpatient/transitional care planning to confirm that the hospital is optimistic about the patient's future.

Peer Evaluation of Hospital Services

People who use psychiatric services deserve and desire high-quality services to assist them in their individual recovery path toward meaningful and productive lives. In addition to having their basic needs (e.g., safety, nutrition) met, people who are in a hospital environment need compassionate care and individualized services in coercion-free settings. Although many psychiatric institutions have at least one person responsible for quality and risk management, the peer leadership movement has identified former patients themselves as catalysts for system transformation. The existence of peer organizations that understand the power of hope and provide peer support has led directly to the creation of organizations focused on the evaluation of psychiatric services and improvement in the quality of the programs being evaluated. These are designed to be peer-run organizations whose boards of directors consist of a minimum of 51% people in recovery and that primarily hire people in recovery for positions as directors of mental health or addictions care. The first such team in the United States was created by consumers and family members in Philadelphia, Pennsylvania, in response to the closure of the state-run psychiatric hospital.

By having consumers interview other consumers face-to-face with a qualitative and quantitative instrument, valuable and unique data can be collected; respondents can and do reveal information that they would not share with a nonconsumer staff person or in a sterile survey instrument. Because consumers are the most important stakeholders in hospital quality, consumer researchers are best able to identify areas for improvement and to advocate for needed system transformations. More recently, organizations that started as satisfaction teams have grown to utilize community-based participatory action research, delivering white papers on quality improvement and work on service planning and needs assessment.

Alternatives to Hospitalization

Being proactive about one's life includes preventing hospitalization whenever possible. From their start in the mid-1800s through the modern movement beginning in the 1940s, peer-run self-help and advocacy groups have operated outside the formal mental health system and have been a means to avoid hospitalization. In recent decades, there has been increasing support and pressure to establish and legitimize peer-operated settings as either adjuncts or alternatives to traditional, professionally run services as part of the continuum of care offered by public mental health systems. As professionals continue to accept the involvement of peers, the culture will face significant stresses and outstanding opportunities.

Peer-run respites are a significant alternative to hospitalization. They are ideally in a residential setting and staffed by people with lived experience of mental health treatment. Rose House, which was created in 2001 and is operated by People USA in Poughkeepsie, New York, is a successful model that has been studied and replicated across the United States and internationally. In total, People USA's Rose Houses have diverted more than 20,000 psychiatric hospital days. Rose Houses are short-term crisis respites that are homelike alternatives to hospital psychiatric emergency departments and inpatient units. The service is 100% voluntary. Guests can stay up to 5 nights, and they can come and go for appointments, jobs, and other essential needs. There are many different models of peer-run respites, but they all share peer-staffing models and can be hospital diversionary if desired by the potential guest.

The Living Room is another service that can divert people from emergency departments and inpatient levels of care. Championed by RI International, they are offered in several states. RI's leadership—along with other members of the Crisis Services Task Force of the National Action Alliance for Suicide Prevention (Action Alliance)—created the Crisis Now concept and authored the *Crisis Now* paper, identifying the exceptional practices desired for crisis services (RI International and NHS Clinical Commissioners 2018). RI focuses on these practices, including recovery orientation, trauma-informed care, significant use of peer staff, a commitment to Zero Suicide/Suicide Safer Care, strong commitments to safety of consumers and staff, and collaboration with law enforcement. The Living Rooms provide a homelike, soothing, and comfortable environment known for creating the best possible recovery experience: healing spaces with recliners, soft colors, and a homelike atmosphere. The teams, composed of doctors, nursing staff, and peers with lived experience, weave recovery, clinical, and medical services together to provide comprehensive care. RI makes every effort to eliminate seclusion and restraint and to serve all people regardless of level of acuity, without resorting to physical interventions. Peer-operated Living Room programs ensure that participants are paired with a team of peer support specialists in recovery. Each guest is encouraged to work with the team and empowered to develop their own recovery plan.

It is estimated that more than 25 million Americans have participated in a mutual-help group at some point over their lifetimes and that groups for individuals with mental illness are the second most frequented type of group; only groups for people with substance abuse issues have a higher membership (Kessler et al. 1997). Mutual-help groups function according to a belief system that lived experience with mental illness is paramount (Borkman 1990). As a result of the inherent value placed on lived experience and experiential knowledge, mutual-help groups are structured to reflect the assumption that all group participants have something of value to contribute. Such groups currently offer support to avoid hospitalization in programs such as peer support lines (also called warmlines) and crisis hotlines, peers in the emergency department, personal care assistant services, crisis respite, transitional respite, crisis stabilization units, walk-in urgent care, programs for assertive community treatment teams, and so on. Proactive alternatives such as Mary Ellen Copeland's Wellness Recovery Action Plan (Copeland Center for Wellness and Recovery 2020) can often decrease reliance on inpatient care and maximize independence for consumers who know their risk factors and supports and have clear communication with their outpatient caregivers. Advance directives for care follow the same guidelines. In recent years, more trainings have developed, such as Whole Health Action Management.

Linking From Hospital Units to the Next Level of Care

Fragmentation of services is among the most common problems associated with trying to obtain care. Too often, people receive good care on an inpatient unit and struggle with the transition to the next level of care. Involving the people who need care in the next step of their recovery journey is essential. Risks for self-harm and suicide are high for people who leave inpatient psychiatric care. The first few weeks following hospitalization put people at a particular risk. A recent review of 48 studies demonstrated increased risk of suicide in the posthospital population (Forte et al. 2019). To minimize this risk, it is essential to engage people proactively in the professional peer and family supports that will be most helpful to the next level of care.

References

Bluebird G: Comfort rooms: reducing the need for seclusion and restraint. Residential Group Care Quarterly 5(4):5–6, 2005

Borkman, TJ: Experiential, professional and lay frames of reference, in Working With Self-Help. Edited by Powell TJ. Silver Spring, MD, National Association of Social Workers Press, 1990 pp 3–30

Champagne T: Creating sensory rooms: environmental enhancements for acute inpatient mental health settings. Mental Health Special Interest Section Quarterly 29(4):1–4, 2006

Commonwealth of Massachusetts: Massachusetts General Laws, Title XVII, Chapter 123, Section 23: Rights of persons receiving services from programs or facilities of department of mental health, 1997. Available at: https://malegislature.gov/Laws/GeneralLaws/PartI/TitleXVII/Chapter123/Section23. Accessed December 6, 2021.

Copeland Center for Wellness and Recovery: What is WRAP? 2020. Available at: https://copelandcenter.com/wellness-recovery-action-plan-wrap. Accessed December 6, 2021.

Corrigan RW, Ralph RO: Introduction: recovery as consumer vision and research paradigm, in Recovery in Mental Illness: Broadening Our Understanding of Wellness. Edited by Corrigan RW, Ralph RO. Washigton, DC, American Psychological Assocation, 2005, p 4

Deegan PE: The lived experience of using psychiatric medication in the recovery process and a shared decision-making program to support it. Psychiatr Rehabil J 31(1):62–69, 2007 17694717

Forte A, Buscajoni A, Fiorillo A, et al: Suicidal risk following hospital discharge: a review. Harv Rev Psychiatry 27(4):209–216, 2019 31274577

Kessler RC. Michelson KD, Zhao S: Patterns and correlates of self-help group membership in the United States. Soc Policy 27(3):27–46, 1997

Mead S, Hilton D, Curtis L: Peer support: a theoretical perspective. Psychiatr Rehabil J 25(2):134–141, 2001 11769979

Mello F. Right to fresh air sought for patients. Boston Globe, July 8, 2007. Available at: http://archive.boston.com/news/local/articles/2007/07/08/right_to_fresh_air_sought_for_patients. Accessed December 6, 2021.

National Alliance on Mental Illness: Cries of Anguish: A Summary of Reports of Restraints and Seclusion Abuse Received Since the October 1998 Investigation by the Hartford Courant. Arlington, VA, National Alliance on Mental Illness, 2000

Rice P: Incommunicado: mental health wards restrict access to email. Spare Change News, February 5, 2007

RI International, NHS Clinical Commissioners: Be the change: ensuring an effective response to all in psychiatric emergency equal to medical care. October 2018. Available at: https://crisisnow.com/wp-content/uploads/2020/02/Be-the-Change.pdf. Accessed December 6, 2021.

Substance Abuse and Mental Health Services Administration: SAMHSA's Concept of Trauma and Guidance for a Trauma-Informed Approach. Rockville, MD, Substance Abuse and Mental Health Services Administration, 2014

Weiss EM: Hundreds of the nation's most vulnerable have been killed by the system intended to care for them. Hartford Courant, October 11, 1998

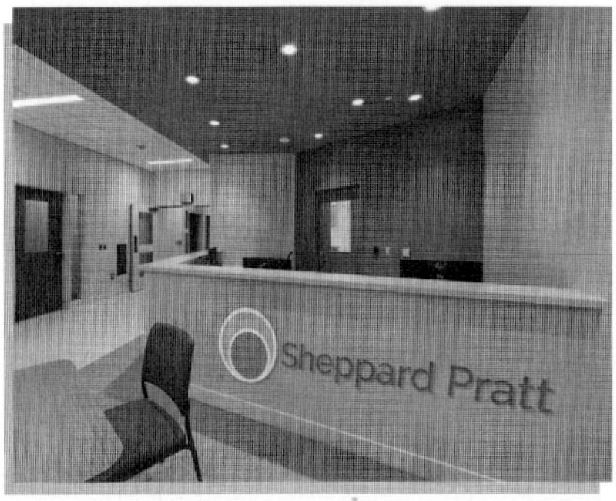

PART 5

The Future of Hospital Psychiatry

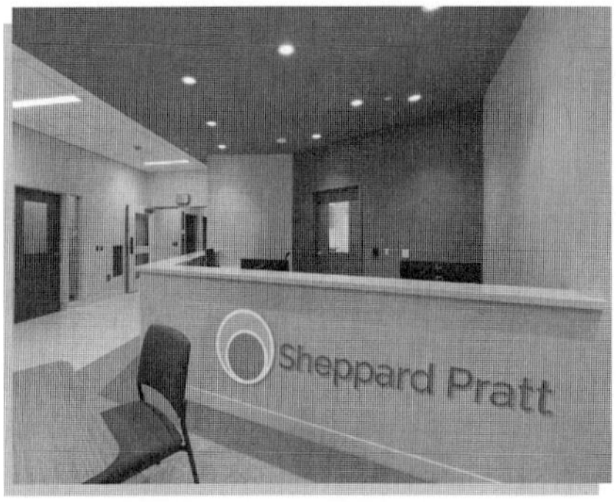

CHAPTER 29

Collaborative Care and Emerging Models

Ken C. Hopper, M.D., M.B.A.
Roger Kathol, M.D., CPE

The journey from traditional hospital psychiatric care to current practice needs to be understood in the context of notoriously poor financing. Mental health *illiteracy* on the part of society at large, health system designers, legislators, physicians, and even mental health workers has led to significant advocacy but has not yielded many impactful innovations that investment-earmarked dollars can multiply and self-sustain (Bhugra et al. 2017). Some common treatment themes have emerged as innovation advocates have chopped through the underbrush of the health care jungle. These themes are repeated and discussed in this chapter as they relate to new and promising methods of behavioral health care service delivery. Successful themes that are taking hold include

- **Proactive, high-fidelity care.** Early detection with assertive and full treatment prevents morbidity and mortality. This has been well known for medical illnesses but, interestingly, has been in the periphery for many patients with mental health conditions. Engineered solutions can be replicated intuitively and improve widespread impact.
- **Longitudinal care.** Since the early 1990s, the treatment mindset of health optimization, maintenance, resilience, and recovery has been applied much more vigorously to medical conditions, such as diabetes, than to mental disorders. Planning

and future treatment models in psychiatry must appreciate this reality to prevent morbidity and mortality.

- **Psychosocial determinants of health solutions and road maps.** Maslow's hierarchy of needs dictates that basic needs (e.g., food, water, shelter) must be met before we can move "up the ladder" and be concerned with issues such as health and personal health management. This argument can resonate with a broad audience.
- **Patient-proximal "touchpoints" for care delivery.** This commonsense, universal concept of place and time efficiency takes us from present to future in health care delivery and health optimization. "Strike while the iron is hot" and many other phrases in the human experience memorialize this principle in a broad sense. Almost all health venues and all varieties of electronic and social communication could be used to create psychiatric impact.
- **Team-based care and clinical pathways.** Medical-context models of team-based care have evolved quite independently from the psychiatry-propagated collaborative care model. An opportunity exists to reframe and reengineer tactics demonstrating value in collaborative care *into* the new, popular medical frameworks of team-care delivery today.
- **Inclusion of society, communities, and patients as stakeholders.** Because human behavior is truly the treatable cause of health outcomes and expenditure, it might be considered our duty professionally to create tools that more clearly describe and communicate our differential psychiatric inputs as well as the tangible value they bring to both patient and health system outcomes. We must move from mystical to tangible, transparent, compelling, and partnered approaches (in both word and deed).

Economic Scarcity: How Has This Differentially Affected Mental Health Services?

Scarcity became the push for innovation over the years. This "survival" backdrop has led to advancements in many areas of human endeavor. In psychiatry, economic scarcity has necessitated innovation as well. For example, the collaborative care model of integrated care—along with its integrated case management (ICM) fortified sibling, TeamCare—has been extremely successful in demonstrating clinical and cost-saving outcomes. The late Wayne Katon referred to the collaborative care model thus: "It wasn't too magical. We had to figure out a way to spread one psychiatrist over way too many patients!" (W. Katon, personal communication, May 2012).

Research since 2000 has demonstrated not only the clinical and cost benefits of newly constructed, total-person approaches but also the multiplier effect of treating in the broader medical context. Said another way, our speculation was found to be *fact*: human behaviors, particularly diagnosable mental health conditions, *do* adversely impact both medical and behavioral outcomes, result in higher crisis-oriented health care utilization, and consequently raise health care expenditures for those patients (Melek et al. 2018). It is wise for both clinical and financial reasons to more broadly invest in proactive behavioral care. Organizations have implemented pilots, hired consultants, and chosen vendors to change the equation toward medical-behavioral integration, but those systems have reaped only a portion of the possible gain through these maneuvers. What is holding us back from greater yield, and what do we need to do to move forward?

Scarcity has also led to innovation in psychiatric care, such as inpatient hospitalization, but financing without downstream planning has created significant functional gaps for patients needing more intensive services. Lack of funding for relatively inexpensive care management is eclipsed by the dramatic costs of crisis-oriented care. These patients, from a financial perspective, can be at the pinnacle of cost-multiplier scenarios. A true unintended consequence of "winning battles at the expense of the war" by financial intermediaries has become clear: increased health expenditures on the medical side due to increased emergency department, medical inpatient, and intensive care unit charges (Figure 29–1) (Kathol 2018; Mitchell 2001).

It is extraordinary for financially oriented companies (i.e., payers) to be blind to the fact that late twentieth-century behavioral health cost-control efforts designed to improve behavioral health spending have in reality *contributed to cost-accelerator and multiplier effects on the medical side*. This contribution comes from the traditional managed behavioral health care organization (MBHO) utilization management belief that providers must orchestrate planning to incorporate "theoretical" resources (particularly psychosocial supports) that allow the "least restrictive" levels of care to be successful. The funding of such psychosocial constructs has traditionally not been considered to be within scope for these payers. Longitudinal patient success considerations have been historically neglected in service of narrowly defined medical necessity decision-making and due to a non-integrated, departmental booking of cost-savings. Silos rule in payer environments. Trends, performance, and bonusing are connected to quality performance, but *only in one's silo*.

Some critical thinkers in the area of integrated care have advocated for a "unified benefit," a health financing model that pulls down the barriers and unintended consequences of separateness (Manderscheid and Kathol 2014). We may be on the verge of sufficient operational paradigms and expected health improvement outcomes (i.e., value-based payment models) to set smart structures in this one-budget environment. Integration at a payer corporate level *without* sufficient operational structures (called "mixed services" protocols in payer environments) has not been effective. What is true within payer environments is likely true elsewhere. Without visible, understandable design elements safeguarding psychiatric and psychological interventions, services tend to degrade. Monies are moved during pressured contract negotiations and in context of other business pressures.

A Historic Case in Point: The Saga of U.S. Psychiatric Inpatient Care

Gaps Created by Incomplete Health System Programming, Historic Reforms, and Redesigns

Psychiatric hospitals carried a variety of names in the nineteenth and early twentieth centuries, including *sanatoriums* and *asylums* (see Chapter 1). These retreats or facilities were structured around healthy eating and living, rest, relaxation, and mindfulness.

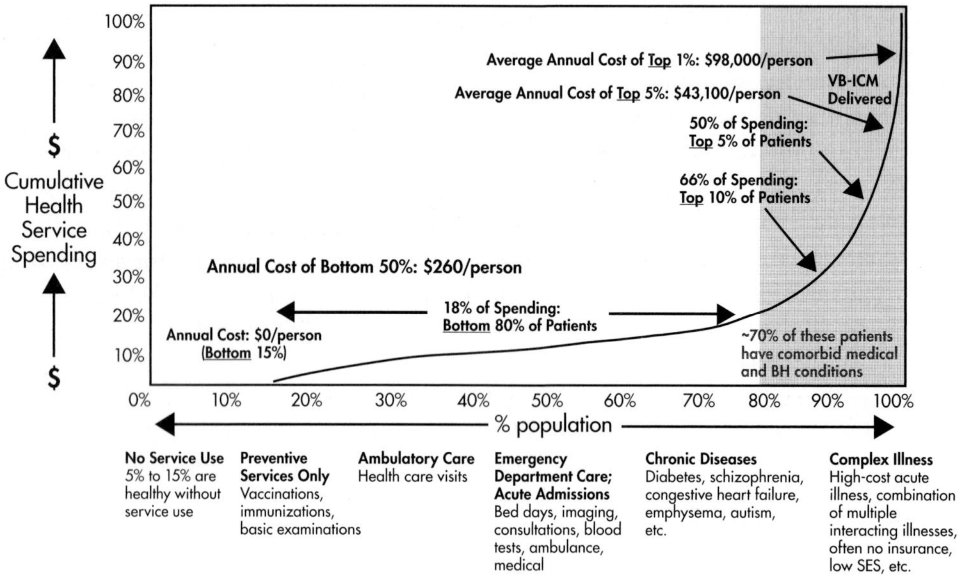

FIGURE 29–1. Driving down costs for complex chronically ill patients.
BH=behavioral health; SES=socioeconomic status; VB-ICM=value-based integrated case management.

They were often located in the country to promote relaxation and well-being. Both people with mental illness and those with chronic medical conditions were treated at these retreats. However, the advent of medications that more effectively treated underlying disease changed the demand for such establishments.

On the medical side, antibiotics for the treatment of tuberculosis eliminated an entire sector of recuperative facilities/hospitals, while on the psychiatric side, psychotropic drugs were being recognized for their ability to reverse depression, psychosis, anxiety, and other conditions. Economic scarcity in the 1930s led to medical-model treatments, and the term *psychopathic hospital* emerged; over time, and even with reductionistic medical-oriented philosophies, psychiatric stays became divergently longer than stays for chronic medical illness. Financial vehicles such as diagnosis-related groups began to significantly change lengths of stay and the settings of recuperation for medical conditions.

The hybrid model of the latter decades of the twentieth century incorporated both of these elements: the retreat-like, milieu-oriented philosophies of sanatoriums and the medical model of care. Legislation for the deinstitutionalization of mentally ill persons was passed, in part, because of the success of this new hybrid model of psychiatric care. However, this legislation also resulted in significant gaps due to some of the underestimated roles psychiatric hospitals served in health and life maintenance. The need for intensive support, including housing and basic needs fulfillment, and the management/oversight of such support were greatly underappreciated.

Adding to the storyline complexity, several large proprietary hospital chains capitalized on the inclusion of unlimited *commercial* behavioral health benefits by major employers to build programs and facilities for behavioral treatment. Some proprietary organizations pushed marketing and hospitalization criteria nearly to the point of unethical interpretation. The ensuing and massive legal challenges and court actions damaged our profession's reputation and set the stage for a polar opposite structure: a compensatory "policing" industry. "Reform" of the psychiatric hospital industry led to yet another wholesale reduction of beds as so-called medical necessity criteria and regulations and the advent of specialty-oriented managed care took hold (i.e., MBHOs). Medical necessity interpreted in the new "MBHO way" was introduced to both Medicare and Medicaid, and managed Medicaid became a rapidly expanding industry included in most payers' portfolios of insurance tactics and products. For patients who had sufficient ego strength, this reform may have led to better venues for addressing their problems and diagnoses, but for others, major treatment inputs and time frames likely shortchanged their chances of recovery. The most vulnerable are often penalized differentially as trends evolve.

The gap formed by this historic reframing of inpatient care revealed an incredible paradox. Intensive supports and behavior change strategies were major contributors to lengths of stay for many patients in psychiatric facilities, but because they were based less on diagnosis or medical models, they were neither fully appreciated nor supported by the medical-necessity continued-stay criteria and funding of the late twentieth century. However, the resulting "alternative levels of care" do not always sufficiently address psychosocial determinants of health, so what we are now emphasizing and *creating funds* to support are health optimization tactics that address the same issues previously eliminated by "medical necessity." Most believe that sufficient lengths of stay, coupled with immediately proximal intensive supports, improve community tenure. Economic scarcity, however, can have longer-term compensatory effects professionally and for the patient, resulting in innovation in treatment approaches.

Innovation in the Face of Scarcity: The Birth and Proliferation of Step-Down Services

Psychiatry and psychiatric hospitals have responded innovatively to the reductions in available beds for treatment. Several alternative levels of care provide intensive therapy while preparing patients for the transition to a real-world environment. Relevant current and important future design elements in the delivery of psychiatric intensive services have been and will be designed in the face of tightened inpatient medical necessity criteria. A number of step-down services have been developed, including the following:

- **Residential treatment and rehabilitative hospitalizations,** which are reserved for the most severe and incalcitrant of patients. In the past, longer-term residential programs were viewed as the pinnacle of psychiatric care. Today, self-funded or exclusionary insurance arrangements dominate the financing of such treatments. As a result, these venues treat only a fraction of the patients who might benefit from their services.
- **Day treatment,** which is often attached to inpatient psychiatric facilities. These services can also be accessed directly (not only as a step-down). Programming and medical monitoring are slated for a significant hour span each day. Staffed by attending physicians, therapists, and nurses, these day treatment facilities conduct psychiatric treatment in much the same way as inpatient units, except patients go home at night.

- **Intensive outpatient programs,** which accept direct admissions as well. These programs are structured to offer at least 5 days per week of care in smaller daily bundles of therapeutic hours.
- **Skilled nursing facilities,** which have recently taken on the position of the chronic, long-term-care institutions of the past. Patients residing in these facilities cannot be acutely psychotic, but they have problems and limitations to the degree that they require a supportive living and care environment.
- **In-home services,** which have been a part of the Medicaid benefit for years. Visiting nurses and supports are becoming more of the home care industry, and with the aging of the American population and the need for supports beyond family, these services will likely continue to grow. One of the many lessons of COVID-19 is that these services can be delivered successfully via electronic platforms. Psychiatric and psychological services can be dialed into an orchestrated array of electronic interventions.

What's Next? Updating Models With Outcomes-Producing Tactics

It is likely that there will be a strong need for these levels of care in any graduated continuum of care and that these models will be part of smart future design. Many of the tenets of collaborative care exist in these delivery constructs: the use of teams, multiple levels of expertise, and credentialed experts to provide orchestrated care to patients. Can even greater structure be inserted for team member roles, systematic case review, escalation, and high-fidelity clinical paths? An elemental gap analysis would be interesting to apply to these traditional constructs compared with the registry core of collaborative care management.

It is noteworthy that 70% of patients with diagnosable mental health conditions do not seek care from specialty behavioral health. The writing thus far has been applicable solely to the 30% of patients willing to separate themselves from the rest of medical care and go to a separate, often costly sector of the medical system. The unwillingness of 70% of patients to seek care in the behavioral sector is at least partially responsible for many ending up in jails and prisons. Outreach, improved understanding, and more "normalized" treatment settings (such as those in the medical sector) can all lead to improved detection, treatment, and maintenance.

Advancing New Models of Care: Improving Reach, Engagement, Impact, and Outcomes

Engineering for Proximal and Convenient Care

It has long been known that patients in primary care settings are not accurately recognized as having behavioral issues. When a diagnosis *is* made, the separateness, perceived stigma, and fear of seeing a psychiatrist make referral difficult. Key developments since 2000 reflect the increasing recognition that integrating behavioral and psychiatric services into medical treatment locations more often visited by patients makes tremendous sense. The entire medical-behavioral integration movement is built around this concept (Figure 29–2).

Engineering Critical Inputs, Outputs, and Outcomes: Key Considerations in Design

Increased access to funding and structures for operating (i.e., high-fidelity models) must exist for improved care to be sustainably realized. This high-fidelity performance aspect is, in fact, our best hope for creating a virtuous cycle of funding increase. Performance and outcomes can justify further creativity, and tests to improve outcomes yield even more as the benefit of our approaches and talent becomes more visible. Another unknown for most branches of medicine is the experience of high-fidelity operations and the expression of high-fidelity clinical maneuvers. As a group of providers, we tend to think and design "to the exceptions," allowing our fear of exceptions to prevent standards—or, in this case, high-fidelity pathways. We also have not embraced the reality that our *operational staff* are a part of the team. When both operations and clinical care exist on the same clinical and administrative team, a different type of shared duty begins to form. This performance environment, as well as an environment that embraces problem identification, is as important as any specification noted for the emerging models outlined later. Unfortunately, such operating aspects are not business as usual in health care or psychiatry. These "total team" models need to be developed and promulgated as clinical change occurs (Delizonna 2017).

Defining, Describing, and Communicating Patients' Conditions and Circumstances in Different Ways

Does overreliance on the disease model truncate behavioral interventions? Any psychiatrist trained in the past 30 years knows that DSM is a product of consensus committees (Möller 2018; Regier et al. 2013; van Heugten-van der Kloet and van Heugten 2015). DSM was an extraordinary advancement at inception, but does it need updating in approach and as a living tool? Many are rallying for a manual that is more frequently updated and includes a matrix of iteratively tested and refined tactics for key patient presentations and circumstances (e.g., use of dimensional rather than categorical diagnoses, many of which are poorly characterized by the primary diagnostic frames we have now). In a period of greater analytic power and real-time testing, is it possible to decrease the "uncontrollable" factors leading to poor outcomes or relapses? Many would argue that we have not tried very hard to test this approach, which is used exclusively in the highly successful software and electronics industries. The well-known physician, researcher, and author Atul Gawande, M.D., has written several books on adopting logical engineering techniques in health care while elevating the quality of therapeutic dialogue with patients (Gawande 2009, 2014).

Defined inputs can drive specific outputs. Professionally, we should be interested only in those outputs—whether alone or in constellation with other inputs—that create outcomes. We should embrace a broad view of potential interventions in order to customize what the patient needs. If, for example, housing appears to be the critical foundational failure in a patient's care, no-fail housing resources should be employed with the same certainty as any treatment. If proactive interventions are strung together with

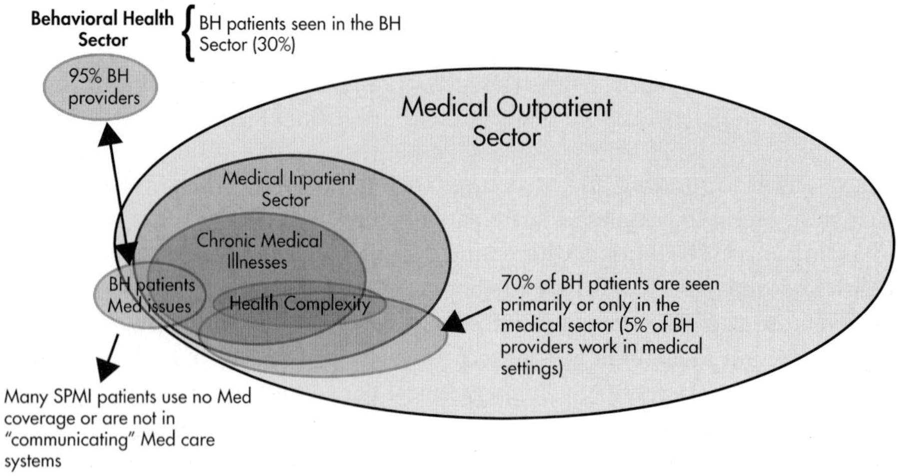

FIGURE 29–2. Where patients go for care.
To view this figure in color, see Plate 14 in Color Gallery.
BH=behavioral health; SPMI=severe and persistent mental illness. (Cartesian Solutions Inc. ©)

optimal inputs and insights, the patient becomes engaged, health is optimized longitudinally, and with tangible inputs, outputs, and outcomes, funding is far more likely.

Getting in Front of, Preventing, and Rapidly Responding to Disease: The Basics of Proactive Care

As a consequence of the new emerging models and constructs, proactive care can have significant impact on health maintenance and chronic condition management. *Proactive care* means that there is urgency in treating emerging conditions and in motivating patients to embrace (and, therefore deal with) their ailments and, oftentimes, their humanity. This is the same eyes-wide-open "conversion" experienced by persons in *true recovery*. Assistance and "motivational push" are all in scope and are actually part of our role in behavioral health. We have long abandoned the belief that providers should be hands-off on discharge planning to allow patients to develop self-reliance, because the data simply do not support this belief (Smith et al. 2017; Steffen et al. 2009).

As an example, patients who demonstrate elevated liver function test results, for example, come out of their behavioral health appointments and into the arms of staff who arrange same-day consultation at a hepatologist's office. Staff check to confirm whether the patient attended this important appointment, and the consultant uses a well-constructed, templated letter while assessing the patient that is sent to the referring clinic. Questions collaboratively prompt answers and allow the specialist to give efficient input on the advisability of continuing psychotropic medications, the suspected etiology of liver laboratory value elevations, and any other salient topics. An invitation to talk via phone is always included on our collaboration templates and yields a response rate of about 20% (beyond the specialist's written response). The outcome of such proximal, intensive case management is a near-100% turnaround in specialist collaboration within 2 days. The patient's treatment is continued or changed (with intensified next steps) in quick order. No patient begging or cajoling is needed in this patient-partnered, provider-collaborative process.

In the future, with proactive care delivery, higher levels of care, such as emergency services and inpatient treatment, might correspondingly *drop* as critical mass is achieved with outcomes-producing proactive care in the community. Would new, widespread proactive care really lead to a "bed surplus" rather than a bed shortage in future-world? This is speculative, and even hypothesizing may be dangerous given our professional *scarcity* experiences of the past. The bottom line is that we will continue to need whatever emerges as the next improved version of standard care delivery (e.g., inpatient psychiatric services in medical settings). The *venues* (locations) for these services and the *surrounding proactive and preventive services* may change the types of patients entering traditional specialty care, and some of the tasks applied also may need to change.

Moving Further Toward an Outcomes-Producing, Integrated Model of Care

Outpatient Treatment and Health Maintenance

Collaborative care (as described on the Advancing Integrated Mental Health Solutions website; https://aims.uw.edu) is a specific type of integrated care developed at the University of Washington that not only treats common mental health conditions, such as depression and anxiety, but also requires systematic follow-up because of the persistent nature of behavioral health conditions prior to symptom resolution. Based on principles of effective chronic illness care, collaborative care focuses on defined patient populations tracked in a registry, measurement-based practice, and treatment to target (Figure 29–3). In collaborative care, achievement of a PHQ-9 score less than 10 or a reduction in the PHQ-9 score by 50% over the span of 2 months would be an example of a "target." Trained primary care providers and embedded behavioral health professionals provide evidence-based medication and psychosocial treatments, supported by regular psychiatric case consultation and treatment adjustment for patients who are not improving as expected.

Collaborative care originated in a research culture and has now been tested in more than 80 randomized controlled trials in the United States and abroad. Several recent meta-analyses make it clear that collaborative care consistently improves upon care as usual and leads to better patient outcomes, better patient and provider satisfaction, improved functioning, and reductions in total medical and behavioral health care costs. It achieves the quadruple aim of health care reform. Collaborative care necessitates a practice change on multiple levels and is nothing short of a new way to practice medicine, but it works; patients get better when these techniques are applied with fidelity. However, there are qualifiers. In a Cochrane review, Archer et al. (2012) noted that clinical improvement with collaborative care lasted for 2 years (was persistent); however, Katzelnick and Williams (2015) noted high variability in outcomes and challenges in deploying collaborative care as the outcomes literature describes.

In what some see as interim steps toward appropriate funding, the Centers for Medicare & Medicaid Services approved the collaborative care Current Procedural Ter-

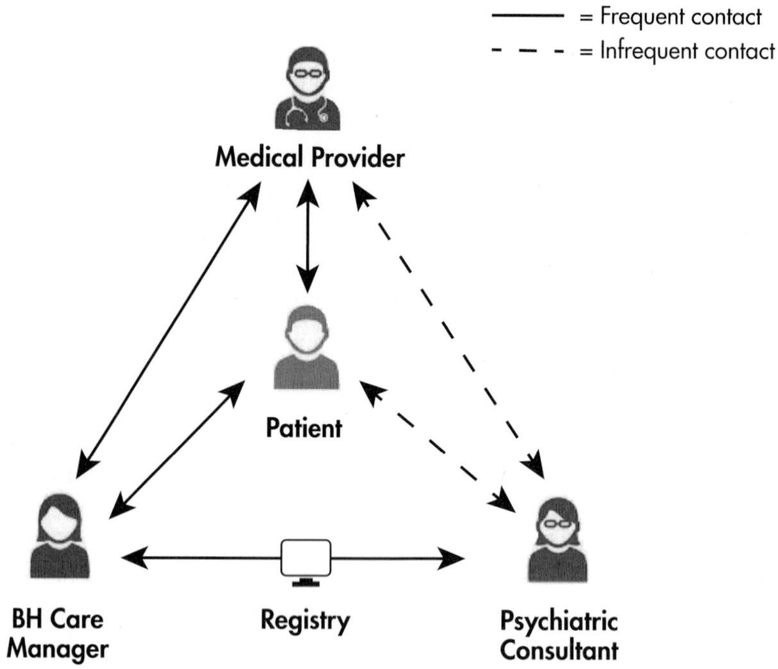

FIGURE 29–3. The collaborative care model pathways of care.
BH = behavioral health.

minology (CPT) codes for use as of January 1, 2018. Additionally, Medicare recognizes CPT codes that have been in existence for some time, which are known as "interprofessional codes" and include such activities as phone or electronic consultations with shared patients. Documentation and appropriate billing are required, and patients can be responsible for the bill if a deductible is part of their plan design. Although this represents a positive step forward, most agree that a myriad of complex CPT codes applied in the correct way is not a long-term solution. More eloquent funding models are needed.

The registry aspect of collaborative care and TeamCare is a key differential because systematic case review introduces an organized, dynamic review and escalation process headed by a psychiatrist. This core element, among several others, is speculated to create both clinical and financial results when manual-based collaborative care is initiated. TeamCare is a variant of collaborative care that incorporates integrated care management (Katon et al. 2010). For populations and clinics serving patients with complex health issues, including deficits in psychosocial supports, the addition of ICM can directly and acutely help health maintenance. Katon, when launching a series of pilot collaborative-care initiatives, noticed that psychosocial needs were significant for portions of several clinics' populations. ICM was added to the core clinic initiative (Kathol 2018), and this not only catalyzed clinical outcomes but also reduced expenditures in a shorter time frame.

Team-based care is a very broadly defined primary care and medical professional construct for managing chronicity and complexity in medical settings. A golden opportunity exists to structure behavioral interventions with key elements from collaborative care or TeamCare. The barriers are fewer and less "foreign" when brought in as add-ons or edits. Nonetheless, the engineering fidelity and behavioral health voices on the team *must be preserved* to ensure positive outcomes.

Medical Inpatient Care Constructs

In addition to traditional psychiatric facility–based inpatient care, *intensive psychiatric services provided in other inpatient facility venues* make good sense. Many Americans spend significant time in medical emergency departments, inpatient units, and outpatient clinics. Chronic disease burden has multiplied significantly over the years as health status has plummeted. Why not use the opportunity of these medical touchpoints to deliver psychiatric care? Data demonstrate improved recovery time and, as a consequence, better financial performance in our diagnosis-related group–based funding context.

Complexity intervention units and *medical psychiatric units* make tremendous sense by almost any yardstick. The increasing load of chronic medical conditions in the American populace, coupled with higher prevalence of depressive disorders with these conditions, is just one example of this perfect comanagement opportunity. Gaps exist between the medical complexity accepted by most psychiatric facilities and the psychiatric complexity that medical facilities feel comfortable treating. Often, patients receive little to no cross-disciplinary care in the separate medical and behavioral health inpatient settings. It is this "Whose patient is this?" conundrum that must be resolved. Data suggest that medical (and behavioral) inpatient population numbers and population characteristics justify the development of such units (Duffy et al. 2018; Jansen et al. 2019; Lobo et al. 2015).

Expertly determining which patients might be best served by psychiatric consultation requires *proactive psychiatric consultation*. Psychiatric consultations are commonly ordered near patient discharge. This timing is unfortunate because psychiatric recommendations are rarely followed when the consultation occurs the day before the patient leaves. Oldham et al. (2019) conducted a systematic review of the impact of proactive consultation on lengths of stay; their observations were similar and in line with those of Sledge et al. (2015) in that consultation was associated with reduced lengths of stay, enhanced staff satisfaction, and (in two studies) favorable return on investment. Sledge and colleagues also described other key elements of the behavioral intervention team conducting multidisciplinary proactive consultation:

1. A trusted and stable procedure for the screening of all medical admissions by a mental health professional through record and staff contacts
2. Rapid intervention from the behavioral intervention team that *anticipates* impending problems before a cascade effect in the hospitalization is triggered
3. Collaborative, multidisciplinary team engagement, with the medical team sharing the burden of care for a psychiatrically complex, medically ill inpatient and transmitting critical behavioral skills to all caregivers, including the ability to recognize patients who may benefit from a psychiatric consultation
4. Daily contact between the behavioral team and medical team so that treatment recommendations are effectively understood, enacted, and reinforced; ineffective treatments are discontinued; and new psychiatric problems are addressed before there are complicating consequences

Mentioned also was the helpful work of Kathol (2018) in defining complex patients and characterizing their needs.

Medical emergency department psychiatric interventions represent a gap like no other. It is fairly common to have very little psychiatric treatment applied in medical emergency departments, including medication, therapy, and individualized case management. At the same time, "sitter use" is so commonplace (unpaid by insurance and invisible) that it is not actually booked as a "cost of not providing psychiatric intervention." Providing intensive, behaviorally geared case management and psychiatric consultation with treatment or treatment recommendations (often delivered in smaller facilities via telemedicine platforms) can dramatically change emergency department patients' status and outcomes; the facility's emergency department throughputs; and the risks to patients, staff, and the facility.

Other Clinical Care Support Services

Telepsychiatry, and some very interesting email- and text-based therapies, were slowly gaining a foothold prior to the COVID pandemic but were catalyzed tremendously by the great need to provide care during the crisis. The American Psychiatric Association (2021) has published about the appropriate uses and methods for telepsychiatry in their Telepsychiatry Toolkit. The tool kit, used to bring a level of expertise impossible (or difficult) to supply, can dramatically change the bottlenecks that exist in medical emergency departments and other difficult-to-staff locations. As in all care, good program design is critical. The provider and health system should have high-fidelity clinical pathways, well-defined roles for both the telepsychiatrist and on-site staff, clear delineation of what is being delivered with the telepsychiatry tool, and realistic and implementable procedures for any emergency.

Value-based integrated case management is a commonsense tool that attempts to bridge many gaps in our system of care (Kathol 2018). Value-based ICM provides a step-by-step interdisciplinary approach for helping complex patients. This approach can maximize clinical and functional value while reducing health-related costs. Uniquely, a standardized complexity assessment grid and communication tool can help identify barriers to improvement in four domains: biological, psychological, social, and health system. Holistic care plans based on "anchored barriers" are monitored to document ongoing targeted outcomes.

Housing and psychosocial supports are part of value-based ICM. As noted in the earlier sections of this chapter, the principles set forth by Maslow define a hierarchy of needs. A gap in solutions is created when attempting to supply resources to those who have few. Is this the accountability of the city, county, state, or national government? Is it possible for health care financing institutions to fund these foundational "needs" so that patients' medical and behavioral health conditions can be more fully treated within and outside a hospital's walls? Some insurers contribute to trusts empowered to fund resources such as housing. The Pathways to Housing initiative, organized and facilitated by the Tarrant County Homeless Coalition, has a multiparty stakeholder mix that brings energy in several dimensions. Individual stakeholders bring expertise, services, and teamwork to the task of converting temporary housing into permanent arrangements (Office of Policy Development and Research 2019). "In situ" medical care by staff from the John Peter Smith Health System, psychiatric care from the state mental health system's local providers, and technical expertise, data, and low-barrier service funding by Amerigroup all contribute to improved patient outcomes. Other programs targeting individuals who do not have permanent housing have been successful in reducing hospitalizations while improving health status. This particular area of endeavor might provide a functional bridge to the communities in which we live and practice. Many communities are attempting to improve the health status of their citizens. Efforts along these lines, done in a citywide fashion, could pay dividends.

In a sense, value-based ICM creates a systematic intervention approach to "health care hotspotting" (Camden Coalition of Healthcare Providers 2016), a related activity coined and popularized by Dr. Jeffrey Brenner (Gawande 2011). Hotspotting alludes to an activity map that "lights up" (appears "hot") where a particular activity is more concentrated. High utilization of medical crisis services "lights up" when plotted geographically. This simple display can begin a process of analytic inquiry and the creation of targeted interventions. "Hot spots" correlate highly with a full array of psychiatric and psychological service needs. This approach is noteworthy because it illustrates how observation, curiosity, and creativity can come together simply by asking, "Why is that patient's chart so much thicker than the charts of others?" Dr. Brenner was in solo family practice, treating a significantly portioned Medicaid population, when he founded the Camden Coalition of Healthcare Providers. The techniques employed are very similar to those designed around the psychosocial interventions of proactive integrated consultation and value-based ICM.

Use of SWOT Analyses and Leveraging Perceived Threats as Opportunities

Psychiatry and mental health services have weathered multiple storms. Two notable hurricanes have been *financial* and *reputational* (which links to mental health literacy and society's understanding of what we do professionally). One approach to help better operationalize our profession's strengths and weakness in practice, including financing, and psychiatry's reputation—and potentially leverage these into learning opportunities—is use of a strengths-weaknesses-opportunities-threats (SWOT) analysis (Figure 29–4).

A clear *strength*, professionally, has been our innovation in the face of scarcity and adversity. Alternative facility-based levels of care, value-based ICM, collaborative care, TeamCare, proactive integrated consult services, and combined medical and behavioral inpatient units highlight just a few of the developments our profession has created or refined over the past 30 years. One obvious *weakness*, however, is the lack of a unified voice, philosophically and functionally, to advocate for both the 30% of patients seen in the behavioral health sector and the 70% of patients largely untreated for behavioral health issues in the medical sector. This lack of unified advocacy makes reference to what, at times, can be politicized positions around private versus public sector or biological versus psychosocial, but it largely has to do with the lack of understanding about models of care that include behavioral interventions and the competing medical and behavioral health dollars used for care by managed care organizations and MBHOs. From a functional perspective, well-engineered and tested integrated medical and behavioral treatments for the most part have not been implemented. How can we expect the public to understand what integrated medical and behavioral health

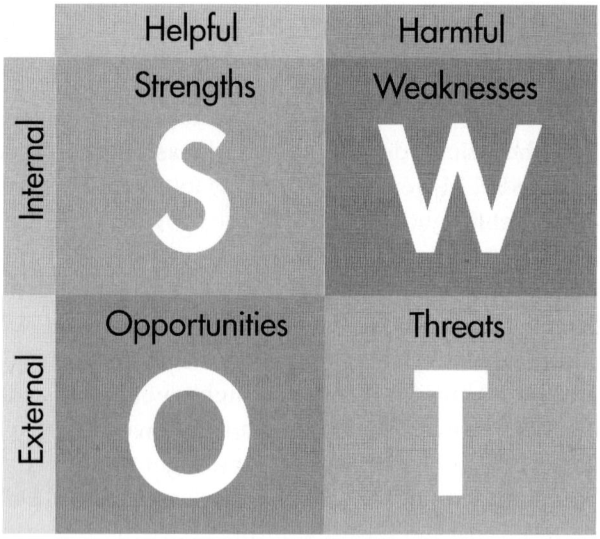

FIGURE 29–4. Components of a strengths-weaknesses-opportunities-threats (SWOT) analysis.
To view this figure in color, see Plate 15 in Color Gallery.

service delivery can do if we cannot institute effective unified medical and behavioral health payment procedures that would allow deployment of engineered, high-fidelity services? This lack of financial support for a best-standard approach to care needs to be understood and corrected for value-based services to be implemented. Dr. Gawande's paradigm-shifting work noted previously gives context to this phenomenon.

Threats continue to come in many forms, including those obvious and less obvious. Mental health literacy has improved, but misinformation remains a threat to the advocacy and support needed for the truly lifesaving activities applied to patients by our profession, especially in the medical setting. The perennial threat of insufficient financing impacts almost every level of design and functioning.

Economic scarcity has been so persistent that it has created a chronic disequilibrium. As in the old fable about a frog in boiling water, we have personally and professionally taken on the burden of unpaid services to the degree that it is now somewhat institutionalized. Individual heroism deserves celebration. Going above and beyond is what we all should aspire to when the times and situations arrive in our professional careers. We must be mindful that if these perspectives become woven into our standard operational procedures, we risk diluting the true picture of the resource needs of our patient populations. Our profession, unwittingly, can shift the burden of accountability from the supplier of resources to ourselves personally. This is a natural compensatory move related to years of scarcity and "back corner" status.

Consider this example: A surgeon would not attempt a heart transplant with the same sterile tray and staff used to remove a sebaceous cyst. Necessary tools and professional staff inputs are required (and accepted by payers and society) for a successful transplant procedure. Consider now the presentation of complex behavioral circumstances, such as a patient with childhood trauma, a major depressive disorder partially responsive to treatment, and continued substance misuse. These providers also need a "tray of tools," such as unhampered frequent visits, case management, the ability to apply dialectical behavior therapy (by the same provider or via a collaborative professional), team meetings, a simple way to advocate for work accommodations during the acute phase of treatments, and fluid access to facility care for significant downturns in treatment. With no-gap transitions and longitudinal case management, necessary resourcing would support outcomes and thus be available when required. Using these options should be as routine as ordering up several surgeons, multiple operating rooms and nursing staff, recovery, intensive care, and any other support required for the successful complex surgical outcome. The cost of multi-input behavioral care *at the highest extreme* is dwarfed in comparison. Further *downstream* multiyear savings in health expenditures and workplace impact (i.e., revenue) are magnitudes higher than those for many surgical procedures. Our own behavioral health professional "trauma" can hold us back from demanding what is required for successful outcomes. Multiple speeds in the funding throttle should reflect not only the setting (i.e., inpatient or outpatient) but also the number, type, and costs of inputs, regardless of patient location or setting/venue. It is our professional duty to make visible the necessary inputs and how they produce change and to provide the materials for improving society's mental health literacy. Funding will follow if citizens demand change.

One *relative* or *mixed threat* (i.e., having both threat and strength potential) is the highly democratized communication and advocacy platform of our times—most visibly represented by social media. How can communication possibly be a threat to a profession *founded on* communication? There has been an undeniable, increasing crescendo of promotional activities, presented in sound bites, both by the population at large and within professional circles. This rapid, uncontrolled, evangelical thought advocacy feels at times like a threat to both evidence-based innovation and a hierarchy that many are familiar with and able to navigate within. It is not an error that there is no "user's manual" for Twitter. The self-discovery and incremental mastery that come with frequent use, "likes," and retweets represent forms of facilitation (and barriers) in this new communication age. One's experimentation, trials, flops, and successes are on display for all.

We paint this backdrop to ask the following: Will medicine or health care delivery remain the same, or will it become more patient-convenient, patient-centric, innovative, and credential-independent? For various reasons, medicine needs to change. The *threat* of significant change can create *opportunity*. Patients (and members of society) are hungry for empowerment. Facilitating the journey to their objectives should be within our professional wheelhouse, and streamlined, democratized communication may change our image to one of a "helpful partner." Some of the new platforms of care delivery discussed (e.g., video chat, email, text) now exist. With refinement, might they become the preferred tools and venues for rapid, convenient communication and expert treatment in the future?

Recommendations for Moving Forward

To promote creativity broadly and expansively, we need more current research and effective models. Creativity will be required in order to improve adoption and the creation of new models of outcomes-producing care. Being reminded of successful models of care in the context of the principles discussed in the SWOT analyses earlier may assist with creative solutions.

1. **Involving communities, families, and patients as thought leaders, stakeholders, and advocates.** Can we jump into the democratized streams of communication to improve mental health literacy? The answer is "yes" if we create a sufficiently sized like-minded "interest group." The message must be clear, simple, visualizable, and patient-helpful and must "grab the spirit." Community involvement means not only use of social media but also stakeholder involvement in solutions designed in the communities at risk. Joint solutions avoid the "imperialistic" importation of solutions not embraced by the communities they target. Conversely, joint problem identification and joint solutions always improve the chances of success and sustainability.
2. **Changing both the approach and the eventual role of health plans and monolithic institutions.** This is the truest justice of all. No profit should be made, no power should be grabbed, off the backs of those who are at the root of the solutions. For examples, if communities come together to create a citywide, longitudinal case management program to improve patient community tenure and outcomes, that community—not the insurer—should reap the rewards for such effort. Dual-track arguments to states and employers can be compelling as a new generation of self-empowered advocates tackles social issues. The global issue of health finance can become quickly politicized. In whatever form budgets are to be arranged, they must support the behavioral/psychiatric inputs necessary to create the outputs that lead to improved outcomes and, where possible, cost reduction. Eliminating barriers and artificial silos of medical versus behavioral while creating a unified pool of resources, as well as mandating sufficient funding for outcomes-lined behavioral resources and treatments, must occur. As illustrated in Figure 29–5, updating would indicate a further evolution to a more integrated solution.
3. **Changing our conceptualization of human behavior and behavioral conditions.** Moving beyond the disease model and fully back to the biopsychosocial model of care makes tremendous sense. This frame resonates with the population at large. The "total person" frame also mirrors recent medical-side conceptualizations of chronic conditions, such as diabetes. Behavioral health professionals need to see and connect to the totality of a patient's needs, desires, and person for sustainable patient improvements. Remaining in polarized philosophies will not serve this goal well.
4. **Providing engineering and team solutions.** Designing techniques and treatments that are visible and understandable, produce outcomes, mitigate patient risk, and constantly and iteratively improve will be imperative. The patient and interested parties must visualize and understand how solutions will produce outcomes. If positioned correctly, ordinary citizens can become partners with medical and behavioral providers and administrators in iterative problem identification and solving. Treatments in these broad, integrated behavioral-medical settings are *their* solutions. We as providers are the custodians of foundational knowledge and human dynamics. Bringing operational flows and professional inputs together fits the reality of how care is delivered. Best practices done "the same way each time" is an

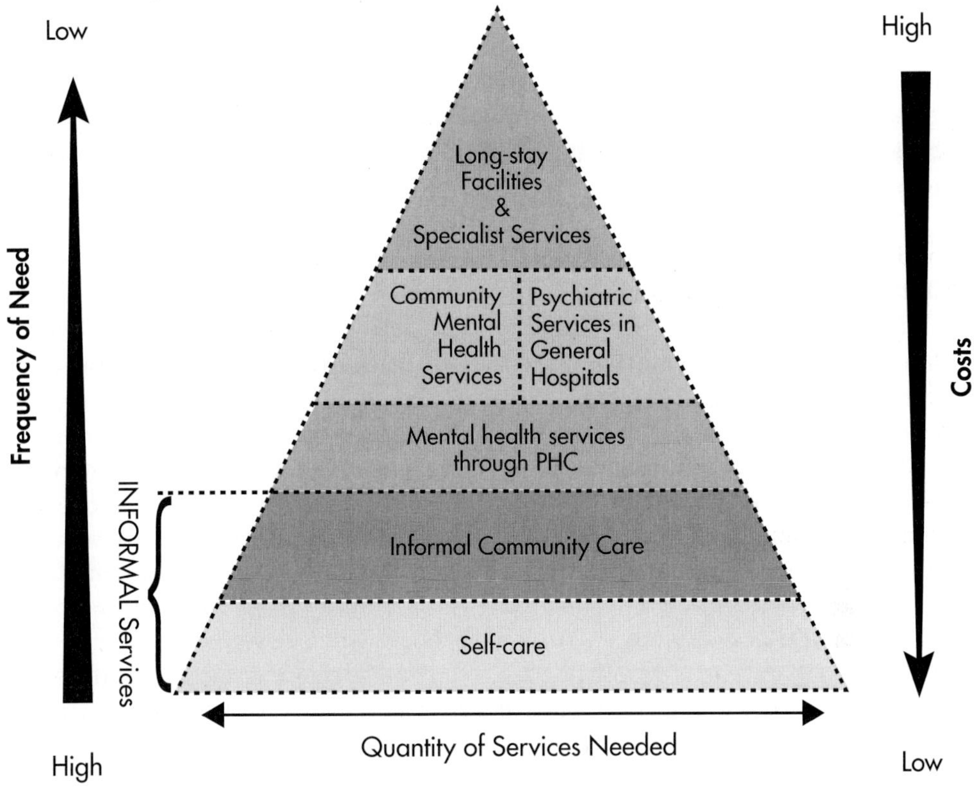

FIGURE 29–5. World Health Organization's optimal mix of services pyramid.
PHC=primary health care.
To view this figure in color, see Plate 16 in Color Gallery.

attainable goal if exception paths are well defined and used as learning experiences. Our personal perfectionism sometimes prevents rigorous critical examination of what we do on a day-to-day basis. This same trait can prevent us from full team participation. The successful models of integrated care mentioned in this chapter are examples of engineered solutions.

5. **Focusing our professional assets and attributes for the future.** Redefining professionalism as technique fidelity rather than blind individualism will change much that challenges the medical profession and will be necessary as we attempt to establish best practices. We must come together as a profession on these standards or risk fragmented, unreliable outcomes attached to our professional identities. Considering ourselves to be members of several teams, including the "big team" of the psychiatric profession, is a critical anchor. Being a contributing team member, and potentially leading teams, is a skill we need to learn. Other professions have recognized the importance of this perspective, as illustrated in Lencioni's *The Five Dysfunctions of a Team* (Lencioni 2002). The ability to negotiate without undue compromise is another skill of great importance in moving forward in a multistakeholder environment. Fisher and Ury (1981), in the book *Getting to Yes*, described this approach in great detail. We should serve as entrepreneurs, not simply with sound bites and slogans but with incremental, rapid, iterative contributions to

improved, replicable processes and techniques. To do less in the consumer-driven world of the future will surely erode the impact of those with the greatest ability to help. Promoting personal leadership in high-functioning teams (even if following and not leading) will be incredibly catalytic to continuously improving patient care. As a tangible next step, advocacy for the application of the models of team-based integrated care (to high-fidelity standards) can create an experiential bedrock for future creativity.

Conclusion

We are facing challenges to the status quo in a way never experienced, but this presents a great opportunity to lead this charge as psychiatrists. In the historic account of hospitals (both medical and psychiatric), wellness-oriented sanatoriums were oriented toward the mind and body. Will we, in many dimensions, circle back to these principles of the past? It certainly makes sense that we consider such a move to improve our collective health and well-being.

References

American Psychiatric Association: Telepsychiatry Toolkit (online). Washington, DC, American Psychiatric Association, 2021. Available at: www.psychiatry.org/psychiatrists/practice/telepsychiatry/toolkit.

Archer J, Bower P, Gilbody S, et al: Collaborative care for depression and anxiety problems. Cochrane Database Syst Rev 10:CD006525, 2012 23076925

Bhugra D, Tasman A, Pathare S, et al: The WPA-Lancet Psychiatry Commission on the Future of Psychiatry. Lancet Psychiatry 4(10):775–818, 2017 28946952

Camden Coalition of Healthcare Providers: Healthcare Hotspotting (online). Camden NJ, Camden Coalition of Healthcare Providers, 2016. Available at: https://hotspotting.camdenhealth.org.

Delizonna L: High-performing teams need psychological safety. Here's how to create it. Harvard Business Review, August 24, 2017. Available at: https://hbr.org/2017/08/high-performing-teams-need-psychological-safety-heres-how-to-create-it.

Duffy RM, Sadlier M, Van Der Ploeg AH, Sheehan J: The case for shared medical and psychiatric units: are they needed and how they could run? Ir Med J 111(9):823, 2018 30556671

Fisher R, Ury WL: Getting to Yes. New York, Penguin, 1981

Gawande A: The Checklist Manifesto. New York, Henry Holt, 2009

Gawande A: The Hot Spotters. The New Yorker, January 16, 2011. Available at: www.newyorker.com/magazine/2011/01/24/the-hot-spotters.

Gawande A: Being Mortal: Medicine and What Matters in the End. New York, Henry Holt, 2014

Jansen L, Hunnik F, Busschbach JJV, Lijmer JG: Measuring outcomes on a medical psychiatric unit: HoNOS, CANSAS and costs. Psychiatry Res 280:112526, 2019 31445422

Kathol R: The Integrated Case Management Manual: Value-Based Assistance to Complex Medical and Behavioral Patients, 2nd Edition. Berlin, Springer, 2018

Katon WJ, Lin EH, Von Korff M, et al: Collaborative care for patients with depression and chronic illnesses. N Engl J Med 363(27):2611–2620, 2010 21190455

Katzelnick DJ, Williams MD: Large-scale dissemination of collaborative care and implications for psychiatry. Psychiatr Serv 66(9):904–906, 2015 26030320

Lencioni P: The Five Dysfunctions of a Team. New York, Jossey-Bass, 2002

Lobo E, Ventura T, Navio M, et al: Identification of components of health complexity on internal medicine units by means of the INTERMED method. Int J Clin Pract 69(11):1377–1386, 2015 26271926

Manderscheid R, Kathol R: Fostering sustainable, integrated medical and behavioral health services in medical settings. Ann Intern Med 160(1):61–65, 2014 24573665

Melek S, Norris DT, Paulus J, et al: Potential Economic Impact of Integrated Medical-Behavioral Healthcare: Updated Projections for 2017. Seattle, WA, Milliman, 2018. Available at: www.milliman.com/en/insight/potential-economic-impact-of-integrated-medical-behavioral-healthcare-updated-projections. Accessed DATE.

Mitchell EM: Concentration of health expenditures and selected characteristics of high spenders, U.S. civilian noninstitutionalized population, 2016, in Statistical Brief (Medical Expenditure Panel Survey). Rockville, MD, Agency for Healthcare Research and Quality, 2001

Möller HJ: Possibilities and limitations of DSM-5 in improving the classification and diagnosis of mental disorders. Psychiatr Pol 52(4):611–628, 2018 30368532

Office of Policy Development and Research: Housing is healthcare for homeless patients in Tarrant County, Texas. HUD User, 2019. Available at: www.huduser.gov/portal/casestudies/study-072919.html. Accessed DATE.

Oldham MA, Chahal K, Lee HB: A systematic review of proactive psychiatric consultation on hospital length of stay. Gen Hosp Psychiatry 60:120–126, 2019 31404826

Regier DA, Kuhl EA, Kupfer DJ: The DSM-5: classification and criteria changes. World Psychiatry 12(2):92–98, 2013 23737408

Sledge WH, Gueorguieva R, Desan P, et al: Multidisciplinary proactive psychiatric consultation service: impact on length of stay for medical inpatients. Psychother Psychosom 84(4):208–216, 2015 26022134

Smith TE, Abraham M, Bolotnikova NV, et al: Psychiatric inpatient discharge planning practices and attendance at aftercare appointments. Psychiatr Serv 68(1):92–95, 2017 27582241

Steffen S, Kösters M, Becker T, Puschner B: Discharge planning in mental health care: a systematic review of the recent literature. Acta Psychiatr Scand 120(1):1–9, 2009 19486329

van Heugten-van der Kloet D, van Heugten T: The classification of psychiatric disorders according to DSM-5 deserves an internationally standardized psychological test battery on symptom level. Front Psychol 6:1108, 2015 26300808

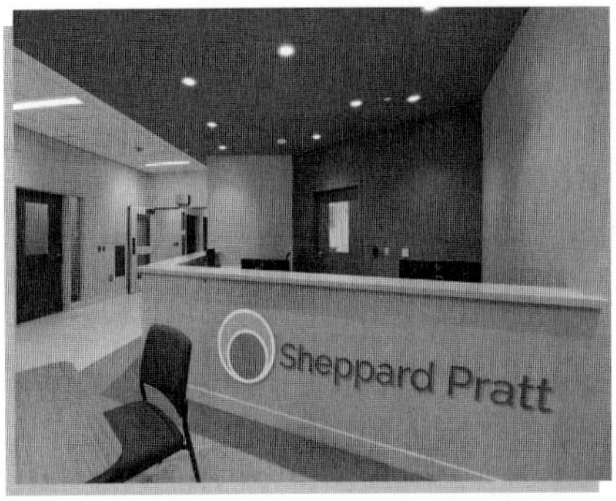

CHAPTER 30

The Future of Hospital Psychiatry

Harsh K. Trivedi, M.D., M.B.A.
Jennifer Weiss Wilkerson, M.H.S.A., FACHE
Thomas Glenn, M.S.F.

Over the past decade, the United States health care system has undergone immense change because of new technologies, better understanding of disease conditions, and pressure to reduce rising costs of care. The COVID-19 pandemic is accelerating change in health care, and most predict that life will never quite return to what it was during the pre-COVID days. Although much of the early focus has gone to respirators and personal protective equipment, the prolonged nature of the pandemic means that lasting mental health impacts will be seen through rising suicide rates, overdose deaths, and mental health sequelae of COVID-related stressors. No other field has as much potential to improve the health and well-being of society at large, which means significant attention will turn to us in the search for substantive, progressive change, and a potentially critical eye will seek the things that do not work well. With this call to action, either the field of mental health care will make meaningful advances or disruptive forces will consume the few areas in which there is still some margin to be had.

Although many aspects of hospital psychiatry are unique to the specialty, the field is undeniably impacted by broader changes in the health care landscape. In general, recent trends in health care that are pertinent include the following:

- **Shrinking inpatient capacity and emphasis on outpatient treatment.** As a result of cost-saving efforts, modern health care has placed an emphasis on reducing or avoiding inpatient stays and effectively treating conditions in outpatient settings. As mild and moderate cases are better managed outside the hospital, inpatient settings are pressed to specialize (Eastaugh 2015). A combination of financial pressures, a shrinking supply of doctors, and growing patient demand for services will lead to different types of workforce and optimization of care coordination (Wishner and Burton 2017). Patients beginning their health care journey with an inpatient stay will see shorter lengths of stay, and case managers will actively work to decrease readmissions along with the high costs associated with them.
- **Value-based care and new reimbursement models.** Commercial and government payers have increasingly favored reimbursement models that prioritize value over volume. In a reversal of fee-for-service models, value-based care and similar models often entail lump-sum payments for a patient's care journey, with payments scaling according to the efficacy and quality of care provided. Other alternative payment models emphasize lowering patient costs of care by incentivizing reductions in potentially avoidable utilization.
- **Focus on populations and social determinants of health.** Traditionally tasked with addressing medical needs of patients, health systems have begun to probe the underlying issues within their patients' communities. Social factors, such as economic stability, education, and food security, have been shown to play a major role in health outcomes from one community to another (Braveman and Gottlieb 2014). In an effort to reduce local socioeconomic disparities, many health systems are implementing creative community-based programs, including fresh food deliveries, job training courses, and housing initiatives.
- **Partnerships and systemization.** Seeking economies of scale, health systems are blazing toward horizontal integration through mergers and acquisitions as independent hospitals dwindle in number (Kacik 2019). Some health systems choose to pursue vertical integration by moving into new aspects of health care, such as surgery centers, senior living facilities, urgent care centers, and insurance plans. The need to capture more components of the patient care continuum drives further consolidation. In cases in which direct acquisition is not feasible, partnerships fill in missing service gaps and create new opportunities.
- **New technologies and competition.** Devices continue to creep into every aspect of daily living for health monitoring, automating the home, and collecting a plethora of data to feed artificial intelligence engines. Telehealth in particular has increased access, expanding providers' reach and better catering to patients' preferences of when and where to see their providers. Data analytics tools in health care aid medical image processing, early disease detection, and selection of treatment protocols (Davenport and Kalakota 2019). Biotech and scientific research continue to uncover novel treatments, while direct-to-consumer advertising helps create markets for products of marginal health benefit. When profitable, new entrants will take advantage of these emerging technologies to redefine entire aspects of the health care market.
- **Consumerism.** As technologies trend toward convenience and bringing care closer to home, consumers have more choices than ever for seeking care, including from big-name brands not typically associated with health care. A rise in virtual con-

sultations, online therapy, and modifications to existing retail space will surely continue to open up new doors. Walmart, Walgreens, and Amazon have already made their first forays into primary care, creating referral networks linked through employee benefit models, and although some such as Haven have not fared so well in this complex landscape, the sheer size of the health care market will attract many more disruptors. The solutions that cater to the needs and preferences of the patients will win the day. Those who lag in adapting or do not evolve quickly enough will be left behind.

- **Lasting impacts of the COVID-19 pandemic.** At the time of this writing, the COVID-19 pandemic is still ongoing and is already regarded as the defining health-related event of the century (Farzan et al. 2020). Because society hopes to avoid another health crisis of such scale, its collective response to this event is likely to define health care for decades to come. In March 2020, individual insurance claims for telehealth jumped 4,347% as compared with the same month the previous year (Gelburd 2020). Going forward, we can expect an increased focus on sanitation and supply chain security and an enduring prominence of telehealth.

The Role of Hospital Psychiatry

There is a significant role for psychiatric hospitals and psychiatric units in general hospitals in meeting mental health needs nationally. The impact of the COVID-19 pandemic on mental health and predicted increases in suicides and overdoses will only exacerbate availability and access issues for inpatient psychiatric beds. The Well Being Trust has projected 75,000 additional mortalities from mental health sequelae due to COVID (Petterson et al. 2020)—these are in addition to the nearly 70,000 deaths from overdoses and nearly 50,000 deaths by suicide annually as reported by the Centers for Disease Control and Prevention (2020a, 2020b; Petterson et al. 2020).

We fundamentally believe that through the work of behavioral health integration, greater understanding of the impact of untreated and undertreated mental health on health outcomes, and the national need to better manage spiraling health care costs, psychiatric care will be thrust forward for the integral role it plays in overall health and as a driver of reducing the total cost of care. As these shifts occur, we are confident that a new national resource will emerge: the role of a specialty psychiatric hospital such as Sheppard Pratt. This comprehensive national resource will be a beacon of hope and a guiding force for best practice implementation, similar to the role of a specialty cancer hospital, a specialty orthopedic hospital, or a specialty cardiac hospital. Throughout the nation, a handful of dedicated comprehensive specialty psychiatric hospitals will emerge that are expert at managing all diagnoses, for all comers, with a comprehensive continuum of services and able to manage the most complex cases in the nation.

There will also be growth of inpatient psychiatric units in general hospitals. As with other hospital-based services, there will be a greater emphasis on developing well-functioning verticals that can track with the patient's care journey and help to move meaningful outcomes and better overall health. As these verticals form, greater collaboration will occur among nontypical partners and, we hope, between hospitals and local community providers. The focus will increasingly be on population health and impacting social determinants in local communities. This will also include a vertical for crisis assessment services that spans emergency departments, urgent care centers, crisis centers, and mobile crisis programs. We already see some health systems that are implementing their own mobile crisis teams and partnering with ride-sharing companies to ensure that an appropriate care team can meet patients in the setting most comfortable for them. Virtual crisis assessment clinics provide another resource for patients to connect with professionals in order to determine an appropriate course of treatment.

At the time of this writing, the worldwide COVID-19 pandemic is in full swing. The coming months will help better define the winning strategies and provide greater perspective on the lessons learned. What we know is that the disease was quick to disrupt global society and will have long-lasting social, emotional, and economic impacts. The future is uncertain and will remain so for the coming years. There will be greater environmental and social impacts on health care. Whether severe weather, racial health disparities, the next global pandemic, or disruptions in our global supply chain for personal protective equipment, health care and behavioral health will be more impacted by these external forces.

Much of the change that has resulted from COVID was likely to have occurred anyway, but the pace of change has only accelerated. Perhaps the most notable change is the shift in location of care, not only from inpatient to outpatient but also to care at home. The post-COVID recovery period will be marked by continued financial stressors and a deeper emphasis on cost control with reduction in capital spending. Those organizations that performed well during COVID will hit the ground running and will be better poised to evolving to new realities and new opportunities. In addition to the shift in location of care, the patient has also experienced the benefits of greater scheduling flexibility and care delivered to the comfort of home. Patients will want more on-demand services and will resist returning exactly to how things worked pre-COVID.

Going forward, organizations will be expected to pivot quickly to respond to future crises. Health care systems of the future must be able to adjust quickly to the first signs of incoming emergencies. Hospitals will need to ensure functionality in supply chains to the best of their ability and be able to think of creative solutions if those chains break down. Successful organizations were able to implement social distancing measures, develop new care protocols, and rapidly expand telehealth capacity. This operational flexibility will be the hallmark of emergency action plans for years to come.

Technology Cures for All

Traditionally, outpatient community mental health providers, medication management appointments, and primary care offices have been the destinations for routine care and ongoing treatment. However, ongoing advances in telepsychiatry and video-based medication-assisted treatment (teleMAT) demonstrate the potential to continue evolving the care delivery system. Whether through online therapy services or a video appointment with providers sitting in traditional settings, individuals struggling with mental illness have more access than ever, assuming they have access to a stable internet connection. In the same vein, technology-enabled medication adherence aims to ensure patients are taking their medications as recommended, while long-acting injectables provide long-term solutions for patients who have traditionally struggled with daily pill intake.

Drug overdoses have spiked even as individuals struggle to remain off substances (Mann 2020). Chief among recent viable technology is the practice of telemedicine and teleMAT for substance use disorders. Telepsychiatry has proved effective as a means of therapy, medication management, and group-based work (Hubley et al. 2016). In community and hospital settings, videoconferencing can extend the capacity for providers to care for patients and convey clinical knowledge. Patients in rural communities can benefit from direct conversation with a specialist located miles away, while their local provider facilitates a warm handoff to the next level of care. Individuals with opioid dependency demonstrate higher retention when receiving teleMAT services than when receiving the same services in person (Eibl et al. 2017). Some providers prefer in-person patient consultation, but the technology's usefulness is undeniable. Virtual health care companies have already established a market by providing access to licensed providers through smartphone applications (apps).

An equally accessible form of technology comes in the form of smartphone apps. There is no telling what the smartphone of 2030 will look like, but it is certain to be able to access mental health solutions. In addition to being conduits for telepsychiatry, applications will dictate the interface through which patients and providers interact. Consumer-facing products will offer direct tools, often with no interaction with a provider or an office visit. This includes automated bots that send daily affirmations and manualized therapies such as cognitive-behavioral therapy delivered through an app (and without a provider). On the provider side, the percentage of acute care hospitals that adopted an electronic health record rose from 9.4% in 2008 to 83.8% in 2015 (Henry et al. 2016). We will see a similar adoption of patient portals across practices. As this occurs, these will take on increasing responsibility for managing patient workflows, data collection, and claims processing. We will also see greater utilization of e-solutions for basic items such as scheduling patient appointments, billing for services rendered, and collecting electronic payments.

Patient data will form the bedrock for patient care quality, outcomes measurement, and cost analysis. The most cost-effective means of treating disease states over the long term will become the future best practices of care. A concern is that health systems are slow to adopt changes in their information technology structures, and data security will be an ever-present concern in the years to come. Despite these challenges, longitudinal access to patients' care journeys will feed machine learning algorithms and power artificial intelligence tools. These systems will be able to detect crises from user data and seamlessly facilitate appropriate care. Genetic testing opens up a world of possibilities for early disease detection and pharmaceutical efficacy on a personalized basis. Wearable devices and internet-connected appliances, such as Wi-Fi scales and smart refrigerators, will feed data to systems capable of responding to patients' needs before they become critical health issues.

Specialization, Diversification, and the Need to Swim Upstream

As a direct result of the pandemic and subsequent social distancing, behavioral health issues will reach greater levels of urgency. Greater awareness of mental health issues and younger generations being more willing to openly talk about their mental health will help people understand that *mental health* is not a vanilla term. People will understand and demand specific and efficacious treatment for their depression, obsessive-compulsive disorder, or PTSD from the outset. Programs will be defined more by type of population served than by age group or level of care, which will allow for greater cross-program comparison of outcomes.

An area of focus will need to be treatment-resistant or difficult-to-treat conditions. Although many individuals with major depressive disorders have benefited from antidepressant treatment, 10%–30% show partial or no improvement (Al-Harbi 2012) and often demonstrate a decline in physical health, increased health care utilization, and increased suicidality. In response to these challenges, the field of treatment-resistant depression continues to be explored in new ways. Neurostimulation, including transcranial magnetic stimulation, electroconvulsive therapy, and vagus nerve stimulation, demonstrates promise in offering respite from an otherwise persistent condition. Emerging pharmaceutical treatments, such as ketamine and psilocybin, offer additional hope to individuals with difficult-to-treat depression.

There will also need to be greater diversification of service availability. It will no longer be viable for a provider to only be in the acute detox space or to rely on simply one funding stream. Diversification will be seen as a hedge to fiscal uncertainty. Not relying too much on any one payer or type of service means that psychiatric services will achieve greater sustainability, particularly by having a more diverse set of programs and increasing the scale of services provided.

As advances occur in all of these areas, basic questions will need to be tackled regarding underpayment for psychiatric services compared with other medical specialties, discriminatory reimbursement policies, and insurance abuses. From mental health parity violations, to unilaterally redefining medical necessity criteria, to limiting access through phantom networks—insurers will need to be held accountable. There will also be a need to swim upstream to where the payment is first received. Clinically integrated networks, accountable care organizations, capitation, and value-based payment arrangements will require providers to work themselves higher up the food chain before administrative and overhead expenses are taken out. They will also require providers to have more robust data management capacity and better ability to manage risk and to follow the patient's care journey longitudinally over time and vertically across levels of care.

The Graying of America and Its Workforce

Our nation is aging. This will lead to an increased burden of multiple chronic diseases within individual patients. As the U.S. population ages, the number of chronic diseases will also increase dramatically. Individuals with chronic diseases, such as congestive heart failure, chronic obstructive pulmonary disease, and diabetes, are also dealing with depression and anxiety (Turner and Kelly 2000). The impact of disease burden and poorer health outcomes in those with increasing numbers of chronic diseases yields the need for more efficacious chronic disease management. This is one area in which value-based contracting may take hold more quickly due to the significant opportunity to reduce potential health care costs. Dementia and delirium are hallmark issues in geriatric psychiatry, and an aging population will only drive future demand for treatment. Elderly patients with behavioral issues are often shunned from nursing homes. More effective solutions will be needed for elder care and for managing those with behavioral issues within long-term-care settings.

Likewise, as providers leave the workforce, there will need to be an even greater emphasis on the workforce of the future. What activities can be completed by an unlicensed, even nonclinical, worker? How can we train the next generation of providers in every discipline? Who will be the psychiatrists of tomorrow? How do we ensure racial and ethnic equity and train those from communities of color? Substantial, deliberate, and meaningful work will need to be done to meet these needs.

The Future Is for Our Children

At the intersection of neurology and psychiatry, neuropsychiatry plays an important role in the evaluation of complex brain-based diseases. With hospitals serving as the hub for treatment and referrals, new centers of excellence are emerging as sites for initial evaluation of diseases related to brain and behavior. Traditionally linked with memory disorders, Parkinson's disease, and stroke care, neuropsychiatry also finds crucial links to diagnosis and treatment of autism spectrum disorders (Zwick 2017). Attention in this area will be bimodal: the ability to identify, diagnose, and begin treating kids at younger ages will be a focus because it predicts better outcomes. Likewise, the aging of individuals with autism will lead to a middle-aged cohort and increasing needs for older adults with autism.

The number of children and adolescents presenting for emergency consultations increased nearly fourfold between 1981 and 2017 (Benarous et al. 2019). Although fewer of these consultations resulted in inpatient admissions, it is clear that youth will continue to seek care at a hospital when other treatment options are not immediately available in their community. Growing knowledge of the impacts of childhood trauma on the development of psychiatric issues will continue to fuel a rise in trauma-informed care, particularly for youth admissions. Youth struggling with behavioral challenges may find themselves receiving care through partial hospitalization and intensive outpatient programs.

Conclusion

Although there is much uncertainty in our world at this moment in time, periods of tremendous change are also marked by incredible opportunities. We can either succumb to external forces or define our strategic path forward. Our patients need us to put our professional passion into yielding greater access, better care, and improved outcomes. There is a bright future for hospital psychiatry, and we look forward to documenting the advances on the horizon in future editions of this textbook. We hope that you will utilize the knowledge and insights contained herein and work as we do each day to make the impossible truly possible.

References

Al-Harbi KS: Treatment-resistant depression: therapeutic trends, challenges, and future directions. Patient Prefer Adherence 6:369–388, 2012 22654508

Benarous X, Milhiet V, Oppetit A, et al: Changes in the use of emergency care for the youth with mental health problems over decades: a repeated cross sectional study. Front Psychiatry 10:26, 2019 30787886

Braveman P, Gottlieb L: The social determinants of health: it's time to consider the causes of the causes. Public Health Rep 129 (suppl 2):19–31, 2014 24385661

Centers for Disease Control and Prevention: About Underlying Cause of Death, 1999–2020. Atlanta, GA, Centers for Disease Control and Prevention, 2020a. Available at: https://wonder.cdc.gov/controller/saved/D76/D123F347. Accessed August 25, 2020.

Centers for Disease Control and Prevention: Drug Overdose Deaths (online). Atlanta, GA, Centers for Disease Control and Prevention, 2020b. Available at: www.cdc.gov/drugoverdose/data/statedeaths.html. Accessed August 25, 2020.

Davenport T, Kalakota R: The potential for artificial intelligence in healthcare. Future Healthc J 6(2):94–98, 2019 31363513

Eastaugh SR: Hospital specialization: benefits-focused product line planning. J Health Care Finance 41(3):1–9, 2015

Eibl JK, Gauthier G, Pellegrini D, et al: The effectiveness of telemedicine-delivered opioid agonist therapy in a supervised clinical setting. Drug Alcohol Depend 176:133–138, 2017 28535455

Farzan AN, Hassan J, Bellware K, et al: U.S. was 'unprepared' for 'greatest public health crisis' in a century, CDC director says. Washington Post, August 13, 2020. Available at: www.washingtonpost.com/nation/2020/08/13/coronavirus-covid-live-updates-us. Accessed August 20, 2020.

Gelburd R: The coronavirus pandemic and the transformation of telehealth. U.S. News and World Report, June 2, 2020. Available at: www.usnews.com/news/healthiest-communities/articles/2020-06-02/covid-19-and-the-transformation-of-telehealth. Accessed August 20, 2020.

Henry J, Pylypchuck Y, Searcy T, Patel V: Adoption of electronic health record systems among U.S. non-federal acute care hospitals: 2008–2015. ONC Data Brief, May 2016. Available at: https://dashboard.healthit.gov/evaluations/data-briefs/non-federal-acute-care-hospital-ehr-adoption-2008-2015.php. Accessed August 25, 2020.

Hubley S, Lynch SB, Schneck C, et al: Review of key telepsychiatry outcomes. World J Psychiatry 6(2):269–282, 2016 27354970

Kacik A: Fewer independent hospitals can weather operating headwinds. Modern Healthcare, February 23, 2019. Available at: www.modernhealthcare.com/article/20190223/NEWS/190229993/fewer-independent-hospitals-can-weather-operating-headwinds. Accessed August 28, 2020.

Mann B: U.S. sees deadly drug overdose spike during pandemic. NPR, August 13, 2020. Available at: www.npr.org/sections/coronavirus-live-updates/2020/08/13/901627189/u-s-sees-deadly drug-overdose-spike-during-pandemic. Accessed August 26, 2020.

Petterson S, Westfall JM, Miller BF: Projected Deaths of Despair From COVID-19. Oakland, CA, Well Being Trust, 2020. Available at: https://wellbeingtrust.org/wp-content/uploads/2020/05/WBT_Deaths-of-Despair_COVID-19-FINAL-FINAL.pdf. Accessed August 26, 2020.

Turner J, Kelly B: Emotional dimensions of chronic disease. West J Med 172(2):124–128, 2000 10693376

Wishner JB, Burton RA: How Have Providers Responded to the Increased Demand for Health Care Under the Affordable Care Act? Washington, DC, Urban Institute, 2017. Available at: www.urban.org/sites/default/files/publication/94396/2001576-how-have-providers-responded-to-the-increased-demand-for-health-care-under-the-affordble-care-act_0.pdf. Accessed August 27, 2020.

Zwick GP: Neuropsychological assessment in autism spectrum disorder and related conditions. Dialogues Clin Neurosci 19(4):373–379, 2017 29398932

Index

Page numbers printed in **boldface** *type refer to tables or figures.*

ABC (antecedent-behavior-consequence) analysis, 167, 171
Abnormal Involuntary Movement Scale (AIMS), **72**
Abstinence, and substance use disorders, 259, 281–282
Acceptance and commitment therapy (ACT), 199, 201
Access, to mental health care
  as critical issue, xxv
  emergency departments and, 399
  quality in psychiatry and, 452
Accreditation, of state hospitals, 300–301
Acetylcholinesterase inhibitors, 128
Activities of daily living (ADLs), and geriatric patients, 117, 135. *See also* Instrumental activities of daily living
Acute units, in state hospitals, 293
Adaptation to Mental Health and Addictive Disorders: Improving the Quality of Health Care for Mental and Substance-Use Conditions (Institute of Medicine 2006), 484
Adaptive functioning, and intellectual disability, 154
Addictive personality, concept of preexisting, 258
Adherence, to medication
  adult crisis stabilization unit and, 98–99
  psychotic disorders unit and, 238–239
Administration. *See also* Finances; Leadership; Quality; Risk management
  corporate governance and, 415–416
  corporate structure and, 411–415
  funding of psychiatric services and, 417
  health care operations and functions of, 426, 427
  organizational structure and, 419–423
  prevention of violence and, 481–482, 483–484, 491–497
  required hospital reporting and, 416–417
  translating strategy into action, 417–419
  trauma-informed systems of care and, 486–491
Admission criteria. *See also* Involuntary admissions
  adolescent unit and, 68–69
  adult crisis stabilization unit and, 88–89
  child unit and, 48
  developmental disabilities co-occurring unit and, 164–167
  forensic unit and, 212–213
  geriatric unit and, 114
  psychotic disorders unit and, 232–233
  residential treatment and, 383–384
  substance use disorders co-occurring unit and, 266–267
Adolescent(s). *See also* Adolescent unit
  frequency of admission to private psychiatric hospitals, 436
  increase in emergency consultations for, 631
  residential treatment centers for, 357
  social workers and care for, 561–565
  state hospitals and, 297
Adolescent unit
  admission criteria for, 68–69
  assessment and, 69–72
  biopsychosocial formulation and treatment planning, 72
  current trends in, 68
  discharge planning and, 81–82
  family therapy and psychoeducation, 78–79
  future directions and, 82–83
  group therapy and, 77–78
  individual therapy and, 76–77
  management of aggressive and suicidal behaviors in, 80–81
  milieu therapy and, 79–80
  psychotherapy and, 75–76, **77**
  psychotropic medication and, 72–75
Adult crisis stabilization unit
  criteria for admission to, 88–89
  diagnostic workup in, 90–96
  discharge planning and, 103–104, 106
  family as partner in treatment, 90
  goals of treatment in, 96

Adult crisis stabilization unit (*continued*)
  management of suicidal and aggressive behavior in, 101–103
  milieu management and, 100–101
  specific treatment interventions in, 96–100
  timeline for treatment in, **110–112**
Adult day care, 136
Advanced Alternative Payment Model, **454**
Advance directives, 135, 296, 349
Advancing Integrated Mental Health Solutions (website), 613
Adverse childhood experiences (ACE). *See also* Trauma
  fetal alcohol spectrum disorder and, 157
  trauma in children and, 56
  treatment resistance and, 379
Advertising, and history of hospital psychiatry, 12
Advocacy movement. *See also* Consumers; Patient rights
  state hospitals and, 303–304
  prevention of violence and, 495
  use of restraints and seclusion, 485
Affordable Care Act (2010), 377, 436, 449, 464
Aftercare. *See also* Discharge planning
  geriatric unit and, 136–137
  residential treatment centers and, 371
  social workers and planning of, 560–561
  substance use disorders co-occurring unit and, 264–265
Age. *See also* Adolescents; Children; Geriatric psychiatry
  anorexia nervosa and, 188
  range of in forensic units, 215
  state hospital populations and, 293
Aggression
  adolescent unit and, 80–81
  adult crisis stabilization unit and, 101–103
  developmental disabilities co-occurring unit and, 165, 167, 171, 173
  evaluation of children and, 49
  forensic unit and, 213, 215, 219–221
  geriatric unit and, 132–133
  psychotic disorders unit and, 234, 249–250
  residential treatment and, 362, 364, 390–391
  substance use disorders co-occurring unit and, 268
  target symptom prescribing for adolescents and, **74**
Agitated catatonia, 168
Agitation
  antipsychotics for delirium and, 131
  dementia and, 127, 128–129
  developmental disabilities co-occurring unit and, 173
  target symptom prescribing for adolescents, **74,** 75
Alameda Model, of emergency psychiatric service, 403
Alcohol, and alcohol use disorders. *See also* Substance use disorders
  eating disorders and, 188
  intellectual disability and, 156
  management of withdrawal from, 276–278, 281
  veterans hospitals and, 323
Alcoholics Anonymous, 104, 284, 285, 286
Almshouses, and history of hospital psychiatry, 2–3
Alpha-adrenergic agonists, 277, 278
Alzheimer's disease, 127
American Academy of Child and Adolescent Psychiatry (AACAP), 47–48, 68, 79, 359, **360,** 540
American Art Therapy Association, 569
American Association for Emergency Psychiatry, 115
American Hospital Association, xix, xxi, 22, 442–443, 473
American Journal of Psychiatry, 18
American Medical Association, 464, 539–540
American Occupational Therapy Association, 570, 572
American Psychiatric Association (APA), 1–2, 19, 22, 28, 98, 193, 194, 459, 470, 616. *See also* DSM-5
American Psychiatric Nurses Association, 547
American Society of Addiction Medicine (ASAM), 259, 261–262, 273, 275–276, 286
American Society for Health Care Engineering, 473
Americans with Disabilities Act, 29–30, 302
America's Health Insurance Plans (AHIP), 380
Angelman syndrome, 156, **160**
Anorexia nervosa (AN), 184–185, 188, 190–192. *See also* Eating disorders; Eating disorders unit
Anticonvulsants, and withdrawal from alcohol, 277
Antidepressants. *See also* Psychopharmacology; Selective serotonin reuptake inhibitors; Tricyclic antidepressants
  black box warning for suicide in adolescents, 75

depression in geriatric patients and, 121–122
Anti-kickback statute, and risk management, 477–478
Antipsychotics. *See also* Clozapine; Psychopharmacology
delirium in geriatric patients and, 131
dementia in geriatric patients and, 129
depression with psychotic features in geriatric patients, 123
forensic unit and, 214, 215
guidelines for use of, 98
introduction of in 1950s, 16
psychotic disorders and, 239–242, 244
quality measures and management of, 456
schizophrenia in older adults and, 126
Anti-war movement, and Vietnam War, 328
Anxiety
ADHD in children and, 54
child unit and, 59
developmental disabilities co-occurring unit and, 169
psychosocial treatment modalities for adolescents with, **77**
residential treatment centers and, 363
target symptom prescribing for adolescents and, **74**
Applied behavior analysis (ABA), 245
Architecture. *See also* Environment
design of care environments and, 519–525
renovations of existing spaces, 526–530
Army Nurse Corps, 313
Art therapy
forensic unit and, 217
psychotic disorders unit and, 247
rehabilitation services and, 569–570
trauma in children and, 55, 57–58
ASD. *See* Autism spectrum disorder
Assertive outpatient treatment (AOT) programs, 29
Assessment. *See also* Diagnosis; Evaluation; Psychosocial assessment
adolescent unit and, 69–72
adult crisis stabilization unit and, **110–112**
developmental disabilities co-occurring unit and comprehensive, 162, 165–166
discharge planning in residential treatment centers and, 370–371
rehabilitation services and, 573
substance use disorders co-occurring unit and, 269–274
of suicide and suicidal behavior, 468–470, **471, 472,** 472–473
Assisted living facility, 136
Assisted outpatient treatment (AOT), 296, 348
Association of Medical Superintendents of American Institutions for the Insane (AMSAII), 2, 4–5, 33
Attention-deficit/hyperactivity disorder (ADHD), 50–55, 157
Audits, of financial statements, 417
Austen Riggs Center, 376, 379, 381–392, 393
Autism spectrum disorder (ASD), 82, 153, 154–155, 364
Autonomy, and eating disorders unit, 203
Avoidant/restrictive food intake disorder (ARFID), 186–187, 189

Balanced Budget Act of 1997, 437
Balanced Budget Refinement Act of 1999, 437–438
Banner Psychiatric Center (Arizona), 403
Baseline exaggeration, and behavioral changes, 168
"Battle fatigue," and World War II, 328
Beck Scale for Suicide Ideation (BSI), 469
Beers criteria medication list, 116
Behavior. *See also* Aggression; Agitation; Behavioral interventions; Self-injurious behavior; Suicide; Tantrums; Threats
dementia with behavioral disturbance in geriatric unit, 127
developmental disabilities co-occurring unit and, 159, 162
psychiatric nurse practitioners and allowing or tolerating problematic, 554
psychosocial treatment modalities for adolescents with disruptive, **77**
psychotic disorders unit and, 248
residential treatment and, 383
Behavioral Health Coverage Transparency Act (2019), 31
Behavioral Health Design Guide, The (Hunt et al. 2019), 519
Behavioral interventions. *See also* Behavioral therapists; Cognitive-behavioral therapy; Dialectical behavior therapy
adolescent unit and, 80
developmental disabilities co-occurring unit and, 171–172
eating disorders unit and, 198–199
forensic unit and, 216, 219
residential treatment centers and training in, 369–370
Behavioral phenotype, of intellectual disability and autism spectrum disorder, 155

Behavioral therapists, and developmental disabilities co-occurring unit, 162. *See also* Behavioral interventions
Bell, Luther Vose, 2, **4**
Beneficence, as ethical principle, 203
Benzodiazepines, 268, 276–277, 280, 281
Binge eating, and bulimia nervosa, 185
Binge-eating disorder (BED), 186, 189, 202
Binge-eating/purging type, of anorexia nervosa, 184
Biophilic design, of hospital interiors, 525
Bipolar disorder
  ADHD in children and, 54–55
  developmental disabilities co-occurring unit and, 168, 169
  geriatric unit and, 123–124, 135
  Prader-Willi syndrome and, 156
  psychosocial treatment modalities for adolescents with, **77**
Bloomingdale Hospital (New York), 6, **8,** 9, 434
Blue Cross/Blue Shield, 21
Boards, and corporate governance, 415
Body image, and eating disorders, 185
Body weight, and anorexia nervosa, 184
Borderline personality disorder, 379
Boston Resource Center, 594
Boundary training, for staff of residential treatment centers, 370
Boys Town Family Home Program, **362,** 372
Brain, anorexia nervosa and abnormalities of, 191–192
Brain imaging, and geriatric patients, 115. *See also* Functional magnetic resonance imaging
Brattleboro Retreat (Vermont), 6, 9, 10
Brief Alcohol Withdrawal Scale, 277
Brief Psychiatric Rating Scale, Child Version, **72**
Brief-stay observation units, 404
Brigham, Amariah, 4, **7**
Brown, Nicholas, 6
Brush, Edward, 15
Bulimia nervosa (BN), 185, 189, 192–193. *See also* Eating disorders; Eating disorders unit
Buprenorphine, 278
Butler, Cyrus, 6
Butler, John S., 13–14, **14**
Butler Hospital (Rhode Island), 6, 9, **9**, 13, 19

California Health Benefits Review Program, 31
Calming box, 63
Camden Coalition of Healthcare Providers, 617
Cannabis, 281, 287. *See also* Marijuana
Capacity. *See* Competency; Decision-making
Carbamazepine, 124
Caregivers
  developmental disabilities co-occurring unit and, 162, 171–172
  geriatric unit and, 120, 136, 137
Carve-outs, and managed behavioral health care organizations, 438–440
Case examples
  of ADHD in child unit, 50–51, 52, 53–54
  of aggression in adult crisis stabilization unit, 102–103, 104
  of coding for treatment of suicidal patient, 477
  of comprehensive team-based dialectical behavior therapy, 352
  of diagnostic workup in adult crisis stabilization unit, 93–94, 95–96
  of discharge planning in developmental disabilities co-occurring unit, 174–175
  of evaluations in child unit, 49, 50
  of family role in residential treatment, 388–389
  of long-acting injection clinics for psychotic disorders, 351
  of quality of care issues, 505–506, 509–510
  of rehabilitation services, 572–573
  of residential treatment for treatment-resistant disorders, 384–386
  of risk management for suicidal patients, 467–468
  of roles of social workers in inpatient care, 564–565, 566–568
  of self-injurious behavior in child unit, 59
  of substance use disorders, 258, 260, 265–266, 267, 268, 271
  of suicidal behavior and psychiatric nurse practitioners, 552
  of team-based care for treatment-resistant depression, 349–350
  of trauma in child unit, 56, 57
  of violence in mental health care setting, 485–486
Case managers, and case management
  adult crisis stabilization unit and, 90
  eating disorders unit and, 205
  geriatric unit and, 137
  hospital-based outpatient services and, 343
  social workers and, 559–560
Casey Foundation, 361, 373
Catatonia, 168, 244–245
Center for Mental Health Services, 22, 491

Center for Risk Analysis (Harvard University), 482
Centers for Disease Control and Prevention, 31–32, 155, 466, 469, 627
Centers for Medicare & Medicaid Services (CMS), 28–29, 220, 301, 414, 437, 443, 449, **453, 454,** 542, 549, 613–614
Central State Hospital (Virginia), 30
Cerebrospinal fluid (CSF), and eating disorders, 191
Cerebrovascular disease, and depression, 121
Chains, of private psychiatric hospitals, 24, 26
Charter Medical Corporation, 24
Checklists, and safety plans, 269
Chesapeake Connections, 235
Chief executive officers (CEOs), 415, 421
Child and Adolescent Needs and Strengths (CANS), 362, 373
Child Protective Services (CPS), 61
Children. *See also* Adolescents; Child unit; Development
  increase in emergency consultations for, 631
  residential treatment centers for, 357, 361–364
  seclusion and restraints for, 482
  social workers and care for, 561–565
  in state hospitals, 297
Children's Depression Inventory, **72**
Children's Global Assessment (CGI), **72**
Children's Health Insurance Program (CHIP), 297
Children's Yale-Brown Obsessive Compulsive Scale, **72**
Child unit, and inpatient care. *See also* Children
  anxiety in, 59
  complicated ADHD in, 50–55
  depression and self-injurious behaviors in, 58–59
  evaluation of children in, 48–50
  future of, 65
  gender dysphoria and, 59
  government agencies and, 61
  interface of with schools, 60–61
  milieu therapy and, 61–65
  obsessive-compulsive disorder and, 59
  outpatient providers and, 61
  psychotic disorders in, 60
  reasons for hospitalization of children, 47–48
  role of family in treatment, 60
  trauma and, 55–58
Chlorpromazine, 16
Cigarette smoking
  discharge from adult crisis stabilization unit and, 104, **105**
  psychotic disorders unit and, 241, 243–244
  substance use disorders co-occurring unit and, 280–281
  use of term *ex-smoker,* 259
  veterans hospitals and, 324
Citalopram for Agitation in Alzheimer Disease Study (CitAD), 128
Civil Rights Division (Department of Justice), 302
Civil Rights of Institutionalized Persons Act of 1980 (CRIPA), 29, 302, 597–598
Civil status population, in state hospitals, 296–297
Clinical Antipsychotic Trials of Intervention Effectiveness (CATIE), 128–129, 379
Clinical care delivery, and hospital operations, 427
Clinical Dementia Rating (CDR) Scale, 117
Clinical Global Impression (CGI), **72**
Clinical Institute Withdrawal Assessment for Alcohol—Revised (CIWA-Ar), 269, 277
Clinical interviews
  assessment of adolescents and, 70
  diagnostic workup in geriatric unit and, 116
  suicide risk assessment and, **471**
Clinical Opiate Withdrawal Scale (COWS), 269, 278
Clinical service delivery, and health care operations, 426
Clonidine, 52
Clozapine, 99, 129–130, 243, 351–352. *See also* Antipsychotics
Cocaine, 323
Code of Medical Ethics (American Medical Association), 464
Code response, and risk management, 474–475
Coercion, and involuntary treatment, 204
Cognition, and cognitive deficits
  developmental disabilities co-occurring unit and disintegration of, 164
  geriatric patients and evaluation of, 117, 125, 130
  relapse process in substance abuse and distortions of, **283,** 285
Cognitive-behavioral therapy (CBT)
  adolescents and, 76
  eating disorders unit and, 197, 198–199, 201

Cognitive-behavioral therapy (CBT) (*continued*)
  social workers and, 559
  substance use disorders co-occurring unit and, 283
Collaborative care model, of integrated care, 606, 613–615
Collaborative Longitudinal Personality Disorders Study (CLPS), 379
Collateral information
  assessment of adolescents and children, 69, 166, 562, 568
  assessment in substance use disorders co-occurring unit and, 270
  diagnostic workup in forensic unit and, 213–214
  evaluation in eating disorders unit and, 195
Columbia-Suicide Severity Rating Scale (CSSRS), **72,** 469
Comfort rooms, and prevention of violence, 494–495
Commission on Accreditation of Rehabilitation Facilities (CARF), 414
Communication. *See also* Language
  developmental disabilities co-occurring unit and, 163, 166
  psychiatric nurse practitioners and, 553–554
Community. *See also* Community mental health
  forensic unit and reintegration into, 217, 222
  leadership and, 426
  state mental health agencies and services in, 300
Community-based outpatient clinics (CBOCs), 315
Community Living Centers (CLCs), 325
Community mental health, history of, 341–342
Community Mental Health Act (1963), 342, 400
Community Psychiatric Centers, 24
Comorbidity, of psychiatric disorders
  of ADHD, 51
  of autism spectrum disorder, 155
  cost of care and, 436
  of eating disorders, 188
  treatment-resistant disorders and, 378–379
Compensation models, for staff, 542–543
Competency. *See also* Decision-making
  assessment of in geriatric patients, 134–136
  forensic patients and restoration of to stand trial, 212, 221–222, 298, 299
Complexity intervention units, 615
Comprehensive Psychiatric Emergency Program (CPEP), 402
Computerized Patient Record System (CPRS), 315
Conditional release, and outpatient civil commitment, 298, 348–349
Confidentiality. *See also* Informed consent
  assessment of adolescents and, 70
  family and, 582–583
  individual therapy for adolescents and, 76–77
  substance use disorders co-occurring unit and, 273
Conflict. *See* Aggression; Violence
Confusion Assessment Method, 130
Connecticut Medical Society, 6–7
Conners' Rating Scales—Revised, **72**
Consolidated Appropriations Act (2020), 377
Consultation-liaison psychiatric services, 405, 414–415, 538–539, 615
Consumers, and consumer movement. *See also* Advocacy movement; Patient rights
  future of mental health care and, 626–627
  narrative on patient experience with psychiatric hospitals, 592–596
  peer recovery movement and, 596–601
  reduction of seclusion and restraint use, 495
  reform of mental health care and, 485
Contingency discharge, from forensic unit, 221–222
Continued-care certification, 439
Continuing care units, in state hospitals, 293, 296
Continuous Performance Test, 237
Continuum of care. *See also* Emergency services; Hospital-based outpatient services; Residential treatment
  impact of state hospitals on overall, 299–300
  organization of current volume, xxvi
  substance use disorders co-occurring unit and computerized version of, 286
Co-occurring unit, use of term, 257, 262. *See also* Developmental disabilities co-occurring unit; Substance use disorders co-occurring unit
Cost-effectiveness research, and adolescent units, 82–83
Countertransference, and psychodynamic psychotherapy, 388, 389
Court orders, and outpatient civil commitment, 349
COVID-19 pandemic, xix, xx, xxv, 305, 323, 513, 610, 616, 625, 627, 628

Cravings, and relapse process in substance use, **283,** 284–285
Cries of Anguish (National Alliance on Mental Illness 2000), 598
Crisis. *See* Adult crisis stabilization unit; Crisis stabilization
Crisis Now (Arizona), 403, 600
Crisis Prevention Institute, 370
Crisis Residential program, 346
Crisis stabilization, and residential treatment, 380
Critical incidents, and risk management, 465
Crossing the Quality Chasm (Institute of Medicine 2001), 448, 504
Cultural Formulation Interview (DSM-5), 580
Culture
  evaluation of children and, 50
  family and, 579–580
  hospital-based outpatient services and, 347
Current Procedural Terminology (CPT) codes, 476, 542, 613–614
Cutter, Nehemiah, 2
Cybersecurity, and risk management, 475–476

Daily huddles, and quality of care, 511–515
Dangerousness, and admission criteria for adolescent unit, **69.** *See also* Safety; Violence
Danvers State Hospital (Massachusetts), 32–33
Data collection, on problem behaviors in developmental disabilities co-occurring unit, 173
Day hospitals
  initiation and promotion of, 16
  psychotic disorders and, 252
  step-down services and, 609
Debriefings
  prevention of violence and, 495–496
  use of restraints or seclusion and, 81
Decision-making
  assessment of capacity in geriatric patients, 134–136
  eating disorders unit and, 203
  geriatric care for veterans and, 325
Deinstitutionalization
  beginnings of movement in 1950s, 17, 152, 435
  increasing use of emergency department for psychiatric care, 400
  of individuals with intellectual and developmental disabilities, 152–153
  psychotic disorders and, 230
  veterans hospitals and, 313, 315
Delirium
  developmental disabilities co-occurring unit and, 170
  geriatric unit and, 130–132
  mental status changes in older patients and, 115
  secondary to substance use or medical illness, 92
Delusions, and schizophrenia, 249
Dementia
  assessment of capacity and, 134
  geriatric unit and, 114, 119, 121, 125–126, 127, 128–132
  veterans hospitals and, 325
Dementia with Lewy bodies, 125, 127, 129
Demographics, and future of geriatric care, 137, 630–631
Demoralization, and psychotic disorders unit, 242–243
Department of Defense, 469
Department of Health and Human Services, 301, 358, 400, 440
Department of Housing and Urban Development (HUD), 321
Department of Justice (DOJ), 26, 29, 30, 302, 441–442, 597–598
Department of Social Services (DSS), 61, 166
Depersonalization, and studies of violence, 490
Depot medications, for psychotic patients, 239–240
Depression. *See also* Major depressive disorder
  ADHD in children and, 53
  child unit and, 58–59
  developmental disabilities co-occurring unit and, 168
  geriatric unit and, 120–123
  psychosocial treatment modality for adolescents with, **77**
  residential treatment centers and, 363
  target symptom prescribing for adolescents and, **74**
  team-based care for treatment-resistant, 349–350
Depression and Bipolar Support Alliance, 97
Depression-executive dysfunction syndrome, 121
Detoxification, and substance use disorders, 96

Development. *See also* Developmental disabilities co-occurring unit
 assessment of adolescents and, 69–70
 diagnostic workup for psychotic patients and history of, 237
 evaluation of young children and, 50
 residential treatment centers and, 364, 369
Developmental Disabilities Administration, 166
Developmental disabilities co-occurring unit. *See also* Autism spectrum disorder; Development; Intellectual disability
 admission to, 164–167
 diagnosis and, 167–169
 discharge planning and, 174
 genetic and neuropsychiatric syndromes and, 155–159, **160–161**
 treatment team and, 158–159, 162–164
Dextroamphetamine, 51
Diagnosis. *See also* Assessment; Collateral information; Differential diagnosis; Evaluation
 adolescent unit and, 71–72
 adult crisis stabilization unit and, 90–96
 child unit and, 48–50
 forensic unit and, 213–214
 geriatric unit and, 116–118, 130
 psychiatric labels and, 490
 psychotic disorders unit and, 234, 235–238
 quality in psychiatry and, 452, 454
 residential treatment centers and holistic approach to, 366–367
 substance use disorders co-occurring unit and, 262–263, 270, 271
Diagnosis-related groups (DRGs), 436–437
Diagnostic Criteria for Psychiatric Disorders for Use With Adults With Learning Disabilities/Mental Retardation (DC-LD), 154
Diagnostic Manual—Intellectual Disability, 2nd Edition (Fletcher et al. 2017), 154
Dialectical behavior therapy (DBT)
 comprehensive team-based in outpatient setting and, 352–353
 eating disorders unit and, 199, 201
 forensic unit and, 216
 social workers and, 558
Dietitian, and eating disorders unit, 197
Differential diagnosis
 of behavioral changes in developmental disabilities co-occurring unit, 168
 diagnostic workup in psychotic disorders unit and, 236
 traumatic brain injury and, 333
Dining room, of eating disorders unit, 202
Directors, and organizational structure, **420,** 421
Disability Law Center, 303–304
Discharge planning. *See also* Aftercare
 adolescent unit and, 81–82
 adult crisis stabilization unit and, 99, 103–104, 106, **110–112**
 developmental disabilities co-occurring unit and, 174–175
 eating disorders unit and, 205
 family and, 586–587
 forensic population in state hospitals and, 298
 forensic unit and, 212, 221–222
 geriatric unit and, 136–137
 psychotic disorders unit and, 250–253
 quality of care improvement and, 508–509, **510**
 residential treatment centers and, 370–372
 social workers and, 561, 563
 substance use disorders co-occurring unit and, 264–265, 286
Disproportionate Share Hospital (DSH) program, 304
Disruptive mood dysregulation disorder, 54–55
Dissociative identity disorder (DID), 57, 58, 235
Dix, Dorothea, 6, 434, 570
Documentation, of patient elopement, 474
Dopamine, and anorexia nervosa, 191, 192
Dosages, of medications
 adult crisis stabilization unit and, 98
 antipsychotics for older adults and, 126
 antipsychotics for psychotic disorders and, 240–241
Down, John Langdon, 155
Down syndrome, 155, **160**
Drug Addiction Treatment Act of 2000, 278
Drug-drug interactions, and antipsychotics, 126, 215
Drug screening, and substance use disorders, 272–273
DSM-5
 adaptive functions and intellectual disability in, 154
 assessment of adolescents and, 70
 classification of eating disorders in, 184–188
 Cultural Formulation Interview in, 580
 delirium and, 130
 elements of comprehensive diagnosis, 91

impact of on inpatient psychiatry, 30
major depressive disorder and, 120
relapse of substance use disorders and, 284
tobacco use disorder and, 259
Dunton, William Rush, Jr., 17, 570
Dysphagia, in geriatric patients, 119

Earle, Pliny, 2, **3**
Eastern Lunatic Asylum of Virginia, 519
Eating disorder not otherwise specified (EDNOS), 189
Eating disorders. *See also* Anorexia nervosa; Bulimia nervosa; Eating disorders unit
adolescent unit and, 80
comorbidity and, 188
DSM-5 classification of, 184–188
epidemiology of, 188–189
pathogenesis of, 189–193
prevalence of, 183
psychosocial treatment modalities for adolescents with, **77**
Eating disorders unit
clinical evaluation and, 194–196
discharge planning and, 205
levels of care in, 193–194
models of inpatient care in, 196–202
physical structure of, 202
treatment consent, coercion, capacity, and commitment as issues in, 202–204
treatment outcomes and, 204–205
E-cigarettes, 280
Education. *See also* Psychoeducation; School(s)
adolescent unit and, 79
continuing for social workers, 558
developmental disabilities co-occurring unit and, 163–164
for families of psychotic patients, 246
forensic unit and, 216–217
psychiatric nurse practitioners and, 541
staff of residential treatment centers and, 369–370
veterans and, 321–322
Electrocardiography115, 131, 236
Electroconvulsive therapy (ECT)
adult crisis stabilization unit and, 99–100
forensic unit and, 215
geriatric inpatients and, 122, 123, 124
psychotic disorders unit and, 244–245
Electronic health records (EHR), 315, 316, 475–476, 504
Emergency department (ED). *See also* Emergency services
agitation and transfer of patients to adult crisis stabilization unit, 89
"boarding" of psychiatric patients in, 88
hospital-based outpatient services and, 345–346
integrated care and, 405, 616
referrals to developmental disabilities co-occurring unit from, 164–165
role of in managing psychiatric needs, 399, 400, 401, 414, 435–436
substance use disorders co-occurring unit and, 266, 272
Emergency Medical Treatment and Active Labor Act (1986), 293, 400, 412, 449, 464
Emergency operations plan, and risk management, 474
Emergency psychiatric assessment, treatment, and healing (EmPATH) service, 402–403
Emergency psychiatric services, 402–405. *See also* Emergency department
Emotional dysregulation, and psychosocial treatment modalities for adolescents, **77**
Employee Retirement Income Security Act (ERISA), 440
Environment. *See also* Architecture
access to outdoor space as human right, 598
design of geriatric unit and, 118
milieu management of forensic unit and, 218
occupational therapy and, 572
risk management and, 473
Environmental factors model, of violence, 489
Environmental rounds, 549
Epilepsy, and autism spectrum disorder, 155
Equity and Fiscal Responsibility Act of 1982, 437
Erikson Institute for Education and Research, 391, 392
Evaluation. *See also* Assessment; Diagnosis
child unit and, 48–50
eating disorders unit and, 194–196
of hospital services by peers, 599–600
"Examined living," and behavior in residential treatment, 383
Exceptional Leadership: 16 Critical Competencies for Healthcare Executives (Dye and Garman 2006), 424, **425**
Executive leader, and organizational structure, 421–422
Exercise, and forensic unit, 217

Exposure therapy, for eating disorders, 199
Expressive therapy. *See also* Art therapy; Music therapy
  for adolescents, 76
  eating disorders unit and, 201
  rehabilitation services and, 569–570

Facility operations, and health care services, 426, 427
Failure to treat, 452
Falls, and geriatric patients, 122, 132, 331
Family. *See also* Family history; Family therapy; Parents
  adult crisis stabilization unit and, 90, 96, 103
  barriers and challenges for clinicians working with, 581–586
  developmental disabilities co-occurring unit and, 162, 172
  discharge planning and care transitions, 586–587
  eating disorders and, 190
  emotional responses of, 578–579
  expectations of, 580–581
  forensic unit and, 216–217
  future directions in psychiatric care and, 588
  geriatric unit and, 137
  messages of hope and recovery for, 587–588
  psychotic disorders unit and, 246, 251
  residential treatment and, 365–366, 371–372, 388–389
  role in lives of persons with mental illness, 577
  social workers and, 565–569
  substance use disorders co-occurring unit and, 264
  treatment of children and, 60
  use of term in context, 578
Family-based therapy (FBT), for eating disorders, 199
Family history
  of bipolar disorder, 123, 124
  diagnostic workup of geriatric inpatients and, 116
  evaluation of children and, 49
Family therapy
  adolescent unit and, 78–79
  eating disorders unit and, 199, 201
Federal Employees Health Benefits Program, 21
Federal financial participation (FFP), and IMD exclusion, 21
Fetal alcohol spectrum disorder (FASD), 156–157, **161**
Fiduciary, and board responsibilities, 415
Finances, and financing. *See also* Insurance
  coding and fraudulent billing, 476–477
  design of mental health facilities and, 529–530
  effects of changing reimbursement systems, 441–442
  funding challenges and, 417
  future of inpatient psychiatric services and, 442–443
  history of, 433–434
  managed behavioral health care organizations and, 438–440
  Medicaid reimbursement and, 440–441
  psychiatric units in general hospitals and, 434–438
  residential treatment and, 389–390
  revenue sources by type of hospital, 442
  staff recruitment and, 543
  state hospitals and, 304–305, 441
  value-based care and, 626
"Fitness for imprisonment," concept of, 213
Five Dysfunctions of a Team, The (Lencioni 2002), 621
Five Fundamental Rights Act (Massachusetts 1997), 598
Fluoxetine, 202
Food and Drug Administration (FDA), 75, 469
Forensic population, in state hospitals, 297–299
Forensic units
  admission criteria for, 212–213
  diagnostic workup in, 213–214
  discharge planning and, 212, 221–222
  dual mandate of, 211–212, 222
  milieu management of, 218–219
  psychotic disorders unit and, 234
  recruitment and retention of staff, 224
  special challenges of, 222–224
  in state hospitals, 296
  suicidal and aggressive behaviors in, 219–221
  treatment in, 214–217
4-A's Test, 130
Fragile X syndrome, 157–158, **161**
Franklin, Benjamin, 5
Free appropriate public education (FAPE), 61
Friends Asylum (Pennsylvania), 7, 10, 13, 434
Functional magnetic resonance imaging (FMRI), and eating disorders, 192, 193
Furniture, and interior design, 525

Future, of hospital psychiatry
adolescent unit and, 82–83
child unit and, 65
families and, 588
financial viability of inpatient services and, 442
geriatric unit and, 137–138
history of hospital psychiatry and, 32–33
hospital-based outpatient services and, 353
organization of current volume, xxvii
recent changes in health care landscape and, 625–627
residential treatment centers and, 373
social work and, 569
state hospitals and, 305–306
substance use disorders co-occurring unit and, 287

Gender, of state hospital populations, 293. *See also* Women
Gender dysphoria, in child unit, 59
General adult units, use of term, 229
General hospitals. *See also* Emergency departments
financing of psychiatric units in, 434–438
history of hospital psychiatry and, 18
role of in psychiatric care, 400–402
General mental abilities, and intellectual disability, 153
General residential treatment centers, 360
Genetics
autism spectrum disorder and, 155
eating disorders and, 190
Genogram, and psychotic patients, 238
Genome-wide association study (GWAS), of eating disorders, 190
Geriatric Depression Scale (GDS), 116
Geriatric psychiatry, 324–325, 630–631
Geriatric unit
admission criteria for, 114
assessement of capacity and competency in, 134–136
bipolar disorder and, 123–124
delirium and, 130–132
dementia and, 127, 128–132
depression and, 120–123
diagnostic workup and, 116–118
discharge planning and, 136–137
future of, 137–138
medical clearance and, 115–116
schizophrenia and, 125–127
treatment considerations for, 118–120, 132–134
GI Bill of Rights, 321–322
Global Assessment of Functioning (GAF), **72**
Goals, of treatment
in adult crisis stabilization unit, 96
in developmental disabilities co-occurring unit, 170–171
in substance use disorders co-occurring unit, 262–266
Group therapy
adolescent unit and, 77–78
adult crisis stabilization unit and, 97
child unit and, 62–63
eating disorders unit and, 199, 200, 201
forensic unit and, 216
veterans hospitals and, 327
Guanfacine, 52
Guardianship
outpatient civil commitment and, 349
surrogate decision-makers and, 136
Guidelines
for antipsychotic use, 98, 126–127
for documentation of seclusion and restraints, 553
for electroconvulsive therapy, 100
for high-quality health care, 448
for milieu therapy, 248–249
for referrals to substance use disorders co-occurring unit, 266
for residential programs, 359, **360**
for standards of care in class action lawsuits, 377–378
for telepsychiatry, 539–540
for trauma-informed systems of care, 487–488
for treatment of children with autism spectrum disorder and intellectual disability, 165
for withdrawal from substance use, 275–276
"Guidelines for Design and Construction of Hospitals" (Facility Guidelines Institute 2018), 519

Hallucinations
dementia and, 127
psychotic disorders in children and, 60
schizophrenia and, 125
Haloperidol, 241
HALT, and relapse of substance abuse, 284
Hamilton Depression Rating Scale (HDRS), 116
Handoff communication, between nurses and shifts, 554
Hardwiring excellence. *See* Administration
Harm reduction, and substance use disorders, 259

Hartford Courant (newspaper), 482, 484, 598
Hartford Retreat (Connecticut), 6–7, 9, 10, **10**, 13
Harvard University, 482
Health care. *See also* Medical conditions
  assessment of capacity for medical decisions, 135
  patients with schizophrenia and, 125
  residential treatment centers and, 365
Healthcare Effectiveness Data and Information Set (HEDIS), 452, **453, 455**
Healthcare Leadership Alliance (HLA), 423–424
Health Catalyst, 426
Health Insurance Plan of Greater New York, 21
Health Related Behaviors Survey (HBRS), 323
Helping Families in Mental Health Crisis Act, 29
Heroin, 323
Hierarchical Taxonomy of Psychopathology (HiTOP), 378
High Point Hospital (New York), 25
Hill-Burton Act, 19
Hippocrates, 447
Hiring incentives, for staff, 543
History, of hospital psychiatry
  changes in from 1921 to 1970, 16–22
  community mental health and, 341–342
  early years of through 1920, 2–15
  financing of psychiatric care and, 433–434
  gaps in inpatient care and, 607–609
  of hospitalization of individuals with intellectual and developmental disabilities, 152–153
  modern era of from 1971 to 2019, 22–32
  moral treatment movement and, 518–519, 570
  neuropsychiatry and, 151–152
  occupational therapy and, 570
  psychotic disorders unit and, 230
  state hospitals and, 3–5, 9–15, 17–18, 28, 291–293, **294–295**
  veterans hospitals and, 311–316
Homelessness, and veterans hospitals, 320–321. *See also* Housing
Homeless Veterans Reintegration Program, 322
Hopelessness, as risk factor for suicide, 470, 473
Hormonal therapy, for sex offenders, 214–215, 223
Hospice, 137, 138
Hospital-Based Inpatient Psychiatric Services, 301, **453**
Hospital-based outpatient services. *See also* Outpatient services
  care teams and, 349–353
  civil commitment and, 348–349
  definition of, 342
  diversity and, 346–347
  future of, 353
  integration of with other hospital programs, 345–346
  levels of care and, 342–345
  peer support services and, 353
  residential and housing support in, 346
  virtual care and, 347–348
Hospital and Community Psychiatry (Pottash et al. 1982), 23
Hospital Consumer Assessment of Healthcare Providers and Systems survey, 418
Hospital Corporation of America, 24
Hospital Elder Life Program (HELP), 131
Hospital psychiatry. *See also* Administration; Continuum of care; Future; General hospitals; History; Inpatient care; Private psychiatric hospitals; Rehospitalization; State hospitals; Veterans hospitals
  advances in new models of care, 610–613
  challenges of last decade, xix–xx
  changes in after introduction of new medications in 1950s, 87
  economic scarcity and, 606–607
  emergence of common treatment themes in, 605–606
  guiding principles of, xxiii–xxiv
  organization of current volume, xxiv–xxvii
  outcome-producing integrated model of care, 613–617
  recommendations for moving forward, 619–622
  redefinition of "hospital" and, xxiv
  SWOT analysis and leveraging of perceived threats as opportunities, 617–619
Hotspotting, and value-based integrated care, 617
Housing, and psychosocial support services, 346, 616. *See also* Homelessness
Hub and spoke model, of emergency psychiatric service, 403
HUD-VASH program, 321
Human rights, and consumer movement, 597–599
Hypoactive delirium, 130

ID. *See* Intellectual disability
IMD (institution for mental diseases) exclusion, xxv, 21, 25–26, 28–29, 304, 417, 440
Immunoassays, and substance use disorders, 273
Improving the Quality of Health Care for Mental and Substance-Use Conditions (Institute of Medicine 2006), 449
Independent ownership, of psychiatric hospitals, 413
Individualized education plans (IEPs), 164, 365, 371
Individuals with Disabilities Education Act (1990), 152, 365
Individual therapy. *See also* Psychotherapy
  adolescent unit and, 76–77
  adult crisis stabilization unit and, 96–97
  eating disorders unit and, 200–201
  residential treatment and, 387–388
Information technology (IT) systems, 315
Informed consent
  adult crisis stabilization unit and, 95
  antipsychotics for geriatric patients and, 129
  treatment of eating disorders and, 204
In-home services
  innovations in step-down care and, 610
  monitoring of geriatric patients and, 137
Inpatient care. *See also* Adolescent unit; Adult crisis stabilization unit; Child unit; Developmental disabilities co-occurring unit; Eating disorders unit; Forensic unit; Geriatric unit; Hospital psychiatry; Integrated care; Psychotic disorders unit; Staff; Substance use disorders co-occurring unit
  crisis stabilization as guiding principle of treatment, 90
  evolution of for children and adolescents, 358
  involvement of family in treatment process, 577
  organization of current volume, xxiv–xxvi
  step-down services and, 609–610
  trend toward increasing patient turnover and acuity of illness, 87–88
  variability of settings for, 88
Inpatient Psychiatric Facility Quality Reporting (IPFQR) program, 438, **453, 455,** 456
Insanity defense, and forensic unit, 212, 222
Insomnia, and target symptom prescribing for adolescents, **74.** *See also* Sleep
Institute for Healthcare Improvement, 505
Institute of Medicine, 448, 484, 485, 488
Institute of the Pennsylvania Hospital (Pennsylvania), 5, **12**
Instrumental activities of daily living (IADLs). *See also* Activities of daily living
  geriatric patients and, 117
  psychotic disorders unit and, 231–232
Insurance. *See also* Finances; Managed care
  accountability and, 630
  expansion of in 1960s, 20–21
  financing of psychiatric services and, 417, 434, 436, 438–440
  impact of on psychiatric care, 26–27, 594–596
  psychotic disorders unit and, 235, 252
  residential treatment and, 377
Integrated care
  collaborative care model of, 606, 613
  emergency departments and, 405
  geriatric unit and, 119
  outcomes-producing model of, 613–617
  roles of psychiatrists in, 539
  substance use disorders co-occurring unit and, 261
Intellectual disability (ID)
  developmental disabilities co-occurring unit and, 152–154, 156–157
  psychotic disorders unit and, 233–234
Intelligence, and intellectual disability, 153–154
Intensive outpatient programs, and hospital-based outpatient services, 344
Interior design, of mental health facilities, 523–525
International Society of Psychiatric Nurses, 547
International Work Group for Therapeutic Residential Care, 359
Internet
  access to in forensic unit, 217
  education on psychotic disorders and, 246
  residential treatment centers and, 363
  resources for families, 588
  resources on neuropsychiatric manifestations of rare diseases, 159
Interpersonal psychotherapy for cognitive impairment (IPT-CI), 136
Intrusive thoughts, and trauma in children, 57
Involuntary admissions
  debate on in 1980s, 24
  legal requirements for, 68

Involuntary admissions (*continued*)
substance use disorders co-occurring unit and, 260
suicide assessment and, 469–470
veterans hospitals and, 318
Involuntary treatment
as legal issue, 203–204
substance use disorders co-occurring unit and, 273
IRS Form 990, 416

Jarvis, Edward, 8–9, 13, 33
Joint Commission on Mental Illness and Health
creation of, 342
quality measures and, 453, **455**
regulatory oversight of psychiatric facilities, 414
renovation of existing facilities, 526
requirement of comprehensive diagnosis, 91
requirements for prevention of suicide in psychiatric hospitals, 32, 437
restrictions on use of restraints and seclusion, 81, 220, 483, 553
risk management and, 466, 467–468, 473
standards for certification of residential facilities, 359
state hospitals and, 300–301
Joint Legacy Viewer (JLV), 315

Ketamine, 215
Kirkbride, Thomas Story, 2, 13, 15, **16**
Korean War, 328
Kubie, Lawrence, 21–22

Laboratory tests
adult crisis stabilization unit and, 92–93
assessment of adolescents and, 71–72, **73**
developmental disabilities co-occurring unit and, 169
eating disorders unit and, 196
geriatric patients and, 115, 117, 130–131
psychotic disorders unit and, 236
substance use disorders and, 266, 272
Language. *See also* Communication; Sign language
developmental disabilities co-occurring unit and, 159
family and, 580
hospital-based outpatient services and cultural diversity, 347
person-first strategy of, 597
recovery-oriented care and, 549
Leadership. *See also* Administration
development and succession planning, 429–430
essential activities of, 428–429
models of, 423–428
organizational structure and, 419–423
prevention of violence and, 492
psychiatrists and, 538
Lean (quality improvement methodology) program, 503, 506–515, 530
Least restrictive alternative, for psychiatric care, 27, 88
Legal issues. *See also* Forensic unit; Informed consent; State(s)
anti-kickback statute and physician self-referral laws, 477–478
assessment of capacity and competency in older adults, 134–136
definition of patient rights, 464
diagnostic workup and competence or ability, 95
involuntary treatment and, 203–204
outpatient civil commitment and, 348–349
state hospitals and, 292, 300–302
veterans hospitals and, 318
Leisure activities. *See also* Recreational activities
adolescent unit and, 80
forensic unit and, 217
Length of stay
effect of shortened on rates of readmission, 441
in emergency department, 400, 401
residential treatment and, 385
substance use disorders co-occurring unit and, 260
Lesch-Nyhan syndrome, 155
LGBTQ+ individuals, and assessment of adolescents, 70
Ligature risk. *See* Suicide
Lighting strategies, and interior design, 525
Lincoln, Abraham, 311–312
Lisdexamfetamine, 202
Lithium, 99, 124, 242
Living Rooms (RI International), 600
Loan repayment benefits, for staff, 543
Long Island House (New York), 12
Longitudinal care, 605–606
Lorazepam, 277
Lumbar puncture, and catatonia or delirium, 236

MacArthur Competency Assessment Tool for Treatment, 135, 203

Major depressive disorder. *See also* Depression
comorbidity of eating disorders with, 188
in geriatric patients, 120, 121–123
Managed behavioral health care organizations (MBHOs), 438–440
Managed care. *See also* Insurance
antipsychotics for psychotic patients and, 241, 242
emergence of in 1990s, 25, 26–27
residential care and, 376
Management, and corporate governance, 415. *See also* Administration; Managers
Management on the Mend: The Healthcare Executive Guide to System Transformation (Toussaint and Adams 2015), 512
Managers, and organizational structure, 420–421. *See also* Management
Mandt System, 370
Mania
secondary in geriatric patients, 123
target symptom prescribing for adolescents and, **74**
Marijuana, 323, 363–364. *See also* Cannabis
Massachusetts Psychiatric Society, 24
Maudsley Emergency Clinic, 402
Mayo Clinic, 418
McLean, John, 6
McLean Hospital (Massachusetts), 6, 12–13, 25, 434
Measurement-based care (MBC), and quality, 457–459
Media, adolescent unit and access to, 80
Medicaid. *See also* Centers for Medicare and Medicaid Services
financing of psychiatric services and, 417, 434, 435, 440–441, 442, 609
hospital-based outpatient services and, 345
IMD exclusion and, xxv, 27, 28–29, 304
psychotic disorders unit and, 252
Medical conditions. *See also* Health care
assessment of adolescents and, 71
consultation in geriatric unit and, 119
cost of treating comorbid in psychiatric patients, 440
delirium and, 92–93, 130–131
developmental disabilities co-occurring unit and assessment of, 169–170
diagnostic workup in psychotic disorders unit and, 236
eating disorders unit and evaluation of, 196
evaluation of children and, 49
evaluation of geriatric patients and, 115–116, 117, 130–131
substance use disorders co-occurring unit and assessment of, 265, 266, 269–270
Medical directors, psychiatrists as, 538
Medical psychiatric units, 615
Medicare. *See also* Centers for Medicare and Medicaid Services
coding and fraudulent billing, 476
establishment of, 21
financing of psychiatric services and, 417, 434–435, 437, 438, 442, 609
hospital-based outpatient services and, 345
psychotic disorders unit and, 252
required cost reports and, 416
Medicare Access and CHIP Reauthorization Act of 2015, 449, **454**
Meetings. *See* Team(s)
Memantine, 128
Menninger Clinic Residential Treatment Program, **362,** 391
Menninger Foundation, 25
Mental Health America, 303
Mental Health Environment of Care Checklist, 318
Mental Health Facilities Design Guide (U.S. Department of Veterans Affairs 2017), 519
Mental Health Parity and Addiction Equity Act of 2008 (MHPAEA), xx, 28, 30–31, 376–377, 436, 449
Mental Health Parity Compliance Act (2020), 377
Mental health service lines, and veterans hospitals, 317
Mental Health Study Act of 1955, 342
Mental status examination
assessment of suicide risk and, 473
eating disorders unit and, 195
Merit-based Incentive Payment System (MIPS), **454, 455**
Methadone, 268–269, 278–279
Methylphenidate, 51
Metro Boston Recovery Learning Community, 594
Milieu therapy
adolescent unit and, 79–80
adult crisis stabilization unit and, 100–101
child unit and, 61–65
eating disorders unit and, 201
forensic unit and, 218–219
introduction and establishment of, 16
psychotic disorders unit and, 229–230, 247–249
residential treatment and, 364, 380
veterans hospitals and, 318

Military. *See* Veterans hospitals
Military sexual trauma (MST), 320, 329–331
Mini-Mental State Examination (MMSE), 117, 130, 135
Mission, and corporate governance, **416, 419**
Mobile crisis intervention, 404
Modern Hospital, The (journal), 18
Montreal Cognitive Assessment (MoCA), 117
Mood stabilizers. *See also* Lithium
  forensic unit and, 214
  psychotic disorders unit and, 242
Moral injury, and military experience, 326–327
Moral treatment movement, and history of mental health care, 518–519, 570
Mortality rate
  anorexia nervosa and, 188, 196
  bipolar disorder in geriatric patients and, 123
  dementia and, 119
  hypoactive delirium and, 130
Motivational interviewing
  adolescents and, 76
  psychiatric nurse practitioners and, 554
  substance use disorders and, 273, 282
Mount Hope Institution (Maryland), 7
Music therapy, and psychotic disorders unit, 247
Multifunctional Treatment in Residential and Community Settings, **362**
Mutual-help groups, 600–601. *See also* Peer support services
Mutual help meetings, and substance use disorders co-occurring unit, 265
MyHealthVet ("My Healthy Vet"), 315–316

Naloxone, 279
Naltrexone, 279
NAMI (National Alliance on Mental Illness), 97, 104, 246, 303, 581, 594, 598–599
Narcotics Anonymous (NA), 285, 286
National Academy of Sciences, 448
National Action Alliance for Suicide Prevention, 600
National Alliance on Mental Illness (NAMI), 97, 104, 246, 303, 581, 594, 598–599
National Association for Behavioral Healthcare, 467
National Association for Mental Health, 22
National Association of State Mental Health Program Directors, 220, 299, 484, 553
National Board for Certification in Occupational Therapy, 569
National Cemetery Administration (NCA), 312
National Center for Injury Prevention, 469
National Center for PTSD (NCPTSD), 329
National Child Traumatic Stress Network, 361
National Committee for Mental Hygiene, 17, 19
National Committee for Quality Assurance (NCQA), 452, **453, 455**
National Comorbidity Survey Replication, 188
National Consensus Statement on Mental Health Recovery, 491
National Council for Behavioral Health, 540
National Epidemiologic Survey on Alcohol and Related Conditions, 183
National Institute for Health and Care Excellence, 98
National Institute of Mental Health, 22, 378
National Medical Enterprises, Inc., 24
National Mental Health Act, 19
National Mental Health Registry (American Psychiatric Association), 459
National Mental Health Services Survey, 358–359
National Patient Safety Goals (Joint Commission), 301, **453,** 467, 549–550
National Quality Forum (NQF), **453, 455,** 457
National Technology Transfer and Advancement Act of 1995, **453**
Natural disasters, and code response, 474–475
Neurobiology. *See also* Neuropsychiatry; Neurotransmitter systems
  of eating disorders, 190–193
  neuropsychiatric symptoms of dementia, 127, 128–132
  traumatic events and, 488
Neurocognitive disorders, in veterans, 325
Neurological examination, and psychotic disorders, 236
Neuropsychiatry, 151–152, 175. *See also* Neurobiology
Neurostimulation, for treatment-resistant conditions, 630
Neurotransmitter systems, and anorexia nervosa, 191
New Freedom Commission on Mental Health, 308, 484, 488
Nicotine replacement therapy, 104, 280. *See also* Cigarette smoking
Nortriptyline, 52
Norway Foundation (Indiana), 19
Not-for-profit organizations
  corporate structure and, 412–413
  tax-exempt status and, 415

"Not otherwise specified" diagnosis, 95
Nurses, and nursing. *See also* Psychiatric nurse practitioners; Staff
  adult crisis stabilization unit and, 101
  developmental disabilities co-occurring unit and treatment team, 159
  forensic unit and, 224
  psychotic disorders unit and, 233
Nursing homes, 136
Nursing-intensive residential programs, 385
Nutritional rehabilitation, for eating disorders, 200
Nutritional status, of geriatric patients, 117, 119

Observation, and suicidal behavior in adult crisis stabilization unit, 101
Obsessive-compulsive disorder, 59, 188
Occupational therapy
  developmental disabilities co-occurring unit and, 163, 172
  eating disorders unit and, 201
  geriatric unit and, 119
  history of hospital psychiatry and, 17
  psychotic disorders unit and, 246, 253
  rehabilitation services and, 570–573, **574**
Office of Juvenile Justice and Delinquency Prevention, 360
Olmstead v. L.C. (1999), 29–30, 302, 303, 304
One Flew Over the Cuckoo's Nest (movie), 592
Open setting, and residential treatment, 386–387
Opioid abuse, and opioid crisis, xix, 268, 278, 281, 323, 324, 440
Organisation for Economic Co-operation and Development (OECD), xxv, 30
Organizational structure, and leadership of behavioral health services, 419–423
"Origins of Addiction Behavior: Evidence From a Study of Stressful Childhood Experiences" (Felitti 2003), 487
ORYX initiative (Joint Commission), 300–301, **453**, 454, 456
Other specified/unspecified feeding or eating disorder, 186
"Other than honorable" (OTH) discharges, 313
Outcomes. *See also* Recovery
  of hospitalization for adolescents, 82
  quality measures and, 450, 457–459
  of treatment for eating disorders, 204–205
  of treatment for intellectual disability and autism spectrum disorder in children, 153
Outdoor space, access to as human right, 598
Outpatient care. *See also* Hospital-based outpatient services; Residential treatment
  adult crisis stabilization unit and, 103
  child unit and, 61
  civil commitment and, 348–349
  decline in capacity of inpatient care and, 626
  eating disorders and, 193, 205
  intensive programs and step-down services, 610
  process of recovery and, 375
Overt Aggression Scale—Modified, **72**
Oxazepam, 277

Pain
  neuropsychiatric symptoms of dementia and, 128
  veterans and chronic, 324
Palliative care, in geriatric unit, 119, 138
Parallel treatment, of substance use disorders, 261
Parkinson's disease, 127, 129
Parents. *See also* Family
  admission criteria for adolescent unit and, 68–69
  adolescent unit and psychoeducation for, 78
  pharmacotherapy for adolescents and, 73
Partial hospitalization. *See also* Day hospitals
  eating disorders and, 205
  hospital-based outpatient services and, 344–345
  psychotic disorders and, 252, 253
Pasero Opioid-Induced Sedation Scale, 268
Pathways to Housing initiative, 616
Patient-centered care
  culture of inpatient care and, 548
  forensic unit and, 214
  institution leadership and, 422, **423**
Patient flow, and leadership of psychiatric facilities, 428
Patient Health Questionnaire–9 (PHQ-9), 116
Patient Protection and Affordable Care Act (PPACA), 413
Patient-proximal "touch points," for care delivery, 606
Patent-reported outcome measures (PROMs), 457–459
Patient rights, and patient rights movement. *See also* Advocacy movement; Patient rights; Peer empowerment movement
  risk management and, 464–465
  self-determination and, 558
  state hospitals and, 301–302

Patient Safety and Quality Improvement Act, 449
Patient Safety Standards, Materials and Systems Guidelines (New York State Office of Mental Health 2021), 519
Pediatricians, and treatment teams in developmental disabilities co-occurring unit, 159, 162
Peer empowerment movement, 594, 599. *See also* Patient rights
Peer support services, 353, 485, 595, 596, 600
Pennsylvania Hospital, 9, 23, 230, 433–434
People USA, 600
Performance measures, and quality indicators, 448
Personality disorders, and residential treatment, 381, 382
Person-environment-occupation (PEO) model, 572–573, **574**
Person-first language, 597
Phishing, and cybersecurity, 476
Physical therapy, and geriatric unit, 119
Physician self-referral laws, 477
Pica, 187
Picture Exchange Communication System, 166
Pierce, Franklin, 32, 434
Pimavanserin, 130
"Plan-do-check-act" (PDCA) method, 507
Play therapy, 55
Polypharmacy
  adult crisis stabilization unit and, 98
  antipsychotics in forensic unit and, 215
  antipsychotics in psychotic disorders unit and, 241–242
  children or adolescents and, 368
Polytrauma/TBI System of Care, 331
Positive Peer Culture (PPC), **362**
Post-9/11 GI Bill, 322
Posttraumatic stress disorder (PTSD)
  hallucinations in children and, 60
  psychotic disorders unit and, 235
  trauma prevalence rates and, 487
  veterans hospitals and, 325, 329, 331
Power dynamics, in psychiatric hospitals, 597
Practice Guideline for the Assessment and Treatment of Patients With Suicidal Behaviors (American Psychiatric Association 2003), 470
Practice Guideline for the Treatment of Patients with Eating Disorders, 3rd Edition (Yager et al. 2006), 193–194, 200
Prader-Willi syndrome, 155, 156, **160**
Pratt, Enoch, 8
Preadmission reviews, 27, 439
Predominantly restricting type, of anorexia nervosa, 184
Pregnancy, and substance use disorders, 267, 279
President's New Freedom Commission on Mental Health, 485
Prevention. *See also* Safety
  of delirium in geriatric unit, 131
  of patient elopement, 474
  of violence, 491–497
Prevention and Management of Disruptive Behavior program, 319
Principles of Care for Treatment of Children and Adolescents With Mental Illnesses in Residential Treatment Centers (AACAP), 359
Principles for the Protection of Persons With Mental Illness and for the Improvement of Mental Health Care (United Nations 1991), 484
Prisons
  forensic units and, 212–213, 223
  frequency of mental illness in, 442
Private psychiatric hospitals
  chains of, 24, 26
  financing of psychiatric care and, 436
  history of hospital psychiatry and, 5–15, 17–18, 23–24, 30
  systems of ownership of, 413
Privatization, of public mental health services in 1990s, 27
Proactive care, 605, 612–613, 615
Problem adaptation therapy for cognitively impaired disabled elderly (PATH), 136
Process improvement, and leadership, 424, 426
Process literary, and quality of care, 508
Process measures, of quality, 450
Productivity-based systems, for staff compensation, 542–543
Professional Crisis Management, 370
Profit, influence of on facility goals and operations, 412
Prospective payment system (PPS), 437–438
Protection and Advocacy for Individuals with Mental Illness Act (PAIMI), 301–302, 599
Pseudodementia, 121
Pseudopatients, and studies of violence, 489–490
Psychiatric advance directives, 296, 349
Psychiatric beds
  decline in numbers of, xxv, 22, 28, 88, 413–414, 439, 441, 504

financing and numbers of in general hospitals, 435
numbers of in state hospitals, 292–293, **294–295**
Psychiatric consultations, and emergency care, 405
Psychiatric nurse practitioners. *See also* Nurses; Staff
care models including, 540–541
communication and, 553–554
culture of inpatient care and, 548–549
nurse-patient therapeutic relationship and, 552–553
safety and, 549–551
seclusion and restraint use, 553
shortage of mental health professionals and, 547
team collaboration and, 551–552
trauma-informed care and, 551
Psychiatric urgent care (PUC), 404–405
Psychiatrists. *See also* Staff
developmental disabilities co-occurring unit and treatment team, 158–159
forensic unit and, 224
impact of utilization management on decision-making, 26
military service and, 328
roles of in hospital setting, 537–540
shortage of, 365, 371, 540
Psychiatry. *See* Consultation-liaison psychiatric services; Hospital psychiatry; Inpatient care; Psychiatric nurse practitioners; Psychiatrists
Psychoanalysis, 16, 17
Psychodynamic psychotherapy, and residential treatment, 387–388
Psychoeducation
adolescent unit and, 78–79
eating disorders unit and, 198
social workers and, 558, 565–566, 568
Psychological testing, for psychotic patients, 237
Psychologists. *See also* Staff
developmental disabilities co-occurring unit and treatment team, 163
roles of in hospital setting, 541–542
Psychopharmacology. *See also* Adherence; Antidepressants; Antipsychotics; Benzodiazepines; Dosages; Drug-drug interactions; Mood stabilizers; Polypharmacy; Side effects
for ADHD, 51–53
adult crisis stabilization unit and, 97–100
alcohol withdrawal and, 276–277
beginning of modern in 1950s, 20
bipolar disorder in geriatric patients and, 124
for delirium in geriatric unit, 131
dementia in geriatric unit and, 128–132
depression in geriatric unit and, 121–122
developmental disabilities co-occurring unit and, 172–173
eating disorders unit and, 201–202
family and, 586
forensic population in state hospitals and, 298
forensic unit and, 214–215, 220
psychiatric nurse practitioners and management of, 550–551
psychiatrists and management of, 538
psychotic disorders unit and, 238–243
quality and management of, 456
residential treatment and, 368–369, 389
schizophrenia in older adults and, 126–127
sexual disinhibition in geriatric patients and, 133
trauma in children and, 56
traumatic brain injury and, 333
treatment-resistant disorders and, 630
Psychosis. *See also* Psychotic disorders; Psychotic disorders unit
dementia and, 127
depression in geriatric patients and, 120, 122–123
developmental disabilities co-occurring unit and, 168
medication-induced in children with ADHD, 55
Prader-Willi syndrome and, 156
psychosocial treatment modalities for adolescents with, **77**
residential treatment centers and, 363
target symptom prescribing for adolescents and, **74**
22q11.2 deletion syndrome and, 157
Psychosocial assessment, and social workers, 558–559, **560,** 562
Psychosocial determinants, of health solutions and road maps, 606
Psychosocial rehabilitation, and forensic unit, 217
Psychosocial treatments
modalities of for adolescents, **77**
substance use disorders co-occurring unit and, 281–285
support services and, 616
veterans hospitals and, 320

Psychotherapy. *See also* Acceptance and commitment therapy; Cognitive-behavioral therapy; Expressive therapy; Group therapy; Psychodynamic psychotherapy
adolescent unit and, 75–76, **77**
adult crisis stabilization unit and, 96–97
eating disorders unit and, 200–201
forensic unit and, 215–216
geriatric unit and, 136
psychotic disorders unit and, 245
Psychotic disorders. *See also* Psychosis; Psychotic disorders unit; Schizophrenia
child unit and, 60
long-acting injection clinics for, 351–352
milieu-based settings for patients with, 229–230
Psychotic disorders unit
admission criteria for, 232–233
diagnostic workup in, 235–238
discharge planning and, 250–253
dissociative identity disorder and PTSD in, 235
dual diagnosis in, 234
intellectual disabilities and, 233–234
milieu management of, 247–249
mission of specialized, 230
psychopharmacology and, 238–243
structure of, 231–232
suicidal and aggressive behaviors in, 249–250
PsychPRO, 459
Public Law 98-21 (1983), 437

Quadruple aim, and quality of care, 505
Quakers (Society of Friends), 7, 433, 434
Quality
current state of in behavioral health care, 456–457
definition of *health care quality,* 448
health care quality in psychiatry, 452, 454, 456
improvement efforts, 448–449
Lean program and, 503, 506–515
measurement-based care and patient-reported outcomes, 457–459
overview of issues in, 504–506
quality measures and, 449–450, **451, 453–454, 455**
residential treatment centers and quality-of-care, 373
state hospitals and monitoring of, 301
Quality Payment Programs (Centers for Medicare and Medicaid Services), **453, 454**
Quetiapine, 129
Quit lines, and tobacco use, 104, 281

Radically open dialectical behavior therapy (RO-DBT), 199
Rapid process improvement (RPI) events, 508–510
Rating scales. *See* Structured instruments
Ray, Isaac, 14, **15**
Readjustment Counseling Centers, 333
Recovery. *See also* Outcomes; Recovery-oriented care
definition of, 375, 591
as goal of treatment for substance use disorders, 259
messages to family on, 587–588
residential treatment and, 392
Recovery Library, 588
Recovery-oriented care
culture of inpatient care and, 548
in forensic unit, 214
Recovery support community, and substance use disorders co-occurring unit, 285–286
Recreational activities. *See also* Leisure activities
forensic unit and, 217
geriatric unit and, 118
psychotic disorders unit and, 247
Re-ED (Re-Education of Children with Emotional Disturbances), **362**
Refeeding syndrome, and anorexia nervosa, 200
Referrals. *See also* Consultation-liaison psychiatric services
developmental disabilities co-occurring unit and, 164–165
family and, 587
physician self-referral laws and, 477–478
Regulatory oversight, of psychiatric facilities, 414. *See also* Joint Commission; State(s)
Rehabilitation services. *See also* Occupational therapy; Rehabilitation therapy
adolescent unit and, 79–80
expressive therapies and, 569–570
forensic unit and, 217
psychotic disorders unit and, 246
state hospitals and, 297
Rehabilitation therapy, 574
Rehospitalization, discharge planning and risk of, 82
Reinforcement strategies, for behavioral intervention in developmental disabilities co-occurring unit, 171

Relapse prevention, and treatment of substance use disorders, 274, 275, 282–285
Relationships, leadership and building of, 428–429
"Release of information" form, 582
Religion. *See also* Quakers
  adolescent unit and, 79
  recovery support groups for substance use disorders and, 285
Repetitive transcranial magnetic stimulation (RMS), 122
Reproductive health services, and medical care for adolescents, 70
Research
  history of hospital psychiatry and, 15
  quality of care and, 505
  residential treatment and, 373, 391–392
  Veterans Administration and, 315
Residential treatment, and residential treatment centers (RTCs)
  children and, 361–364
  components of care in, 364–372
  development of, 357–358
  eating disorders and, 205
  emergence of, 376–378
  future of, 373
  indications for, 378–379
  psychodynamic systems of care and, 381–392
  for psychotic patients, 252
  regulation and oversight of, 358–359
  step-down services and, 609
  types of programs and varieties of, 359–360, 380–381
Resilience-informed care, 488
Resource managers, and residential treatment, 390
Respiratory depression, and withdrawal from substances of abuse, 268, 281
Rest homes, 18
Restraints and seclusion
  adolescent unit and, 81
  adult crisis stabilization unit and, 101
  calls for reform of use, 484–485
  child unit and, 64
  consequences of use, 482–483
  definition of, 481–482
  executive management and oversight of, 492
  forensic unit and, 220–221
  geriatric unit and, 132–133
  human rights and, 598–599
  psychiatric nurse practitioners and, 553
  psychotic disorders unit and, 250
  quality measures and, 456
  residential treatment centers and, 369
  risk management and, 466
  strategies for reducing use of, 492–493, 494–495
  trauma-informed systems of care and, 486–491
  veterans hospitals and, 319
Rett syndrome, 158
"Revolving door" scenario, for severely psychotic chronic patients, 231
Reward-based systems, and milieu therapy in child unit, 61–63
Reward-centered model, of anorexia nervosa, 192
RI International, 600
Risk adjustment, and quality measures, 450
Risk factors
  for fetal alcohol spectrum disorder, 157
  for suicide and suicidal behaviors, 132, 468
Risk management
  anti-kickback statute and physician self-referral laws, 477–478
  code response and, 474–475
  coding and fraudulent billing, 476–477
  electronic health records and cybersecurity, 475–476
  importance of, 463
  patient elopement and, 473–474
  patient rights and, 464–465
  physical environment and, 473
  safety and, 465–466
  sexual harassment and assault, 474
  suicide and suicidal behavior, 466–473
Rockefeller Foundation, 434
Rockwell, William, 9
Root cause analysis
  behavior in developmental disabilities co-occurring unit, 173
  quality monitoring for state hospitals and, 301
  risk management and, 466
Rorschach Inkblot Test, 237
Rose House (New York), 600
Rounds and rounding
  psychiatric nurse practitioners and, 549
  visibility of leadership and, 429
Rumination disorder, 187–188

Safety, and safety plans. *See also* Suicide; Violence
  adolescent unit and, 69, 80–81
  child unit and, 48
  developmental disabilities co-occurring unit and, 173

Safety, and safety plans (*continued*)
design of mental health care facilities and, 520–521, 522
forensic unit and, 217, 218
health care operations and, 427
psychiatric nurse practitioners and, 549–551
psychotic disorders unit and, 235–236
quality measures and, 456
risk management and, 465–466
social workers and, 562, 566
strategies to improve, 491–497
substance use disorders co-occurring unit and, 262, 267–269
veterans hospitals and, 318
St. Jude's Children's Hospital, 418
Same-day crisis clinics, and hospital-based outpatient services, 343
San Antonio State Hospital (Texas), 30
Sanctuary model, **362**
Scale for Suicide Ideation—Worst (SSI-W), 469
Schizophrenia. *See also* Psychotic disorders unit
aggressive behavior and, 249
in children, 60
clozapine and treatment-refractory, 243
electroconvulsive therapy for, 244
geriatric unit and, 125–127, 134
psychoeducation for families and, 566
School(s). *See also* Education
adolescent unit and reentry meetings, 82
developmental disabilities co-occurring unit and, 164
interface of with child unit, 60–61
residential treatment centers and, 365, 371
School refusal, 59, 363
Screen for Child Anxiety Related Emotional Disorders (SCARED), **72**
Screening, for PTSD in veterans hospitals, 329
Seclusion, definition of, 481. *See also* Restraints and seclusion
Section 1115 waiver (Medicaid), 28, 29
Security, and residential care, 359–360
Seizure disorder, and stimulants for children with ADHD, 52
Selective serotonin-norepinephrine reuptake inhibitors (SNRIs), 122, 123
Selective serotonin reuptake inhibitors (SSRIs), 122, 123, 128
Self-determination, patients' right to, 558
Self-esteem, and anorexia nervosa, 185
Self-injurious behavior. *See also* Suicide
adolescent unit and, 81
child unit and, 58–59
developmental disabilities co-occurring unit and, 164, 165, 167, 173
Self-reports, of violence in mental health settings, 485–486
Semistructured interviews, and eating disorders, 203
Sensory interventions
developmental disabilities co-occurring unit and, 173–174
prevention of violence and, 494–495
Sentinel Event Alert, 467
Sequential treatment, of substance use disorders, 261
Serotonin, and anorexia nervosa, 191
Service-connected (SC) benefits, 312
Sex offenders, and forensic units, 214–215, 223, 299
Sexual abuse, and military sexual trauma, 320, 329–331
Sexual disinhibition, and dementia in geriatric patients, 133
Sexually transmitted diseases, and substance use disorders, 272
"Shell shock," 328, 570
Sheppard, Mose, 8
Sheppard Pratt (Maryland)
architecture of, 517–518, 526–530
continuum of care and, xxvi
description of, xxiii
history of hospital psychiatry and, 8–9, **11**
measurement-based care and patient-reported outcome measures, 458–459
new facilities of, xxvi
psychotic disorders unit and, 230, 232, 234, 246, 252
quality of care programs, 503, 504, 507, 513
substance use disorders co-occurring unit and, 267
Sheppard Pratt Suicide Risk Assessment Instrument (SPSRAI), 470, 472, 473
Shouting, and behaviors in geriatric unit, 133–134
Side effects, of medications
ADHD and, 51–52
adolescents and, 75
antipsychotics for older adults and, 126, 127, 128
antipsychotics for psychotic patients and, 243, 244
developmental disabilities co-occurring unit and, 173
forensic unit and, 215

Signing bonuses, for staff, 543
Sign language, and nonverbal patients with intellectual disability or autism spectrum disorder, 166
Sign outs
  developmental disabilities co-occurring unit and, 172
  residential treatment centers and, 371–372
Situational model, of violence, 489
Six Core Strategies to Prevent Conflict and Trauma in Behavioral Health Settings (Huckshorn et al. 2021), 489
Six Sigma (process improvement methodology), 514
Skilled nursing facilities, and step-down services, 610
Skills training, and substance use disorders co-occurring unit, 266
Sleep, and children with ADHD, 52. *See also* Insomnia
Smartphone applications, 629
Smith-Magenis syndrome, 155
Smith's Recognizable Patterns of Human Malformations (Jones et al. 2013), 159
Social determinants of health, 626
Social history, and diagnostic workups of geriatric patients, 116–117
Social learning programs, in forensic unit, 219
Social norms, and children in residential treatment centers, 362–363
Social script, and children, 63–64
Social Security Act (1965), 21, 434
Social Security Disability Insurance, 252
Social service agencies, 61
Social work, and social workers
  developmental disabilities co-occurring unit and, 162, 172
  families and, 565–569
  future directions in, 569
  infrastructure of, 557–558
  interventions with patients, 558–565
  residential treatment and, 385
  role of in inpatient care, 557
  substance use disorders co-occurring unit and, 264
Society for Adolescent Health and Medicine, 193–194
Soldier, use of term in context, 312
Somatic complaints, and depression in geriatric patients, 120
Specialty Outpatient Treatment programs, 329
Specialty programs, and residential treatment centers, 361, 372
Specialty settings. *See* State hospitals; Veterans hospitals
Speech and language pathologists (SLPs), 163
Sports programs, and forensic unit, 217
Staff. *See also* Nurses; Psychiatrists; Psychologists; Social workers
  abuse of power by, 488
  compensation models and, 542–543
  forensic unit and, 218–219, 224
  future of hospital psychiatry and, 631
  partial hospital programs and, 344
  prevention of violence and, 493–494
  psychotic disorders unit and, 232
  ratio to patients in eating disorders unit, 202
  residential treatment centers and, 369–370
  safety and retention of, 483–484
  substance use disorders co-occurring unit and, 260
  use of restraints and seclusion, 483
Stage-based treatment, of substance use disorders, 264
Standardized testing, of intellectual ability, 154
Standards of care, and *Wit v. United Behavioral Health/Optum*, 377–378
Stanford-Binet Intelligence Scale, 154
STAR*D study, 378
Stark Law violations, 477–478
"Start low and go slow" approach, to antipsychotics for older patients, 126
START NOW (evidence-based skills therapy), 216
State(s)
  legal requirements for involuntary commitment, 68
  legislatures and funding of state hospitals, 304–305
  Medicaid and, 29
  outpatient civil commitment and, 348–349
  patient rights and laws of, 464
  privatization of mental health services in 1990s, 27
State hospitals
  accreditation of, 300–301
  budget and legislative issues, 304–305
  child and adolescent population in, 297
  civil status population in, 296–297
  consumers, advocates, and providers, 302–304
  court oversight of, 302
  financing of psychiatric services in, 441
  forensic population in, 297–299
  future of, 305–306

State hospitals (*continued*)
history of hospital psychiatry and, 3–5, 9–15, 17–18, 28, 291–293, **294–295,** 434
impact of on overall continuum of care, 299–300
for individuals with intellectual and developmental disabilities, 152
patient rights and, 301–302
types of units in, 293, 296
State mental health agencies (SMHAs), 299, 300, 301
Step-down levels of care
adolescent unit and, 82
birth and proliferation of, 609–610
social workers and, 561
Stigma, of mental illness, 18, 347
Stop Gap Model, **362**
Strategy, and corporate governance, 415, **416,** 417–419
Strengthening Behavioral Health Parity Act (SBHPA), 31
Strength-weaknesses-opportunities-threats (SWOT) analysis, 617–619
Stress, and psychosocial treatment modalities for adolescents, **77**
Structural measures, of quality, 450
Structured instruments
assessment of adolescents and, 71, **72**
diagnosis of geriatric patients and, 116
response of target symptoms to medications, 99
suicide risk assessment and, 469
Study of the Pharmacotherapy of Psychotic Depression (STOP-PD), 123
Substance abuse disorders (SUDs). *See also* Alcohol; Opioid abuse; Substance use disorders co-occurring unit
adult crisis stabilization unit and, 96
delirium and, 92
Medicaid and, 440–441
psychosocial treatment modalities for adolescents with, **77**
psychotic disorders unit and, 234
residential treatment and, 363–364, 382
telemedicine and treatment of, 629
therapeutic pessimism about, 258
veterans hospitals and, 322–324
Substance Abuse and Mental Health Services Administration (SAMHSA), 358, 375, 401, 452, 469, 540, 599
Substance use disorders co-occurring unit
admissions to, 266–267
assessments and, 269–274
conceptual framework of, 258–259
decription of, 259–262
discharge planning and, 264–265, 286
future of, 287
goals of treatment, 262–266
importance of long-term follow-up, 286–287
recovery support community and, 285–286
safety and, 267–269
psychosocial interventions in, 281–285
treatment planning and, 274–275
withdrawal management and, 275–281
Succession planning, and leadership, 430
Suicide, and suicidal behaviors. *See also* Safety; Self-injurious behaviors
adolescent unit and management of, 80–81
adult crisis stabilization unit and management of, 101–103
antidepressants for adolescents and, 75
design of facilities and, 526–530
eating disorders and, 188, 195
forensic unit and, 218, 219–221
geriatric unit and, 114, 117, 122, 132
hospital operations and, 427
increased risk of in posthospital population, 601
Joint Commission on prevention of, 31–32
psychotic disorders unit and, 249–250
quality measures and failure to report, 454
residential treatment and, 390–391
risk management and, 466–473
veterans hospitals and, 325
Sullivan Day Hospital, 232
Supervisors, and organizational structure, 420
Supportive counseling, by social workers, 559
Supportive therapy, and developmental disabilities co-occurring unit, 162
Support networks. *See also* Peer support services
adult crisis stabilization unit and, 90, 96
family and, 583
psychotic disorders unit and, 238
Support programs, for caregivers, 120, 137
Surrogate decision-makers, and capacity, 135–136, 203
Symptom reduction, and substance use disorders co-occurring unit, 262
Syndrome of inappropriate secretion of antidiuretic hormone (SIADH), 122
System ownership, of psychiatric hospitals, 413

Tantrums
ADHD and medication-induced psychosis, 55
child unit and, 50, 55–58
developmental disabilities co-occurring unit and, 167–168
Target symptom prescribing, for adolescents, 73, **74–75**
Tarrant County Homeless Coalition, 616
Tax-exempt status, and non-profit organizations, 415
Team(s), and team members
developmental disabilities co-occurring unit and, 158–159, 162–164
eating disorders unit and multidisciplinary, 197
geriatric unit and, 118–119, 137
hospital-based outpatient services and care teams, 349–353
milieu management in adult crisis stabilization unit and, 100
milieu therapy in child unit and, 64–65
psychiatric nurse practitioners and collaboration of, 551–552
residential treatment centers and multidisciplinary, 367–368
substance use disorders co-occurring unit and multidisciplinary, 261
team-based care as emerging theme in hospital psychiatry, 606, 614–615
TeamCare, 617
Technology, and future of mental health care, 628–629. *See also* Cybersecurity; Electronic health records; Internet; Telepsychiatry; Videoconferencing
TeleMAT services, 628, 629
Telepsychiatry
future of mental health care and, 616, 626, 628–629
geriatric patients and, 137
hospital-based outpatient services and, 347
psychiatrists and, 539–540
Telepsychiatry Toolkit (American Psychiatric Association), 616
Tetrahydrocannabinol (THC), 281
Texas Implementation of Medication Algorithms (TIMA), 98, 241–242
Therapeutic alliance. *See also* Therapeutic relationship
adolescent unit and, 76
residential treatment and, 383, 384, 391
suicidal ideation and, 470
Therapeutic Crisis Intervention, 370
Therapeutic environment, design of, 519–520
Therapeutic relationship, nurse-patient, 552–553. *See also* Therapeutic alliance
Threats, and threatening behavior in adult crisis stabilization unit, 103
3-Minute Diagnostic Assessment, 130
Tics, and stimulant medications, 52
Time-outs, in forensic unit, 220
TJC. *See* Joint Commission
Tobacco use. *See* Cigarette smoking
To Err is Human: Building a Safer Health System (Institute of Medicine 2000), 448, 504
Toyota Motor Corporation, 503
"Tradition of Toughness: A Study of Nonprofessional Nursing Care in Psychiatric Settings, The" (Morrison 1990), 490–491
Transdisciplinary teams, and geriatric unit, 118, 137
Transtheoretical model, and treatment of substance use disorders, 274–275, 281–282
Trauma. *See also* Adverse childhood experiences; Military sexual trauma
ADHD in children and, 53–54
children in residential treatment centers and, 361, 362
events defined as, 486–487
psychosocial treatment modalities for adolescents with, **77**
substance use disorders and, 271–272
veterans hospitals and, 326–333
Trauma-informed systems of care, 486–491, 548, 551, 599
Traumatic brain injury (TBI), and veterans, 325, 331, **332,** 333
Treatment. *See* Behavioral interventions; Electroconvulsive therapy; Goals; Group therapy; Individual therapy; Inpatient care; Involuntary treatment; Milieu therapy; Motivational interviewing; Psychopharmacology; Psychosocial treatments; Psychotherapy; Sensory interventions; Treatment plans
"Treatment mall" care model, 523
Treatment plans
adult crisis stabilization unit and, 95
developmental disabilities co-occurring unit and, 170–171
substance use disorders co-occurring unit and, 274–275
Treatment refusal, and eating disorders, 203

Treatment-resistant disorders
future of mental health care and, 630
team-based therapy for depression and, 349–350
residential treatment and, 382–383, 393
Treatment team. *See* Team(s)
Tricyclic antidepressants (TCAs), and depression in geriatric patients, 122
Triggers, and relapse process in substance abuse, **283,** 285
Tuke, Samuel, 434
12-step groups, and substance use disorders, 285–286
21st Century Cures Act (2016), 29
22q11.2 deletion syndrome, 157, **161**

Unemployment, of veterans with psychiatric issues, 321–322
"Unified benefit" health financing model, 607
Unions, and state hospital employees, 303
United Auto Workers, 21
United Nations, 484
U.S. Census Bureau, 17
U.S. General Accounting Office, 482, 484
U.S. News & World Report, xxiii
U.S. Office of Personnel Management, 315
U.S. Public Health Service, 19
Universal precaution, and trauma-informed care, 486
University of Washington, 613
Utica State Hospital (New York), 10, **13**
Utilization management, and managed care, 26–27

Valproic acid, 242
Value(s)
corporate governance and, **416, 419**
eating disorders and, 203
quality of care and concept of, 506–507
Value-based integrated care management, 616–617, 626
Vascular depression, 121
Vascular disease, and late-onset bipolar disorder, 123–124
VA Supported Housing (VASH), 321
VA Women Veterans Health Care program, 313
Veteran Readiness and Employment (VR&E) program, 322
Veterans Administration medical centers (VAMCs), 312, 316–319, 333–334. *See also* Veterans hospitals
Veterans Benefits Administration, 312
Veterans Health Administration (VHA), 312
Veterans hospitals
clinical challenges in, 319–333
history of, 311–316
VA medical centers and, 312, 316–319, 333–334
Veterans Integrated Service Networks (VISNs), 313, **314,** 315
Veterans Justice Outreach (VJO), 321
Videoconferencing, 251, 629
Video games, and residential treatment centers, 363
Vietnam War, 328–329
Vineland Adaptive Behavior Scales, 2nd Edition, 154
Violence. *See also* Aggression; Safety; Suicide
adult crisis stabilization unit and past history of, 101
consumer and staff experiences of, 485–486
factors in causality, 483–484
forensic unit and potential for, 218, 223
issues and costs of in mental health settings, 481–482
portrayal of in literature, 488–489
psychotic disorders unit and, 234, 249–250
trauma-informed systems of care and, 486–491
veterans hospitals and, 318–319
Virtual care, and hospital-based outpatient services, 347–348
Visibility, of leadership, 429
Vision, and corporate governance, **416**
Vitamin deficiencies, and substance use disorders, 272, 278
Vocalizations, management of in geriatric unit, 133–134
Vocational rehabilitation program, for veterans, 322

Walk-in clinical appointments, and hospital-based outpatient services, 343
Wechsler Adult Intelligence Scale, 154
Weight gain, and eating disorders, 205
Weinberg Residential Crisis Program, 232
Welcome folder, and adult crisis stabilization unit, 100
Well Being Trust, 627
Wellness Recovery Action Plan, 595, 601
White, Samuel, 2
Whole Health Action Management, 595, 601
Wide Range Achievement Test, 237
Willard Asylum for the Chronic Insane (New York), 4, **6**
Wisconsin Card Sorting Test, 237

Withdrawal, and substance use disorders
co-occurring unit, 275–281
Wit v. United Behavioral Health/Optum (2020), xxv, 377, 380
Women. *See also* Gender
military sexual trauma and, 320, 329–331
service of in military, 313, 326
12-step groups for substance use disorders and, 286
Women's Army Auxiliary Corps, 313
Woodward, Samuel Bayard, 2, **2**
Worcester Recovery Center and Hospital (Massachusetts), 30
Worcester State Hospital (Maryland), 3, **5**
Workforce. *See* Staff
Workplace Behavioral Risk Assessment, 319
World Health Organization, **621**
World War I, and "shell shock," 328, 570
World War II, and psychiatric care for veterans, 20, 328
Wyatt v. Stickney (1971), 21, 302

York Retreat (England), 434
Young Mania Rating Scale, **72**
Youth Risk Behavior Survey (2017), 183

Zero Suicide/Suicide Safer Care, 600